Clinical Studies in Medical Biochemistry

SECOND EDITION

Edited by

ROBERT H. GLEW
Professor and Chairman
Department of Biochemistry
University of New Mexico

YOSHIFUMI NINOMIYA
Professor and Chairman
Department of Molecular Biology
and Biochemistry
Okayama University Medical School

New York   Oxford
OXFORD UNIVERSITY PRESS
1997

Oxford University Press

Oxford   New York
Athens   Auckland   Bangkok   Bogota
Bombay   Buenos Aires   Calcutta   Cape Town
Dar es Salaam   Delhi   Florence   Hong Kong   Istanbul
Karachi   Kuala Lumpur   Madras   Madrid
Melbourne   Mexico City   Nairobi   Paris
Singapore   Taipei   Tokyo   Toronto

and associated companies in
Berlin   Ibadan

Copyright © 1997 by Oxford University Press

Published by Oxford University Press, Inc.
198 Madison Avenue, New York, New York 10016

Oxford is a registered trademark of Oxford University Press

Library of Congress Cataloging-in-Publication Data
Clinical studies in medical biochemistry /
edited by Robert H. Glew, Yoshifumi Ninomiya. — 2nd ed.
p. cm.   Includes bibliographical references and index.
ISBN 0-19-509928-1 (cloth). — ISBN 0-19-509929-X (paper)
1. Clinical biochemistry—Case studies.
I. Glew, Robert H.   II. Ninomiya, Yoshifumi.
[DNLM: 1. Biochemistry.   2. Diagnosis, Laboratory—case studies.
RB112.5.C57   1997   616—dc20
DNLM/DLC   for Library of Congress   96-22249

1 3 5 7 9 8 6 4 2

Printed in the United States of America
on acid-free paper

Preface

Since the first edition of this collection of clinical studies was published in 1987, there has been a widespread movement in medical schools to integrate the teaching of basic science knowledge, including biochemistry, into the clinical world. In fact, it is rare today to find a medical school curriculum in which biochemistry is taught in isolation as a vast array of reactions and metabolic pathways dissociated from the normal and pathophysiologic processes involved in human health and disease. As such, many departments of biochemistry, particularly those located in or associated with medical schools, are in need of teaching materials in which biochemical facts and concepts are articulated and developed through presentations of specific examples of human disease.

This book is intended to fill that need. Whereas it certainly can serve as a companion text to many of the 900-page plus standard textbooks of biochemistry, experience with the first edition of *Clinical Studies in Medical Biochemistry* has shown that the 12- to 20-page chapters that constitute this collection of actual case reports are sufficiently comprehensive and self-contained to stand on their own. In fact, the book has been and can be used as the primary resource in 'biochemistry of disease' courses at the advanced undergraduate level or in M.S. or Ph.D. graduate programs.

Each chapter begins with a detailed case report that includes the relevant history, pertinent clinical laboratory data, and physical findings. In some cases, the patient about whom the chapter is developed was the very same case that was the first of its kind described in the medical literature. The contributors to this book have been careful to define medical terms with which the reader might be un-

familiar and to minimize their need to resort to a medical dictionary. The case presentation is followed by a brief "Diagnosis" section, which includes a brief discussion of differential diagnosis and criteria needed for establishing the diagnosis. In addition, this section of each chapter usually explains the principle behind key laboratory and diagnostic tests. "Molecular Perspectives" forms the heart of each chapter and is the longest section; it goes into considerable detail in explaining the fundamental defect that lies at the core of each case. Because there has been such an explosion of knowledge in the last decade about the molecular biology aspects of most of the diseases this book describes, this section provides molecular biological as well as classic biochemical-enzymologic explanations of pertinent pathophysiologic mechanisms. The fourth section of each chapter, entitled "Therapy," provides a concise account of how the disease in question is treated. Finally, each chapter ends with a list of references and set of questions that are intended not only to test the reader's comprehension of the case in all its dimensions but also to stimulate group discussions if the book is being used in a tutorial setting.

During the past 10 years, a new approach to medical education called the "new pathway" has been conceived, developed, and implemented at many medical schools in North America and elsewhere. Namely, several medical schools embarked on a fundamental reform of the content and method of its medical curriculum. The motivation for such reform arose for the two considerations: one, that the traditional educational system may not adequately prepare physicians for the increasing complexity of medicine in the future; the other, that the educational process itself did not adequately recognize medical students as being adult learners capable of self-learning. One of the factors influencing the shape of medical care today is the ongoing, rapidly advancing pace of scientific discovery and technological invention, challenging physicians to keep abreast of new departments and to manage information effectively.

The diseases and disorders chosen for discussion and the order of presentation should parallel subject matter taught in most first-year medical biochemistry courses. Chapters in the first part of the book, "Nucleic Acids, Viruses, and Protein Structure and Function," illustrate basic aspects of DNA and RNA structure and synthesis in the context of viruses ("Human Immunodeficiency Viruses and the Acquired Immunodeficiency Syndrome" and "Fulminant Hepatitis B"), and bacteria ("Pertussis"). The chapter on "Creatine Kinase Isoenzymes and the Diagnosis of Myocardial Infarction" demonstrates the usefulness of enzymes as markers of disease that affect particular organs. The role of structural proteins in cells is presented in the context of "Hereditary Spherocytosis," and the relationship between protein structure and function is illustrated in the chapter on "Sickle Cell Anemia."

The second part of the book deals with "Metabolism and Energetics." Important pathways and enzymes involved in carbohydrate metabolism ("Neonatal Hypoglycemia," "Pyruvate Dehydrogenase Complex Deficiency"), the hexose monophosphate shunt ("Glucose 6-Phosphate Dehydrogenase Deficiency"), and fatty acid metabolism and transport ("Biotin and Multiple Carboxylase Deficiency," "Systemic Carnitine Deficiency") are discussed. Finally, the second part concludes with a discussion of "Diabetes Mellitus" so that many of the concepts of intermediary metabolism can be integrated.

Various aspects of the "Metabolism of Complex Molecules" constitute the third part of the book. The synthesis of glycoproteins (α_1-Antitrypsin Deficiency"), packaging of lysosomal enzymes into lysosomal granules ("I-Cell Disease"), hereditary nephritis caused by a defect in basement membrane collagen ("Alport Syndrome"), disorders of glycolipid ("Gaucher Disease: A Sphingolipidosis") and amino acid ("Phenylketonuria") metabolism and urea synthesis ("Inborn Errors of Urea Synthesis") are all discussed. The chapter on "Inborn Errors of Urea Synthesis" not only discusses the pathophysiology of these disorders but also serves to point out that different metabolic defects can result in a similar clinical syndrome.

The short fourth part on "Steroids" discusses aspects of cholesterol ("Low-Density Lipoprotein Receptors and Familial Hypercholesterolemia"), calcium and vitamin D ("Rickets Caused by a Vitamin D Deficiency"), and glucocorticoid and mineralocorticoid synthesis and function ("Cushing's Syndrome").

Finally, the fifth part ("Aspects of Infection and Pharmacology") discusses several diverse topics, including defects in phagocytic cells ("Chronic Granulomatous Disease") and the use of enzyme inhibitors as pharmacological agents ("Management of Hypertension with Particular Attention to the Renin-Angiotensin System").

This book could not have been put together without the assistance of the skilled and patient investigators who contributed chapters to this second edition of *Clinical Studies in Medical Biochemistry,* most of whom have had firsthand experience with the clinical disorders they describe. Furthermore, most of the authors of these chapters are themselves engaged in educating medical students in North America and the Far East. Whatever success this book enjoys we owe to these contributors and to our skilled editor at Oxford, Mr. Jeffrey House.

Contents

PART III   METABOLISM OF COMPLEX MOLECULES

Contributors

ROBERT M. AMORY, Ph.D.
Allegheny General Hospital
Pittsburgh, Pennsylvania

SANJEEV AURORA, M.D.
Department of Medicine
University of New Mexico School of Medicine
Albuquerque, New Mexico

ERNEST BEUTLER, M.D.
Molecular and Experimental Medicine
The Scripps Research Institute
La Jolla, California

SAUL W. BRUSILOW, M.D.
Division of Metabolism
Department of Pediatrics
The Johns Hopkins Medical Institutions
School of Medicine
Baltimore, Maryland

CATHERINE M. BULEY, M.D.
University of Minnesota Medical School
Minneapolis, Minnesota

JAMES P. CHAMBERS, Ph.D.
The Brain Research Laboratory of Biochemistry
The Division of Life Sciences
The University of Texas at San Antonio
San Antonio, Texas

SAMUEL CHARACHE, M.D.
Department of Medicine and Pathology
The Johns Hopkins University School of Medicine
Baltimore, Maryland

RUSSELL W. CHESNEY, M.D.
Department of Pediatrics
University of Tennessee
College of Medicine
Memphis, Tennessee

SHERMINE DABBAGH, M.D.
Department of Pediatrics
Wayne State University
School of Medicine
Detroit, Michigan

K. DAKSHINAMURTI, M.D.
Department of Biochemistry
University of Manitoba
Winnipeg, Manitoba
Canada

GINGI ENDO, M.D.
Department of Preventive Medicine
and Environmental Health
Osaka City University Medical School
Osaka, Japan

JOSEPH N. FISHER, M.D.
Division of Endocrinology & Metabolism
Department of Medicine
University of Tennessee Center for the Health Sciences
Memphis, Tennessee

WILLIAM R. GALEY, Ph.D.
Department of Physiology
University of New Mexico School of Medicine
Albuquerque, New Mexico

ROBERT H. GLEW, Ph.D.
Department of Biochemistry
University of New Mexico School of Medicine
Albuquerque, New Mexico

WILLIAM S. HAYS, Ph.D.
Department of Biochemistry
University of New Mexico School of Medicine
Albuquerque, New Mexico

IAN R. HOLZMAN, M.D.
Department of Pediatrics
Mount Sinai School of Medicine
The Mount Sinai Hospital
New York, New York

BRIAN HJELLE, M.D.
Department of Pathology
School of Medicine
University of New Mexico
Albuquerque, New Mexico

HIROSHI IDEGUCHI, M.D.
Department of Clinical Chemistry and Laboratory
  Medicine
Fukuoka University, School of Medicine
Fukuoka, Japan

DAVID W. JACKSON, B.S.
Department of Biochemistry
University of New Mexico School of Medicine
Albuquerque, New Mexico

STEVEN JENISON, M.D.
New Mexico Department of Health
Santa Fe, New Mexico

GORO KAJIYAMA, M.D.
First Department of Internal Medicine
Hiroshima University School of Medicine
Hiroshima, Japan

KOICHI KANAI, M.D.
Department of Gastroenterology
Toshiba General Hospital
Tokyo, Japan

HARVEY, R. KASLOW, Ph.D.
Department of Physiology and Biophysics
University of Southern California School of Medicine
Los Angeles, California

MINEO KOJIMA, M.D.
Kojima Internal Clinic
Gifu, Japan

ABBAS E. KITABCHI, Ph.D., M.D.
Division of Endocrinology & Metabolism
Department of Medicine
University of Tennessee Center for the Health Sciences
Memphis, Tennessee

KEVIN LAUBSCHER, Ph.D.
Molecular and Experimental Medicine
The Scripps Research Institute
La Jolla, California

SIMEON MARGOLIS, M.D.
Endorcrinology and Metabolism
The Johns Hopkins University School of Medicine
Baltimore, Maryland

DENIS M. MCCARTHY, M.D., Msc.
Division of Gastroenterology and Hepotology
Department of Medicine
University of New Mexico School of Medicine
Albuquerque, New Mexico

DONALD MERCER, Ph.D.
Allegheny General Hospital
Pittsburgh, Pennsylvania

J. ROSS MILLEY, Ph.D.
Division of Neonatology
Department of Pediatrics
The University of Utah School of Medicine
Salt Lake City, Utah

SHUNJI MISHIRO, M.D.
Department of Medical Sciences
Toshiba General Hospital
Tokyo, Japan

KAZUHARU MURAKAMI, M.D.
Central Hospital Tamashima
Kurashiki, Japan

KOJI NARAHARA, M.D.
Department of Pediatrics
Okayama University Medical School
Okayama, Japan

YOSHIFUMI NINOMIYA, M.D., Ph.D
Department of Molecular Biology and Biochemistry
Okayama University Medical School
Okayama, Japan

TADAO ORII, M.D.
Chubu Women's College
Seki, Japan

HARBHAJAN S. PAUL, Ph.D.
Biomed. Research & Technologies, Inc.
Wexford, Pennsylvania

MICHAEL E. PICHICHERO, M.D.
Elmwood Pediatric Group
University of Rochester Medical Center
Rochester, New York

ALAN T. REMALEY, M.D., Ph.D.
National Institutes of Health
Clinical Center
Clinical Pathology Department
Bethesda, Maryland

PHILIP REYES, Ph.D.
Department of Biochemistry
University of New Mexico School of Medicine
Albuquerque, New Mexico

JOHN K. SCARIANO, B.S., M.Sc.
Department of Biochemistry
University of New Mexico School of Medicine
Albuquerque, New Mexico

SARAH JANE SCHWARZENBERG, M.D.
Division of Gastroenterology
Department of Pediatrics
University of Minnesota Hospitals
Minneapolis, Minnesota

AJOVI B. SCOTT-EMUAKPOR, M.D., Ph.D.
Department of Pediatrics and Human Development
School of Medicine
Michigan State Univesity
East Lansing, Michigan

ANTHONY W. SEGAL, M.D.
Department of Medicine
University College London Medical School
Rayne Institute
London, England

GAIL SEKAS, Ph.D.
Department of Molecular Genetics and Biochemistry
University of Pittsburgh School of Medicine
Pittsburgh, Pennsylvania

ALVIN P. SHAPIRO, M.D.
Department of Medicine
Shadyside Hospital
and
the University of Pittsburgh School of Medicine
Pittsburgh, Pennsylvania

HARVEY L. SHARP, M.D.
Division of Gastroenterology
Department of Pediatrics
University of Minnesota Hospitals
Minneapolis, Minnesota

YASUYUKI SUZUKI, M.D.
Department of Pediatrics
Gifu University School of Medicine
Gifu, Japan

SHIGERU TAKETANI, Ph.D.
Department of Hygiene
Kansai Medical University
Moriguchi, Japan

SUSUMU TAZUMA, M.D.
First Department of Internal Medicine
Hiroshima University School of Medicine
Hiroshima, Japan

ADRIAN J. THRASHER, M.D.
Molecular Immunology Unit
Division of Cell and Molecular Biology
Institute of Child Health
London, England

YEHUDA TRAUB, M.D.
Department of Medicine
Shadyside Hospital
and
the University of Pittsburgh School of Medicine
Pittsburgh, Pennsylvania

BARBARA TRIGGS-RAINE, M.D.
Department of Molecular Biology
University of Manitoba
Winnipeg, Manitoba
Canada

KARL TRYGGVASON, M.D., Ph.D.
Division of Matrix Biology
Department of Medical Biochemistry and Biophysics
Karolinska Institute
Stockholm, Sweden

DOROTHY J. VANDERJAGT, Ph.D.
Department of Biochemistry
University of New Mexico School of Medicine
Albuquerque, New Mexico

MURRAY A. VARAT, Ph.D.
Allegheny General Hospital
Pittsburgh, Pennsylvania

B. SYLVIA VELA, M.D.
Division of Endocrinology
Department of Medicine
University of New Mexico School of Medicine
Albuquerque, New Mexico

JULIAN C. WILLIAMS, M.D., Ph.D.
Division of Medical Genetics
Children's Hospital Los Angeles
Los Angeles, California

BEULAH M. WOODFIN, Ph.D.
Department of Biochemistry
University of New Mexico School of Medicine
Albuquerque, New Mexico

YUJI YOKOYAMA, M.D.
Department of Pediatrics
Okayama University Medical School
Okayama, Japan

Part I

Nucleic Acids, Viruses, and Protein Structure and Function

Creatine Kinase Isoenzymes and the Diagnosis
of Myocardial Infarction

DONALD W. MERCER, MURRAY A. VARAT, AND ROBERT M. AMORY

CASE REPORTS

Case 1

PS, a 59-year-old man, was admitted on November 20, 1991, with a chief complaint of a cold and painful right leg for the previous 24 hours. He had a long history of peripheral vascular disease, with intermittent claudication for 10 years. During that time he had three separate bypass grafts and required amputation of one leg (left).

His medical history was strongly indicative of coronary artery disease. An acute myocardial infarction following the most recent surgery in 1991 was attributed to intraoperative hypotension. His subsequent chest pain was thought to be angina pectoris, and he began receiving digoxin for atrial fibrillation in 1989.

Physical examination revealed an alert man with moderately severe leg pain. His blood pressure was 140/80 mm Hg, and his pulse was 115 beats per minute and irregular. There was no neck vein distension. The lungs were clear. The apical pulse was palpable at the fourth left interspace along the midclavicular line. A grade II/VI murmur that continued throughout systole was audible at the cardiac apex, indicating moderate regurgitation of blood through an incompetent mitral valve. There were no gallops. The left leg had been amputated just above the knee. The right leg was cold and cyanotic. No lower extremity pulses were palpable.

The presumptive diagnosis was a thrombosed axillopopliteal graft with early ischemic changes. Thrombectomy was carried out 2 days after admission using local anesthesia. During surgery his ventricular rate increased to 150 beats per minute and he complained of chest tightness. Two days later, on repeat thrombectomy, his ventricular rate increased to 180 beats per minute, although he had no chest discomfort. Intravenous (i.v.) digoxin and propranolol were required to control his heart rate.

Cardiac isoenzymes drawn the evening of November 24 indicated a myocardial infarction. He developed mild heart failure the next day but subsequently did well. On recognition of the acute infarction, the patient was treated with i.v. xylocaine to prevent potentially lethal ventricular arrhythmias. Digoxin therapy was continued to control his heart rate and to increase myocardial contractility when heart failure occurred. Intravenous diuretics were also used for the episode of heart failure. He was discharged on December 6, 1991, and he remains free of chest and leg pain.

Because the patient experienced chest tightness during the first operation, serial blood samples were obtained for determination of creatine kinase (CK) and its cardiac-specific isoenzyme (MB). Serum CK was markedly elevated in the first two samples and subsequently declined (Fig. 1-1). The initial MB values were also high (up to 16 U/L). When expressed in relation to total CK, however, MB was always <1% in these first few samples, indicating skeletal muscle necrosis rather than myocardial damage as the

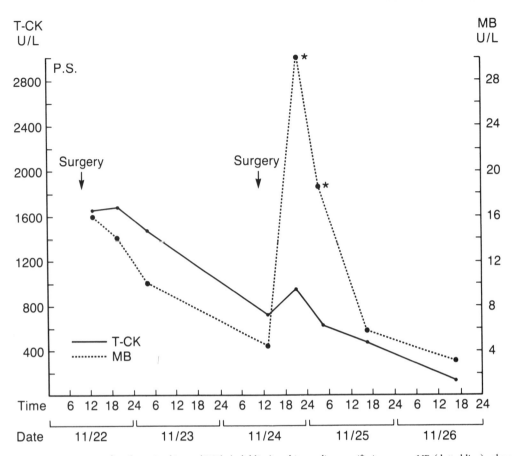

Figure 1-1. Time course of total creatine kinase (T-CK) (solid line) and its cardiac-specific isoenzyme MB (dotted line) values in patient PS (case 1); *elevated percentage MB.

source of the elevated enzyme level. Ischemic necrosis of muscle in the leg, secondary to the clotted graft, was the most likely cause. Surgery itself also results in skeletal muscle damage and causes release of CK into the blood.

The pattern of enzyme level changes following the second operation indicates an acute myocardial infarction, despite the absence of chest pain and electrocardiographic (ECG) changes. The precipitating event was probably the episode of a very rapid ventricular rate at the initiation of surgery. Serum CK and MB values obtained shortly after surgery were elevated but not impressively so in light of the prior high values. Twelve hours after surgery, total CK levels had risen but not enough to suggest strongly that acute muscle necrosis had occurred; however, there was a sharp rise in MB to 30 U/L, which is >3% of total CK and is diagnostic of an acute myocardial infarction.

Case 2

RS, an 82-year-old woman, was admitted on February 21, 1994, with a 12-hour history of bilateral shoulder pain. Her cardiac history dated from July 1992, when she was hospitalized with similar pain and found to have suffered an acute anterior-wall myocardial infarction. In January 1994, she had a similar pain episode. There was a small rise in her cardiac isoenzyme values, and a diagnosis of non-Q wave infarction was made. Otherwise, she had had no exertional chest or shoulder discomfort. She had never experienced symptoms of heart failure.

Physical examination revealed an alert but fatigued woman, free of pain. Her blood pressure was 160/84 mm Hg, and her pulse was 60 beats per minute and regular. The neck veins were flat. There were no carotid bruits. Her lungs were clear to auscultation and percussion. The first heart sound was muffled, and second one sharp. There was a loud S-4 gallop, but no murmurs were present. There was trace pitting ankle edema bilaterally. The peripheral pulses were both palpable. The admitting ECG showed sinus rhythm, left-axis deviation, left ventricular hypertrophy, and changes in the precordial leads consistent with an old anterior myocardial infarction. The tracing was unchanged from that of the previous month.

Her hospital course was characterized by recurrent episodes of chest and shoulder pain. The pain on admission was initially relieved by i.v. morphine. An episode of mild pain 2 days later was alleviated by sublingual nitroglycerin. Two days after that she had more severe pain, again requiring morphine. The following day she had a prolonged episode of severe pain requiring morphine and a 16-hour infusion of i.v. nitroglycerin. No significant ECG changes were noted following any of these episodes, but a two-dimensional echocardiogram revealed poor contraction of the inferior wall of the left ventricle in addition to the expected poor function of the anterior wall. Surprisingly, she never developed major signs of heart failure and subsequently did well in the

hospital, with only occasional mild pain; however, 6 weeks after discharge she died at home.

Values for serial enzyme determinations in this patient are illustrated in Figure 1-2. Following admission, there was a slight rise in total CK, but the values remained within normal limits. In the third, fourth, and fifth samples, however, MB was mildly but definitely elevated. There were no enzyme level rises following the next two episodes of pain. Eleven hours after the severe episode of December 27, there was a sharp rise in both total CK and MB. When the next sample was taken 10 hours later, the MB percentage had dropped to normal (1.5%), although the total CK was peaking. Total CK did not return to normal until 48 hours after the onset of chest pain.

There was a definite, albeit small, myocardial infarction on admission; total CK levels remained within normal limits, whereas values for raw MB nearly quadrupled. In calculating percentage MB, total CK is the denominator. When total CK is low, percentage MB is necessarily unreliable. Therefore, elevations in the absolute MB values are used. In this case the rise in the absolute MB value above normal (normal in

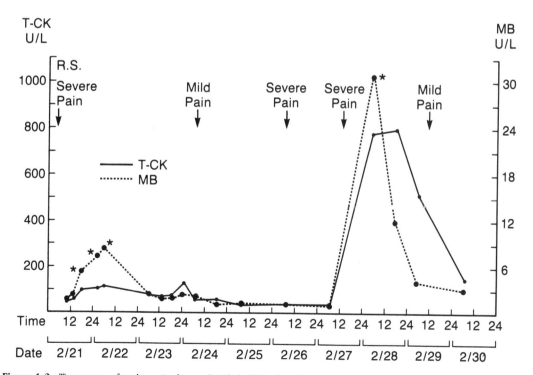

Figure 1-2. Time course of total creatine kinase (T-CK) (solid line) and its cardiac-specific isoenzyme MB (dotted line) values in patient RS (case 2); *elevated percentage MB.

this laboratory is >3.0 U/L) was diagnostic of myocardial necrosis. Such small infarctions are frequently called "non-Q wave," a term that is applied to clinical situations in which there is a small amount of myocardial necrosis and only ST-T wave changes (or no changes at all) in the ECG. Non-Q wave infarctions frequently presage a larger infarction and are associated with a poor long-term prognosis.

There was no significant change in the MB value following the next two chest pain episodes, indicating that they did not result in myocardial necrosis. Following the next very severe episode, however, the MB level rose abruptly to $\sim$30 U/L, which was $\sim$4% of total CK. This is consistent with a transmural (or Q wave) infarction, although in this case the diagnosis was confirmed by the echocardiogram rather than the ECG. The peak CK was 800 U/L, indicating a moderate-sized infarction. The size of the infarction has traditionally been estimated using total CK rather than MB, partly because of the very rapid rise and fall in MB values following an infarction. The slower time course of total CK allows construction of a more accurate curve for estimating, or even predicting, infarct size.

On admission the patient was begun on long-acting nitrates and calcium channel-blocking drugs, but they did not avert the larger infarction. Because of her poor left ventricular function, she began to receive digitalis and to participate in a slowly progressive activity schedule.

Case 3

SM, a 72-year-old man, was admitted on July 23, 1994, with a chief complaint of chest pain. His symptoms had begun approximately one month before and had progressively worsened over the few days before admission. They included chest pain and shortness of breath while ambulating, but recently they had begun to occur while he was sleeping and this would awake him during the night. He had a past medical history of coronary artery disease and stable angina pectoris, which had been treated with medications since January 1992. He stated that his symptoms were similar to the previous angina attacks.

SM's past medical history also included non-insulin-requiring diabetes mellitus, hypertension, and a smoking history of one pack per day for the last 30 years. His medications at the time of admission included a transdermal nitrate patch and a calcium channel blocker for coronary vasodilatation along with one aspirin per day to reduce platelet aggregation.

Physical examination revealed a well-developed, alert, and oriented male with no current complaint of chest pain. His blood pressure was 160/90, his pulse 86, and he was afebrile. No neck vein distension, thyromegaly, or corotid bruits were found. He had a normal first and second heart sound. He did not have a third heart sound, but a fourth heart sound was present and best in the left lateral position. There were no murmurs. Lungs were clear to auscultation. No clubbing, cyanosis, or edema were noted, and pulses were symmetric bilaterally of both upper and lower extremities.

The working diagnosis was unstable angina, which required admission to the hospital for further cardiac workup. Serial CK and MB values were done every 8 hours from admission, and they were all within normal limits. A cardiac catheterization was performed on July 24, 1994, and showed a 90% stenosis of the midportion of the left anterior descending artery (LAD) that involved the proximal first diagonal branch. There was only mild diffuse disease of the left circumflex and right coronary arteries. Percutaneous transluminal coronary angioplasty (PTCA) of the LAD was decided on.

On July 25, 1994, at 3:00 PM the PTCA was performed on the LAD but was complicated by the acute onset of chest pain and complete occlusion of the first diagonal branch during the procedure. The diagonal branch was occluded and the patient had chest pain for 30 minutes. The diagonal branch was subsequently opened using the same PTCA procedure with less than 20% residual stenosis.

Because the patient had chest pain and an occluded coronary artery, CK, MB, and MB isoforms were drawn at 7:00 PM on the evening of the procedure and again at 6:00 AM the following day. The cardiac enzyme results are depicted in Table 1-1. The initial CK and MB results drawn at 7:00 PM were within normal limits; however, the first MB isoform sample was positive at 1.72. The second samples drawn at 6:00 AM revealed a normal CK but an abnormal MB and MB isoform suggestive of a small myocardial infarction during the time the diagonal coronary artery was occluded. The electrophoretic curves are shown in Figure 1-3. The patient was

Table 1-1. Cardiac Enzyme Results[a]

	Total CK	CK-MB	MB Isoforms
7:00 PM	64	2.5	1.72
6:00 AM	115	13.1	2.76

CK, creatine kinase; MB, the cardiac-specific isoenzyme of CK.

[a] Cardiac enzyme results after acute occlusion of the diagonal branch of the left anterior descending artery at 3:00 PM. Blocked numbers are elevated above the normal values.

discharged 2 days later in stable condition and on the same medications.

This case is a good example of MB isoforms rising earlier than total CK and MB. It also demonstrates that MB and MB isoforms can be elevated during an infarction despite normal levels of total CK.

DIAGNOSIS

The diagnosis of acute myocardial infarction was difficult to make in PS (case 1) because of the complicating skeletal muscle damage, the confusing clinical picture, and the unremarkable ECGs. CK-MB determination provided a precise clarification, ruling out an infarction initially and then substantiating it for the second, quite similar, clinical episode.

Determining the MB level in RS (case 2) facilitated the diagnosis of a small myocardial infarction, despite normal levels of total CK and an unchanged ECG. The reliability of MB level determination allowed the patient's physicians to rule out infarctions with confidence following the next two clinical episodes. Unfortunately, a large infarction then ensued, confirmed by a rise in both MB and total CK levels. Subsequent myocardial necrosis was ruled out, de-spite postinfarction pain, by observing no change in the MB curve.

These two cases illustrate several different examples of the clinical benefit to be obtained by using isoenzyme determinations to diagnose specific organ damage. The first case demonstrates the specificity of MB determination in contrast to total CK. Creatine phosphokinase is found in skeletal muscle, cardiac muscle, and brain tissue. The form of the enzyme that occurs in the brain (BB) does not usually get past the blood–brain barrier and is therefore not normally present in the serum. There are two additional isoenzymes: MM and MB. Skeletal muscle contains mainly MM, with only 0 to 2% of its CK in the MB form. A similar ratio of MM to MB occurs in normal serum. MM is also the predominant myocardial CK but not to as great an extent; MB makes up 10 to 15% of CK in heart muscle. When skeletal muscle necrosis occurs, virtually all the increased CK in the serum is MM. Although there may be a small absolute rise in serum MB, as a percentage of total CK, MB remains unchanged.

Skeletal muscle necrosis occurs in many clinical situations in which myocardial infarction is a likely diagnosis. Probably the most common occurrence is the requirement for external defibrillation to correct a life-threatening ventricular tachyarrhythmia; the electric current passing through the body may de-stroy muscle cells in the chest wall and release CK, although it is interesting that defibrillation does not damage cardiac muscle. Shock complicating an acute myocardial infarction decreases blood flow to the extremities, sometimes leading to ischemic ne-crosis of the limb muscles. In case 1, ischemic ne-crosis caused the elevated CK, although here the blood flow was decreased by arterial obstruction rather than by shock. One or more of these causes of

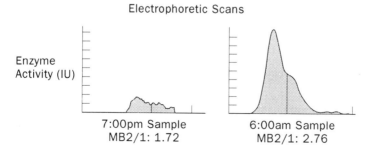

Electrophoretic Scans

Enzyme Activity (IU)

7:00pm Sample
MB2/1: 1.72

6:00am Sample
MB2/1: 2.76

Figure 1-3. Time course of creatine kinase isoenzyme MB isoforms as described in case 3.

skeletal muscle necrosis may be present in as many as 25% of all patients admitted to a coronary care unit with the presumptive diagnosis of acute myocardial infarction.

An elevation in total CK level thus has a low *specificity* in the diagnosis of myocardial infarction. On the other hand, because significant amounts of MB are found only in the heart, a rise in percentage MB above normal levels is very specific for acute infarction.

Total CK determination is also not as *sensitive* as MB measurement. The relatively large amount of CK present in the normal serum may mask the CK released from small amounts of myocardial necrosis; however, because MB is present in only minute amounts in normal serum (0–2% of total CK), even minimal degrees of myocardial necrosis will increase serum MB. Therefore, MB determination identifies many cases of acute myocardial infarction that would not have been diagnosed using total CK determination. So small an infarction would not be immediately life-threatening, but it does confirm the presence of coronary artery disease in previously undiagnosed patients. In other patients, as in our case 2, small infarctions may be a prelude to a much more serious clinical course. The high sensitivity of MB determination is also illustrated in case 1. Following this patient's myocardial infarction, the rise in total CK did not stand out from the previous high values, but the MB elevation was striking. This situation is more commonly encountered when a small infarction follows a larger one. A second peak in the MB values will be present while total CK continues its uninterrupted decline.

MOLECULAR PERSPECTIVES

The enzyme creatine kinase [CK, CPK, adenosine triphosphate (ATP):creatine *N*-phosphotransferase, EC 2.7.3.2] is an energy transfer enzyme that catalyzes the reversible biochemical reaction shown in Figure 1-4.

The highest CK activity in the body is found in skeletal and heart muscle. Muscle CK appears to function within the cytoplasmic and mitochondrial compartments of the cell. Mitochondrial CK, which is bound to the outer surface of the inner mitochondrial membrane, reacts with creatine and with ATP produced via oxidative phosphorylation to form adenosine diphosphate (ADP) and creatine phosphate (CP). ADP is recycled into the mitochondria and CP diffuses into the cytoplasm, where it serves as a substrate for cytoplasmic CK. Here cytoplasmic CK, associated with the M-line of myofibrils, catalyzes the reaction between CP and ADP to form ATP, which provides the immediate source of energy for muscle contraction. CK has been also detected in other tissues, such as colon and brain, in lesser amounts than muscle. Here its physiological function is thought to be related to the production of ATP for cellular transport processes.

CK is one of several blood or serum enzymes that have become useful clinical tools in the diagnosis of various diseases (Mercer, 1996). It exists primarily intracellularly as a result of its large molecular size (80,000 Da), which prevents it from readily crossing healthy cell membranes. The use of CK as a diagnostic test is based on the premise that CK can be released and appear in blood whenever cell membrane damage occurs. Trace amounts of CK can be detected in the blood of healthy individuals as a result of normal cell breakdown and turnover. When muscle cells are damaged, however, above-normal amounts of CK rapidly appear in the circulation.

CK was first recognized in the early 1960s as a potential diagnostic indicator of heart damage or myocardial infarction. Generally, above-normal CK activity occurs 4 to 6 hours following the onset of chest pain, reaches its peak by 24 to 36 hours, and returns to baseline levels within 72 hours. CK was found to be more sensitive than other diagnostic

Creatine Phosphate (CP) + Adenosine Diphosphate (ADP)

⇅

Creatine (C) + Adenosine Triphosphate (ATP)

Figure 1-3. The biochemical reaction of creatine kinase.

enzymes, such as glutamic-oxaloacetic transaminase (GOT) and lactate dehydrogenase (LDH), as peak CK values often reached 10 to 20 times the upper limit of normal. Enhanced tissue specificity was also observed, as the hepatic congestion and liver disorders that sometimes accompany cardiac disease did not elevate serum CK levels.

Although techniques for CK assay have been developed, most were nonkinetic and cumbersome and required serum blanks to eliminate the interference of endogenous substrate. In 1967 a spectrophotometric kinetic method, originally introduced by Oliver for measurement of tissue CK and adapted for serum CK by Rosalki (1967), emerged as the most widely accepted method. The Rosalki assay is based on the following three reactions:

Reaction 1, creatine kinase (CK):

$$ADP + creatine\ phosphate\ (CP) \rightarrow creatine\ (C) + ATP$$

Reaction 2, hexokinase:

$$ATP + glucose \rightarrow ADP + glucose\ 6\text{-phosphate}\ (G6P)$$

Reaction 3, glucose 6-phosphate dehydrogenase:

$$G6P + NADP^+ \rightarrow 6\text{-phosphogluconate} + NADPH + H^+$$

The above procedure is based on the formation of ATP by the action of CK in Reaction 1 with subsequent coupling to the hexokinase and glucose 6-phosphate dehydrogenase reactions. A thiol compound is added to reactivate CK that may have been oxidized during storage of sera. Adenosine monophosphate (AMP) is also added to prevent a second source of ATP formation from adenylate kinase (myokinase), which catalyzes the following reaction:

$$2ADP \rightarrow ATP + AMP$$

The net result of the assay mixture is the formation of the reduced form of nicotinamide adenine dinucleotide phosphate (NADPH), a compound easily detected spectrophotometrically at 340 nm. To simplify preparation of the reaction mixture, Rosalki (1967) lyophilized and distributed the dried powder into capsules. Introduction of bulk, freeze-dried substrate in kit form (commercially available) has made this procedure rapid and easy to perform.

Creatine Kinase Isoenzymes

With the use of more sensitive and convenient CK assays, it soon became apparent that CK was not as specific an indicator of acute myocardial infarction as initially thought. Numerous reports began to appear of CK elevations resulting from noncardiac conditions, such as chronic alcoholism, cardioversion, cerebrovascular disease, hypothyroidism, intramuscular injections, and surgical trauma.

In the early 1970s, attempts to enhance the diagnostic specificity of CK assays focused on the isolation and identification of tissue-specific isoenzymes (Lott and Stang, 1980). *Isoenzymes* are multiple forms of an enzyme family that catalyze the same biochemical reaction but differ in their physical and chemical properties.

Three cytoplasmic and one mitochondrial CK isoenzymes (Table 1-2) have been identified in CK-rich tissues. Each isoenzyme is a dimer composed of two subunits of the M, Mt, or B type. Cytoplasmic extracts of skeletal muscle contain CK consisting of two subunits of the M type, namely, the MM isoenzyme. Cytoplasmic CK in brain and colon extracts consists of two subunits of the B type, namely, the BB isoenzyme. CK in cytoplasmic cardiac extracts reveal two isoenzymes, the MM and MB. MB isoenzyme, a hybrid of M and B subunits, is found in significant amounts only in heart muscle. Considering the unique tissue distribution of CK isoenzymes, it is apparent that differential analysis of these isoenzymes can reveal diagnostic information.

CK isoenzymes MM, MB, and BB catalyze the same reaction with minimal differences in kinetic properties, such as pH optimum and substrate affinity; however, marked differences do exist with regard to other properties, such as thermal stability, chromatographic behavior on ion-exchange columns, electrophoretic mobility, and immunological properties.

Mitochondrial preparations of all CK-rich tissues contain the CK-Mt isoenzyme which, like MM, MB,

Table 1-2. Creatine Kinase (CK) Subunits and Isoenzymes

CK Subunits	CK Isoenzymes		Major Tissue Site
M	M	M	Skeletal muscle
B	M	B	Heart muscle
	B	B	Brain and colon
Mt	Mt	Mt	Muscle, brain, and colon

and BB, is also a dimer composed of two identical subunits of the Mt type. The molecular mass of CK-Mt is identical to that of the cytoplasmic isoenzyme, but the amino acid composition, electrophoretic mobility, and chromatographic and immunological properties all differ. A unique property of CK-Mt is its ability to form aggregates of high molecular mass.

Methods of Isoenzyme Measurement

Measurement of CK isoenzymes in clinical laboratories has focused on CK-MB because of its unique specificity for the diagnosis of myocardial injury. The methods of CK-MB determination fall into three general groups: electrophoretic, chromatographic, and immunochemical. Currently, clinical laboratories are using one of these three methods to perform CK-MB assays. Routine use of these procedures has been made possible by development of kit methods by various manufacturers.

Isoenzyme Separation by Electrophoresis

Electrophoretic techniques separate CK isoenzymes in an electrical field by taking advantage of differences in their net charge. Successful CK isoenzyme separations on support media, such as cellulose acetate, agarose, and polyacrylamide gels, have been achieved. Figure 1-5 illustrates the rapid anodic migration of BB isoenzyme and the slow anodic mobility of the MM isoenzyme. The MB isoenzyme, which is found in significant amounts only in cardiac tissue, migrates with intermediate mobility. CK-Mt migrates in the opposite direction

(cathodic). Infrequently in serum a CK band of activity appears midway between the MM and MB isoenzymes, but this atypical CK is not another isoenzyme. Instead, it has been shown by several investigators to be a CK-linked macromolecular complex composed of immunoglobulin G (IgG) and CK-BB isoenzyme.

Quantitation of the electrophoretically separated isoenzymes is usually accomplished by incubating the support media with CK reagent system (Rosalki, 1967) and measuring the amount of fluorescent NADPH produced. Although electrophoresis provides a means for separation of all CK isoenzymes including the CK-BB macrocomplex, the technique is more qualitative than quantitative. In addition, routine use is limited, as special technical skill is required to obtain reproducible results.

Resolution of CK-MB Isoforms by High-Voltage Electrophoresis

CK-MB exists in two other forms, called isoforms 1 and 2, that result from postsynthetic modification of the primary protein structure of CK-MB (Fig. 1-6). Synonymous terms for these forms are subbands, subforms, subtypes, and variant forms. CK-MB2 originates from cardiac tissue and is named according to its relatively slow anodic migration in electrophoresis (Fig. 1-7). CK-MB1 is a product of CK-MB2 and results from the enzymatic action of a serum protease, namely, carboxypeptidase-N. The proteolytic action of serum carboxypeptidase-N removes a terminal positively charged amino acid (lysine) to produce a more negatively-charged CK-MB with greater anodal mobility.

Clinical studies have shown that the CK-MB isoforms have greater diagnostic value, especially as cardiac markers during early periods after myocardial infarction, in the range of 3 to 6 hours after the onset of chest pains. Automated high-voltage electrophoresis is the method of choice for CK-MB isoform isolation and quantitation, but special technical skills are required to obtain reproducible results, especially in the lower CK activity range (2–10 U/L) (Talamo et al., 1985). Densitometric scans of typical patient samples are illustrated in Figure 1-7. Note the increased amount of CK-MB isoform 2 in the sample from a typical patient with myocardial infarction collected shortly after the onset of chest pain.

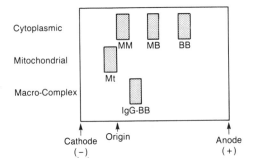

Figure 1-5. Typical electrophoretic separations of creatine kinase isoenzymes on thin-layer agarose gels.

CK-MB ISOFORMS

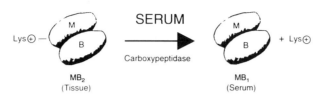

Figure 1-6. Enzymatic transformation of creatine kinase isoenzyme 2 (CK-MB$_2$) to isoenzyme 1 (CK-MB$_1$).

Isoenzyme Separation by Ion-Exchange Column Chromatography

Ion-exchange chromatography also takes advantage of isoenzyme charge differences. Here the CK isoenzymes are separated on the basis of their differential affinity for an ion-exchange resin (Galen, 1975; Mercer, 1974; Mercer and Varat, 1975). The procedure involves the use of columns filled with the anion resin, DEAE-Sephadex. The long elution times usually associated with conventional column chromatography are eliminated by the use of mini-

ELECTROPHORETIC SEPARATION OF CK-MB ISOFORMS

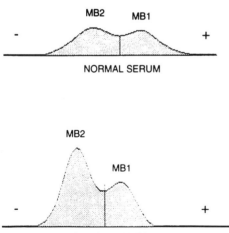

Figure 1-7. Typical densitometic scans of normal and acute myocardial infarction (AMI) patient samples.

columns the size of a pencil and stepwise elution instead of gradient elution procedures. Need for pretreatment of the sample (e.g., dialysis) is also eliminated by setting the column's exchangeable chloride concentration equal to that of serum. Thus, with a positively charged column, the noncharged MM isoenzyme and positively charged Mt isoenzyme pass through the ion exchanger while negatively charged MB and BB isoenzymes remain attached to the resin until a specified increase in chloride concentration decreases their ionic interaction with the ion exchanger. Quantitative assay of column effluents by the Rosalki CK assay completes the CK isoenzyme analysis. Figure 1-8 shows the ion-exchange elution patterns for tissue extracts of skeletal muscle, cardiac muscle, and brain.

Column-chromatographic separation of the CK-MB isoenzyme in serum and subsequent CK assay by a quantitative method has been shown to be an extremely sensitive and specific method. Routine use of the column method has been made possible by the commercial availability of ready-made columns and rapid elution procedures. Problems can arise, however, as a result of carryover of the MM isoenzyme into the MB column fraction when column separation procedures are not followed exactly. In addition, the occasional presence of the CK-BB macrocomplex in cardiac patients can lead to a false-positive MB measurement. This is not a major disadvantage, provided serial time-course patterns are observed and the typical rise and fall (spiked pattern) of CK-MB for myocardial infarction is considered.

Isoenzyme Separation by Immunoassay

In the 1970s immunochemical CK detection methods using the ability of inhibiting antibodies to block selectively the activity of the CK-M subunit began to appear. When CK-inhibiting antibodies are added to serum, the enzymatic activities of all the CK-M subunits in CK-MM and CK-MB are inhibited, and only the enzymatic activity of the B component of CK-MB and CK-BB remains intact. The chief advantage of the immunochemical method is the ease and rapidity with which CK-MB activity can be measured, as the use of only a conventional spectrophotometer is required. There is a serious disadvantage, however, because CK-BB and CK-Mt are not inhibited by anti-CK-M antibodies. Thus, clinical use of this type of immunochemical method results in false-positive CK-MB results because of the frequent presence of CK-BB and CK-Mt (low levels) in patient sera.

For many years no one was successful in raising an antibody specific to CK-MB, but in the early 1980s such an antibody was developed. Since then, improved monoclonal antibody-based immunoassays have allowed the clinical laboratory to provide timely, sensitive, and specific CK-MB assays for the rapid diagnosis of myocardial infarction.

Immunoassays measure mass isoenzyme concentration and differ from column and electrophoretic methods that measure enzymatic activity. Mass measurements using monoclonal antibodies to CK-MB correlate well with enzymatic CK-MB assays (Wu and Schwartz, 1989; Puleo et al., 1989; Puleo et al., 1990).

Initially, radioimmunoassays and enzymeimmunoassays required long incubations (2–3 hours) and were very expensive. Newly developed second-generation assays are now fully automated and quite fast (15–30 minutes). A typical enzyme immunoassay involves the following steps:

1. Addition of patient sample to an incubation well coated with anti-CK-MB antibody.
2. After incubation and washing of the well, enzyme-labeled anti-CK-M antibody is added to form an immunocomplex between CK-MB and the two antibodies.
3. Washing the sample well removes unbound CK-MM and CK-BB, but immunobound CK-MB remains.
4. Enzyme substrate is added and a reaction between the enzyme-labeled immunocomplex takes place, which results in a product that is highly fluorescent.
5. Measurement of the intensity of fluorescent is quantitatively related to the concentration of CK-MB in the patient's serum.

Several commercially available immunoassays for CK-MB are listed in Table 1-3. The newly automated immunoassays have results similar to those obtained in the 1970s by the time-consuming column and electrophoretic techniques.

Clinical Significance

The symptom of chest pain is a common complaint with many possible causes. Although in many cases, the ECG is used to distinguish trivial disorders from coronary disease, it is well known that a normal ECG does not necessarily exclude acute myocardial infarction, as in some cases ECG changes may be absent, minimal, or slow to develop. Moreover, in patients with previous heart disease, old ECG changes may obscure the current ECG picture. Measurement of the serum enzyme CK is of value in the above situations but, as indicated in other sections of

Table 1-3. Commercially Available Automated CK-MB Immunoassays

Instrument	Detection	Antibody Anchor	Antibody Tag
Abbott IMx	Fluorescence	Anti-CK-MB, Latex microparticles	Anti-CK-M Alkaline phosphatase
Baxter Stratus	Fluorescence	Anti-CK-MB, Glass fiber paper	Anti-CK-B Alkaline phosphatase
Ciba-Corning Magic Lite	Chemiluminescence	Anti-CK-B, Paramagnetic particles	Anti-CK-MB Acridinium ester
Johnson & Johnson Amerlite	Enhanced luminescence	Anti-CK-B, Microtitration plate	Anti-CK-M Peroxidase

this chapter, CK enzyme elevations are sensitive but not cardiac specific. Evidence that diagnostic accuracy for myocardial infarction is enhanced by quantitatively measuring the cardiac-specific CK-MB isoenzyme was first demonstrated in a 1975 study by Varat and Mercer. Here, ion-exchange column-isolated MB was quantitatively determined in 100 consecutive admissions to a coronary care unit. Table 1-4 lists the results obtained for total CK, MB isoenzyme, and percentage MB.

In 47 patients with proven acute myocardial infarction, including three with normal total CK, the MB peak accounted for >2% of total CK. In 49 patients without acute myocardial infarction, including 15 with elevated total CK due to trauma, injections, or cardioversion, the MB peak constituted <2% of total CK. The isoenzyme MB was elevated but did not peak in four patients with chronic atrial fibrillation.

Consideration of percentage MB is required for accurate diagnosis of myocardial infarction because cardiac tissue, although the richest in the MB isoenzyme, is not the only source. Trace amounts of CK-MB ($\leq$2% of the total CK activity) are detected in skeletal muscle extracts. MB is found in normal serum ($\leq$2%), and its origin is most likely skeletal muscle. Thus, serum samples with increased total CK activity as a result of skeletal muscle damage would be expected to show slightly elevated amounts of MB

activity, as demonstrated in the 15 patients without acute myocardial infarction but with elevated serum total CK, probably from skeletal muscle necrosis. Although raw MB levels were elevated, peak percentage MB levels never exceeded 2%, which is the lowest percentage level observed in patients with myocardial infarction.

Thus, a clear separation between patients with and without acute myocardial infarction is possible when data are expressed as percentage MB values. There was no overlap between the two groups in 96 of 100 cases when 2% MB was used as the cutoff point. There were no false-negative determinations with clinically diagnosed acute myocardial infarction. The four patients with elevated percentage MB from prolonged atrial fibrillation did have characteristics that could help identify them and clarify their diagnosis. In addition to prolonged atrial fibrillation, increased levels of MB have recently been detected in several patients with congestive heart failure, cardiomyopathy, muscular dystrophy, and polymyositis. Although all these conditions give MB values that could lead to misdiagnosis of myocardial infarction, they appear to be easily distinguishable when daily determinations of MB isoenzyme are performed and changes with time are followed (Fig. 1-9).

For practical purposes, serial measurements of cardiac-specific CK-MB isoenzyme or CK-MB iso-

Table 1–4. Total Creatine Kinase (CK) and Cardiac-Specific CK in Sera of 100 Patients Admitted to Coronary Care

	No. of Patients	Peak Total CK^a (U/L)	Peak MB U/L^b	Peak MB %^{c}
AMI	47			
↑ CK (abnormal)	44	144–4125	6.8–336	2.0–19
CK (normal)	3	64–114	3.6–25	2.0–22
No AMI	49			
↑ CK (abnormal)	15	135–1521	0.1–9.5	0–1.9
CK (normal)	34	9–113	0–1.8	0–3.3
No AMI, AF	4	17–114	3.4–8.7	4.0–16

AF, atrial fibrillation; AMI, acute myocardial infarction; ↑ CK, total creatine kinase (> 130 U/L).

^{a} Range of the single highest CK value in each patient.

^{b} MB isoenzyme.

^{c} MB isoenzyme expressed as a percentage of the simultaneously determined total CK.

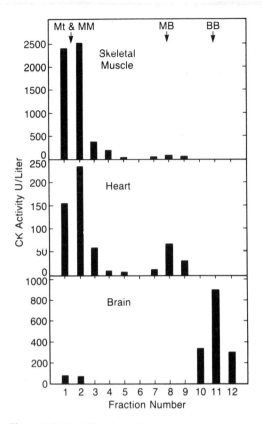

Figure 1-8. Typical column-chromatographic separations of creatine kinase (CK) isoenzymes (Mt, MM, MB, and BB). A stepwise elution was performed with three Tris-buffered sodium chloride solutions; 100 mmol/L (fractions 2–6); 200 mmol/L (fractions 7–9); and 300 mmol/L (fractions 10–12).

THERAPY

Treatments designed to salvage infarcted myocardial tissue are now commonly used. Measurement of MB levels would seem to be an excellent way to monitor the effectiveness of such treatment, as changes in infarct size would be expected to influence serum MB levels. The finding of persistent elevations of MB in the serum of patients with chronic atrial tachyarrhythmias suggests that under certain conditions myocardial necrosis may not be an abrupt event but may be continuous. There may be other conditions, such as congestive heart failure or cardiomyopathy, in which a small but continuous degree of myocardial destruction occurs.

Serial MB measurement would appear to provide

forms are recommended, especially for patients with chest pain of unknown origin in the emergency department or coronary care unit. Table 1-5 summarizes the clinical utility of total creatine kinase, total CK-MB isoenzyme, and CK-MB isoforms. Results should enhance the diagnosis of myocardial infarction and recurrent infarction, thus aiding in the timing of further diagnostic or operative procedures and in providing more certain psychological reassurance to patients. Moreover, cardiac-specific CK determinations should also enable cardiologists to make better use of available beds in coronary care units, as patients exhibiting normal levels can be transferred to other areas of the hospital as soon as possible.

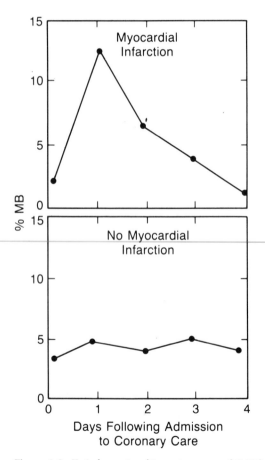

Figure 1-9. Typical creatine kinase isoenzyme (CK-MB) time course patterns for coronary care patients with and without myocardial infarction.

Table 1-5. Creatine Kinase (CK) Cardiac Markers

Marker	Diagnostic (AMI)	Sensitivity	Specificity	Assay
Total CK	No	High	Low	Enzymatic
CK-MB	Yes	High (4–10 h after onset of chest pain)	High	Electrophoresis, column, immunochemical
CK-MB isoforms	Yes	High (3–6 h after onset of chest pain)	High	Electrophoresis

AMI, acute myocardial infarction; CK-MB, the cardiac-specific isoenzyme of creatine kinase.

an effective way to monitor treatment for both acute and chronic myocardial necrosis. In addition, the isoforms of CK-MB are receiving attention as potential markers for assessing the success of balloon angioplasty or thrombolytic therapy with drugs such as tissue plasminogen activator (t-PA), streptokinase, and urokinase. For thrombolytic therapy or balloon angioplasty to be maximally effective, therapy must be initiated in the initial hours of infarction. Thus, the use of earlier markers such as CK-MB isoforms appears to be ideal for monitoring this type of clinical situation.

Although this chapter has centered on the isolation and quantitation of CK-MB isoenzyme, CK-BB and CK-Mt isoenzymes should not be neglected. Both CK-BB and CK-Mt have been detected in cancer patients and show considerable promise as potential markers for management of tumors.

QUESTIONS

1. Describe the serum CK isoenzyme column and electrophoretic patterns that exclude the diagnosis of myocardial infarction.
2. Three patients exhibit the following data:

	Total CK (U/L)	CK-MB (ng/mL)
Patient A	400	40
Patient B	50	6
Patient C	400	4

Identify the patients with results characteristic of myocardial infarction.

3. The value of any laboratory test depends on both its specificity and its sensitivity. Considering both criteria, why is determination of serum total CK superior to serum glutamic-oxaloacetic transaminase (SGOT) in the diagnosis of acute myocardial infarction? Why is determination of CK-MB superior to total CK?

4. CK-MB determination can reveal very small myocardial infarctions. List three reasons why knowledge of such limited amounts of myocardial necrosis is clinically important.
5. CK-MB isoforms appear to be earlier markers of acute myocardial infarction. True or False?
6. The following total CK and CK-MB data were obtained from the emergency department on three patients admitted with chest pain and a nondiagnostic ECG. Based on the CK data listed below, what is the best diagnosis?

	Time	TCK (U/L)	CK-MB (ng/mL)
Patient 1	0300	60	3.3
	0500	65	7.2
	0700	70	10.9
Patient 2	1000	650	4.5
	1200	700	5.0
	1400	675	5.2
Patient 3	1320	950	6.7
	1520	1005	8.6
	1720	1200	10.2

REFERENCES

Galen RS: The enzyme diagnosis of myocardial infarction. *Hum Pathol* **6:**141–155, 1975.

Lott JA, Stang JM: Serum enzymes and isoenzymes in the diagnosis and differential diagnosis of myocardial ischemia and necrosis. *Clin Chem* **26:**1241–1250, 1980.

Mercer DW: Separation of tissue and serum creatine kinase isoenzymes by ion-exchange column chromatography. *Clin Chem* **20:**36–40, 1974.

Mercer DW: A historical background of cardiac markers. *Med Lab Observ* **28:**45–51, 1996.

Mercer DW, Varat MA: Detection of cardiac-specific creatine kinase isoenzymes in sera with normal or slightly increased total creatine kinase activity. *Clin Chem* **21:**1088–1092, 1975.

Puleo PR, Guadagno PA, Roberts R, Perryman B: Sensitive, rapid assay of subforms creatine kinase MB in plasma. *Clin Chem* **35:**1452–1455, 1989.

Puleo PR, Guadagno PA, Roberts R, et al.: Early diagnosis of acute myocardial infarction based on assay for subforms of creatine kinase-MB. *Circulation* **82:**759–764, 1990.

Roberts R, Sobel BE, Parker CW: Radioimmunoassay for creatine kinase isoenzymes. *Science* **194**:855–857, 1976.

Rosalki SB: An improved procedure for serum creatine phosphokinase determination. *J Lab Clin Med* **69**:696–705, 1967.

Talamo TS, Losos FJ, Mercer DW: Interpretative reporting of cardiac profile data by microcomputer. Update. *Comput Med Imaging Graph* **3**:10–13, 1985.

Varat MA, Mercer DW: Cardiac specific creatine phosphokinase isoenzyme in the diagnosis of acute myocardial infarction. *Circulation* **51**:855–859, 1975.

Wu AHB, Schwartz JG: Update on creatine kinase isoenzyme assays. *Diagnostics and Clinical Testing* **27**:16–18, 1989.

2

Hereditary Spherocytosis

HIROSHI IDEGUCHI

CASE REPORT

A 25-year-old Japanese man was admitted to the hospital because of fever, sore throat, and general malaise. He had been febrile for several days and had noticed that the color of his urine was unusually dark. On admission, his temperature was 37.8°C. The physician noted anemic conjunctiva, infected pharyngeal mucosa, cervical lymphadenopathy, and mild splenomegaly. There were no constitutional anomalies. Hematological data showed a moderate anemia (hemoglobin 95 g/L; normal, 136–172 g/L), reticulocytosis (reticulocytes 7.8%; normal, <2.4%), and leukocytosis (leukocytes 12 × 10^9 /L; normal, 3.2–9.8 × 10^9 /L) with increased lymphocytes (62% of total leukocytes). The blood film showed a moderate anisocytosis (variability of size of erythrocytes), increased spherocytes (small, globular erythrocytes without the usual central pallor), and a scatter of atypical lymphocytes. Urine tests revealed no abnormality except an increase in the level of urobilinogen. The erythrocyte sedimentation rate was increased (45 mm/hr; normal, <20 mm/ hr). Biochemical data of his serum were as follows: total bilirubin, 99.2 μmol/L (normal, 3.4–20.5 μmol/L), conjugated bilirubin, 15.4 μmol/L (normal, 0–6.8 μmol/L), alanine aminotransferase, 125 U/L (normal, 0–40 U/L), and lactate dehydrogenase, 570 U/L (normal, 120–250 U/L). Serological examinations for Epstein-Barr virus confirmed that he had infectious mononucleosis. He was kept in bed for 2 weeks, by which time the signs of inflammation and hepatocellular damage entirely disap-

peared. Mild anemia (hemoglobin 110–120 g/L) with reticulocytosis (5.0–6.0%), increased serum unconjugated bilirubin and splenomegaly still remained, suggesting the presence of persistent hemolysis.

The physician therefore performed additional examinations to confirm the diagnosis of hemolytic anemia. Bone marrow aspirates from the sternum showed marked erythroid hyperplasia (increased number of erythroid cells in bone marrow); the granuloid-to-erythroid ratio was 1:1.5. The antiglobulin (Coombs') test failed to detect autoantibodies to red blood cells. Hemoglobin electrophoresis showed no abnormally migrating hemoglobins, and the levels of both hemoglobin F and hemoglobin A$_2$ were normal. The isopropanol test did not reveal any unstable hemoglobins. The sugar water test and Ham test, the diagnostic tests for paroxysmal nocturnal hemoglobinuria, were negative. In contrast, the osmotic fragility of the patient's erythrocytes was increased and was enhanced by incubating the cells at 37°C for 24 hours. These results were consistent with a diagnosis of hereditary spherocytosis (HS). The half-life of the ^{51}Cr-tagged erythrocytes was 14 days (normal, 25–32 days). Ultrasonic tomography of the abdomen revealed moderate splenomegaly and gallstones.

The patient had an episode of transient jaundice of unknown etiology at the age of 22 years. His parents had been in apparent good health; however, his father had also experienced repeated episodes of mild jaundice since childhood. Laboratory examinations of his family members revealed that the father's erythrocytes were also spherical and osmotically fragile. From these findings, he was finally diagnosed as having: (1) HS with gallstones and (2) infectious mononucleosis. To define the underlying molecular lesion, the physician tried to analyze red-cell membrane proteins by sodium dodecyl sulfate-polyacrylamide gel electrophoresis (SDS-PAGE) but did not detect any obvious quantitative defect of the major membrane proteins.

The patient underwent splenectomy and cholecystectomy (surgical removal of the gallbladder) at the age of 26 years. An enlarged spleen weighing 530 g and a gallbladder containing numerous small stones were removed. Two months after the operation, all previous findings reflecting accelerated hemolysis disappeared.

DIAGNOSIS

Hereditary spherocytosis is a congenital hemolytic disorder caused by an intrinsic defect of the red cell membrane (Palek and Lux, 1983; Palek and Sahr, 1992). It is now clear that the molecular basis of HS is heterogeneous and that the primary defect involves one of the red cell membrane proteins. In general,

patients with HS have mild anemia, intermittent jaundice, and splenomegaly. Common complications include neonatal jaundice, gallstones, and intermittent hemolytic or aplastic crises.

Symptoms and Signs

A typical HS patient is relatively asymptomatic (Palek, 1987; Palek, 1991). As already noted in one of the first descriptions of the disorder, mild jaundice may be the only symptom. Bilirubin (i.e., unconjugated bilirubin), a breakdown product of heme formed mainly in the reticuloendothelial cells, circulates in plasma as a complex with albumin and is taken up by liver cells and conjugated to form bilirubin diglucuronide (conjugated bilirubin), the water-soluble pigment excreted in bile. Serum unconjugated bilirubin is generally increased but seldom exceeds 85 μmol/L (normal <14 μmol/L). Anemia is usually mild or even absent owing to compensatory erythroid hyperplasia in bone marrow. Spherocytosis, or more correctly microspherocytosis, is a characteristic feature of the stained blood films (Fig. 2-1). The microspherocytes are small cells, usually with perfectly round contours, which stain relatively densely with Romanowsky dyes. The

(a)   **(b)**

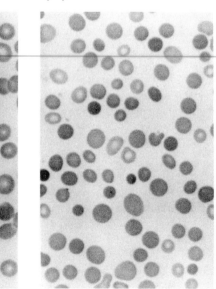

Figure 2-1. Photomicrographs of blood films of a normal subject **(a)** and a patient with hereditary spherocytosis **(b).** Note the small, densely staining microspherocytes in (b).

Romanowsky stain, a combination of eosin with a saturated methanol solution of methylene blue, is the basis for the most commonly used stains for blood, such as the Wright and Giemsa stains. The reticulocyte count is usually increased (5–20%) and remains high throughout the patient's life unless splenectomy has been carried out. Anisocytosis and polychromasia are elevated compared with normal films, and the small densely staining microsphero-cytes contrast well with the relatively larger, paler staining reticulocytes.

The osmotic fragility test, particularly that examined in incubated cells, is the most sensitive and useful test for the diagnosis of HS (Fig. 2-2). The test measures *in vitro* lysis of red cells suspended in solutions containing various concentrations of sodium chloride. In hypotonic solutions, the red cell progressively increases its volume by the rapid movement of water across the membrane until a critical hemolytic volume is reached. At this point, the red-cell membrane ruptures and hemoglobin escapes into the supernatant. Cells with a decreased surface-to-volume ratio, such as occurs in hereditary spherocytes, can tolerate less swelling than normal, leading to increased susceptibility to rupture (osmotic fragility). Although the fresh red cells of about 20% of HS patients have a normal or near-normal osmotic fragility, the test performed with cells incubated at 37°C for 24 hours is more often positive in association with an increased rate of spontaneous hemolysis (*autohemolysis*).

Patients with HS, like individuals with other hemolytic conditions, are occasionally subject to a sudden exaggeration of their anemia; this is the so-called *crisis.* Two types of crises, the *hemolytic* and *aplastic,* are known. As in the patient described herein, hemolytic crises usually occur with common viral syndromes and are characterized by a manifestation of accelerated destruction of red cells, such as a mild, transient increase in jaundice, anemia, reticulocytosis, and splenomegaly. Aplastic crises, on the other hand, are less frequent but usually more serious, as they can result in severe life-threatening anemia. They also develop in association with viral infections and typically present with fever, vomiting, abdominal pain, headache, and symptoms of anemia. During the aplastic phase, the counts of red cells and reticulocytes rapidly fall and marrow erythroblasts disappear. It is now generally agreed that aplastic crises are brought about by a temporary failure of erythropoiesis, resulting in insufficient supply of red cells to compensate for hemolysis. Recent observations have indicated that a common cause of aplastic crisis may be an infection of human parvovirus B19 (*erythema infectiosum*).

Gallstones are a common complication of HS, and most patients eventually develop them; they are rarely found in children, and their incidence increases with age. The stones are characteristically small, multiple, and of the pigmented variety. Because gallstone colic and cholecystitis are quite common, it is desirable that HS patients be periodically examined by abdominal ultrasonic tomography.

Differential Diagnosis

The following are the most important diagnostic features of HS: (1) a congenital hemolytic anemia;

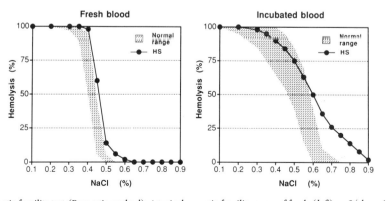

Figure 2-2. Osmotic fragility test (Parpart's method). A typical osmotic fragility curve of fresh (*left*) or 24-hour incubated (*right*) erythrocytes from a patient with hereditary spherocytosis (HS). The hatched area represents the normal range.

(2) microspherocytosis on the peripheral blood film and increased osmotic fragility, particularly in incubated red cells; (3) negative antiglobulin (Coombs') test; and (4) a favorable response to splenectomy. The antiglobulin (Coombs') test is used in the evaluation of autoimmune and drug-induced hemolytic anemia and hemolytic disease of the newborn. The direct antiglobulin test detects antibodies bound to red cells *in vivo,* and the indirect antiglobulin test detects serum antibodies that bind to red cells in an *in vitro* incubation step. Because of the relatively asymptomatic presentation of HS, this diagnosis should be considered during evaluation of unexplained splenomegaly, unconjugated hyperbilirubinemia of unknown etiology, gallstones at a young age, anemia during pregnancy, or transient anemia during acute infections. In general, HS is easily diagnosed and differentiated from other causes of spherocytosis, but there are several situations in which diagnosis may be difficult. In the neonatal period, it is not easy to differentiate HS from ABO incompatibility because both disorders are accompanied by microspherocytosis and the antiglobulin (Coombs') test is frequently negative in ABO disease. The diagnosis may not be finally settled until it becomes clear that the microcytosis and possibly other signs of hemolysis persist.

Sporadic HS in the adult or elderly patient may be confused with Coombs'-negative autoimmune hemolytic anemia. Erythrocyte survival studies, sensitive antiglobulin test with the use of radioactive antiglobulin reagents, and the clinical effect of corticosteroids may help the physician to arrive at the correct diagnosis. Diagnostic difficulties also arise when the patient is seen for the first time in an aplastic crisis. Early in the crisis the acute nature of the symptoms and severe anemia without reticulocytosis may divert the physician from a diagnosis of hemolytic anemia. The physician may have to bear in mind that in the young patient HS red cells initially emerging in the recovery phase are much less spherocytic and osmotically fragile than usual and acquire their typical microspherocytic form only with age and reticuloendothelial conditioning.

MOLECULAR PERSPECTIVES

History

Hereditary spherocytosis was first described in 1871 by Vanlair and Masius. The patient was a young woman who had repeated attacks of abdominal pain and jaundice; in addition, some of her erythrocytes were spherical and much smaller than normal. They named the condition *la microcythémie.* In 1893 Wilson and Stanley confirmed the inherited nature of the disease and described the spleen at autopsy as being grossly firm and dark and microscopically engorged with red cells. In 1907 Chauffard demonstrated increased osmotic fragility of erythrocytes as the hallmark of the disease. A membrane lesion was first suggested by the observation of Bertles in 1957 that HS red cells are unusually permeable to sodium ions. Since then, many abnormalities have been reported in HS red cells, but most are believed to be secondary and do not represent primary defects, which include changes in energy metabolism, alterations in cation transport, abnormal membrane protein phosphorylation, and altered membrane lipid composition. It is now clear, however, that the molecular basis of HS is heterogeneous and that several red cell membrane proteins are involved in the pathogenesis of HS.

Red-cell Membrane Organization

The red cell membrane is principally composed of a lipid bilayer and membrane proteins (Benz, 1994). The red cell membrane has been well characterized biochemically and the topological organization of various lipids and proteins has been delineated (Fig. 2-3). The major lipid components are cholesterol and phospholipids, and they are present in nearly equimolar amounts. Cholesterol and the phospholipids, phosphatidylcholine and sphingomyelin, are mostly found in the outer monolayer of lipid bilayer; the phospholipids, phosphatidylethanolamine and phosphatidylserine, are localized in the inner monolayer. The lipid composition of the membrane is

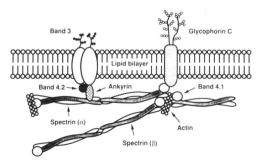

Figure 2-3. Structure of the red cell membrane.

responsible for the fluidity of the membrane matrix in which transmembrane proteins reside. The 12 major membrane proteins are conventionally separated by SDS-PAGE, and these proteins are classified into two groups: *integral* and *peripheral* proteins (Fig. 2-4; Table 2-1). The integral proteins penetrate into or are embedded in the lipid bilayer and are tightly bound to the membrane lipids through hydrophobic interactions; the peripheral proteins are located on the cytoplasmic surface of the lipid bilayer and associate with each other to form a flexible, filamentous network that provides mechanical stability of the membrane and a major determinant of red-cell shape and deformability. This filamentous network is generally referred to as the *membrane skeleton*.

The major components of the membrane skeleton are spectrin, actin, and band 4.1. Spectrin is a highly flexible, rodlike molecule composed of two nonidentical polypeptides: band 1 (spectrin α-chain; 240,000 Da) and band 2 (spectrin β-chain; 220,000 Da). These chains are aligned side by side in the form of an $\alpha\beta$ heterodimer. Spectrin heterodimers in turn join head to head to form $(\alpha\beta)_2$ tetramers. The tail ends of spectrin tetramers are associated with short actin filaments composed of 12 actin monomers. Although the spectrin-actin interaction itself is weak, each spectrin-actin junction is greatly stabilized by the formation of a ternary complex with the band 4.1 protein. This stabilization occurs

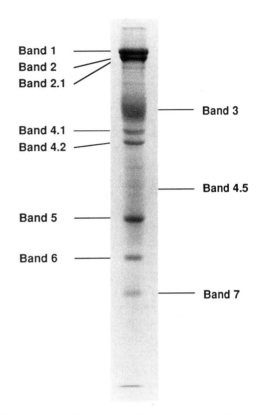

Peripheral   **Integral**

Band 1, Band 2, Band 2.1, Band 3, Band 4.1, Band 4.2, Band 4.5, Band 5, Band 6, Band 7

Figure 2-4. Sodium dodecyl sulfate-polyacrylamide gel electrophoresis (SDS-PAGE) pattern of normal red cell membrane proteins with Coomassie blue staining.

Table 2-1. Red-Cell Membrane Proteins

Band	Designation	Molecular Weight (Kd)	Protein	Function
Band 1	Spectrin-α	240	P	Membrane skeleton
Band 2	Spectrin-β	220	P	Membrane skeleton
Band 2.1	Ankyrin	210	P	Anchoring skeleton to bilayer
Band 3	Anion Exchanger	95	I	Anion transport; binding sites for ankyrin, band 4.2
Band 4.1		80	P	Membrane skeleton; association with GPC
Band 4.2		72	P	Stabilizing ankyrin-band 3 interaction(?)
Band 5	Actin	43	P	Membrane skeleton
Band 6		35	P	Glyceraldehyde 3-phosphate dehydrogenase
Band 7		29	I	(Unknown)
GPA	Glycophorin A	31	I	MN blood group
GPB	Glycophorin B	23	I	Ss blood group
GPC	Glycophorin C	29	I	Gerbich blood group; association with band 4.1

P, peripheral protein; I, integral protein

through direct interaction of band 4.1 with the spectrin β-chain at sites close to the region where spectrin interacts with actin oligomers. Thus, six spectrin termini complex with each actin oligomer to form a network with an approximately hexagonal lattice (Fig. 2-5). This structural model for the organization of the membrane skeleton has been confirmed by high-resolution electron micrographs of isolated membranes.

The major integral proteins include band 3 and the glycophorins. These proteins span the membrane and have distinct structural and functional domains, both within the bilayer and on either side of the membrane. Band 3, the anion exchanger, is the major integral protein, constituting about 25% of total membrane protein. The two clearly established functions of band 3 are: (1) the mediation of $Cl^--HCO_3^-$ exchange across the membrane, which is essential for the transport of CO_2 from the tissues to the lungs; and (2) the anchorage of the underlying membrane skeleton to the membrane by binding to ankyrin (band 2.1) and possibly band 4.2. The four sialic-acid–rich glycoproteins (glycophorins A–D) also belong to the class of integral proteins. The glycophorin A molecule carries the MN blood group specificity, glycophorin B the Ss specificity, and glycophorin C the Gerbich blood group specificity. The presence of sialic acids imparts a strong net negative charge to the erythrocyte surface, which is functionally important in reducing the interaction of red cells with one another as well as with other blood cells or the vascular endothelium.

The physiological linkage of the membrane skeleton to the lipid bilayer is thought to be mediated by two important interactions. As described above, the first linkage is provided by ankyrin (band 2.1), which simultaneously interacts with both spectrin and band 3. The interaction of ankyrin with band 3 is presumably stabilized by band 4.2. The second linkage is thought to result from the association of glycophorin C with band 4.1. Through these interactions, the lipid bilayer is mechanically coupled to the membrane skeleton, thereby providing the composite structure responsible for the unique properties of the red-cell membrane. The red cell constantly undergoes cycles of deformation and relaxation during its time in the circulation, requiring the membrane skeleton to accommodate to extensive and dynamic changes in cell shape, probably by the dynamic regulation of the interactions between various proteins, although the regulatory mechanisms still remain unclear.

Molecular Lesions in HS Erythrocytes

As knowledge of the membrane skeleton and its contribution to red-cell shape and stability emerged during the 1970s, investigators sought evidence of a skeletal protein defect in HS (Lux and Becker, 1989). The search was given impetus by the finding of a marked spectrin deficiency in the common house mouse. The spectrin-deficient red cells of the mouse were found to be spherocytic and osmotically fragile and to vesiculate spontaneously in the circulation. In several mutants, the ja/ja, sph/sph, and nb/nb mutants, the severity of hemolysis varies in proportion to the degree of spectrin deficiency. The ja/ja mutant completely lacks both α and β spectrins and has severe hemolytic anemia with massive splenomegaly and reticulocytosis exceeding 90%. Thus, investigators have focused on spectrin as the possible primary lesion of HS. Subsequent biochemical studies of spectrins and other membrane proteins in human HS red cells have led to the identification of several distinct molecular defects (Table 2-2).

In a subset of HS patients, the primary molecular lesions were in their spectrin. In 1982 Agre and coworkers first described two patients with severe HS inherited autosomal recessively and whose red cells had only about half the normal spectrin content. On the other hand, Goodman's group and Wolfe's group reported patients with autosomal dominant HS

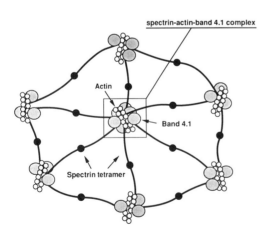

Figure 2-5. The hexagonal lattice structure of the membrane skeleton.

Table 2-2. Molecular Basis of Hereditary Spherocytosis

Responsible Gene	*Chromosome Locus*	*Phenotype and Molecular Lesion*		*Inheritance*	*Clinical Expression*	*Prevalence*
Spectrin-α	1	Spectrin deficiency		AR	Severe	Rare
Spectrin-β	14	Defective binding to band 4.1		AD	Mild to moderate	~10%
		Spectrin Kissimmee	(202Trp→Arg)			
Ankyrin	8	Ankyrin and spectrin deficiency		AD or AR	Mild to severe	40–50%
		Ankyrin gene deletion				
		Promoter region mutations				
		Ankyrin Prague (fast migrating)				
		Ankyrin Stuttgart	(329: 2nt del)			
		Ankyrin Einbeck	(572: 1nt ins)			
		Ankyrin Marburg	(797/798: 4nt del)			
		Ankyrin Bovenden	(1436Arg→ter)			
Band 3	17	Band 3 deficiency		AD or AR	Mild to moderate	?
		Band 3 Prague	(10 nt duplicate)			
		Band 3 Coimbra	(488Val→Met)			
		Band 4.2 deficiency		AD or AR	Mild to moderate	Rare
		Band 3 Tuscaloosa	(327Pro→Arg)			
		Band 3 Montifiore	(40Glu→Lys)			
		Band 3 Fukuoka	(130Gly→Arg)			
Band 4.2	15	Band 4.2 deficiency		AR	Mild to moderate	Rare; (more common in Japan)
		Band 4.2 Nippon	(142Ala→Thr)			
		Band 4.2 Fukuoka	(119Try→ter)			
		Band 4.2 Komatsu	(175Asp→Tyr)			
		Band 4.2 Tozeur	(310Arg→Gln)			
		Band 4.2 Shiga	(317Arg→Cys)			
		Band 4.2 Notame	(Int.6 nt1G→A)			

AD, autosomal dominant; AR, autosomal recessive

whose red cells were mildly deficient in spectrin and whose β-spectrin bound poorly to band 4.1. In one well-studied instance, spectrin Kissimmee, there is a single amino acid change (β202Trp→Arg) in a conserved region near the N-terminus of β-spectrin, which probably forms part of the band 4.1 binding site. In most HS patients, however, spectrin deficiency may not represent the primary molecular defect, as revealed by recent cytogenetic studies that failed to link HS with polymorphisms of both α- and β-spectrins.

It is now clear that a deficiency or dysfunction of ankyrin, the protein that anchors the spectrin-based skeleton to integral protein band 3, may represent a common membrane lesion in autosomal dominant HS. A combined deficiency of spectrin and ankyrin was first found in two unrelated patients with unusually severe, morphologically atypical HS. The synthesis of ankyrin and its assembly on the membrane were reduced; as a consequence, assembly of spectrin was also reduced despite normal spectrin synthesis. Either interstitial deletion of chromosome 8

(which contains the ankyrin gene) or its translocation to chromosome 3 and 12 has been reported in a subset of patients with combined spectrin-ankyrin deficiency. It was shown that the HS phenotype was genetically linked to the ankyrin gene in one large family with typical, mild HS. Moreover, a fast-migrating ankyrin (ankyrin Prague) resulting from a defect in a regulatory domain of ankyrin was found in mild, dominantly inherited HS. More recently, eight ankyrin mutations were discovered in 34 unrelated German HS patients.

A missing or partially reduced quantity of the band 4.2 protein was also noted in several patients with HS, particularly in the Japanese population. Although the physiological role of band 4.2 is still unclear, this protein binds to both band 3 and ankyrin, presumably stabilizing their association. In 1992 two Japanese HS patients with band 4.2 deficiency were reported to be homozygotes for a missense mutation in codon 142 of band 4.2 gene with the alanine-to-threonine amino acid substitution (band 4.2 Nippon). Subsequently, several other mutations in the band 4.2 gene were reported in Japanese patients with band 4.2 deficiency. Figure 2-6 shows an example of SDS-PAGE analysis of a family carrying the band 4.2 Nippon mutation. Patients 1, 2, and 3 are homozygotes for the mutation and have hemolytic anemia with an apparently complete deficiency of band 4.2, whereas patients 4 and 6, who are heterozygotes for the mutation, are healthy and have a normal amount of the band 4.2 protein.

In patients with a partial deficiency of band 4.2, several mutations have been found in their band 3 gene. These mutations include band 3 Tuscaloosa (327Pro→Arg), band 3 Fukuoka (130Gly→Arg), and band 3 Montefiore (40Glu→Lys), which are located in the cytoplasmic domain of band 3 where the skeletal network anchors through ankyrin and possibly band 4.2.

Another putative primary lesion appears to involve the band 3 protein. A partial deficiency of band 3

was reported in several patients with autosomal dominant HS. Moreover, it was shown by restriction fragment length polymorphism analysis that the primary defect is linked to the band 3 gene in one large family with HS.

Because of the heterogeneous molecular nature of HS, as shown in Table 6-2, the "HS genes" can be assigned to several chromosomes: chromosome 1 (α-spectrin), chromosome 8 (ankyrin), chromosome 14 (β-spectrin), chromosome 15 (band 4.2), and chromosome 17 (band 3). The inheritance is both autosomal dominant (in most HS patients) and autosomal recessive.

Recently, several rapid and sensitive methods were developed to detect mutations in cDNA and genomic DNA, including RNase protection analysis, denaturing gradient gel electrophoresis (DGGE), and single-strand conformation polymorphism (SSCP) analysis. These methods can be used in conjunction with the polymerase chain reaction (PCR) technique to detect small deletions or insertions and single base substitutions. RNase protection is used to detect the RNase-sensitive site in a synthetic RNA probe that has been hybridized with the DNA fragment to be examined. If a particular mutation lies within the DNA fragment, the RNA probe is mismatched at the site of the mutation where RNase digestion occurs. DGGE is used to detect the change in mobility of DNA fragments run on a polyacrylamide gel formed with an increasing gradient of the denaturant (urea, formamide, and so on). It is based on the principle that different DNA fragments begin to undergo regional denaturation at different points in the gradient, and the rate of migration is markedly slowed (Fig. 2-7a). SSCP analysis is the more popular method because of its simplicity and wide applicability to many different genes. This method makes use of sequence-dependent folding of single-stranded DNA, which alters the electrophoretic mobility of the fragments to reveal sequence differences between closely related molecules. In brief, regions of DNA thought to contain mutations are amplified using the PCR technique and rendered single-stranded by heating in a denaturing buffer. The separated strands are then fractionated on polyacrylamide gels under conditions that can resolve two molecules differing by a single base (Fig. 2-7b). If by one of these methods the DNA fragment appears to be abnormal, the specific change can then be determined by subsequent nucleotide sequence analysis.

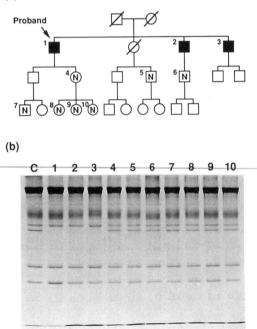

Figure 2-6. Sodium dodecyl sulfate-polyacrylamide gel electrophoresis (SDS-PAGE) analysis of a family with band 4.2 Nippon. Family pedigree **(a)**. ■ = Hereditary spherocytosis with band 4.2 deficiency. N = Healthy subjects without hemolytic anemia. SDS-PAGE of membrane proteins with Coomassie blue staining **(b)**. Lane C is from a control subject, and lanes 1–10 are from patients 1–10 shown in (a), respectively.

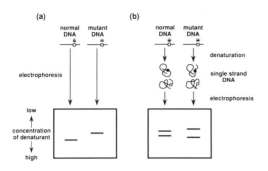

Figure 2-7. Rapid and sensitive methods for detecting mutations in DNA: denaturing gradient gel electrophoresis **(a)**; and single-strand conformation polymorphism **(b)**.

Pathophysiology of Hemolysis in HS Erythrocytes

The importance of the spleen in the pathophysiology of the hemolysis of HS was appreciated even in the original description of the disease and has been substantiated by subsequent studies. Two factors determine the selective destruction of the HS cells in the spleen: (1) a poor HS red cell deformability, which is a reflection of a decreased surface-to-volume ratio resulting from the loss of membrane; and (2) the unique anatomy of the splenic vasculature, which acts as a "microcirculation filter." As shown in Table 2-2, the underlying molecular basis of HS is heterogeneous and the primary molecular lesion in HS is likely to involve several membrane proteins, including spectrin, ankyrin, band 3, and band 4.2. These molecular lesions may finally lead to a reduced density of the submembrane skeletal network, presumably causing lipid bilayer destabilization and microvesiculation (Fig. 2-8). This hypothesis is supported by the following findings: (1) the degree of spectrin deficiency is proportional to the cellular spheroidicity and lipid bilayer instability; (2) under some *in vitro* conditions, the lipid bilayer is detached from the underlying skeleton, leading to formation of microvesicles, which contain integral proteins but no skeletal proteins; and (3) the density of the skeletal network is reduced and vesiculation is markedly enhanced in severe spectrin deficiency.

The principal sites of red-cell entrapment in the spleen are fenestrations in the endothelial wall of splenic sinuses, where blood enters the venous circulation. In contrast to normal discocytes, which have an abundant surface that allows red cells to deform and pass through narrow slits, the HS red cells lack the extra surface needed to permit deformation. It is actually visualized on electron micrographs of spleen specimens that few HS red cells

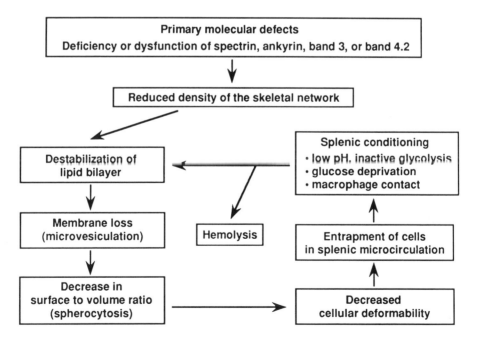

Figure 2-8. Pathophysiology of hemolysis of hereditary spherocytosis red cells.

transverse these endothelial slits. Consequently, the nondeformable spherocytes accumulate in the red pulp and become grossly engorged. Once entrapped by the spleen, HS red cells incur additional damage. Because of the stagnant circulation, lactic acid accumulates and the extracellular pH falls, probably to between 6.5 and 7.0. Intracellular pH must also decline, inhibiting hexokinase and phosphofructokinase, the rate-limiting enzymes of glycolysis, thereby retarding glucose utilization and adenosine triphosphate production. Contact of red cells with macrophages may inflict additional damage on the red cell membrane. Thus, the spherocytes detained in the splenic cords are severely stressed by erythrostasis in a metabolically threatening environment and are subject to further loss of surface area and an increase in the density of the cells. This process is known as *splenic conditioning* (Fig. 2-8). The conditioning effect of the spleen is likely to represent a cumulative injury. Conditioned red cells appear as microspherocytes in the peripheral circulation and are particularly susceptible to recapture and destruction in the spleen and other parts of reticuloendothelial system.

THERAPY

Patients with mild cases of HS often do not need any treatment; however, these patients should be watched carefully for the development of hemolytic or aplastic crisis. Splenectomy is the treatment of choice in moderate to severe HS cases. In general, splenectomy is indicated in patients who are continuously anemic or who have a history of a gallstone colic or repeated crises. The clinical results of splenectomy for HS are almost uniformly excellent. Although the spleen can be removed successfully in infancy, splenectomy in very young children should be postponed to later in childhood, if possible, because splenectomized infants are more susceptible to serious and potentially lethal infections than are older children and adults. At the time of splenectomy, it is important to identify and remove any accessory spleen; otherwise, the operation will result in an unfavorable outcome. Patients who experience an episode of gallstone colic or cholecystitis may have to simultaneously undergo cholecystectomy (removal of the gallbladder).

Within days following splenectomy, jaundice fades, the hemoglobin concentration rises, and red cell survival usually returns to near normal. High-normal values for reticulocytes and serum bilirubin reflect on ongoing but modest increase in red cell turnover. Although the numbers of peripheral blood microspherocytes remain unchanged, the morphological features of accelerated erythropoiesis are not observed.

Blood transfusion is rarely indicated except during aplastic crisis. At such times, red cell replacement may be lifesaving.

QUESTIONS

1. What are the essential findings for the clinical diagnosis of hereditary spherocytosis (HS)?
2. Patients with HS may occasionally undergo two types of "crises." Describe the mechanisms causing these crises.
3. The osmotic fragility of HS red cells is a reflection of a decreased surface-to-volume ratio (spherocytosis). Why are spherocytes osmotically fragile?
4. The HS red cells are hemolysed *in vivo* principally in the spleen. Explain why HS red cells are trapped by the spleen and describe the process of "splenic conditioning."
5. Describe the structural organization of the membrane skeleton that provides the mechanical stability of the membrane and is a major determinant of red-cell shape and deformability.
6. Hereditary spherocytosis is a group of disorders caused by heterogeneous intrinsic defects of the red-cell membrane proteins. It is usually difficult to define these molecular defects only by protein chemical methods such as SDS-PAGE. Describe other methods that can be used to detect these defects at the molecular level.

REFERENCES

Agre P, Orringer EP, Bennett V: Deficient red-cell spectrin in severe recessively inherited spherocytosis. *New Engl J Med* **306:**1155–1161, 1982.

Benz EJ: The erythrocyte membrane and cytoskeleton: structure, function, and disorders, *in* Stamatoyannopoulos G, Nienhuis AR, Majerus PW, Varmus H (eds): *The Molecular Basis of Blood Diseases*, 2nd ed. Philadelphia, WB Saunders Company, 1994, pp. 257–292.

Bertles JF: Sodium transport across the surface membrane of red cells in hereditary spherocytosis. *J Clin Invest* **36:**816–824, 1957.

Chauffard A: Pathogéne de l'ictére congenital de l'adulte. *Sem Med (Paris)* **27:**25–29, 1907.

Goodman SR, Schiffer KA, Casoria LA, Eyster ME: Identification of the molecular defect in the erythrocyte membrane skeleton of some kindreds with hereditary spherocytosis. *Blood* **60:**772–784, 1982.

Lux SE, Becker PS: Disorders of the red cell membrane skeleton: Hereditary spherocytosis and hereditary elliptocytosis, *in* Scriver CR, Beaudet AL, Sly WS, Valle D (eds): *The Metabolic Basis of Inherited Disease,* 6th ed., vol II. New York, McGraw-Hill Information Service Company, 1989, pp 2367–2408.

Palek J: Hereditary elliptocytosis, spherocytosis and related disorders: Consequences of a deficiency or a mutation of membrane skeleton proteins. *Blood Rev* **1:**147–168, 1987.

Palek J: Red cell membrane disorders, *in* Hoffman R, Benz EJ, Shattil SJ, Furie B, Cohen HJ (ed): *Hematology Basic Principles and Practice.* New York, Churchill Livingstone, 1991, pp. 472–504.

Palek J, Lux SE: Red cell membrane skeletal defects in heredi-tary and acquired hemolytic anemias. *Semin Hematol* **20:**189–224, 1983.

Palek J, Sahr KE: Mutations of the red cell membrane proteins: from clinical evaluation to detection of the underlying genetic defect. *Blood* **80:**308–330, 1992.

Vanlair CF, Masius JB: De la microcythémie. *Bull Acad Roy Med Belg,* 5, **3rd series:** 515–613, 1871.

Wilson C, Stanley DA: A sequel to some cases showing hereditary enlargement of the spleen. *Trans Clin Soc Lond* **26:**163–171, 1893.

Wolfe LC, John KM, Falcone JC, Byrne AM, Lux SE: A genetic defect in the binding of protein 4.1 to spectrin in a kindred with hereditary spherocytosis. *New Engl J Med* **307:**1367–1374, 1982.

3

Fragile X Syndrome

KOJI NARAHARA AND YUJI YOKOYAMA

CASE REPORT

The patients were brothers, aged 2 years 9 months and 1 year 8 months, and were referred to the hospital for evaluation for developmental delay.

The Elder Brother

The elder brother was born at term when his mother was 22 years old and his father 33. Pregnancy and delivery were uneventful. The birth weight was 3260 g. Neonatal screening for metabolic diseases and hypothyroidism did not show any abnormalities. He had gross psychomotor retardation: He controlled his head at the age of 5 months, sat alone at 12 months, and began to walk at 20 months, but he never spoke any meaningful words. Physical examination showed a hyperactive boy with a height of 94.5 cm, weight of 13.2 kg, and head circumference of 47.8 cm (Fig. 3-1a). His face was somewhat long and square-shaped with a high forehead. His ears were large and prominent. His left lower incisor was absent; the testes were not enlarged. Psychometric testing revealed a developmental quotient (DQ) that was 38% that of a normal child of the same age. He had unique behavioral abnormalities characterized by hyperactivity, short attention span, poor eye contact, and excessive withdrawal response to strange persons or environments; however, these behaviors did not meet the *Diagnostic and Statistical Manual of Mental Disorders* (DMS)-IV criteria for childhood autistic disorders. Electroencephalography (EEG) and acoustic brainstem response (ABR) were normal.

The Younger Brother

The younger brother was born at the 36th week of gestation with a birth weight of 2780 g. His psychomotor development was moderately retarded: He controlled his head at the age of 4 months, sat alone at 10 months, and could stand up holding onto furniture at 20 months, but he had not acquired any meaningful words yet. Physical examination showed a hyperactive boy with normal height and head circumference. His face was somewhat square-shaped with a prominent forehead, everted ears, and absent left lower incisor, like his elder brother (Fig. 3-1b). His DQ was assessed as 47% of normal. He had a short attention span but no social aversion or hand mannerisms. At the age of 20 months, his EEG and ABR were not remarkable, but massive epileptic discharges during sleep had become evident on the bilateral parieto-occipital regions since 1 year and 6 months of age.

The Family

The family pedigree of the patients (Fig. 3-2) revealed the presence of mental retardation in one maternal aunt (II-6, closed circle). She was born at term with a birth weight of 3080 g. The pregnancy was complicated by upper gastrointestinal (GI) radiographic exposure in the first trimester. Her motor development was reported to be almost normal, but speech was grossly delayed. She attended special educational schools. Anticonvulsant drugs were administered for EEG abnormalities. Physical examination at age 20 years showed a shy and mentally

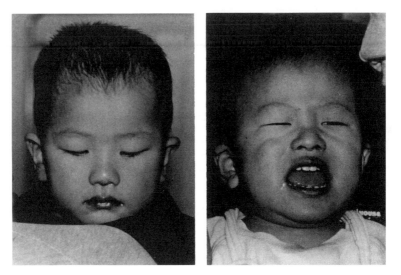

Figure 3-1. The two patients, the older brother, aged 2 years 9 months (**a**), and the younger brother, aged 1 year 8 months (**b**) showing the square-shaped faces, high forehead, and large everted ears.

retarded girl with a normal height and head circumference. She had a somewhat long face with prognathism; however, her ears were not malformed. Menstruation started at the age of 13 years and remained regular. Her speech disturbance was characterized by lack of fluency, echolalia, and inappropriate grammatical usage. Psychometric testing showed an intelligent quotient (IQ) of 45 (normal range, 77–124). The remaining maternal sibs appeared to be intellectually normal, although psychometric tests were not performed. They had no school problems except for one uncle (II-1) who left high school to work as a truck driver. The mother's IQ

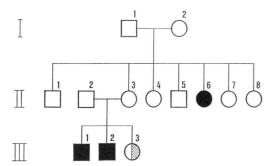

Figure 3-2. Family pedigree of the patients. Solid squares and circles indicate subjects with mental retardation, and circle with hatched lines denotes a person with borderline intelligence.

was assessed to be 92 by the Wechsler Adult Intelligence Scale test (WAIS). The maternal grandmother (I-2) was the sixth of seven sibship, and she denied the presence of mental retardation in her brothers and sisters.

The mother became pregnant again 6 months after the first visit regarding her two sons. Prenatal diagnosis of a fetus was refused on religious grounds. A female infant weighing 3462 g was delivered at term by cesarean section. Except for speech, her psychomotor development was almost normal. She began to speak a few meaningful words at the age of 18 months. Physical examination at age 2 years 10 months showed a child with normal height and head circumference. She had a somewhat square face but otherwise appeared normal. Her intelligence score was assessed at 85% that of a normal child.

DIAGNOSIS

The two probands presented moderate to severe developmental retardation, which was not associated with any recognizable malformation syndromes. Their dysmorphic features included a long, square-shaped face, large prominent ears, and a prominent forehead. The elder brother showed unique behavioral abnormalities and seemed to show an autistic trait. The younger sister also showed borderline mental retardation. Although the existence of mental retardation in one maternal aunt was difficult to explain, the familial disease could be consistent with X-linked inheritance with low *penetrance* (the frequency with which a heritable trait is manifested by persons carrying the affected gene) in females. Because fragile X syndrome represents about 40 to 50% of all forms of X-linked familial mental retardation, diagnostic workup should be initiated on this disorder.

Fragile X syndrome is associated with a rare fragile site at Xq27.3 (Fig. 3-3) in cytogenetic studies and is caused by a mutation in the fragile X mental retardation-1 (*FMR1*) gene. Although diagnosis of the disorder should be based on molecular studies, cytogenetic studies are useful to exclude sex chromosome and subtle autosomal abnormalities frequently associated with nonspecific mental retardation. The fragile site, fra(X)(q27.3), can be induced under specific culture conditions (e.g., medium deficient in folate or medium supplemented with methotrexate, fluorodeoxyuridine, or excess thymidine during the final 24 hours of cultures can perturb folate metabolism). As shown in Table 3-1, the two patients (III-1 and III-2), the sister (III-3), the mother (II-3), and the aunt (II-6) all had the fra(X)(q27.3) expression, whereas the remaining family members did not have the fragile site. To test whether the selective inactivation of X chromosomes could be related to the difference in phenotypes of the female carriers with fra(X)(q27.3), we studied DNA replication patterns of the X chromosome using bromodeoxyuridine (thymidine analogue) incorporation during the final 7 hours of the incubation. These studies demonstrated that the ratio of inactivated late-replicating X chromosomes (those incorporating much bromodeoxyuridine into DNAs) carrying fra(X)(q27.3) was not significantly different among the three female carriers.

The fragile X mutation involves an expansion of a CGG repeat stretch in the 5′ encoding region to *FMR-1*. *Hypermethylation* (a chemical alteration of DNA introduced by the attachment of a methyl group to deoxycytidine, thereby producing 5-methyl-deoxycytidine, in the CG sequence where cellular regulation of gene expression or X-inactivation is believed to occur) of a regulatory CpG island (a DNA

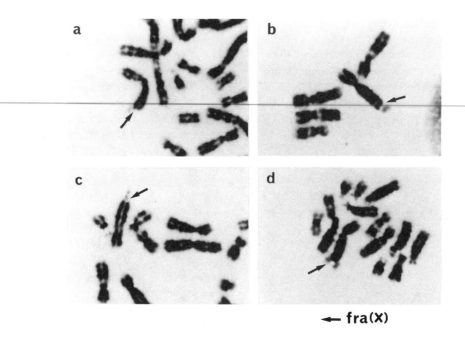

Figure 3-3. Partial karyotypes of Giemsa-stained human chromosomes showing various manifestations of the fragile X site (arrows): a chromatid break **(a)**, an isochromatid gap **(b)**, a chromosome break **(c)**, and endoreduplication **(d)**.

Table 3-1. Cytogenetic Studies of the Family

Subject	Sex	Age (yr)	Intelligewnce Quotient	Fra(X)(q27.3) Expression	Ratio of Inactivated fra(X) Positive X
I-1	M	59	Normal[a]	0%	ND
I-2	F	53	Normal	0%	ND
II-1	M	27	Normal	0%	ND
II-2	M	35	Normal	0%	ND
II-3	F	25	92	9%	48%
II-4	F	23	Normal	0%	ND
II-5	M	21	Normal	ND	ND
II-6	F	20	45	19%	53%
II-7	F	18	Normal	0%	ND
II-8	F	16	Normal	0%	ND
III-1	M	2	38	28%	ND
III-2	M	1	47	32%	ND
III-3	F	2	85	18%	58%

ND, not determined.

[a]Normal range: 77–124.

region of high deoxycytidine and deoxyguanosine content linked by a phosphodiester located near the protein coding region of a gene and related to its regulation of gene expression) just upstream of the CGG repeat segment and nonexpression of FMR-1 protein. We studied the length of the CGG repeat segment and the methylation status of the CpG island in the family of the patients, using Southern blot hybridization with pPCRFX1 (a kind of Pfxa3) as a DNA probe which detects restriction fragments containing the CGG repeat (Fig. 3-4). Digestion with a methylation-insensitive restriction enzyme, *EcoR1*, will generate a 5.2-kilobase (kb) fragment containing the mutable region. This fragment may be further digested by a methylation-sensitive restriction enzyme, *Eag1*, into 2.4 kb and 2.8 kb fragments if the *Eag1* site is not methylated. Normal males will have a 2.8-kb band, whereas normal females will have a 2.8-kb band and a 5.2-kb band. The two patients (III-1 and III-2) had a nondistinct smear band (meaning a dispersed expansion) ranging from 6 to 9 kb (0.7–4 kb expansion of the CGG repeat segment), and the aunt (II-6) also had a nondistinct smear band ranging from 6 to 9 kb in addition to the 2.8- and 5.2-kb normal bands. The grandmother (I-2) and the mother had additional 2.9-kb and 3.8-kb bands, respectively. The maternal uncle (II-1) also had a 3.1-kb band instead of a normal 2.8-kb

band. Intriguingly, the sister (III-3) had 4.0-kb and 6.4-kb bands in addition. It is conceivable that the CpG island did not undergo hypermethylation despite the CGG repeat expansion in a full mutation range (approximately 370 copy number of CGG repeats). The other family members showed normal blotting patterns. We diagnosed the two patients, the sister and the aunt, as having fragile X syndrome, and the mother, the uncle, and the maternal grandmother as being fragile X premutation carriers.

MOLECULAR PERSPECTIVES

Fragile X Syndrome

It is well known that the incidence of mental retardation is higher in males than in females. In 1943 Martin and Bell (1943) reported on familial mental retardation consistent with X-linked inheritance, and this family has now been demonstrated to be the first example of fragile X syndrome. The increasing medical interest in the causation and biological mechanisms of mental retardation has stimulated much research in the past three decades. In 1969 Lubs (1969) described a *marker X* (a constriction in the distal long arm of the X chromosome) present in affected males and obligate carrier females of a fami-

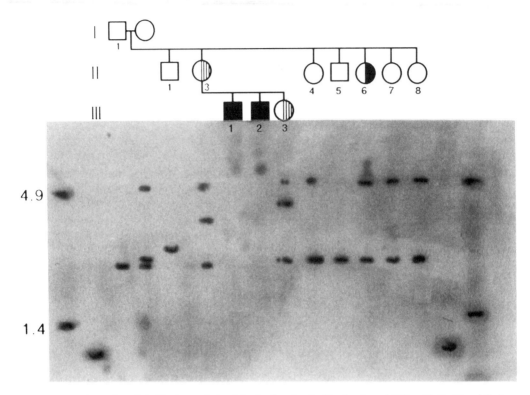

Figure 3-4. Southern hybridization analysis of the family using double-digestion of DNAs with *EcoRI* and *EagI*.

ly with X-linked mental retardation; however, it was not readily reproduced by standard cytogenetic techniques. It was not until 1977 that Sutherland (1977) reported that the induction of rare fragile sites, including marker X, is dependent on the composition of medium used for culturing peripheral blood lymphocytes. Because only the expression of the fragile site in band Xq27.3 (FRAXA) is associated with clinical disease among all rare fragile sites, the term *fragile X syndrome* was given to this condition (Sutherland and Richards, 1994).

The establishment of cytogenetic methods for detecting fragile X syndrome prompted epidemiologic studies on its prevalence in various populations. The syndrome occurs in all ethnic groups and affects approximately one in 1250 males and one in 2500 females. It accounts for about 20% of all familial mental retardation. This estimate is comparable to that of Down syndrome (one in 800–1000) as a cause of mental retardation. Ascertainment of the frequency in these studies has been based on cytogenetic detection, however, and the true prevalence

may be even higher using a newly available molecular test for population screening.

The phenotypic features of fragile X syndrome in relation to puberty are summarized in Table 3-2. Although the syndrome is apparent from birth in affected patients, it is difficult to diagnose during early infancy. Prepubertal males tend to exhibit only nonspecific clinical findings, and characteristic physical features become obvious with age. Typical postpubertal males with fragile X syndrome have a clinical triad of the so-called Martin-Bell syndrome: mental retardation, long face with large everted ears, and *macro-orchidism* (abnormally large testes). Other craniofacial features include prominent jaws, large forehead, and relative macrocephaly. Other symptoms are suggestive of connective tissue dysplasia: hyperextensible joints, mitral valve prolapse (falling down to the left atrium), and dilatation of the ascending aorta (aortic root dilatation). Developmental delay and mental retardation are the most significant and prominent symptoms of fragile X syndrome. Most male patients have IQ scores in the 20

Table 3-2. Clinical Features in Males
with Fragile X Syndrome

Prepubertal
  Birth weight: a mean at the approximately the 70th percentile
  Height: mostly between 50th and 97th percentile
  Head circumference: slightly increased
  Developmental delay: sit alone at 10 months, walk at 20.6
    months, first meaningful words at 20 months
  Abnormal behavior: hyperactivity, hand mannerisms, excessive
    shyness, tantrum, autism

Postpubertal
  Mental retardation
  Craniofacial features: prominent forehead, prominent jaw, large
    prominent ears, long face
  Macro-orchidism

Additional Features
  Orthopedic: joint hyperextensibility, flat feet, torticollis (a
    contracted state of the neck), *kyphoscoliosis* (backward and
    lateral curvature of the spinal column)
  Ophthalmologic: myopia and strabismus
  Cardiac: mitral valve prolapse and dilatation of ascending aorta
  Dermatologic: fine velvety skin with striae
  Genitourinary: *cryptorchidism* (failure of the testes to descend
    into the scrotum) and inguinal hernia
  Others: epilepsy, hyperreflexia, *gynecomastia* (excessive
    development of the male mammary glands)

to 60 range, with an average between 30 to 45. In particular, prepubertal fragile X boys have characteristic behavioral abnormalities, including hyperactivity, short attention span, emotional instability, hand mannerisms, and autistic features.

The physical and behavioral features of the disease in female patients are usually milder than those of affected males. Somatic features may be absent or mild, although the faces of mentally retarded females tend to resemble those of male patients with advancing age. The intelligence defect of female patients is less severe, with most patients belonging to the mild to borderline range. There is evidence of an increase in emotional or psychotic problems among female patients.

The inheritance pattern of fragile X syndrome is unusual. About 80% of males who inherit the mutation have mental retardation and a more or less definitive phenotype, but the remaining 20% of carrier males have a normal phenotype. Such clinically normal hemizygous males are termed *transmitting males* because the mutation is transmitted through their unaffected daughters to grandchildren, who often manifest this syndrome. The risk of mental retardation in grandchildren is 74% for males and 32% for females, whereas sibs of transmitting males have a much lower risk of mental retardation (18% for males and 10% for females). Male offspring of mentally impaired carrier mothers have a higher risk of being mentally retarded (100%) than do mentally normal carrier mothers (76%). The large variation in recurrence risk for mental retardation in fragile X families containing transmitting males cannot be explained by classic genetics and is termed the *Sherman paradox* after its discoverer (Sherman et al., 1985).

Because the cytogenetic approach is of limited value in detecting transmitting males and carrier females, efforts to identify and characterize a putative fragile X gene were undertaken in many molecular genetic laboratories during the past decade. The association of the fragile site at Xq27.3 with this form of X-linked mental retardation indicated that the putative gene may be located at or near the fragile X site. How positional cloning of the fragile X site was achieved is described by Tarleton and Saul (1993). New molecular tools, such as pulsed field gel electrophoresis and the yeast artificial chromosome (YAC), were used to define and isolate this region in addition to conventional analysis of restriction fragment length polymorphisms (RFLPs). The YACs can accommodate large DNA fragments from species other than yeasts, facilitating the cloning of a gene of interest; RFLPs provide useful molecular landmarks on chromosomes, enabling segregation analysis and risk assessment of the probability of inheriting a disease (linkage analysis).

The *FMR-1* Gene

In 1991 several groups of investigators reported almost simultaneously that the mutation responsible for fragile X syndrome is an expansion of the trinucleotide sequence CGG (or CCG) within a gene termed fragile X mental retardation-1 (*FMR-1*) (Oberle et al., 1991; Yu et al., 1991; Verkerk et al., 1991). The *FMR-1* gene encompasses 38 kb on the X chromosome at the position of the fragile site and is comprises 17 exons. The triplet repeat of sequence CGG lies within the 5' untranslated region of the first exon, 69 base pairs (bp) upstream from the initiating codon and 250 bp downstream from the CpG island, a regulatory gene (Fig. 3-5). This micro-

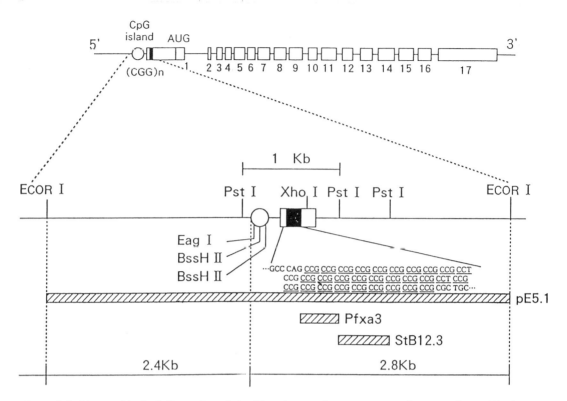

Figure 3-5. Diagram of the fragile X mental retardation (*FMR-1*) gene with restriction map and *FMR-1* probes used for diagnostic Southern blots. The circle indicates the CpG island, and the box represents the first exon. The dark region shows the location of triplet repeats.

satellite repeat is polymorphic in normal humans, ranging from 6 to 52 repeats, with a mean of 30 repeats. In affected patients with fragile X syndrome, however, this repeat contains many times the normal number of triplet repeats: between 230 and several thousand copies of CGG. When the trinucleotide repeats exceed 230 copies, the repeats are chemically modified in such a way that the *FMR1* gene will no longer function. The deoxycytidines within the repeats become derivatized with a methyl group, producing 5-methyldeoxycytidines. These methylation events extend upstream into the regulatory CpG island, which is normally unmethylated, and prevents the gene from being expressed. Virtually all affected patients lack detectable *FMR-1* mRNA, and the loss of *FMR-1* function as a result of the suppression of transcription is believed to be the cause of fragile X syndrome. Three instances of non-CGG mutations of the *FMR-1* gene, including deletions of the *FMR-1* locus and a missense mutation involving the critical domain of *FMR-1* in patients with apparent fragile X

syndrome, have provided further supporting evidence for this hypothesis. It should be emphasized that the mutation resulting from triplet expansion is unprecedented as a cause of human genetic disease.

Although its complete sequence is known, the exact function of the *FMR-1* gene has not been defined yet. The *FMR-1* gene has properties of a housekeeping gene because it is expressed in diverse tissues and has DNA sequences that are highly conserved in other species. Alternate splicing produces a considerable number of mRNAs. As would be expected, the gene is most intensely transcribed in both the brain and testes. Its protein product (FMRP), which is predominantly cytoplasmic, has some motifs characteristic of RNA-binding proteins (Siomi et al., 1993). It is thought that the extinction of an interaction between FMRP and a subset of brain mRNA in neurons could play an important role in the neurological manifestation of fragile X syndrome.

There are two types of mutations for the *FMR-1*

gene within fragile X families. The repeat expansion of more than 230 copies with the subsequent methylation of the CpG island is referred to as a *full mutation*. All males and about half of the females who carry full mutations are mentally retarded. Mosaic males with full mutations are almost always affected to the same extent as fully affected males. Mosaic females vary in clinical phenotype. The mosaic state is thought to be due to different degrees of expansion or DNA methylation in somatic cells. The other mutation in which the copy number of the repeat ranges from 50 to 230 is termed *premutation*. Because premutations are not methylated and are transcriptionally active, none of the male or female carriers with this type of mutation has any phenotypic abnormalities; however, it should be understood that no precise number of copies marks the transition from the normal chromosome to premutation or from premutation to full mutation. In general, geneticists have agreed to define a copy number between 50 and 230 as premutation and more than 230 as full mutation.

The most prominent characteristic of the CGG repeat is the instability of its length. Because expansion occurs after conception, the range of repeat expansion varies in different cells from the same tissue in the same affected person. This instability is especially enhanced when the expanded repeat is transmitted from mother to child. When women transmit the repeat to offspring of either sex, the sequence usually increases in size (although it has been known to decrease); however, when transmitted by males, the size of the sequence either stays the same or decreases. Males do not transmit more than 230 copies of the repeat, so their daughters do not have fragile X syndrome. This means that even an affected male with a full mutation in nearly all of his cells may be essentially within the premutation range of the repeat number in his sperm. No new mutation from the normal number of repeats has been seen in fragile X syndrome. A complete family investigation always identifies a premutation in one of the available ancestral generations. It is likely that small premutations may have segregated through many generations before a further repeat expansion occurs.

The Sherman paradox (Sherman et al., 1985; Sherman, 1991) was resolved by analyzing of the *FMR-1* gene in fragile X families with transmitting males (Fu et al., 1991). Transmitting males always have premutations, and the daughters of transmitting

males inherit about the same number of CGG repeats as found in the fathers. The premutations become unstable after *oogenesis* (the process of formation of the gametes) in the daughters, leading to full mutations with more than hundreds of CGG repeats in their offspring. Because the mothers of transmitting males have copy numbers of CGG repeats in the lower end of the carrier range (50–70), brothers of transmitting males are much less likely to have full mutations than premutations. Premutations larger than 80 repeats of CGG, however, almost always expand into the full mutation range when passed through mothers. Therefore, the Sherman paradox indicates that the variation in the propensity of premutations to become full mutations may be related to the size of a premutation and the gender of the carrier.

The fragile X site is expressed when the CGG repeat is expanded to a copy number higher than 230. The expression of the fragile site is thought to be a result of incomplete DNA replication in the expanded region caused by depletion of intracellular pools for dCTP and dGTP under specific culture conditions; however, the enormous expansion of CTG triplets in myotonic dystrophy, another genetic disease of trinucleotide repeat expansion, has never been known to be associated with any visible fragile site, suggesting that the nucleotide composition of the amplified repeats is crucial to the expression of the fragile site as well. In contrast to CTG repeats, CGG repeats undergo methylation, which might stabilize tetraplex DNAs formed by CGG tracts. These stable tetrahelical structures could suppress transcription, replication, and chromatin condensation, leading to generation of the fragile site.

Now that the molecular basis of the fragile X syndrome has been defined and characterized, exclusion of this disorder on clinical or cytogenetic grounds is no longer warranted. Once a child is identified with this syndrome, family members should be evaluated to detect individuals at risk of having affected children and to facilitate decisions about future reproduction.

Southern Blotting

Molecular diagnosis of fragile X syndrome is now possible using Southern hybridization and polymerase chain reaction (PCR) methods (Rousseau et al., 1991; Brown et al., 1993). Southern hybridization is the diagnostic method of choice because it can determine the extent of CGG repeat expansion as well as the methylation status of the CpG island. The choice between a restriction enzyme and a probe depends on the diagnostic information expected (Table 3-3). Cleavage with *PstI* and hybridization with a *Pfxa3* probe is suitable for detecting small premutation alleles. To examine the methylation status and CGG repeat length simultaneously, double-digestion with a methylation-insensitive enzyme, *EcoRI,* and a methylation-sensitive enzyme, such as *BssHII* or *EagI,* can be used (see Fig. 3-5). A 5.2-kb band is observed from the inactive X, and two smaller bands (2.8 and 2.4 kb) are observed from the active X of the female and the single X of a normal male. As the CGG repeat lies in the 2.8-kb band, males with premutations show a band slightly larger than 2.8 kb, corresponding to an increase in the size of the repeat length. Males with full mutations show a band larger than 5.2 kb, reflecting the methylated and expanded *FMR-1* mutation. Females with premutations have three bands of a normal female pattern (unmethylated active state of 2.4 and 2.8 kb, and methylated, inactive state of 5.2 kb) plus two additional premutation bands, which sometimes merge into the normal bands. In full-mutation females, the expanded CGG repeat is always overmethylated, and a smear band in excess of 5.7 kb can be seen in addition to the normal female bands. The interpreta-

tion of data in mosaic female patients is more complex because the pattern of bands reflects the methylated and unmethylated states of both normal and abnormal X chromosome alleles.

Polymerase Chain Reaction (PCR)

The PCR approach is particularly useful when a more accurate determination of CGG repeat numbers is necessary in normal or premutation carriers. Initial attempts to analyze the fragile X mutation by PCR were not successful because of the difficulty in amplifying DNA regions with a high CG content, the preferential amplification of the smallest allele in females, and the failure to amplify full mutations. These disadvantages have been partially corrected by the substitution of 7-deaza-dGTP for dGTP, the use of improved primers, and the introduction of sequencing acrylamide gels. The advantages of PCR are that it is rapid and requires only minimal amounts of DNA. It will likely become the technique of choice in the diagnosis of fragile X syndrome if a method that can reliably amplify full mutations is devised.

Prenatal Diagnosis

Because no effective therapy is available, prenatal diagnosis of fragile X is of prime importance in pregnancies of female carriers at risk of having af-

Table 3-3. RFLP Patterns by Southern Blot Analysis from Normal Individuals, Premutation Carriers, and Patients Affected with Fragile X Syndrome[a]

| | DNA digestion with Ecori + Eagl or BssHII | | PstI |
| | Hybridization with | | |
	pE5.1	Pfxa3 or StB12.3	Pfxa3
Normal (6–50 repeats)			
Male	2.4 + 2.8	2.8	1.0
Female	2.4 + 2.8 + 5.2	2.8 + 5.2	1.0
Premutation carriers (50–230 repeats)			
Male	2.4 + (2.9–3.3)	(2.9–3.3)	(1.1–1.6)
Female	2.4 + 2.8 + (2.9–3.3) + 5.2	2.8 + (2.9–3.3) + 5.2	1.0 + (1.1–1.6)
Patients with full mutations (>230 repeats)			
Male	>5.7	>5.7	>1.6
Female	2.4 + 2.8 + 5.2 + >5.7	2.8 + 5.2 + >5.7	1.0 + >1.6
Mosaic patients			
Male	(2.9–3.3) + >5.7	(2.9–3.3) + >5.7	(1.1–1.6) + >1.6
Female	2.4 + 2.8 + (2.9–3.3) + 5.2 + >5.7	2.8 + (2.9–3.3) + 5.2 + >5.7	1.0 + (1.1–1.6) + >1.6

RFLP, restriction fragment length polymorphisms.

[a] Sizes of bands are expressed in kilobases.

fected children. Cytogenetic analysis no longer has a place in the prenatal diagnosis of fragile X syndrome. Prenatal diagnosis can be accomplished by analyzing DNA obtained by chorionic villus (a villus on the external surface of the chorion: fetal tissue) sampling (CVS) using Southern blot analysis or, more recently, using PCR, which can detect the copy number of the CGG repeat. Male fetuses with 50 to 230 copies of the repeat should be asymptomatic, whereas those with more than 230 copies will have fragile X syndrome. Female fetuses with 50 to 230 copies will be also asymptomatic; however, it is difficult to predict the extent of mental retardation in female fetuses with more than 230 copies of the repeat. Although hypermethylation of the CpG island is a poor prognostic indicator, it is not always present in DNA extracted from CVS (Sutherland et al., 1991). Empiric data showing that female carriers with full mutations have nearly a 50% risk of mental impairment should be considered reliable.

Genetic Diseases Associated with Dynamic Mutations

Fragile X syndrome is the first example among eight human genetic diseases wherein dynamic mutation of the trinucleotide repeat has been shown to be the cause (Table 3-4). The sequence of the trinucleotide repeat and the effect of the expansion on the function of the gene in which it resides can differ. *Genetic anticipation* (a phenomenon in which the disease has an earlier age of onset and becomes increasingly severe in succeeding generations) is a common feature in these diseases and can be explained by the expansion of the repeat when transmitted from parent to child. The gender bias of the parent contributing severe forms of the disease is evident in some of these diseases. The form of myotonic dystrophy that is apparent from birth occurs only in children who have inherited the mutation from their mother. The juvenile-onset forms of Huntington disease and spinocerebellar ataxia type I develop primarily when the mutation is transmitted from the father. It should be noted that another fragile site, FRAXE (Fragile site, X chromosome, E site), has a similar genetic mechanism to fragile X syndrome, an expansion of the CGG repeat, and methylation of the CpG island, resulting in mental retardation. In contrast to the repeats in fragile X syndrome, the repeat in the FRAXE can expand or contract and is equally unstable when passed through the mother or father.

The molecular mechanism of the repeat expansion in fragile X syndrome is not known. Linkage analyses of microsatellite markers flanking the CGG repeat have suggested a founder effect in fragile X

Table 3-4. Genetic Diseases Associated with Dynamic Mutations

Disease	Chromosome Location	Repeated Sequence	Sex Bias of Parent Contributing Severe Form	Normal no. of Copies	No. of Copies Associated with the Disease	Change in Gene Function
Fragile X syndrome	Xq27.3	CGG	Maternal	6–50	Premutation: 50–230 Full mutation: 230–2000	Loss
Spinobulbar muscular atrophy (Kennedy disease)	Xq11–12	CAG	?	11–31	40–62	Gain
Myotonic dystrophy	19q13.3	CTG	Maternal	5–35	Premutation: 50–80 Full mutation: 80–2000	mRNA stability
Huntington disease	4p16.3	CAG	Paternal	9–37	Premutation: 30–38 Full mutation: 37–121	Gain
Spinocerebellar ataxia type 1	6p22–23	CAG	Paternal (possibly)	25–36	43–81	Gain
Fragile XE mental regardation	Xq28	CGG	?	6–25	Premutation: 25–200 Full mutation: >200	Loss
Dentatorubral-pallidoluysian atrophy	12p12.13	CAG	Paternal (mainly)	7–23	49–75	Gain
Machado-Joseph disease	14q32.1	CAG	?	13–36	68–79	Gain

Modified and reproduced with permission from Sutherland and Richards (1994).

syndrome: Prevalent full fragile X mutations are derived from a few ancestral premutations that could increase in the genetic pool because of their being relatively stable and selectively neutral. There is other evidence that the CGG repeat of the *FMR-1* gene in normal individuals has AGG interruptions and the repeat with documented unstable transmissions has lost AGG interruptions (Eichler et al., 1994), which means that either DNA sequences flanking the repeat or variations in the repeat itself are involved in the mutation mechanism. The massive expansion of triplet repeats associated with fragile X syndrome, when transmitted from a parent with more than approximately 80 copies of the repeat, cannot be explained by simple recombination. *Okazaki fragment slippage* (the tendency for a single-strand DNA with free ends caused by two breaks to slide along a template strand, resulting in a greater likelihood of mutation after DNA replication) has been proposed as a possible mechanism for such rapid expansion (Fig. 3-6) (Richards and Sutherland, 1994).

Studies of dynamic mutations (i.e., expansion of the trinucleotide repeats) are still in their infancy. A larger number of human genes have been found to contain trinucleotide repeats, and more diseases due to dynamic mutations of the repeat will emerge in the future. Better understanding of how predisposed chromosomes undergo mutational changes will contribute to the development of possible interventions in the disease process.

THERAPY

Because no specific treatment for fragile X syndrome is available, medical, physical, and occupational interventions are directed toward alleviating neurologic and behavioral manifestations of the disorder (Hagerman, 1989). It is also important for parents to be in contact with other fragile X families for further support and information. Medical management in fragile X syndrome includes medical treat-

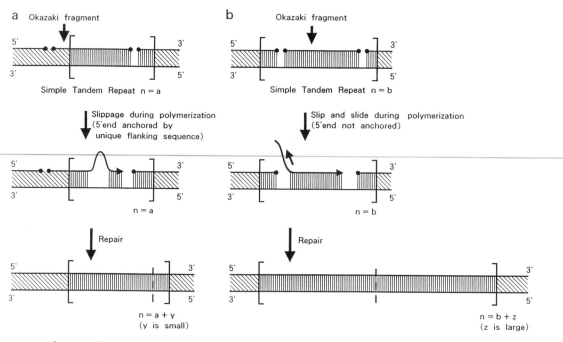

Figure 3-6. Models for instability and hyperexpansion involving Okazaki fragment slippage. For copy number <80 (n = a), only one single-stranded break is likely to occur within the repeat during replication **(a)**. Slippage of the elongated strand during polymerization can result in the addition or deletion of a few copies (y). For copy numbers >80 (n = b), it is possible that two single strand breaks occur within the repeat in the process of replication **(b)**. The strand between these breaks is not anchored at either end by unique sequences and is therefore free to slide during polymerization, enabling the addition of many more copies (z) than were present in the original sequence (b) pending the outcome of the repair process. *Nature Genetics* **6:**115, 1994.

ment for specific behavioral problems and follow-up of complications that are frequently seen in fragile X syndrome. Folic acid supplementation is no longer recommended for treatment of the intellectual and behavioral deficits in fragile X syndrome because several studies have found that it is of no benefit. Central nervous system stimulants, such as methylphenidate and dextroamphetamine, have proved to be effective in improving the attention span and learning performance of some hyperactive fragile X children.

Educational interventions can be instituted after diagnosis of the disorder has been made and extensive genetic counseling of the family has been initiated. Teachers and therapists should create an educational program in keeping with the neuropsychological characteristics of fragile X patients. Fragile X patients have more difficulty with the auditory processing than with visual processing, which relates to their attentional problems, impulsivity, and distractibility, validating the use of central nervous system stimulants in fragile X patients. Calming techniques, such as deep breathing, relaxation, and environmental music, are sometimes effective in avoiding emotional upsets and outbursts of tantrum in new situations or confusing circumstances. The goal of speech and occupational therapies is to help fragile X patients reach their intellectual potentials.

QUESTIONS

1. What clinical features do prepubertal male patients affected with fragile X syndrome have?
2. Why is it important for medical personnel and scientists to understand the molecular basis of fragile X syndrome?
3. What is the Sherman paradox in fragile X syndrome, and how can this paradox be resolved on a molecular basis?
4. How would you go about informing the mother (II-2) and the uncle (II-1) of the patients about the risk of their having children affected with fragile X syndrome in a future pregnancy?
5. Both the aunt (II-6) and the sister (III-3) of the patients had fragile X expression and apparent full mutation. Why was the phenotype of the sister much milder than that of the aunt?
6. What other human genetic diseases have been attributed to dynamic mutation of a trinucleotide repeat?

Acknowledgment: We thank Dr. Grant R. Sutherland (Center for Medical Genetics, Department of Cytogenetics and Molecular Genetics, Women's and Children's Hospital, Adelaide, South Australia) for reading the manuscript and for permission to use Figure 3-6.

REFERENCES

Brown WT, Houck GE, Jeziorowska A, et al.: Rapid fragile X carrier screening and prenatal diagnosis using a nonradioactive PCR test. *JAMA* **270:**1569–1575, 1993.

Eichler EE, Holden JJA, Popovich BW, et al.: Length of uninterrupted CGG repeats determines instability in the FMR1 gene. *Nature Genet* **8:**88–94, 1994.

Fu YH, Kuhl DPA, Pizzuti A, et al.: Variation of the CGG repeat at the fragile X site results in genetic instability: resolution of the Sherman paradox. *Cell* **67:**1047–1058, 1991.

Hagerman R: Behaviour and treatment of the fragile X syndrome, *in* Davies KE (ed): *The Fragile X Syndrome.* Oxford, Oxford University Press, 1989, pp 56–75.

Lubs HA: A marker X chromosome. *Am J Hum Genet* **21:**231–244, 1969.

Martin JP, Bell J: A pedigree of a mental defect showing sex-linkage. *J Neurol Psychiatry* **6:**151–154, 1943.

Oberle I, Rousseau F, Heitz D, et al.: Instability of a 550-base pair DNA segment and abnormal methylation in fragile X syndrome. *Science* **252:**1097–1102, 1991.

Richards RI, Sutherland GR: Simple repeat DNA is not replicated simply. *Nature Genet* **6:**114–116, 1994.

Rousseau F, Heitz D, Biancalana V, et al.: Direct diagnosis by DNA analysis of the fragile X syndrome of mental retardation. *N Engl J Med* **325:**1673–1681, 1991.

Sherman SL, Jacobs PA, Morton NE, et al.: Further segregation analysis of the fragile X syndrome with special reference to transmitting males. *Hum Genet* **69:**289–299, 1985.

Sherman S: Epidemiology, *in* Hagerman RJ, Silverman AC (eds): *Fragile X Syndrome: Diagnosis, Treatment, and Research.* Baltimore, Johns Hopkins Press, 1991, pp 69–97.

Siomi H, Siomi MC, Nussbaum RL, Dreyfuss G: The protein product of the fragile X gene, FMR1, has characteristics of an RNA-binding protein. *Cell* **74:**291–298, 1993.

Sutherland GR: Fragile sites on human chromosomes: demonstration of their dependence on the type of tissue culture medium. *Science* **197:**265–266, 1977.

Sutherland GR, Gedeon A, Kornman L, et al.: Prenatal diagnosis of fragile X syndrome by direct detection of the unstable DNA sequence. *N Engl J Med* **325:**1720–1722, 1991.

Sutherland GR, Richards RI: Dynamic mutations. *Am Sci* **82:**157–163, 1994.

Tarleton JC, Saul RA: Molecular genetic advances in fragile X syndrome. *J Pediatr* **122:**169–185, 1993.

Verkerk AJMH, Pieretti M, Sutcliffe JS, et al.: Identification of a gene (FMR-1) containing a CGG repeat coincident with a break-point cluster region exhibiting length variation in fragile X syndrome. *Cell* **65:**905–914, 1991.

Yu S, Pritchard M, Kremer EJ, et al.: Fragile X genotype characterized by an unstable region of DNA. *Science* **252:**1179–1181, 1991.

Human Immunodeficiency Viruses and the Acquired Immunodeficiency Syndrome

STEVEN JENISON AND BRIAN HJELLE

CASE REPORT

IG, a 34-year-old man from New Mexico, had lived in San Francisco, California, for 14 years. He returned to Albuquerque to live with his family 2 years before his death. He had acquired human immunodeficiency virus (HIV) infection through unprotected sexual contact with men. His previous medical history was notable for recurrent perianal herpes. Five years before his death, he developed a painful erythematous vesicular rash over the right chest in the dermatomal distribution of the sixth thoracic spinal nerve (T6). Varicella zoster virus was isolated from cultures of vesicle fluid. Three well-defined dark purple lesions, two on the left anterior leg and one over the right scapula, were also present. These pigmented lesions were Kaposi's sarcomas based on histologic examination of skin biopsies. The mucosal surface of the right lateral tongue margin had a white thickened, shaggy appearance suggestive of oral hairy leukoplakia.

Because Kaposi's sarcoma is often a manifestation of HIV disease, testing for the presence of HIV-specific antibodies was recommended and the patient's informed consent was obtained. Serum HIV antibodies were detected in the HIV enzyme immunoassay (EIA). The HIV Western blot assay showed antibody reactivities with HIV envelope glycoproteins (gp120 and gp41) and the capsid protein (p24). The CD4-positive T-lymphocyte count was 330 cells/mm^3 (normal, 600–3100 cells/mm^3). Routine peripheral blood cell counts and serum chemistry tests were normal except for an elevated serum total protein of 8.8 g/dL (normal, 6.0–8.0 g/dL) and a serum albumin level of 3.3 g/dL (normal, 3.8 to 4.8 g/dL). Hepatitis B virus (HBV) blood tests were negative for the presence of hepatitis B surface antigen, positive for antibodies to hepatitis B core antigen, and positive for antibodies to hepatitis B surface antigen. These results indicated that an HBV infection had occurred in the past and that chronic HBV infection was not currently present. A delayed-type hypersensitivity reaction to the *Mycobacterium tuberculosis* antigen tuberculin (PPD) was not present by skin testing. Delayed-type hypersensitivity reactions to mumps virus and *Candida albicans* skin test antigens were intact.

The polyvalent *Streptococcus pneumoniae* vaccine and influenza virus vaccine were administered. Antiretroviral chemotherapy was initiated with the nucleoside analogue zidovudine (AZT). The nucleoside analogue acyclovir was given twice daily to decrease the frequency of perianal herpes recurrences. Three months later, the hemoglobin level had dropped from 15.5 g/dL to 13.8 g/dL (normal, 14.0–18.0 g/dL). The red blood cell mean corpuscular volume had increased from 92 fL to 108 fL (normal, 81–94 fL). The absolute neutrophil count was normal.

Over the next 2 years, the CD4-positive T-lymphocyte count decreased gradually to 170 cells/mm^3. The antiretroviral agent dideoxycytidine was added, but it was discontinued 4 months later after a chronic painful mucosal ulcer developed in the oropharynx. The ulcer healed gradually in 2 weeks after dideoxycytidine was stopped. AZT was discontinued also and the antiretroviral agent dideoxyinosine (didanosine) was started. Trimethoprim-sulfamethoxazole (TMP-SMX) was given three times weekly for prophylaxis against *Pneumocystis carinii* pneumonia (PCP). After 10 weeks of TMP-SMX prophylaxis, a diffuse pruritic erythematous skin eruption developed that was presumed to be a hypersensitivity reaction to TMP-SMX ("sulfa allergy"). PCP prophylaxis with the sulfone antibiotic dapsone was started once a normal level of erythrocyte glucose 6-phosphate dehydrogenase (G6PD) was demonstrated.

Kaposi's sarcoma lesions progressed to involve confluent areas of his legs, arms, and torso, and lymphedema (tissue swelling that results from obstruction of normal lymphatic drainage) developed in his feet. The Kaposi's sarcoma was treated intermittently with the chemotherapeutic agents bleomycin and vincristine to provide symptomatic relief from the leg edema.

The patient developed progressive nonproductive cough and fever. Chest radiograms showed a subtle interstitial and alveolar infiltrate involving the right middle lobe of the lung. Three red-purple lesions suggestive of Kaposi's sarcoma were seen in the bronchial mucosa at bronchoscopy. Microscopic examination of bronchoalveolar lavage fluid was negative for the presence of *P. carinii* organisms but showed large acid-fast bacilliform organisms, and cultures were positive for *Mycobacterium kansasii.* Respiratory symptoms and chest radiogram abnormalities resolved following treatment with the antibacterial agents isoniazid, rifampin, and amikacin. One month later, he experienced the abrupt onset of right-sided chest pain and dyspnea. Chest radiogram showed a large right pneumothorax, which was evacuated with a chest tube. *P. carinii, Mycobacterium* spp., and common bacterial pathogens were not detected in samples obtained at a repeat bronchoscopy. Sputum cultures grew many colonies of the yeast *C. albicans,* which were thought to be contaminants derived from the oral cavity.

The Kaposi's sarcoma lesions progressed to involve more than 50% of the skin surface. Lymphedema of the legs and scrotum progressed until he was unable to walk. His weight had decreased from

65 to 50 kg over a year. He developed a large, painful perianal ulcer; cultures were positive for herpes simplex virus type 2 (HSV-2). The ulcer regressed during a 3-week course of intravenous (i.v.) acyclovir, but it gradually progressed during oral acyclovir maintenance therapy. The ulcer failed to regress after treatment with a second course of high-dose i.v. acyclovir. One month before his death, the patient complained of decreased vision in his right eye. Ophthalmoscopic examination showed confluent white retinal infiltrates with areas of hemorrhage involving both eyes, an appearance consistent with cytomegalovirus (CMV) retinitis. Intravenous administration of the nucleoside analogue ganciclovir was begun. The absolute neutrophil count dropped to 350 cells/mm^3, but increased to 5,400 cells/mm^3 in response to daily administration of recombinant granulocyte colony stimulating factor. The CD4-positive T-lymphocyte count was 4 cells/mm^3. The day before his death, he experienced the abrupt onset of left-sided chest pain and severe dyspnea. Chest radiogram showed a complete left pneumothorax. He refused chest tube placement or hospitalization. Opioid analgesics and benzodiazepines were administered to alleviate pain and anxiety. He died at home the following evening with family members in attendance.

At necropsy, a B-lymphocyte lymphoma was found within the right frontal lobe of the brain. The hepatobiliary tract was irregularly dilated. CMV cytopathic effects (CMV inclusion bodies) were seen within cells of the biliary mucosa, and *Cryptosporidium* organisms were adherent to the biliary mucosal surface. In summary, this young man experienced eight major infections and two malignancies during the five years before his death as complications of HIV infection.

THE HUMAN IMMUNODEFICIENCY VIRUSES

Recognition of the HIV Pandemic

In 1981 clusters of cases of *P. carinii* pneumonia and Kaposi's sarcoma among previously healthy homosexual men were reported in the United States. Soon thereafter, other opportunistic infections were described among homosexual men and injection drug users, including oral candidiasis, *Toxoplasma gondii* infections of the brain, *Cryptococcus neoformans* meningitis, *Cryptosporidium* diarrhea, and CMV retinitis. These diseases were associated with markedly low counts of CD4-positive T-lymphocytes in the peripheral blood. The newly recognized disease was called the acquired immunodeficiency syndrome (AIDS). In 1984, HIV type 1 (HIV-1) was identified as the causative agent.

The World Health Organization estimates that over 13 million people have become infected with HIV as of 1993, 8 million of whom are residents of sub-Saharan Africa. In some cities in eastern Africa, a third of all adults are HIV-infected. The HIV pandemic is now sweeping through southern and southeastern Asia (Merson, 1993). The vast majority of HIV cases have been acquired through heterosexual intercourse, and approximately 1 million infected women have transmitted the infection to their newborn infants. Disease treatment gains have been modest, and vaccine development has suffered numerous setbacks. The HIV pandemic has also brought about the worldwide resurgence of another scourge: tuberculosis. Into the twenty-first century, HIV will continue to spread its devastation. Its impact will be felt most among the poor and the politically disenfranchised.

RNA Viruses, DNA Viruses, and Retroviruses

Viruses use the information encoded within a nucleic acid genome to express proteins that promote viral replication and dissemination. Different virus families use either deoxyribonucleic acid (DNA) or ribonucleic acid (RNA) as their genomes. Medically important families of DNA viruses include the herpesviruses (HSV, varicella zoster virus, CMV, Epstein-Barr virus), the papovaviruses (human papillomaviruses, JC virus), the hepadnaviruses (HBV), and the parvoviruses (human parvovirus B19). RNA virus families include the retroviruses (HIV, human T-lymphotropic viruses [HTLV]), the picornaviruses (poliovirus, hepatitis A virus), the flaviviruses (yellow fever virus, Japanese encephalitis virus, hepatitis C virus), the orthomyxoviruses (influenza A virus, influenza B virus), the paramyxoviruses (measles, mumps, respiratory syncytial virus, parainfluenza virus), the bunyaviruses (hantaviruses, California encephalitis virus), and many others. Most RNA viruses replicate their genomes by synthesizing complementary RNAs directly from viral RNA templates through the action of a viral RNA-dependent RNA polymerase. The retroviruses are unique among the RNA viruses in that they first synthesize a complementary DNA (cDNA) from the RNA genome by reverse transcription. The cDNA then serves as the template for the synthesis of viral genomic RNAs and the transcription of viral messenger RNAs (mRNAs). Because reverse transcription is a reaction that is not performed by the nucleic acid polymerases of eukaryotic cells, retroviral replication requires a unique polymerase called reverse transcriptase (RT) (Poeschla and Wong-Staal, 1994; Schnittman and Fauci, 1994). Similarly, the hepadnaviruses (HBV, for example) are unique among DNA viruses in that they replicate their DNA genome through a complementary RNA intermediate (RNA pregenome). The RNA pregenome is then used as the template for synthesis of genomic DNA through the action of the HBV polymerase, which also has a RT activity. Some DNA viruses (the human papillomaviruses, for example) do not express nucleic acid polymerases and rely entirely on cellular polymerases to replicate their genomes.

The retroviruses are subdivided into oncornaviruses, spumaviruses, and lentiviruses. The oncornaviruses include the human T-lymphotropic viruses (HTLV-1, HTLV-2). The lentiviruses include the human immunodeficiency viruses (HIV-1, HIV-2) and several animal immunodeficiency viruses (simian immunodeficiency virus [SIV], feline immunodeficiency virus, bovine immunodeficiency virus, and visna virus of sheep).

The Emergence and Evolution of HIV

Viruses vary greatly in terms of pathogenicity, transmissibility, genetic stability, host specificity, and geographic range. At one extreme are viruses that have achieved an evolutionary equilibrium with their host species, including many of the human papillomaviruses (HPVs) and some oncornaviruses (HTLV-2, for example). These agents often establish chronic infections, cause mild or no disease, are poorly transmissible, display a narrow host range, and have evolved slowly in association with their primary host species. On the other extreme are viruses such as influenza A virus that are prone to genetic instability, are readily transmissible, display a broad species tropism, and can cause severe diseases in humans.

Many viruses that are prone to rapid evolution and antigenic selection are associated with short-term infections.

The lentiviruses do not fall at either of these extremes but rather display some characteristics of both. Genetic variability is common, and member strains are prone to rapid and unpredictable evolution. Many lentiviruses are highly pathogenic to their hosts, but important exceptions exist. Some SIV strains appear to have achieved, at least temporarily, a stable niche within their original primate hosts. For example, the SIV associated with sooty mangabey monkeys (SIV_{SMM}) causes a chronic infection that does not appear to result in disease; however, a rapidly progressive and fatal immunodeficiency disease can ensue when SIV_{SMM} infects other monkey species, such as macaques.

In Africa several different SIV strains are enzootic in each of several distinct primate species. Rough estimates of the time at which two modern-day SIV strains diverged can be made by comparing their current genetic sequence variance. These "molecular clock" estimates suggest that different SIV strains may have diverged from a common ancestor very recently, perhaps within the last 100 years. Taken farther back, some estimates have suggested that a common lentivirus ancestor could have given rise to all of the current lentiviruses (including HIV-1 and visna virus) within the last several hundred years!

In Africa, humans interact extensively with monkeys. Monkeys are hunted and their carcasses are cleaned with bare hands. Several strains of SIV are *sympatric* (share a geographic distribution) with HIV-2, an HIV that is endemic in western Africa. HIV-2, which causes a human immunodeficiency disease similar to that caused by HIV-1, is strikingly similar to SIV. In fact, some genotypes of HIV-2 are not distinguishable from some west African SIV genotypes. The diversity of HIV-2 strains in western Africa suggests that it may have been introduced into the human population on several occasions. Monkey-to-human transmission of SIV has been documented in primate colony workers in the United States, demonstrating that cross-species transmission of SIV to humans is possible. As with monkey-to-monkey transmission of SIV, a primate retrovirus strain that does not cause disease in its native host appears to be capable of causing a devastating disease when transmitted to humans.

The origin of HIV-1 is more enigmatic. HIV-1 is the HIV that is pandemic and responsible for the vast majority of human AIDS cases. Unlike HIV-2, HIV-1 does not have a close homolog among primates, at least not one that has yet been identified. The first known human HIV-1 infections are believed to date to the 1950s. It was not until the 1980s that the massive HIV-1 pandemic was recognized. Molecular clock estimates of an HIV-1/SIV divergence are concordant with these observations, suggesting that the split occurred about 40 to 50 years ago. These estimates chase a moving target, however, as new subtypes of HIV-1 are identified that more closely resemble SIV and new SIV subtypes are identified that are more closely related to HIV-1. Currently, there are six known distinct lineages of HIV-1. The closest recognized simian counterpart to HIV-1 is currently SIV_{CPZ}, a virus of chimpanzees. The recently discovered HIV-1 "subgroup O" is the strain that is believed to have the closest relationship to the SIV_{CPZ}/HIV-1 ancestor.

Many theories have been proposed to account for the origins of HIV-1. Perhaps the most parsimonious hypothesis suggests that one or more lentivirus transmissions occurred from chimpanzees to humans in Africa within the last 40 to 50 years. This "big bang" hypothesis is supported by human seroprevalence data and by molecular clock estimates. Given 40 to 50 years of confinement to the human species, HIV-1 would have had ample time to distance itself from its chimpanzee homolog and to develop into at least six distinct lineages. HIV-1 has been extremely successful at infecting humans, but it is also clear that it has not yet come to occupy a stable niche in our species.

MOLECULAR PERSPECTIVES

Replication of HIV in the Cell

The HIV genome consists of one single-stranded RNA molecule of plus sense (meaning that the genome has the same sense as mRNA). The genome includes three large genes: *gag, pol,* and *env* (Fig. 4-1). The *gag* gene encodes core structural proteins that encase and protect the viral genome, including the major capsid protein (p24) and the matrix protein (p18). The *pol* gene encodes viral replication enzymes, including RT, an integrase, and the HIV protease. The *env* gene encodes envelope-associated

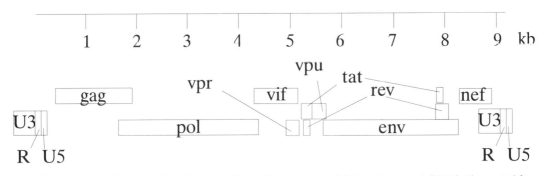

Figure 4-1. Structure of the proviral (DNA) genomic form of human immunodeficiency virus type 1 (HIV-1). The proviral form differs from the viral (RNA) form in that two sequences that are unique to the 3′ and the 5′ ends of the viral form (U3 and U5, respectively) are duplicated in the provirus and are present on both ends of the genome. These sequences flank the repeat (R) sequences that specify the beginning and ending of the transcriptional unit. The U3-R-U5 sequence is collectively known as the long terminal repeat. All three reading frames of the transcript are translated. Those in frame 1 are shown at the top (*gag, vif,* the 3′ end of *tat,* and *nef*). The genes expressed from frame 2 (the 5′ end of *tat,* as well as *vpu* and the 3′ end of *rev*) are shown at the second level. Frame 3 encodes *pol, vpr,* the 5′-end of *rev,* and *env.*

glycoproteins gp120 and gp41, which mediate virus attachment and entry into cells. In addition to the *gag, pol,* and *env* gene products, the HIV genome encodes small regulatory proteins including the *tat, rev, nef, vif, vpr,* and *vpx* products. The functions of *tat, rev,* and *nef* are described below. The HIV genes are flanked by regions called long terminal repeats (LTRs). The 5′-LTR contains transcription promoter and *cis*-acting regulatory elements that bind viral and cellular transcription factors.

The HIV virion is a lipid-enveloped particle with a dense central core containing genomic RNA. The outer envelope is a phospholipid bilayer derived from the cytoplasmic membrane of the host cell. Viral glycoproteins extend from the surface of the virion, where they serve in virus attachment and entry into cells. The viral glycoprotein gp41 is embedded within the phospholipid membrane through hydrophobic interactions. The glycoprotein gp120 lies entirely outside the viral envelope, where it is held in place through noncovalent bonding to gp41. Just inside the viral envelope is a loosely structured protein mantle composed of the matrix protein p18. The viral core, which contains the RNA genome and replication enzymes, lies at the center of the virion. The core is protected by a dense capsid composed of the p24 protein. The capsid encases two copies of genomic RNA, RT, and other enzymes that are necessary for the initial steps of HIV replication.

Free HIV virions attach to human cells through the high-affinity binding of HIV gp120 to cellular CD4 molecules (Fig. 4-2). CD4 molecules are cytoplasmic membrane proteins that participate in the interaction of specific T-lymphocytes (helper/inducer T-lymphocytes) with antigen-presenting cells. Because gp120 binds only to human CD4, animal models of HIV infection have been difficult to develop. Virus binding to cell-associated CD4 induces the fusion of the viral envelope with the cellular cytoplasmic membrane, a process that is mediated by gp41. Membrane fusion releases the viral core into the cytoplasm of the cell. Within the cytoplasm, the viral RNA genome is reverse-transcribed into a single-stranded cDNA and then converted into double-stranded DNA ("provirus") by RT. The provirus enters the nucleus, where a viral integrase protein catalyzes the integration of the proviral double-stranded DNA into the cellular chromosome. A specific integration site is present within the proviral LTR, but cellular chromosomal integration sites are largely random. The integrated provirus behaves similarly to a cellular gene, expressing the RNA genome and viral mRNAs by using cellular transcription machinery. This almost seamless interaction between the HIV provirus and the infected cell confounds efforts to develop antiretroviral therapies.

Early viral gene expression results in synthesis of the HIV *tat* gene product, which is transported to the nucleus. The *tat* gene product (Tat) belongs to a class of regulatory proteins called *transcription factors*. Transcription factor proteins generally bind to specific DNA sites adjacent to transcription promo-

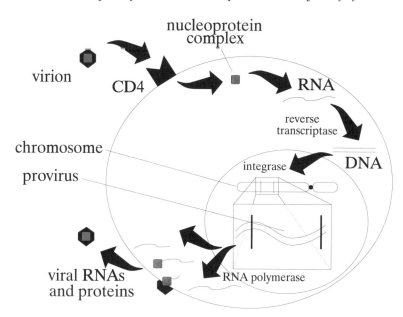

Figure 4-2. Life cycle of retroviruses as exemplified by human immunodeficiency virus type 1 (HIV-1). The entry of HIV-1 into cells involves binding of virion-associated glycoprotein (gp) 120 with the T-lymphocyte cytoplasmic membrane protein CD4. The fusion of virion and cellular membranes facilitates the ingress of viral RNA in the form of a nucleoprotein complex. Viral RNA is then reverse-transcribed into double-stranded DNA through the action of virion-associated reverse transcriptase. The viral DNA (provirus) is then integrated into the cellular chromosome (not drawn to scale). The provirus serves as the template for elaboration of viral RNAs, including genomic (unspliced) RNA and spliced RNAs designed to express specific replicative and structural proteins. The mature virion includes two copies of genomic RNA, a core, and a cell membrane-derived lipid bilayer envelope.

ters. *Transcription promoters* are specific DNA sites that initiate mRNA synthesis by binding and assembling the DNA-dependent RNA polymerase enzyme complex. The binding of transcription factors adjacent to the promoter either upregulates or downregulates the initiation of transcription. Transcription factors provide a mechanism by which organisms can turn genes on or off, according to need. Tat is extremely unusual among transcription factors because it upregulates transcription by acting at the RNA level rather than the DNA level. Its action is mediated via an RNA hairpin sequence known as the transactivation response region, which is found at the start of the HIV transcript. Tat binding upregulates HIV transcription, providing a strong positive feedback loop that accelerates viral expression. Tat also appears to promote polymerase processivity, the ability of cellular RNA polymerases to produce full-length transcripts without terminating synthesis prematurely. The HIV proviral 5′-LTR contains sites that bind cellular transcription factors (i.e., NF-κB and

SP-1) and transcription factors expressed by other viruses. Cytokines, such as tumor necrosis factor alpha, generally activate T-lymphocytes by stimulating the expression of cellular transcription factors. In HIV-infected T-lymphocytes, cellular transcription factors that increase the expression of cellular genes can also increase the expression of HIV genes. Therefore, T-lymphocyte activation is often associated with significant increases in viral expression and replication. The *rev* gene product is an RNA-binding protein that facilitates the efficient transport of unspliced and singly spliced HIV RNAs from the nucleus to the cytoplasm of the infected cell. In the absence of *rev*, only multiply spliced HIV RNA accumulates in the cytoplasm. The *nef* gene product downregulates CD4 expression in HIV-infected cells, perhaps contributing to the dysfunction of CD4-positive T-lymphocytes. Because functions analogous to *tat* and *rev* are not known to be present in HIV-uninfected cells, they are being investigated as targets of antiretroviral therapies.

Retroviruses generally use an unspliced mRNA to express the core proteins and RT and use a spliced mRNA to encode the envelope glycoproteins. Viral mRNAs are translated by cellular ribosomes as polyproteins, which are subsequently cleaved into mature proteins by the HIV protease. Many viruses, most notably the picornaviruses, express more than one mature viral protein as a single polypeptide (*polyprotein*). The polyprotein is subsequently cleaved at specific sites by a viral protease to yield the mature proteins. In HIV replication, protease function is necessary for the post-translational processing of gag proteins. Like Rev and Tat, the HIV protease serves a function that is unique to the HIV life cycle. HIV protease inhibitors are currently being investigated for safety and efficacy as antiretroviral agents in human clinical trials.

HIV virions are assembled within the cytoplasm of the infected cell. The genomic RNA contains a domain that is necessary for its packaging into the maturing virion particle. An RNA-binding core protein recognizes this domain and thus incorporates viral RNA in preference to cellular RNA. Two copies of viral genomic RNA are taken up into each capsid. After assembly of the core, the nascent virion acquires a lipid envelope by budding from the cytoplasmic membrane, which contains the viral envelope glycoproteins. The life span of HIV virions in the blood is quite brief, with a half-life of about 2 days.

The Diagnosis of HIV-1 Infections

Usually HIV infection is diagnosed by detecting virus-specific antibodies in serum samples. B-lymphocytes respond to HIV proteins by secreting immunoglobulin G (IgG) molecules that react with the envelope glycoproteins (gp120 and gp41), the capsid protein (p24), the matrix protein (p18), and other viral proteins. Virus-specific IgG is detected in the serum within 12 weeks of infection in most cases and persists for the life of the host.

A subset of HIV antibodies, called *neutralizing antibodies,* is capable of abrogating virus infectivity both *in vitro* and *in vivo.* These antibodies, once bound to the HIV virion, prevent the virus from infecting T-lymphocyte cultures or infecting experimental animals (such as chimpanzees). HIV-neutralizing antibodies probably interfere with the interaction of gp120 with the CD4 molecule or interfere with the subsequent gp41-mediated fusion of the virion envelope with the T-lymphocyte cytoplasmic membrane. An important HIV-neutralizing epitope has been mapped to a gp120 segment called the V3 loop. Different isolates of HIV-1 show marked amino acid sequence variability within the V3 loop, which could represent a mechanism by which HIV evades containment by the host immune response. Variability within the V3 loop could also confound efforts to develop HIV vaccines if vaccine efficacy is dependent on the generation of neutralizing antibodies.

In serologic testing, HIV-specific antibodies are detected by binding them to viral protein antigens. The HIV protein antigens are derived from purified HIV virions grown in human T-lymphocyte cell cultures. The virions are treated with detergent solutions to form an HIV viral lysate, which is used as a target to detect virus-specific antibodies in two different test formats: EIA and the Western blot assay (Fig. 4-3).

Serum samples are screened for the presence of HIV antibodies in the HIV EIA. In the EIA, the HIV viral lysate solution is placed in a small plastic well, and the HIV proteins adsorb to the plastic much as milk proteins adhere to dishes. The serum sample is then added to the well. If the serum contains HIV-specific antibodies, the antibodies will bind to the viral proteins that are adsorbed to the well. The serum sample is removed, and the well is rinsed to wash away unbound serum proteins. Human antibodies bound to HIV proteins are detected by using goat antibodies that react specifically with human IgG antibodies (goat anti-human IgG antibodies). The goat "secondary antibodies" are chemically conjugated with an enzyme that catalyzes the conversion of chemical substrates to colored chemical products. A test well that changes color after the addition of chemical substrates may contain HIV-specific antibodies.

Positive HIV EIA results are confirmed by using the HIV Western blot assay. In the Western blot assay, the HIV viral lysate is subjected to electrophoresis through a polyacrylamide gel matrix in the presence of the denaturing detergent, sodium dodecyl sulfate. The polyacrylamide gel acts as a fine sieve, slowing the movement of larger molecules and allowing smaller molecules to move more rapidly. As a result, the HIV proteins are separated according to their relative molecular masses. After electrophoresis, the HIV proteins are transferred onto a nitrocellulose membrane. Strips cut from the nitrocellulose mem-

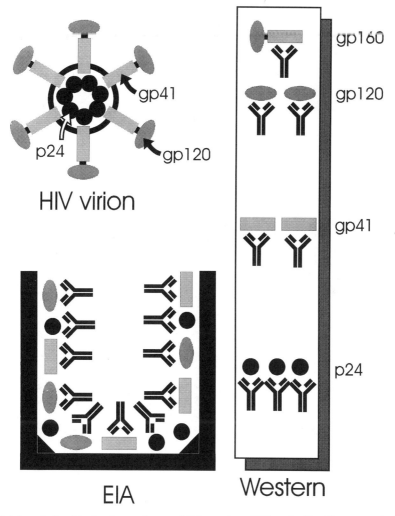

Figure 4-3. Test formats for detecting human immunodeficiency virus (HIV) antibodies. The HIV antibodies in serum are detected by reacting them with HIV proteins in two different test formats, the HIV enzyme immunoassay (HIV EIA) and the HIV Western blot assay. In both cases, HIV proteins are derived from a lysate of purified HIV virions. In the figure, three HIV proteins (gp120, gp41, and p24) are shown. gp160 is a nondissociated complex of the membrane glycoproteins gp120 and gp41. In the HIV EIA, the viral proteins are coated onto the walls of a plastic well. Human HIV antibodies then bind to the HIV proteins. In the Western blot assay, the HIV proteins are separated by electrophoresis onto discrete locations of a nitrocellulose strip. The HIV antibodies specific for each HIV protein can be detected in this way (see Fig. 4-4).

brane are soaked in human serum samples. If HIV-specific antibodies are present, they will bind to their respective viral proteins (gp120, gp41, p24, p18). The viral protein-bound human antibodies are detected by using enzyme-conjugated goat anti-human IgG secondary antibodies. The HIV Western blot test is positive if reactivities to the viral envelope glycoproteins (gp160, gp120, and gp41) and the core protein (p24) are detected. Usually, reactivities to

multiple other virion proteins also are observed (Fig. 4-4).

The HIV EIA is commonly used to screen serum samples for HIV antibodies because it can be run rapidly and inexpensively. Sensitivity is high, but the test specificity of the HIV EIA is suboptimal. False-positive HIV EIA results can occur because: (1) some human serum samples are sticky, and non-HIV antibodies can bind to the plastic wells nonspecifically;

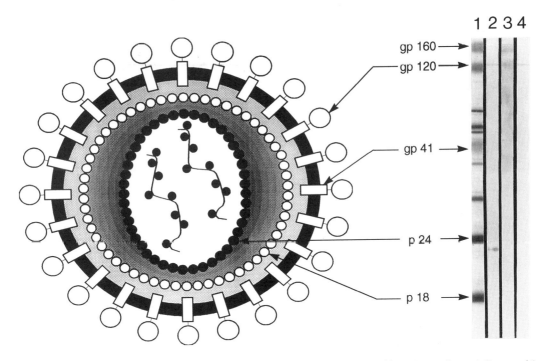

Figure 4-4. Human immunodeficiency virus (HIV) Western blot assays. Four HIV Western blot strips are shown. A diagram of the HIV virion on the left illustrates the locations of the HIV proteins on the nitrocellulose test strip. Strip 1 was reacted with serum from a person infected with HIV. Antibody reactivities to membrane glycoproteins (gp160, gp120, and gp41) and viral core proteins (p24 and p18) are seen. Strips 2 through 4 were reacted with serum samples from people who were not infected with HIV. On strip 2, antibodies can be seen reacting with a contaminating protein that is slightly smaller than p24. Strip 3 illustrates a "sticky" serum sample where serum antibodies adhere nonspecifically to the strip. No antibody binding is seen on strip 4.

(2) some serum samples contain non-HIV antibodies that fortuitously cross-react with one of the HIV viral proteins; and (3) some serum samples contain antibodies that bind specifically to non-HIV contaminants in the viral lysate. Because the HIV viral lysate is prepared from cultures of human T-lymphocytes, T-lymphocyte proteins (including major histocompatibility complex [MHC] class I molecules) can contaminate the lysate. If the test serum contains antibodies that react with allogeneic (non-self) MHC class I antigens contaminating the viral lysate, then a false-positive result can be obtained. False-positive EIA results can be seen in *multiparous* women (women who have had many children) and among recipients of multiple blood product transfusions; people in both groups potentially have been immunized against allogeneic MHC proteins.

The specificity of the Western blot assay is greater than that of the EIA because: (1) antibodies that bind to HIV proteins can be differentiated from antibodies that bind to contaminating cellular proteins because the HIV proteins and the contaminating proteins are present in different locations on the nitrocellulose strip; (2) HIV antibodies bind to discrete viral protein bands on the Western blots, whereas nonspecifically sticky antibodies bind diffusely to the nitrocellulose membrane; and (3) polyclonal HIV antibodies bind to multiple HIV proteins (i.e., gp120, gp41, and p24), whereas non-HIV antibodies that fortuitously cross-react with an HIV protein will bind to only one viral protein (p24, for example).

HIV Infection and the Immune System

HIV virions infect cells that express the CD4 molecule on their cytoplasmic membrane surface. Human cells that express CD4 include the helper/inducer subset of thymus-derived lymphocytes (CD4-positive T-lymphocytes), monocytes and tissue macrophages, and brain microglial cells. CD4 participates in the communication between helper/inducer T-lymphocytes and antigen-presenting cells, an interaction that is vital to the normal functioning of the immune system.

CD4-positive T-lymphocytes are pivotal in the recognition and response to foreign antigens (Fig. 4-5). The CD4-positive lymphocyte population consists of a myriad of different clones that differ in the specificities of their *T-cell receptors* (TCRs), which are cytoplasmic membrane proteins that are members of the immunoglobulin superfamily, a class of related proteins that includes antibodies. The TCR is the T-lymphocyte molecule that recognizes a foreign protein as nonself. The ability to bind to nonself proteins

is "hard-wired" into TCRs while immature T-lymphocytes (thymocytes) are maturing within the thymus. TCRs are heterodimers that consist of disulfide-bonded polypeptide chains. The polypeptide chains have both constant and variable domains. The gene segments that encode the variable domains are generated by complex genetic recombination events during thymocyte maturation in a manner analogous to the generation of antibody variable domains. As a result, a multitude of different TCRs are produced that can bind to different peptides, both nonself and self. Because immune recognition of self-proteins is disadvantageous, thymocytes whose TCRs bind self-peptides are induced to undergo programmed cell death (*apoptosis*). This "education" process allows

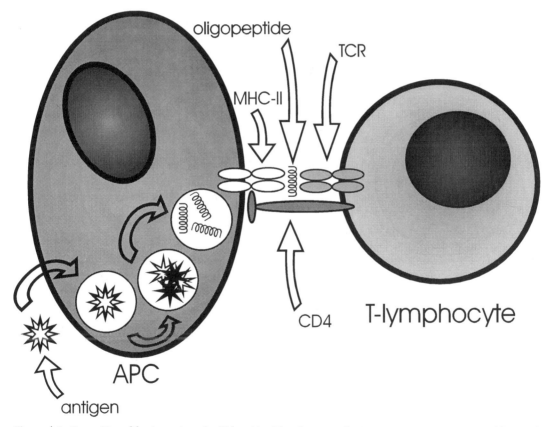

Figure 4-5. Recognition of foreign antigens by CD4-positive T-lymphocytes. A foreign protein antigen is recognized by a CD4-positive T-lymphocyte after processing of the foreign protein by an antigen-presenting cells (APC). The APC ingests the foreign protein into a phagocytic vacuole and then degrades the protein into oligopeptides. A foreign oligopeptide is loaded into an apical groove of major histocompatibility complex (MHC) class II molecule, and the MHC class II molecule is then transported to the cytoplasmic surface. The MHC-II/oligopeptide is bound by an antigen-specific T-cell receptor (TCR) on the cytoplasmic surface of a CD4-positive T-lymphocyte. The CD4 molecule binds the MHC-II molecule in an antigen-independent manner, stabilizing the intercellular interaction and promoting cell adherence.

only those T-lymphocytes that do not recognize self-peptides, and hence recognize nonself-peptides, to reach maturity and proliferate. Therefore, a TCR is not specific for a foreign peptide as the result of a previous exposure to that peptide. Rather, an extensive repertoire of TCRs exists that can alert the immune system to the presence of nonself proteins that have not been encountered previously.

Unlike antibody molecules, TCRs do not bind to native foreign proteins or free peptides; they bind only to foreign peptides that are associated with MHC molecules. Specialized phagocytic cells called antigen-presenting cells (APCs) prepare foreign antigens for presentation to CD4-positive T-lymphocytes in the context of MHC. Macrophages, monocytes, and B-lymphocytes can function as APCs. APCs ingest foreign proteins into phagocytic vacuoles, cleave the proteins into small peptides by proteolysis, and load the foreign peptides into a specialized groove on MHC class II molecules. The peptide-loaded MHC class II complexes are then translocated to the surface of the APC, where they interact with the TCRs of circulating CD4-positive T-lymphocytes.

TCRs that are capable of binding to a foreign peptide-MHC class II complex with high affinity will enable the subsequent stimulation or activation of the T-lymphocyte. The CD4 molecules of T-lymphocytes interact with MHC class II molecules of APCs in an antigen-independent manner. This interaction promotes T-lymphocyte/APC binding, perhaps through the induction of cellular adhesion molecules. Antigen-specific binding of the TCR activates a TCR-associated cytoplasmic membrane protein complex called CD3, which initiates the intracellular biochemical pathways that result in the activated T-lymphocyte phenotype. At least 60 different cellular genes are expressed during the first several hours after the activation signal. An important component of T-lymphocyte activation is the secretion of intercellular signaling proteins called cytokines, which include interleukin-2 (IL-2), interferon-γ, and tumor necrosis factor-β (TNF-β). IL-2 has an autocrine effect by further activating the T-lymphocyte from which it was secreted. IL-2 also exerts a paracrine effect by activating other nearby immune cells. Through cytokine secretion, activated CD4-positive T-lymphocytes recruit a mixed population of specialized immune cells to the site where foreign peptide was recognized. This response is referred to as the *delayed-type hypersensitivity* reaction, which plays an important role in immune responses to intracellular pathogens, including viruses, certain fungi (*P. carinii, Histoplasma capsulatum, Coccidioides immitis*), certain bacteria (*Mycobacterium* spp., *Salmonella* spp.), and eukaryotic parasites (*Toxoplasma gondii, Cryptosporidium*).

CD4-positive T-lymphocytes also provide helper functions to B-lymphocytes, which secrete immunoglobulins (antibodies) that bind specifically to non-self-molecules, including foreign proteins and polysaccharides. Antibody binding can: (1) physically block the infectivity of a pathogen, (2) promote the destruction of a pathogen through activation of the complement pathway, or (3) target an infected cell that displays foreign proteins on its surface for destruction by killer T lymphocytes (antibody-dependent cellular cytotoxicity). B-lymphocytes, in addition to secreting antibodies, embed antigen-specific immunoglobulin in their cytoplasmic membrane. Membrane-bound immunoglobulin binds the foreign antigen to the B-lymphocyte and promotes its internalization. Acting as an antigen-specific APC, the B-lymphocyte presents peptides processed from the foreign antigen in the context of MHC Class II molecules to CD4-positive T-lymphocytes. T-lymphocytes that recognize the same antigen (albeit different epitopes of that antigen) bind to the B-lymphocyte and secrete cytokines (IL-4, IL-6), stimulating B-lymphocyte maturation and Ig secretion. In HIV infection, there is a dysregulation of antigen-specific B-lymphocyte responses as a result of dysfunction of CD4-positive T-lymphocytes. Paradoxically, there is also nonspecific polyclonal B-lymphocyte activation and proliferation, with polyclonal Ig secretion that results in hypergammaglobulinemia. Polyclonal B-lymphocyte activation may result from high circulating levels of IL-6, a cytokine secreted by monocytes and T-lymphocytes in response to continuous antigenic stimulation by HIV proteins. HIV-associated hypergammaglobulinemia manifests on clinical laboratory testing as an elevation in total serum protein in association with a normal or depressed serum albumin level. Serum protein electrophoresis reveals a diffuse increase in the gamma globulin fraction composed of many different types of antibody molecules (polyclonal antibodies).

Natural History of HIV Infection

HIV infection usually remains clinically silent for many years. The median interval between initial infection and the onset of clinical illness is about 10 years. During that time, HIV replicates actively in lymphoid tissues throughout the body, but little or no HIV is detected in circulating T-lymphocytes. The number of CD4-positive T-lymphocytes in the peripheral blood decreases slowly from a normal value of 600 to 3100 cells/mm^3 to a level below 200 cells/mm^3. Decreases in circulating CD4-positive T-lymphocytes are paralleled by a dramatic rise in the levels of circulating HIV virions.

The reasons for the steady decline in CD4-positive T-lymphocytes are not well understood. HIV infection may result in the lysis of some infected cells, and some viral proteins may be directly toxic. For example, intracellular gp120 can bind to intracellular CD4 molecules, forming abnormal complexes that interfere with protein transport pathways. Cell death can result from syncytia formation, a process by which HIV-infected cells fuse with uninfected CD4-positive cells. HIV-infected T-lymphocytes express HIV gp120–gp41 glycoproteins on their cytoplasmic membranes. These cell membrane-bound viral glycoproteins can bind to the CD4 molecules on the surfaces of uninfected T-lymphocytes and induce cell-to-cell membrane fusion. The fused cells (*syncytia*) are dysfunctional and highly labile.

HIV-infected CD4-positive T-lymphocytes are the targets of cellular cytotoxicity mediated by immune cells, including cytotoxic T-lymphocyte (CTL) responses, natural killer cell responses, and antibody-dependent cellular cytotoxicity (ADCC). CTL responses are mediated by CD8-positive T-lymphocytes, which recognize HIV-infected CD4-positive T-lymphocytes and macrophages. HIV-infected T-lymphocytes, like other virally infected cells, process intracellular viral proteins into peptides and present these peptides on the cell surface in association with MHC class I molecules. The HIV peptide-MHC class I molecule is recognized by the TCRs of certain CD8-positive T-lymphocytes. By a mechanism that is analogous to the interaction of CD4 with MHC class II molecules, CD8 probably promotes the adhesion of CD8-positive T-lymphocytes to target cells through an antigen-independent interaction with MHC Class I molecules. The antigen-specific binding of cytotoxic CD8-positive T-lymphocytes to HIV-infected CD4-positive T-lymphocytes stimulates the CTL response, resulting in death of the HIV-infected cell. Natural killer cells are large granular lymphocytes that can recognize and kill virally infected cells by mechanisms that do not involve MHC molecules (MHC-unrestricted). In ADCC, circulating gp120 antibodies

bind to HIV-infected T-lymphocytes. The membrane-bound antibodies are then bound by Fc receptors on certain killer effector cells (large granular lymphocytes, monocytes, macrophages) that direct their cytotoxic responses at the HIV-infected T-lymphocyte.

Recent findings suggest that some HIV-infected T-lymphocytes are lost through the process of programmed cell death, or apoptosis. Apoptosis is an orderly series of cellular events that require specific gene expression and result in cell death. It is the mechanism by which T-lymphocytes that recognize self-antigens are eliminated in early T-cell ontogeny. The evidence suggests that gp120 and gp120 antibodies complex with CD4 molecules (and perhaps other cell-surface molecules), resulting in aberrant intracellular signals that initiate apoptosis (Gougeon and Montagnier, 1993; Weiss, 1993).

Stages of Immunodeficiency

Certain disease manifestations are characteristically seen during early HIV infection (peripheral blood CD4-lymphocyte count greater than 200 cells/mm^3) (Fig. 4-6). HIV infection of lymphoreticular organs is responsible for diffuse lymphadenopathy, recurrent fevers, and night sweats. B-lymphocyte dysfunction can manifest as recurrent pneumonias with encapsulated bacteria, especially *S. pneumonia*. Nonspecific polyclonal B-lymphocyte activation is responsible for HIV-associated *thrombocytopenia*, a condition in which antibody-coated platelets are targeted for clearance from the peripheral blood. Reactivation pulmonary tuberculosis is most likely to develop during this time, as delayed-type hypersensitivity responses that hold latent *M. tuberculosis* infections in check begin to wane. Cellular immune dysfunction allows herpesviruses to emerge from latency and cause diseases like recurrent anogenital herpes (HSV), dermatomal zoster (varicella zoster virus), oral hairy leukoplakia (Epstein-Barr virus) and probably Kaposi's sarcoma (a newly recognized human herpesvirus) (Chang et al., 1994). Superficial oral or genital tract mucosal infections with the yeast *Candida albicans* are common.

As immune function deteriorates further (CD4-positive T-lymphocyte count <200 cells/mm^3), more serious bacterial, viral, fungal, parasitic, and neoplastic diseases are observed. In HIV disease and in other diseases associated with profound cellular immune dysfunction, reactivation of latent human herpesvirus infections is a major cause of morbidity

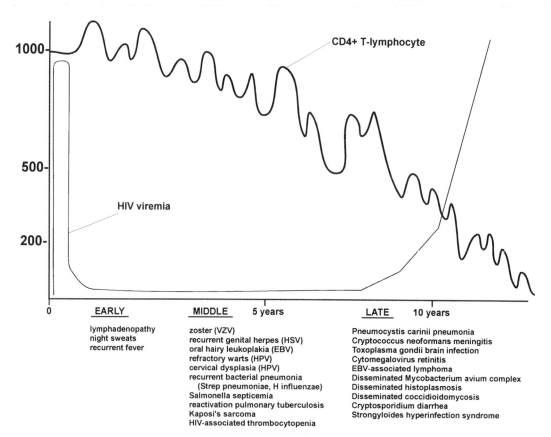

Figure 4-6. Natural history of human immunodeficiency virus (HIV) infection and the HIV-associated acquired immunodeficiency syndrome (AIDS). Declines in CD4-positive T-lymphocyte counts in peripheral blood are shown in relation to levels of HIV viremia. Opportunistic infections and neoplastic diseases characteristic of early, middle, and late stages of HIV disease are listed.

and mortality. Recurrent HSV anogenital lesions can develop into chronic painful ulcers that are refractory to antiviral therapy. CMV emerges from latency to cause severe infections of the retinas, the gastrointestinal tract, and the biliary tract. In particular, CMV retinitis is associated with severe immunodeficiency and is a marker for poor survival. Epstein-Barr virus reactivation can cause rapidly fatal malignant B-cell lymphomas of the brain.

Other DNA viruses that cause disease in late stages of HIV infection include JC virus, HPVs, and human parvovirus B19. JC virus is a polyomavirus that latently infects the brain. In advanced HIV infection, JC virus can reactivate and cause a rapidly progressive viral encephalitis called *progressive multifocal leukoencephalopathy*. Certain HPVs (especially HPV type 16) cause dysplastic proliferative lesions of

anogenital tract epithelium in normal hosts. This tendency is accentuated in HIV disease, predisposing HIV-infected women to cervical dysplasia and carcinoma and predisposing both sexes to perianal neoplasms. Human parvovirus B19 infects erythroid precursor cells in the bone marrow. It is the cause of aplastic crisis in sickle cell disease. Similarly, acute parvovirus B19 infection can result in severe red-cell aplasia in people with HIV disease. HIV-infected people are more likely to develop chronic disease as a consequence of acute HBV infection. Therefore, it is recommended that HIV-infected people without prior HBV infection should receive HBV vaccine.

Life-threatening fungal infections are commonly seen in advanced HIV disease. Often PCP presents with slowly progressive malaise, fever, and dyspnea but can accelerate rapidly to cause severe respiratory insufficiency and death. Smoldering *P. carinii* infections can weaken the pleural surfaces of the lungs and cause recurrent *pneumothorax* (escape of air from the lung into the pleural cavity). Antibiotic prophylaxis against PCP with TMP-SMX, dapsone, and aerosolized pentamidine has significantly reduced the morbidity and mortality of PCP. Unfortunately, chronic TMP-SMX administration often results in the development of drug hypersensitivity skin eruptions (sulfa allergy). The sulfone antibiotic dapsone is an alternative PCP prophylactic agent in sulfa-allergic patients, but it has been reported to cause acute red blood cell lysis (acute hemolytic anemia) in people with congenital deficiencies of G6PD. The yeast *Cryptococcus neoformans* causes a fungal meningoencephalitis, which has a high mortality even when appropriately treated. *H. capsulatum* and *C. immitis* are fungi that are endemic to North America that can cause disseminated infections (histoplasmosis and coccidioidomycosis, respectively) in people with advanced HIV disease.

Opportunistic parasitic infections are hallmarks of HIV disease. Multifocal brain infections caused by reactivation of latent *T. gondii* infections are common and can be difficult to differentiate clinically from Epstein-Barr virus-associated B-cell lymphomas of the brain. Severe diarrheal illnesses caused by the unicellular eukaryotic parasites *Giardia lamblia, Cryptosporidium, Microsporidium,* and *Isospora belli* are common. *Strongyloides* hyperinfection syndrome, caused by the nematode worm *Strongyloides stercoralis,* is a dramatic and dreaded parasitic illness associated with HIV infection. Because of the severe cellular immune dysfunction associated with advanced HIV disease, the worms proliferate freely and invade through the bowel wall, through the diaphragm, and into the lungs. The ectoparasite *Sarcoptes scabii,* a mite that burrows into the epidermis and commonly causes an infestation called scabies, can produce a severe generalized skin infection in people with HIV infection called *crusted scabies* or *Norwegian scabies.*

Abnormal delayed-type hypersensitivity responses predispose people with HIV disease to disseminated infections with intracellular bacteria, including disseminated *Mycobacterium avium*-complex infections, infections with other nontuberculous mycobacteria, and disseminated *Salmonella* infection.

Primary HIV infection of macrophages, monocytes, and brain microglial cells also manifests as disease. HIV infection of macrophages/monocytes causes aberrant secretion of cytokines, including tumor necrosis factor alpha and IL-6. Aberrant cytokine secretion may contribute to HIV-associated chronic wasting syndromes, including "slim disease," a major cause of mortality in Africa. HIV infection of brain microglial cells appears to result in cytokine-mediated or glutamate-mediated damage to surrounding neurons, resulting in progressive HIV dementia.

THERAPY

The proper treatment of viral infections is problematic. Viruses are intracellular molecular parasites that subvert cellular biochemical process to their own expression and replication. It is difficult to interfere with viral processes without subjecting the host cells to significant toxicities. The principal strategy of antiviral therapy is to target viral molecules or biochemical pathways that are unique to the virus relative to its host cell. To date, the only incontrovertible success in antiviral therapy has been the use of the nucleoside analogue acyclovir for the treatment of HSV infections.

HSV-1 and HSV-2 cause acute and recurrent mucocutaneous vesicular and ulcerative eruptions of oral and genital tract epithelium. The HSVs are large, complex viruses that express many proteins required for their replication, including nucleoside kinases and DNA polymerases. In contrast, many smaller DNA viruses (HPVs, for example) use exclusively cellular DNA replication pathways to replicate their genomes. By testing many nucleoside analogues *in vitro,* HSV replication was found to be significantly inhibited by 9-[(2-hydroxy-ethoxy)methyl]guanine, or acyclovir. Acyclovir is an analogue of the nucleoside 2′-deoxyguanosine in which a linear (or "acyclic") side chain has been substituted for the cyclic deoxyribose sugar (Fig. 4-7). HSV thymidine kinase (TK), which normally phosphorylates pyrimidine nucleosides, binds acyclovir with high affinity and converts it to acyclovir monophosphate. Cellular nucleoside kinases convert acyclovir monophosphate to acyclovir diphosphate and then acyclovir triphosphate. Acyclovir triphosphate is bound by HSV DNA polymerases, which incorporate it into replicating HSV DNA instead of 2′-deoxyguanosine triphosphate, resulting in DNA chain termination, be-

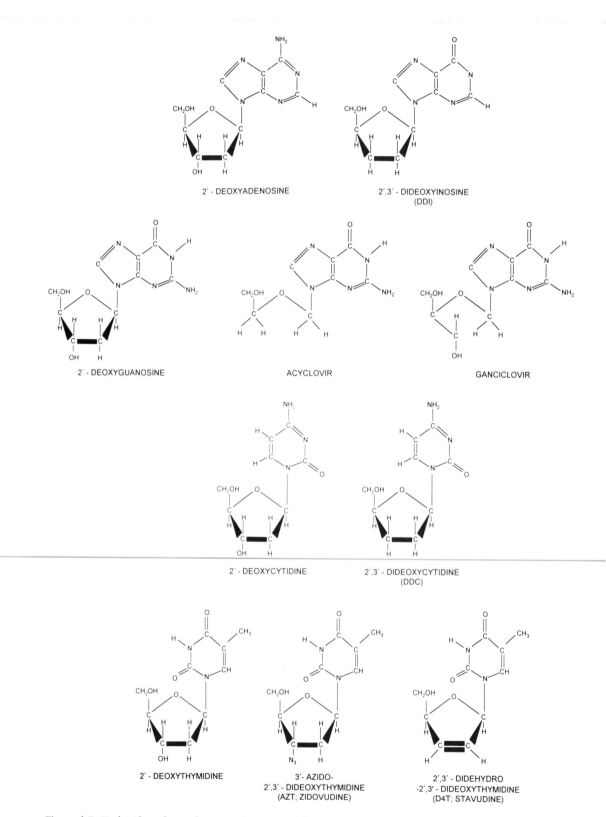

Figure 4-7. Nucleoside analogues that are used in anti-viral therapy. Nucleosides dA, dG, dC, and dT are shown together with nucleoside analogues that are used to inhibit human immunodeficiency virus (HIV) and herpesvirus replication.

cause acyclovir does not have a 3′-hydroxyl group with which to form a phosphate bond with the next nucleoside triphosphate. Cellular nucleoside kinases have a low affinity for the unphosphorylated acyclovir. As a result, acyclovir is preferentially concentrated within HSV-infected cells that express TK.

The widespread clinical use of acyclovir has occasionally resulted in the emergence of acyclovir-resistant HSV stains. These strains have been most commonly observed among chronically immunocompromised hosts who develop severe recurrent HSV infections and are treated repeatedly with acyclovir. The most common mechanism of acyclovir resistance is the emergence of HSV mutants that lack a functional thymidine kinase (TK− phenotype). TK− variants of HSV tend to be less pathogenic than their wild-type ancestors, but they may be entirely resistant to the antiviral effects of acyclovir.

A more modest success has been achieved in the treatment of CMV infections with the nucleoside analogue ganciclovir. Ganciclovir, 9-[[2-hydroxy-1-(hydroxymethyl)-ethoxy]methyl]guanine, is an acyclic analogue of 2′-deoxyguanosine (Fig. 4-7). Its mechanism of action is similar to that of acyclovir. Unlike acyclovir, however, ganciclovir has a significant inhibitory effect on the DNA replication of bone marrow hematopoietic cells, which commonly results in severe neutropenia. During ganciclovir therapy of CMV retinitis, it is often necessary to support blood neutrophil counts by stimulating bone marrow production with recombinant granulocyte colony stimulating factor.

Unlike the herpesviruses, HIV does not express its own nucleoside kinases. One prominent feature of HIV replication unique relative to cellular DNA replication is reverse transcription. Soon after HIV was isolated, many nucleoside analogues were screened for activity against the HIV RT. 3′-Azido-2′,3′-dideoxythymidine (AZT, zidovudine), the dideoxy analogue of 2′-deoxythymidine, significantly inhibited HIV RT function while having a lesser effect on cellular DNA polymerases (Fig. 4-7). When HIV RT incorporates AZT-triphosphate into the growing viral cDNA strand, the chain is terminated. The major dose-limiting toxicity of AZT is its suppression of hematopoietic cell replication. DNA synthesis inhibition of bone marrow precursor cells is manifest as decreased red blood cell production (*anemia*) and decreased polymorphonuclear leukocyte production (*neutropenia*). Like the red blood cell DNA synthesis block that results from folic acid and vitamin B12 deficiencies, AZT toxicity produces an anemia in which the red blood cells are abnormally large (*megaloblastic anemia*). It is often possible to determine whether HIV-infected patients are taking AZT by noting whether the red blood cell mean corpuscular volume is abnormally high.

Three other nucleoside analogues are currently licensed for HIV therapy in the United States. Like AZT, they are 2′,3′-dideoxyribonucleosides that inhibit HIV RT (Fig. 4-7); 2′,3′-dideoxyinosine (ddI or didanosine) is a purine analogue that has a significant inhibitory effect on the HIV RT. Although ddI does not have significant adverse effects upon hematopoietic cells, its use has been associated with acute hemorrhagic pancreatitis. The dideoxy analogue of 2′-deoxycytidine is 2′,3′-dideoxycytidine (ddC), the most commonly observed toxicity of which is peripheral neuropathy, which manifests as abnormal sensations (*dysesthesias*) in the hands and feet. Painful chronic oral ulcers (*aphthous ulcers*) are also seen during ddC therapy and resolve when the agent is discontinued. 2′,3′-Didehydro-2′,3′-dideoxythymidine (d4T, stavudine) is structurally similar to AZT, but it does not appear to suppress bone marrow function to the same extent. Peripheral neuropathy is the dose-limiting toxicity of stavudine.

The RT inhibitors have significant effects on HIV replication *in vitro,* and their clinical use has been associated with slower declines in CD4-positive T-lymphocytes counts; however, the beneficial effects of these drugs appear to be transient. Prolonged administration of the drugs, used individually, has been associated with the emergence of drug-resistant HIV variants. In most cases, drug resistance is conferred by specific RT amino acid changes that result in decreased affinity of RT for the triphosphate form of the drug. RT mutations occur frequently because of the relatively poor fidelity of RT as a polymerase, resulting in frequent nucleotide substitutions in the RT gene. Under the pressure of AZT therapy, RT mutations that confer AZT resistance offer a selective advantage to the mutant virus if the overall functionality of RT is not compromised. Some evidence suggests that the HIV RT may have a limited repertoire for attaining drug resistance while maintaining polymerase function. In HIV-infected people who developed AZT-resistant mutants, treatment with ddI resulted in significant decreases in viral load. Ultimately, ddI-resistant mutants emerged as the predominant HIV population. The ddI-resistant mutants were AZT sensitive. These observations suggest that

RT can incorporate only certain mutations that confer drug resistance without significantly altering polymerase function and provide the rationale for multidrug therapy of HIV, a strategy similar to the use of multiple antibacterial agents for the treatment of tuberculosis. It is thought that HIV may be unable to develop RT mutants that are resistant to multiple antiretroviral drugs while maintaining adequate replication function. This enthusiasm should be tempered by Louis Pasteur's admonition, "The microbes will prevail."

QUESTIONS

1. When HIV infects a human CD4-positive cell, it uses its genetic material and proteins to accomplish certain unique functions. What are some important functions that HIV encodes for itself, and what major function of the HIV life cycle is supplied by the infected cell?
2. Explain the pathways of HIV genomic replication. Which replication functions are performed by the HIV RT, and which are performed by cellular DNA-dependent RNA polymerase?
3. What is the mechanism by which nucleoside analogues (AZT, ddI, ddC, d4T) exert an antiretroviral effect? Which part of the HIV genomic replication pathway is affected, and which part is not? What is the most common mechanism of antiretroviral drug resistance?
4. Acyclovir exerts a strong antiviral effect against herpes simplex viruses and has a high therapeutic index (drug efficacy:drug toxicity ratio). What feature of HSV replication is responsible for the differential effect of acyclovir on HSV-infected cells? What is the most common mechanism of acyclovir resistance?
5. CD4-positive T-lymphocytes are central to normal cellular and humoral immune responses. Explain the role of CD4-positive T-lymphocytes in generating mixed cellular immune responses (DTH responses) and the helper functions provided by CD4-positive T-lymphocytes in generating antibody responses. How do the various effects of HIV infection on immune cells account for the immunodeficiency state, opportunistic infections, opportunistic malignancies, and wasting syndromes seen in HIV infection?
6. Compare the advantages and disadvantages of HIV EIA compared with the HIV Western blot assay for diagnosing HIV infections.

REFERENCES

Chang Y, Cesarman E, Pessin MS, et al.: Identification of herpesvirus-like DNA sequences in AIDS-associated Kaposi's sarcoma. *Science* **266**:1865–1869, 1994.

Gougeon M-L, Montagnier L: Apoptosis in AIDS. *Science* **260**:1269–1270, 1993.

Merson MH: Slowing the spread of HIV: Agenda for the 1990s. *Science* **260**:1266–1268, 1993.

Poeschla E, Wong-Staal F: Molecular biology of HIV: Challenges for the second decade. *AIDS Research and Human Retroviruses* **10**:111–112, 1994.

Schnittman S, Fauci AS: Human immunodeficiency virus and acquired immunodeficiency syndrome: an update. *Advances in Internal Medicine* **39**:305–355, 1994.

Weiss RA: How does HIV cause AIDS? *Science* **260**:1273–1279, 1993.

5

Pertussis

HARVEY R. KASLOW AND MICHAEL E. PICHICHERO

CASE REPORT

A 12-week-old girl was admitted to the hospital with an afebrile peribronchial pneumonia and *paroxysms* (sudden spasms) of cough. The onset of illness was seven days before admission when a mild upper respiratory infection began with symptoms of *rhinorrhea* (excessive mucous secretion from the nose), occasional sneezing, and mild cough but no fever. These coldlike symptoms continued with a persistent and increasing dry, hacking cough. One day before admission, the coughing became more forceful with episodes of paroxysms; she appeared reasonably well between coughing fits. On the day of admission, the patient had 15 coughing paroxysms characterized by a staccato series of brief coughs lasting up to one minute with no effective inspiratory effort between the coughs. An inspiratory whoop was not reported. She was brought by ambulance to the hospital emergency department following a brief generalized seizure. The parents said she had received one dose of whole-cell pertussis vaccine combined with diphtheria-pertussis-tetanus (DPT).

Physical Examination

The examination revealed a well-developed, well-nourished infant in no apparent distress. Temperature was 37.3°C (normal, 36–37°C), respiratory rate 30 (normal, 20), heart rate 100 (normal, 60–90), blood pressure 70/40 (normal, 110/70). On examination of the head, eyes, ears, nose and throat clear rhinorrhea and mild conjunctival (inner eyelid) infection were noted. Chest examination findings were of scattered *rhonchi* (lung sounds detected with a stethoscope). Neurologically, the infant was alert and responsive to her environment; no abnormalities were found.

Laboratory

On admission the patient's white blood cell count was 24,000 per cubic millimeter (normal, 3200–9800/mm^3) with 80% lymphocytes (normal, 15–50%). Electrolytes, blood urea nitrogen, serum creatinine, serum calcium, serum phosphate and liver function tests and an arterial blood gas were all normal. A computerized axial tomography scan of the head was normal. Lumbar puncture was performed due to the occurrence of the seizure. The opening pressure was normal and no cells were found; glucose and protein were normal.

Admitting Diagnosis

On admission, the diagnosis was peribronchial pneumonia. The differential diagnosis of etiologic agents included *Bordetella pertussis, Mycoplasma pneumoniae,* and viral agents, particularly adenovirus. The patient was placed on respiratory isolation precautions. A nasopharyngeal swab for direct fluorescent antibody (DFA) and culture for *B. pertussis* were obtained. Cold agglutinins and mycoplasma acute serology as well as viral cultures were also procured, and the infant was administered a course of erythromycin therapy. The following day, her DFA for *B. pertussis* was reported to be positive. The acute cold agglutinin titer was negative. *Cold agglutinins* are substances that develop in the serum during *M. pneumoniae* infection. They are capable of agglutinating human group O cells at 4°C but not at 20°C or 37°C. Her course was prolonged and marked by severe spells of paroxysmal cough and whoop often associated with *bradycardia* (slow heart rate), severe *hypoxemia* (deficient oxygenation of the blood), and *apnea* (transient cessation of respiration). Hospitalization was maintained in the intensive care unit, where careful monitoring showed that the bradycardia appeared to occur before the hypoxemia and did not appear to be directly associated with the paroxysms of coughing. Episodes of apnea were brief, and intubation with assisted ventilation was therefore not necessary. After 3 weeks in the intensive care unit, the paroxysms of cough diminished in frequency and severity. She was transferred to the regular wards until the paroxysms of cough were no longer a daily occurrence. Discharge from the hospital was after 5 weeks.

During the patient's hospital admission, it was noted that her 16-year-old mother had a cough that was mild in severity but frequent in occurrence. Several days after the child's hospitalization, the mother's cough became persistent, and nasopharyngeal swabs for DFA and *B. pertussis* culture were obtained. The mother's DFA test was negative, but on day 7 of incubation, the culture grew *B. pertussis.* Subsequently, exposed hospitalized infants and hospital staff were tested for *B. pertussis* infection. One house officer, two infants, three nurses, and the husband of one of the nurses were subsequently shown to have acquired *B. pertussis.* All were treated with 14 days of oral erythromycin therapy. During the 3 months following hospital discharge, the mother reported that the child had spells of significant coughing with mild paroxysms in association with three episodes of apparent viral upper respiratory infections.

DIAGNOSIS

The first classic description of pertussis (whooping cough) may be that of de Baillau in 1578 during an epidemic in Paris. "The patient is seen to swell up, and as if strangled holds his breath tightly in the middle of his throat . . . for they are without this troublesome coughing for the space of 4 or 5 hours at a time, then this paroxysm of coughing returns, now so severe that blood is expelled with force through the nose and through the mouth. Most frequently an upset of the stomach follows" [see Major, (1954) for historical review]. The earliest American description of pertussis was not until 1822 by Waterhouse in an essay concerning "tussis convulsiva." The direct proof of the bacterial cause of *B. pertussis* came from the experiments of McDonald and McDonald, who inoculated their own infants with 140 live *B. pertussis* organisms.

B. pertussis, in its classic form, is quite uncommon in the United States as a consequence of widespread use of the DPT vaccine. Milder forms of whooping cough, without the characteristic inspiratory whoop, are probably often misdiagnosed as *M. pneumoniae, C. pneumoniae,* or viral lower respiratory infections. Typical pertussis has three stages: the catarrhal, paroxysmal, and convalescent stages. The incubation period is 7 to 10 days and is usually not more than two weeks (Gordon et al., 1994). The onset of illness resembles a mild upper respiratory tract infection similar to the common cold; however, a mild, dry hacking cough progresses to the paroxysmal stage. The patient typically appears quite well between episodes of paroxysmal cough. Most noteworthy is that the patient is usually afebrile, and physical examination is often not revealing. At the termination of paroxysms of coughing, the patient frequently vomits. The paroxysmal stage lasts 1 to 4 weeks, and then the paroxysms become less frequent and severe. Paroxysms often recur with subsequent upper respiratory viral infections for 4 to 6 months after the acute illness during this convalescent stage.

In smaller infants, pertussis is particularly severe. The greatest morbidity and mortality are seen in infants under one year of age. Seizures, peribronchial pneumonia, apnea, and cyanosis are uncommon, but when these more severe disease manifestations do occur, it is in infants aged less than six months. The *nosocomial* (originating in a hospital) spread of *B. pertussis* as highlighted in the case report is consistent with the epidemiology of whooping cough, which is as contagious as *varicella* (chicken pox). An 80 to 90% attack rate in susceptible persons in the same household and a 20 to 50% attack rate in nurseries are common.

The diagnosis of whooping cough is based on a characteristic history and physical examination; it is unmistakable in a typical case. Most cases are atypical, however, and several laboratory tests are useful. An elevated total white blood cell count with associated lymphocytosis is often present. The absolute lymphocyte count typically exceeds 10,000/mm³; numbers of both B and T cells are elevated. The gold standard for the diagnosis of *B. pertussis* infection is the culture of the organism from a nasopharyngeal swab; however, the organism is fastidious and slow growing, and its culture is complicated by the need for direct plating onto selective media: Regan-Lowe, charcoal agar, modified Stainer-Scholte agar, or fresh Bordet Gengou medium. Prior antibiotic treatment with erythromycin, trimethoprim-sulfamethoxazole, tetracycline, and other antibiotics will reduce the isolation rate. Direct fluorescent antibody testing of nasopharyngeal smears is a useful rapid method of presumptive diagnosis of *B. pertussis*, but both false-positive and false-negative results occur. The technique requires experienced personnel and appropriate controls, including concomitant processing of the smear with a negative control using antisera to *B. parapertussis*.

B. pertussis infection can be diagnosed serologically. The measurement of agglutination antibodies is the classic test; it has been used for more than 45 years. The antigens expressed by *B. pertussis* that produce the agglutination response are primarily fimbriae. More recently, enzyme-linked immunosorbent assay (ELISA) methods have been applied to the serologic diagnosis of pertussis. An elevation of immunoglobulin A (IgA) to a *B. pertussis* cell wall protein, filamentous hemagglutinin (FHA), occurs in modest to high titer in association with infection; it can be used as a single serologic marker in the acutely ill patient. Other serologic tests include determining the IgG and IgA titers for pertussis toxin and the titer of anti-FHA IgG in acute sera. Significant titer rises in IgG antibody to FHA and pertussis toxin (PT) are typically seen during convalescence from acute *B. pertussis* infection.

MOLECULAR PERSPECTIVES

Pertussis Vaccines, and the Continuing Threat from *Bordetella pertussis*

The disease pertussis, characterized by the cough with a whoop that gives the disease its common name, has plagued humans for centuries. The causative organism, *B. pertussis*, was finally isolated in the early 1900s. Today, in the United States, the potential impact of this organism is not widely appreciated. In the 1930s, however, in the United States alone, *B. pertussis* attacked more than 200,000 children per year and killed as many as 12,000. Fortunately, after the introduction of a vaccine containing killed, whole-cell *B. pertussis*, the incidence of serious pertussis dramatically declined: Currently, in the United States, approximately 3,000 cases are reported per year with few or no deaths. Nonetheless, as the preceding case demonstrates, *B. pertussis* remains a real threat. Adults in the United States constitute an infectious reservoir of the bacterium, putting infants at risk. The continuing increase in global travel may well increase this threat: During the 1980s pertussis may have killed between 500,000 to a million persons per year outside the United States, primarily in countries lacking effective vaccination programs.

The vaccine currently most used in the United States is essentially the original "whole-cell" vaccine, consisting of cells and debris of killed *B. pertussis* (Ad Hoc, 1988; Cherry et al., 1988; Pichichero, 1993). Frequently, the preparation is combined with diphtheria and tetanus vaccines and is referred to as the *DTP vaccine;* preparations lacking the pertussis component are termed *DT vaccines.* Compared with CT vaccines, DTP vaccinees are more reactogenic: The pertussis component frequently causes redness, swelling, and tenderness at the site of injection. Systemic effects include fever, fretfulness, drowsiness, vomiting, and anorexia. Particularly noticeable to parents is an unusual and persistent crying that occurs in about 5% of children. Despite these reactions, the vaccine was well accepted when the threat of pertussis was perceived to be frequent and life-threatening.

In the 1980s, media attention to reports that the pertussis vaccine might cause permanent neurologic damage, coupled with the perception that the risk of children contracting severe or fatal disease was small, led to substantial declines in vaccination rates outside the United States, with subsequent epidemics and deaths. The concern was particularly acute for parents whose child had reacted strongly to a previous dose of the vaccine, yet required additional doses to gain good protection. In the United States, the notion that the pertussis vaccine caused harm led to lawsuits with literally billions of dollars at stake.

These lawsuits further intensified parental concerns and prompted federal legislation to compensate putative victims of the vaccine.

The threat to the acceptance of the whole-cell pertussis vaccine arises in part because the contents of the vaccine are undefined, making it difficult to defend as "safe." Thus, considerable effort has been devoted to the development of vaccines based on molecularly defined antigens, termed *acellular vaccines* (Robbins et al., 1993). At this time, acellular vaccines are in clinical trials around the world. Almost certainly, physicians will be called on to make recommendations, to either groups or individuals, as to which vaccine is most appropriate. Unfortunately, a potency assay suitable for acellular vaccines has not yet been firmly established. In fact, even though the whole-cell vaccines has been used for decades, the mechanism underlying its efficacy is not yet defined, and for a potency assay the U.S. Food and Drug Administration (FDA) relies on the empirical observation, reported in 1958, that protection in humans correlated to protection of mice from an intracerebral (ic) challenge from an atypical strain of *B. pertussis*, not from a nasal challenge with typical strains (Standfast, 1958). An additional gap in our knowledge is the absence of a molecularly defined correlate of protection measurable in humans suitable for acellular vaccines.

Molecular knowledge of how responses to specific antigens contribute to protection would certainly help provide a rational basis for recommendations regarding the use of pertussis vaccines, and these "Molecular Perspectives" focus on this issue.

Pertussis Toxin and the Pertussis Vaccine

The success of the diphtheria and tetanus vaccines, based solely on the toxoids of diphtheria and tetanus toxins, respectively, raised the notion that a single toxoid could be found that would be sufficient to confer adequate protection from pertussis. Although this notion is currently held strongly by some, most acellular vaccines contain multiple antigens, indicating that others doubt this notion. To date, however, nearly all candidate acellular vaccines, whether they contain one or more antigens, contain a version of the protein termed *pertussis toxin* (PT) (Pittman, 1979).

The widespread inclusion of a version of PT in acellular pertussis vaccines is not surprising. First, although other strains of *Bordetella* can cause pertussis-like disease, *B. pertussis* is likely the predominant cause of severe pertussis in humans. A feature that clearly distinguishes *B. pertussis* from other *Bordetella* strains is the production and release of PT.[1] Second, transposon-induced mutations that selectively prevent expression of PT markedly increase the median lethal dose (LD_{50}) challenge dose of *B. pertussis* in mice. Third, also in mice, PT causes some of the symptoms specific for pertussis disease: for example, lymphocytosis, which may reflect a mechanism compromising proper anti-*B. pertussis* immune functions, and hypoglycemia, which arises from excessive insulin release in response to glucose.[2] Thus, at the least, antibodies that neutralize PT should reduce the severity of pertussis disease.

Initial studies with vaccines based solely on toxoids of PT using mice were encouraging: Such immunizations protected mice from death, as did passive administration of anti-PT monoclonal antibodies. Unfortunately, in a subsequent human trial, although vaccines based on formalin-treated PT provided substantial protection from severe disease, many considered the protection from infection to be insufficient and less than that afforded by whole-cell vaccines. Furthermore, assays measuring anti-PT antibodies that neutralize its activity[3] did not correlate with protection, and antibodies were detected in vaccines against other antigens of *B. pertussis*, particularly a 69-kd protein, now termed *pertactin*, that apparently contaminated the PT preparation.

The results from the human trial raised many questions. For example, perhaps the configuration of the formalin-treated PT in the vaccine was not optimal. Alternatively, perhaps other factors in *B. per-*

---

[1]Although *B. parapertussis* and *B. bronchiseptica* contain a gene encoding the PT protein, the promoter region of this gene is different from that in *B. pertussis*. This difference causes *B. parapertussis* and *B. bronchiseptica* to fail to produce PT under all conditions studied to date.

[2]Pertussis toxin has gone by many names related to its numerous effects, for example, lymphocytosis-promoting factor (LPF), histamine-sensitizing factor (HSF), and islet-activating protein (IAP), the last of which refers to PT's increase in glucose-promoted release of insulin from pancreatic beta cells. Purification of IAP to homogeneity revealed that a single protein was responsible for the diverse effects. The acronyms have now been largely abandoned in favor of pertussis toxin or pertussigen.

[3]Typically, titers of neutralizing antibodies are determined by measuring inhibition of PT-induction of clumping of cultured CHO (Chinese hamster ovary) cells. Other assays have been developed that measure inhibition of PT ADP-ribosyltransferase activity.

tussis were crucial either as antigens or adjuvants. Finally, *B. pertussis* may express PT not because it is crucial for colonization or growth in the host but because it contributes to the cough that spreads the organism to other humans. Testing this last notion is made difficult by the failure of infected mice and most other animals to exhibit the "whooping" cough typical of human pertussis. Finally, it has been suggested that PT may contribute to the severe undesired reactions associated with the vaccine, including the putative neurological damage. In light of these issues, considerable effort has been devoted to the study of PT.

Pertussis Toxin: Structure and Function

Pertussis toxin consists of six polypeptides held together by noncovalent interactions and arranged in the A-B architecture typical of many bacterial toxins (Kaslow and Burns, 1992). The A protomer consists of a single S1 subunit (molecular mass, or M_r = 26,220) which possesses the toxin's catalytic ADP-ribosyltransferase activity. The B oligomer, which binds the toxin to target cells, contains five subunits: S2 (21,920), S3 (21,860), S4 (12,060), and S5 (10,940) in a 1:1:2:1 ratio. An unusual property of the S1 subunit is a lack of lysine residues, which may protect it from ubiquitin-mediated proteolytic destruction inside target cells. Comparison of sequence and crystal diffraction data indicate considerable structural homology with the *Escherichia coli* heat-labile and cholera enterotoxins, which also possess ADP-ribosyltransferase activity. Site-directed mutagenesis studies have demonstrated that many (but not all) mutations of corresponding amino acids in these three toxins produce similar changes in ADP-ribosyltransferase activity.

The G-protein, termed G_i, was the first protein identified to be a functionally relevant substrate for the ADP-ribosyltransferase activity of PT. G_i derives its name from its first identified function: mediating inhibition of adenylate cyclase by inhibitory hormones such as somatostatin. PT ADP-ribosylates a cysteine residue on G_i, locks the G-protein into a guanosine diphosphate (GDP)-liganded form, and blocks signal transduction. In contrast, cholera toxin ADP-ribosylates an arginine residue on the G-protein, termed G_s, that mediates stimulation of adenylate cyclase, locks G_s into a guanosine triphosphate (GTP)-liganded form, and causes a signal equivalent to persistent stimulation of signal transduction. Figure 5-1 summarizes the general features of G-protein regulation. Figure 5-2 relates these general features to the regulation of adenylate cyclase. It is important to recognize that these figures show the known, but not necessarily all, functions of these proteins and that G_s and G_i may not be the sole targets of these toxins. Particularly for PT, other G protein substrates have been identified, and it is likely that G_i is involved in the *stimulation* of other transmembrane-

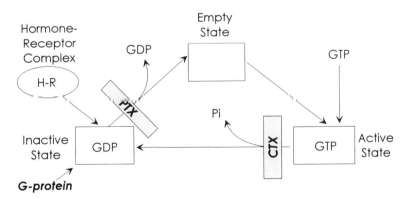

Figure 5-1. The G-protein cycle. In the absence of a hormonal signal, the G-protein binds guanosine diphosphate (GDP) and is in an inactive state. Stimulation by a hormone-receptor (H-R) complex causes the release of GDP; pertussis toxin (PTX) blocks this release. The empty G-protein can then bind guanosine triphosphate (GTP), which puts it into an active state; in this state the G-protein allosterically regulates the function, in either a positive or negative fashion, of another protein. After a while the GTP is hydrolyzed, inorganic phosphate is lost, and the G-protein returns to the inactive state. Cholera toxin (CTX) prevents the hydrolysis of GTP, locking the G-protein in an active state.

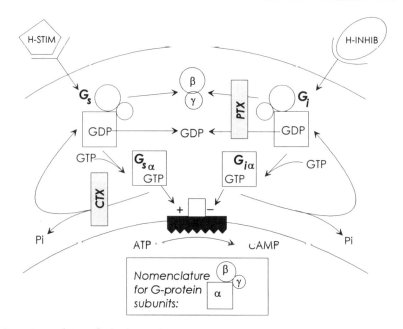

Figure 5-2. G-protein regulation of adenylate cyclase. Two G-proteins regulate adenylate cyclase; the G-protein mediating stimulation is termed G_s, and the G-protein mediating inhibition is termed G_i. Pertussis toxin (PTX) adenosine diphosphate (ADP)-ribosylates the alpha subunit of G_i, and thereby blocks guanosine diphosphate (GDP) release. The result is blockade of hormone action. Cholera toxin (CTX) ADP-ribosylates the alpha subunit of G_s, resulting in persistent activation of adenylate cyclase. Not shown in the figure is the regulation of other cellular functions by the released alpha and beta/gamma subunits. GTP, guanosine triphosphate.

signaling events. The protein transducin has found use as an ADP-ribose acceptor to assess the effects of mutations and chemical treatments on the ADP-ribosyltransferase activity of PT. Transducin is a retinal G-protein that transduces photon activation of rhodopsin into regulation of a cGMP phosphodiesterase.

When released from *B. pertussis*, PT is catalytically silent. The activity of the S1 subunit is demonstrable only after reduction of the subunit's single disulfide bond. The reduction of this disulfide bond is markedly enhanced by the addition of lipids and ATP, which also promote the dissociation of the S1 subunit from the B oligomer. Once reduced, the S1 subunit will not reassociate with the B oligomer to form holotoxin. Current interpretations of these data lead to a model in which, after the toxin is internalized, membrane lipid allows ATP to promote separation of the S1 subunit from the B oligomer. The intracellular reducing environment then breaks the disulfide bond in S1; the subunit then catalyzes ADP ribosylation of G_i (Fig. 5-3). There are, to our knowledge, no reports of other toxins in which al-

losteric actions of ATP promote dissociation and activation.

Knowledge of the ATP-lipid contribution to the activation of PT was crucial for the development of accurate enzymatic assays of the ADP-ribosyltransferase activity of PT. Because the ADP-ribosyltransferase activity of PT may contribute to the undesired reactions to the pertussis vaccine, an obvious goal has been pursued: to create an analog of PT that retains the ability to elicit a protective response but no longer modifies G-proteins. Formalin treatment of PT may not be sufficient to achieve this goal: the lack of lysines in the S1 subunit prevents formalin from covalently modifying S1, and this lack of lysines may account for occasional reversion of formalin-treated PT to an active form. Thus, it has been useful to use enzymatic assays, cultured cells, and mice to demonstrate that specific mutations or chemical treatments remove the ADP-ribosyltransferase activity from PT.

In addition to effects arising from ADP ribosylation, the mere binding of PT to cells can cause biological effects. Carbohydrate moieties, attached either to protein or lipid, are crucial components of

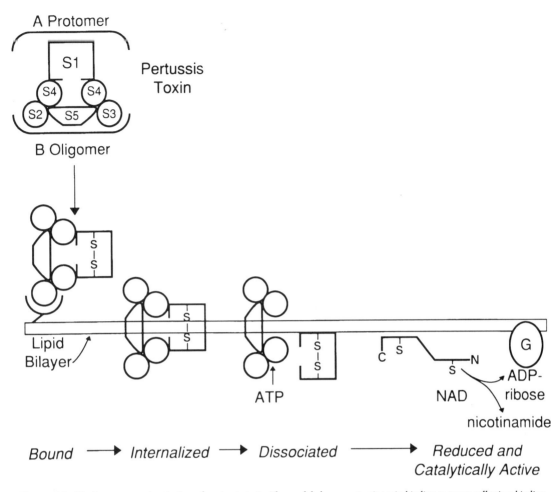

Figure 5-3. Binding, entry, and activation of pertussis toxin. The model shows pertussis toxin binding to target cells via a binding site on the B-oligomer. The initial binding event need not obscure the S1 subunit, and potentially neutralizing antibodies may still bind to it. Other B oligomer binding sites are also exposed, allowing the toxin to bind simultaneously to another host cell or *B. pertussis* itself. After penetration, adenosine triphosphate (ATP) promotes the release of the S1 subunit from the B oligomer, the disulfide bond of the subunit is reduced, and the subunit adenosine diphosphate (ADP)-ribosylates its G-protein targets. It is unlikely that reduced S1 subunits reform holotoxin and intoxicate other cells.

receptors recognized by the B oligomer. Variants of cultured cells that have lost sialic acid residues on their surface glycoproteins and glycolipids are dramatically resistant to PT compared with their parent cell types. The B oligomer contains multiple sites with different receptor specificities and can agglutinate erythrocytes. Although frequently thought of as a systemic toxin, PT may also contribute to the adhesion of *B. pertussis* to the cilia of the lung and the surface of macrophages. It is most likely that it is the B oligomer that contributes to such adhesion by allowing PT to bind not only to eukaryotic cells but to *B. pertussis* itself.

Most of the biological activities of PT arise from ADP ribosylations catalyzed by the S1 subunit and occur at nanogram per milliliter concentrations *in vitro* or from doses of 10 to 400 ng per mouse *in vivo*. The mere binding of the B oligomer can alter eukaryotic cell functions, although such effects are seen only at concentrations in the microgram per milliliter range. The physiologic importance of B-oligomer effects remains to be determined: They could be relevant if high local concentrations of the toxin are reached at the site of infection. Mutations that remove the ability of the B-oligomer to bind to certain receptors have been identified. Incorporating such mutations into the PT analogs of pertussis vaccines may further alleviate concerns regarding the biological activity of this component.

Although PT can modify the G-proteins in target cells within minutes, injecting anti-PT antibodies 1 to 5 days after injection of PT can decrease PT-induced lymphocytosis. Such observations indicate that intact pertussis toxin persists in vivo for days, likely using the multiple binding sites on the B oligomer to hop from one cell to another. Thus, the continued modification of cell function by S1 subunit within cells or holotoxin outside cells may contribute to the persistence of pertussis symptoms even after initiation of antibiotic therapy.

Other Antigens and Toxic Factors of *B. pertussis*

Regardless of the answers to the above questions, the course many physicians take to improve vaccine performance is to include other antigens in the pertussis vaccine. To date, those included in preparations undergoing clinical trial are surface proteins also expressed by other strains of *Bordetella;* however, other toxic factors of *B. pertussis* may be included in future tests (Weiss and Hewlett, 1986). Vaccines containing other antigens effectively protect mice when challenged with strains expressing those antigens. Two commonly used surface proteins are pertactin, a protein with no well-defined crucial function, and FHA, which can promote adherence of the *B. pertussis* to eukaryotic cells. Other antigens under consideration include proteins termed *agglutinogens,* which vary among strains of *B. pertussis* and have been used to type the strains. Some agglutinogens may be structural proteins forming the fimbriae on the bacterium's surface.

B. pertussis also produces a toxic protein with at least two known activities: a calmodulin-activated adenylate cyclase activity and a hemolysin activity. This toxin, termed *ACT/HLY,* is crucial for colonization in mice and is produced by other strains of *Bordetella.* These characteristics distinguish ACT/HLY from PT, which is not a crucial colonization factor, and its expression may be restricted to *B. pertussis.* These distinguishing characteristics of ACT/HLY have caused many to consider it a strong candidate for inclusion in future acellular pertussis vaccines (Goodwin and Weiss, 1990).

Bordetella also produces a *dermonecrotic* (causing skin necrosis), heat-labile toxin (DNT or HLT), but its role in colonization and disease is not well defined. Whether it will prove to be a valuable component in a vaccine is a little-explored topic.

In addition to the above toxic proteins, *B. pertussis* also produces nonprotein toxic factors. One, a 921-Da muramyl peptide, termed *tracheal cytotoxin* (TCT), first causes *ciliostasis* (inhibition of cilial movement), thereby disrupting a key defense mechanism of the lung. Ciliostasis is followed by profound damage to the ciliated cells of the lung, characteristic of *Bordetella* infection. Other toxic factors are derived from *B. pertussis* lipopolysachcharides.

Variation in Expression of Antigens and Toxins

Expression of PT, ACT/HLY, HLT, FHA, and pertactin, but not TCT, is under the control of a gene termed *vir,* which is a genetic switch that turns on expression of virulence factors in an environment like the lung and turns off expression under other conditions that are sufficient to maintain the bacteria in culture. The environment regulation of *vir* by transcription factors is termed *antigenic* or *phenotypic modulation.* Quite clearly, an immune mechanism for protection aimed at factors regulated by *vir* would be of little help if such factors were not expressed. Whether humans are challenged by avirulent-modulated *B. pertussis* is an unresolved question.

In addition to environmental modulation, *vir* is subject to frequent mutations which also cause loss of expression of the virulence factors. When such mutations occur, the lack of expression of virulence factors is relatively stable and is termed *phase variation.* At least two types of mutations are frequently found: (1) frame-shift mutations within a string of C residues; and (2) deletions. The deletion mutants are presumably irreversible, but the frame-shift mutations can be reversed by other frame-shift mutations, and such reversion has been observed. Whether the frequency of such frame-shift mutations meaningfully contributes to the survival of *B. pertussis,* either in the human host or the external environment, is unclear.

Future Molecular Issues

The introduction of acellular vaccines has already begun in Japan, consisting of PT and a few other antigens, primarily FHA. A similar product is now available in the United States. It is worth considering that the introduction of these vaccines may also introduce a new set of problems. An acellular vaccine, containing a limited set of surface antigens, may cause selective pressures that will change the serotypes of *B. pertussis* in the environment. If such changes occur, then previous clinical trials evaluated only in terms of "protection," without evaluation of the response to individual molecular components, may not provide data that reliably predicts future vaccine performance in terms of protection from infection or severe disease.

Recent observations concerning cholera lend plausibility to this concern. For both pertussis and cholera, recovering from disease can protect from a subsequent challenge. Recently, a new strain of *Vibrio cholerae* (strain *0139,* synonym *Bengal*) has emerged and is causing a new pandemic with severe diarrhea. The new strain is a completely new serotype, but it still produces cholera toxin (CT) with conserved amino acid sequence and action. The pandemic is spreading through populations that, because of previous exposures, are resistant to most other strains of *V. cholerae.* Thus, it appears that immunity to previous strains of *V. cholerae* involved responses to proteins other than CT, and mutations have caused the organism to evade this immune response.

Just as there are multiple serotypes of *V. cholerae,* there are multiple serotypes of *B. pertussis.* Although FHA and pertactin serve as protective antigens in mice, the loss of FHA by transposon insertion has little effect on the survival of *B. pertussis* in the mouse, and monoclonal antibodies recognizing pertactin agglutinate one strain *B. pertussis* and protect mice from that strain, fail to agglutinate other strains. Recent outbreaks of pertussis in populations vaccinated with whole-cell preparations may have arisen from selective pressures imposed by such vaccines on such antigens (Mink et al., 1992). The use of acellular vaccines may make it easier for *B. pertussis* to evade a vaccine. If so, the design of future pertussis vaccines will be aided by the continued molecular analysis of *B. pertussis.*

Because acellular vaccines are less reactogenic, and theoretically safer, their use in adult populations will be considered, and the notion that such use could eradicate the disease will be debated. Adult use could also change the effect of the transmission of maternal antibodies to infants in terms of protection from disease and effectiveness of vaccination.

THERAPY

Erythromycin is the agent of choice. It is effective in reducing contagion; if it is administered to the patient early in the course of illness for treatment of *B. pertussis,* preferably during the catarrhal stage or early paroxysmal stage, evidence shows that it can reduce the severity and duration of the illness. Beyond antibiotic therapy, supportive measures, including supplemental oxygen and assisted respiratory ventilation, should be provided as necessary. Quite recently, a new hyperimmune globulin prepared from human sera of adult volunteers vaccinated with a pertussis toxoid vaccine has been described as useful in the treatment of whooping cough. Intravenous infusion of this hyperimmune globulin has been reported to reduce promptly and dramatically the frequency and severity of paroxysmal coughing with associated apnea. The use of pertussis toxoid hyperimmune globulin is currently in preliminary experimental human trials.

QUESTIONS

1. At lunchtime, a child aged 11 weeks receives her first dose of DPT vaccine containing the whole-cell pertussis component. Six hours later, the child begins to cry loudly, and the crying lasts until morning. The concerned parents contact the vaccinating physician, no intervention is done, and the episode passes. A few months later, the parents are reluctant to vaccinate their child again. What advice should the physician offer?

2. A college student who smokes presents with a bothersome cough that began suddenly and has persisted for six weeks; however, the cough has not interfered with the student's work: the only reason the student has sought medical advice is out of concern for some serious underlying disease, such as lung cancer. Given the trouble and expense of the effort needed to determine whether *B. pertussis* is the cause of the cough, is the effort worth expending?

3. Another college student also presents with a cough that has lasted three weeks. The student complains of dizziness and sweating after drinking hot chocolates. How might an infection from *B. pertussis* cause such symptoms?

4. An outbreak of severe respiratory disease, seemingly pertussis, breaks out in a kindergarten class. The school district requires that children present evidence of vaccination with DPT before attending school. What should be done?

5. As a physician, you are called to perform emergency surgery in an underdeveloped country where few are vaccinated against pertussis, and the disease is common. On the return flight, a sick child next to you is coughing with a bit of a whoop. You are returning to your spouse and your 1-month-old infant. Should any action have been taken before the trip? Should any action be taken now? If so, what? If not, why not?

REFERENCES

Ad Hoc Group for the Study of Pertussis Vaccines: Placebo-controlled trial of two acellular pertussis vaccines in Sweden-protective efficacy and adverse effects. *Lancet* **1:**955–960, 1988.

Cherry JD, Brunell PA, Golden GS, Karzon DT. Report of the Task Force on Pertussis and Pertussis Immunization—1988. *Pediatrics* **81:**939–984, 1988.

Goodwin MStM, Weiss AA: Adenylate cyclase toxin is critical for colonization and pertussis toxin is critical for lethal infection by *Bordetella pertussis* in infant mice. *Infect Immun* **58:**3445–3447, 1990.

Gordon M, Davies HD, Gold R: The clinical and microbiological features of children presenting with pertussis to a Canadian pediatric hospital over a 10 year period. *Pediatr Infect Dis J* **13:**617–622, 1994.

Kaslow HR, Burns DL: Pertussis toxin and target eukaryotic cells: binding, entry, and activation. *FASEB J* **6:**2684–2690, 1992.

Major RH: *A History of Medicine,* vol. I. Springfield, IL, Charles C. Thomas, 1954, p. 423.

Mink CM, Cherry JD, Christenson P, et al.: A search for *B. pertussis* infection in university students. *Clin Infect Dis* **14:**464–471, 1992.

Pichichero ME: Pertussis and the pertussis vaccines. *Cur Op Infect Dis* **6:**1–6, 1993.

Pittman M: Pertussis toxin: the cause of the harmful effects and prolonged immunity of whooping cough. A hypothesis. *Rev Inf Dis* **1:**401–412, 1979.

Robbins JB, Pittman M, Trollfors B, Lagergard TA, Taranger J, Schneerson R: *Primum non nocere:* a pharmacologically inert pertussis toxoid alone should be the next pertussis vaccine. *Pediatr Infect Dis J* **12:**795–807, 1993.

Standfast AFB: The comparison between field trials and mouse protection tests against intranasal and intracerebral challenges with *Bordetella pertussis. Immunology* **1:**135–143, 1958.

Weiss AA, Hewlett EL: Virulence factors of *Bordetella pertussis. Ann Rev Microbiol* **40:**661–686, 1986.

6

Fulminant Hepatitis B

SHUNJI MISHIRO, KOICHI KANAI, AND MINEO KOJIMA

CASE REPORT

A 44-year-old man was admitted to the hospital because of evidence of gastrointestinal hemorrhage with acute jaundice. (This patient's case history was initially presented in 1985 at the Gifu Hepatitis Conference by Dr. Mineo Kojima, and the virological characteristics of the virus were later published in detail by Yotsumoto et al., 1992.)

The patient had been well until 4 days earlier, when chills, fever, general malaise, and anorexia developed. He visited another hospital, and medication was prescribed under the diagnosis of "common cold." Two days before admission, the patient noticed that his urine was dark. On the day before admission, he revisited the first hospital, and evaluation there showed the presence of jaundice. Later on the same day, a tarry stool discharge and vomiting of a black coffee-colored material developed. During these preadmission days, malaise and anorexia increased gradually.

The patient, a worker for a newspaper company, had cohabited with his wife for 13 years. She had been under medical care because of persistent infection with hepatitis B virus (HBV) and was seropositive for anti-hepatitis B e antigen (HBe) antibody at the time of her husband's admission. Two children born to these parents were well. The patient had no habit of drinking alcohol, but he did smoke an average of 20 cigarettes per day for about 20 years. He had never traveled to areas where hepatitis was endemic. There was no history of surgery, receipt of blood products, intravenous drug abuse, acupunc-

ture therapy, tattoo, previous jaundice, or gastrointestinal tract disease.

On admission to the hospital he was found to be afebrile; his pulse was 88 beats per minute, blood pressure 130/56 mm Hg. On physical examination, the patient was moderately icteric and appeared acutely ill. Petechiae, ecchymoses, rash, or lymphadenopathy were not found. His head was normal except for jaundiced conjunctiva bulbi. The lungs were clear, and the heart was normal. The lung-liver border on percussion was at the 7th rib level. On abdominal examination, there was tenderness in the lower abdomen; the liver and spleen were not felt; and there was no evidence of ascites. On neurologic examination, consciousness was clear, there was no involuntary movement, and the tendon reflexes were normal. Laboratory findings on admission are summarized in Tables 6-1, 6-2, and 6-3.

Several hours after admission, the patient began to show some signs of consciousness disturbance. Disorientation was one of the first signs to appear; for example, he was unable to find his room after walking outside. Somnolence followed and involuntary movements developed. A flapping tremor was noticed. Viewed together with the laboratory findings (in particular, the elevated serum levels of ammonia, methionine, and liver enzymes and prolonged prothrombin time, shown in Tables 6-1 and 6-2), these neurologic signs were interpreted as being due to hepatic encephalopathy. The intravenous administration of methylprednisolone, glucagon-insulin, and GO-80 (an amino acids mixture) was begun. On the 2nd hospital day, the consciousness disturbance pro-

Table 6-1. Laboratory Findings on Admission: Hematologic Values

Variable	Patient's Value	Normal Range
Hematocrit (%)	47.2	38–52
Hemoglobin (g/dL)	15.8	11–16
Red-cell count (per mm³)	4.99×10^6	4–6×10^6
Erythrocyte sedimentation rate (mm/h)	2	1–7
White-cell count (per mm³)	12,100	3500–9500
Platelet count (per mm³)	132×10^3	150–350×10^3
Prothrombin time (s)	52.4	11–13
Hepaplastin test (%)	<10	65–135
Thrombotest (%)	<5	>70
Fibrinogen (mg/dL)	157	200–400
Fibrin-degradation products (μg/mL)	10	<10

gressed to a grade III coma, and plasma-exchange therapy was initiated. Serum bilirubin and ammonia levels decreased significantly after the plasma exchange but increased again on the 3rd hospital day. On the 4th hospital day, the coma reached a level of grade IV and persisted thereafter. Plasma exchange was repeated daily until the 5th hospital day but without clinical improvement.

On the 7th hospital day (the 11th day from the

Table 6-2. Laboratory Findings on Admission: Blood Chemical Values

Variable	Patient's Value	Normal Range
Bilirubin, total (mg/dL)	10.6	0.1–1.5
Bilirubin, direct (mg/mL)	6.9	0–0.5
Aspartate aminotransferase (U/L)	2027	1–35
Alanine aminotransferase (U/L)	5270	1–40
Lactate dehydrogenase (U/L)	2617	100–220
Alkaline phosphatase (U/L)	434	80–250
Leucine aminopeptidase (U/L)	388	20–60
γ-glutamyl transpeptidase (U/L)	63	0–80
Total cholesterol (mg/dL)	191	125–230
Albumin (g/dL)	4.5	4.1–5.1
Amino acids		
Valine (mM/mL)	242.7	150–310
Leucine (mM/mL)	80.2	78–180
Isoleucine (mM/mL)	34.6	40–110
Phenylalanine (mM/mL)	478.0	43–76
Tyrosine (mM/mL)	499.2	40–90
Methionine (mM/mL)	684.7	19–40
Urea nitrogen (mg/dL)	40	8–22
Ammonia (μg/dL)	216	0–120
Alpha-fetoprotein (ng/mL)	1.4	0–20

Table 6-3. Laboratory Findings on Admission: Virological Values

Variable	Value
Hepatitis A virus	
IgM class anti-HAV antibody (ELISA)	Negative
Hepatitis B virus	
HBs antigen (RPHA & RIA)	Negative
HBe antigen (RIA)	Negative
Anti-HBs antibody (PHA)	+ (2^5)
Anti-HBe antibody (RIA)	+ (95% inhibition)
IgM class anti-HBc (RIA)	+ (cutoff index = 7.1)
Hepatitis C virus	
Anti-HCV antibody (ELISA)	Negative
Hepatitis D virus	
Anti-delta antibody (RIA)	Negative

Ig, immunoglobulin; HAV, hepatitis A virus; ELISA, enzyme-linked immunosorbent assay; HBs, hepatis B surface; HBe, hepatitis Be; RPHA, reverse passive hemagglutination assay; RIA, radioimmunoassay; PHA, passive hemaglutination; HBc, hepatitis B core; HCV, hepatitis C virus.

appearance of symptoms) the patient died. An autopsy was performed.

DIAGNOSIS

Clinically, fulminant hepatitis is characterized by the rapid course of disease progression: only 11 days from the onset of symptoms to death in the present case. The laboratory findings on admission of this patient suggested the presence of: (1) hepatocyte injury (aspartate aminotransferase ast = 2027 U/L; alanine aminotransferase t = 5270 U/L: see Tables 6-1 and 6-2 for normal ranges); (2) decreased metabolic functions of the liver (total bilirubin = 10.6 mg/dL; ammonia = 216 μg/dL); (3) insufficient synthesis by the liver of rapid turnover proteins (prothrombin time = 52.4 s); and (4) acute infection with hepatitis B virus (high-titered immunoglobulin M [IgM] class anti-HBc antibody, rarely observed in chronic infection). Although hepatic failure (or the presence of the first three listed items) can also be observed in cases of acute exacerbation or at the end-stage of long-standing chronic liver disease, such as cirrhosis, several lines of evidence indicate that the present patient was not suffering from such a chronic liver disease. First, the patient had no history of previous liver disease. Second, on physical examination, no enlargement of the liver or spleen or other signs of portal hypertension were seen. Third, normal serum values were obtained from this patient for total cholesterol, albumin, and zinc turbidity test, which might have been abnormal if the patient had had advanced chronic liver disease. Acute infection in this patient was also indicated by the fever at the onset and leukocytosis on admission.

The course of fulminant hepatitis is often devastating, and once profound encephalopathy develops, mortality exceeds 50%. The present patient died 6 days after the development of the initial signs and symptoms of encephalopathy. Hyperammonemia is often associated with hepatic encephalopathy and was present in this patient even before its clinical manifestation in the form of disorientation and flapping tremor followed by deep coma. Changes in the serum aminogram pattern are also of diagnostic value for hepatic encephalopathy; they reflect decreased metabolism of amino acids in the liver.

Pathologically, fulminant hepatitis relates to a massive necrosis of the liver. On autopsy this patient's liver showed atrophy: Its weight was only 630 g, about half the normal weight. The liver surface was smooth, and no nodule formation was observed, suggesting the nonexistence of a chronic inflammatory process. Instead, parenchymal necrosis was prominent on the cut surface of the liver (Fig. 6-1). Microscopically, the liver showed destruction of lobular architecture, massive necrosis of hepatocytes, lymphocyte infiltration, hemorrhage around central veins and portal triads, and formation of pseudo-bile canaliculi; however, there was no evidence of a chronic pathological process, such as fibrosis (Fig. 6-2). The pathological diagnosis was acute liver atrophy (massive hepatocyte necrosis), compatible with the clinical diagnosis of fulminant hepatitis.

The clinical and pathological diagnosis of fulminant hepatitis is relatively easy. A much harder task is virological diagnosis with respect to the causative agent. Hepatitis B and non-A, non-B (NANB) hepatitis account for the majority of patients with fulminant hepatitis, hepatitis A and hepatitis E for a minority, and hepatitis C remains controversial as a possible cause. Routine serologic and virologic examinations,

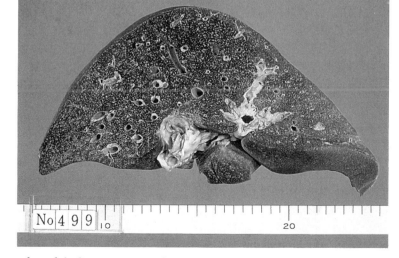

Figure 6-1. *Cut surface of the liver on autopsy.* The liver was significantly atrophic (630 g); parenchymal necrosis was prominent on the cut surface.

Figure 6-2. *Microscopy of the liver on autopsy.* Destruction of lobular architecture, massive necrosis of hepatocytes, lymphocyte infiltration, hemorrhage around central veins and portal triads, and formation of pseudobile canaliculi were observed without evidence of a chronic pathological process, such as fibrosis.

however, do not always reveal the causative virus in patients with fulminant hepatitis, whereas they almost always do in the case of acute hepatitis. It may be that fulminant hepatitis runs too rapid a course for antiviral antibodies to be produced or that the host immune reaction against the causative virus in fulminant hepatitis patients is very different from that in acute hepatitis patients. In the present case, IgM class anti-HB core antibody was positive with relatively high titers, and this was the only serologic evidence indicating HBV as the cause in this patient. A definitive diagnosis of HBV infection in this patient was obtained by detecting HBV DNA in his serum, with an analysis of its nucleotide sequence, as is described in the following section.

MOLECULAR PERSPECTIVES

Sexual transmission is one of the most important modes of horizontal transmission of HBV, to the extent that acute hepatitis B can now be classified into the category of sexually transmitted disease, as is acquired immunodeficiency syndrome (AIDS). Therefore, a strongly suspected source of infection of this patient was his wife. She was aged 40 years at the time of her husband's illness and had received a blood transfusion at age 16 years; when she was aged 37 years, she was diagnosed serologically and histologically with chronic hepatitis B and had continuous medical care thereafter. Her sera, obtained over time during those years from her diagnosis to her husband's illness had been stored in good condition, allowing retrospective analyses for various markers of HBV.

As shown in Figure 6-3, the HBV DNA and DNA polymerase (DNAp) in the sera of the patient's wife showed a sharp spike a month before her husband developed his acute illness in July 1984. This finding implies that for some unknown reason the so-far suppressed rate of replication of HBV suddenly increased in the wife, and the risk of sexual transmission of HBV to the husband increased in this special period. The time lag of 1 month, that is, between the peaking of HBV DNA/DNAp in the wife and the onset of the disease in the husband, is consistent with the incubation time for HBV infection in general. Thus, it is quite possible that the patient was infected by his wife, not by other sources.

Direct evidence supporting this speculation, however, came from extensive analyses of HBV DNA sequences from both the patient's and his wife's sera; this type of analysis is similar to the "DNA fingerprinting" often employed to obtain legal evidence. Because HBV undergoes mutation during persistent infection, the nucleotide sequence of HBV DNA shows some differences among those who are infected as long as they do not share same source of recent infection (i.e., before the mutations occur). In the present case, we detected at least one clone of HBV with a nucleotide sequence that was identical in the patient and his wife. Moreover, this husband-wife identical HBV clone was found in the wife's sample obtained in June 1984 but not in that obtained in January 1984, suggesting that the patient was infected by his wife in June 1984 and not before.

An extensive literature (Kosaka et al., 1991; Liang et al., 1991; Omata et al., 1991; Terazawa et al., 1991) has pointed to the responsibility of so-called *precore-defective* HBV mutants in the etiology of fulminant hepatitis. HBV has a double-stranded DNA about 3.2 kilobases (kb) long as its genome (Fig.

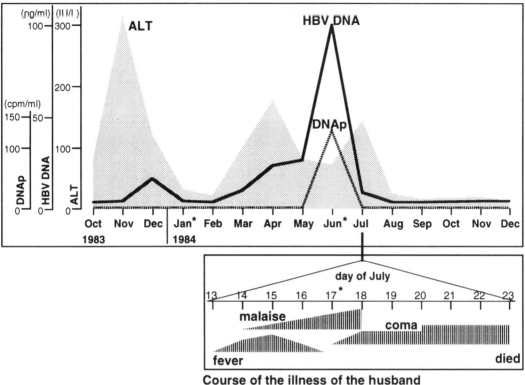

Figure 6-3. *Disease course of the patient and his wife.* Note that hepatitis B virus (HBV) DNA and DNA polymerase (DNAp) in the sera of the patient's wife showed a spike a month before the patient developed acute illness. ALT, alanine aminotransferase.

6-4). *Precore* relates to a region of HBV DNA that encodes 29 amino acids (aa) just upstream of the "core" region that codes for the 185-aa nucleocapsid protein of HBV. When the 3.5-kb mRNA involving both the precore and core regions is translated, there appears a precore-plus-core protein of 211 aa, a precursor protein of e antigen (Fig. 6-5a). HBeAg is a nonstructural protein of HBV and is secreted from infected hepatocytes into the bloodstream, as described later in more detail. In *precore-defective* mutants of HBV, the normal e antigen precursor protein is not produced as a result of one or both of two defect patterns in the precore region of HBV DNA: (1) the generation of a stop codon by a point mutation in the 28th codon of the precore (*nonsense mutation*) (Figs. 6-5b and 6-6); (2) a deletion or insertion somewhere within the precore region that results, mainly by way of a frameshift effect, in the expression of a truncated or misshapen e antigen (*frameshift mutation*). The first pattern relates much more commonly than the second to the

etiology of fulminant hepatitis; indeed, the present patient's HBV DNA showed the first pattern.

The wife of the patient harbored HBV with various patterns of precore defects. It is of special interest, however, that the relative proportion of these patterns changed between January 1984, when viremia was stably at low levels, and June 1984, when an abrupt rise in HBV DNA and DNAp was observed. The most significant change was the increase in the HBV population with mutations at both codon 28 and codon 29. Moreover, the precore mutant population of her husband's HBV was almost exclusively of this type (Table 6-4). These observations suggest that the HBV mutant with G to A mutations at the second bases of both 28th and 29th codons of the precore, or at the -5 and -2 positions relative to core AUG (Fig. 6-6), has some selective advantages over other types of precore mutants as well as over wild-type HBVs.

Indeed, it could have structural advantages. A 137-nucleotide sequence, termed ε, involving the

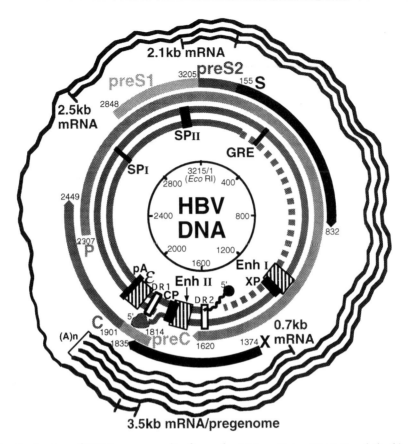

Figure 6-4. *Genetic structure of HBV.* Four open reading frames (preC+C, preS1+preS2+S, P, and X) of hepatitis B virus (HBV) DNA are shown together with four distinct-sized messenger RNAs (3.5 kb mRNA, 2.5 kb mRNA, 2.1 kb mRNA, and 0.7 kb mRNA). Transcription regulation elements are also mapped on the DNA: SP I (preS1 promoter); SP II (preS2/S promoter); CP (preC, C/P, pregenome promoter); XP (X promoter); Enh I (enhancer I); Enh II (enhancer II); GRE (glucocorticoid-responsive element); ϵ (encapsidation signal); and pA (poly-A signal).

precore-core junction of HBV genome has been identified as necessary for encapsidation of the HBV pregenome. The 80 nucleotides within ϵ from -50 to $+27$ relative to core AUG may be important because they are highly conserved among hepadnaviruses as well as among various subtypes of HBV. This sequence contains many indirect repeats, which could form various kinds of secondary structures. Among several possible structures, the one shown in the Figure 6-7 has been proposed as an HBV encapsidation signal in which the CUGU motif shared among hepadnaviruses is exposed as a loop. G to A mutations at the -5 or -2 position would further stabilize this structure by converting the U-G wobbly pairings to stronger U-A pairings. Thus, these mutations would result in accelerated encapsidation of

the HBV pregenome. If the replication cycle of the mutant HBV is shortened, the virus should increase faster and reach a higher titer than wild-type HBV in a given period, thereby leading to a more aggressive course of hepatitis. In addition, if wild-type HBV and mutant HBV coreplicate in a hepatocyte, the pregenome of the latter would preferentially be encapsidated into core particles. This speculation is supported by a previous observation (Okamoto et al., 1990) and by the results of the present case study showing that the -5/-2 precore mutants of HBV prevailed over preexisting wild-type HBV or mutants of other types in persistently infected carriers. There is no certainty that selective encapsidation results in increased virulence of HBV precore mutants; the selective advantage may be extremely small. How-

a) Wild type

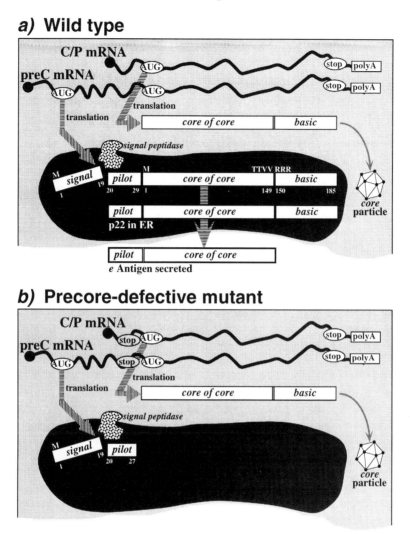

b) Precore-defective mutant

Figure 6-5. *Translation of the preC mRNA with or without nonsense mutation at 28th codon of precore.* (a) In the case of wild-type hepatitis B virus (HBV) infection, the precursor protein of e antigen is translated from preC mRNA (one of 3.5-kb mRNAs) and processed in the lumen of the endoplasmic reticulum (ER) to be secreted as mature e antigen from the hepatocyte into the circulation. (b) In the case of the most common precore-defective HBV mutant with a nonsense mutation at precore codon 28, the e antigen precursor is truncated.

ever, viruses increase geometrically via replication. A 1% advantage during the viral assembly process for the mutant over the wild-type in one cycle would lead to a 170% advantage in 100 cycles. Even a 0.1% advantage per cycle would lead to a 172% advantage in 1000 cycles. The encapsidation mechanism described here, consistent with the above findings of a predominance of G to A mutations at the -5/-2 positions in patients with severe and persistent HBV infections, has also been supported by transfection experiments *in vitro*. The more efficient packaging of pregenome RNA was observed in mutants with the stronger base pairings within the concerned region of the ε structure.

That these precore-defective mutants are incapable of producing HBeAg may be yet another reason why they are associated with the more severe forms of hepatitis, including fulminant hepatitis (see Fig. 6-5b). HBeAg is a unique viral protein in that it is neither a structural protein nor a nonstructural pro-

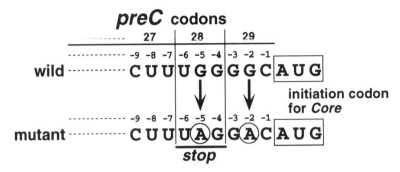

Figure 6-6. *The -5/-2 G to A mutant.* The nonsense mutation at the precore codon 28 due to a G to A replacement at the -5 position is often associated with another G to A mutation at the -2 position relative to the core AUG.

tein with catalytic functions. The e antigen of HBV is unique among viral proteins in that it plays the role of an immunosuppressant. It is secreted from wild-type HBV-infected hepatocytes into the circulation in a free form, not associated with HBV particles, whereupon it suppresses a host immune response, particularly T-cell function. Thus, if e antigen is not secreted, as in the case of precore-defective mutant infection, the host T cells are rid of one suppressive pressure. Hepatocyte degeneration in hepatitis B (and perhaps hepatitis C, too) has been ascribed not to the direct cytopathic effects of the virus but to *apoptosis* (programmed cell death) of infected hepatocytes. An infected hepatocyte presents on its surface a virus-derived oligopeptide with its own HLA molecules. These signals of infection are soon recognized and bound by cytotoxic T lymphocytes (CTL), and the infected hepatocytes then undergo apoptosis triggered by cytokines from the CTL. According to

this widely accepted mechanism, the more active the T cell response of hosts, the more severe the hepatitis. Thus, in the case of precore-defective HBV infection, e antigen is not secreted, CTL response is less suppressed, and eventually hepatitis tends to become more aggressive than in case of wild-type HBV infection.

Last but not least is the question of why the wife of the present patient did not herself contract fulminant hepatitis. The wife and husband shared the same HBV strain that caused a fatal outcome in one but in the other only a transient rise in viremia without clinical significance. This great difference in response may be explained by differences in host factors, rather than viral factors. As described above, hepatocyte degeneration in hepatitis B is induced by CTLs specifically directed to infected hepatocytes. In chronically infected individuals, like the wife, the CTLs, which are able to recognize infected hepato-

Table 6-4. Patterns of Precore Mutations Observed in HBV Clones from the Patient and His Wife

Patterns			No. of HBV Clones Obtained From		
			Wife		Patient
Codon 28	Codon 29	Insertion	Jan 1984	June 1984	July 1984
−	−	−	0	0	0
−	−	+	0	0	0
−	+	−	0	0	0
−	+	+	0	0	0
+	−	−	<u>9</u>	2	1
+	−	+	4	5	0
+	+	−	3	<u>8</u>	<u>19</u>
+	+	+	3	5	0
Total			19	20	20

The most abundant genotypes are underscored.

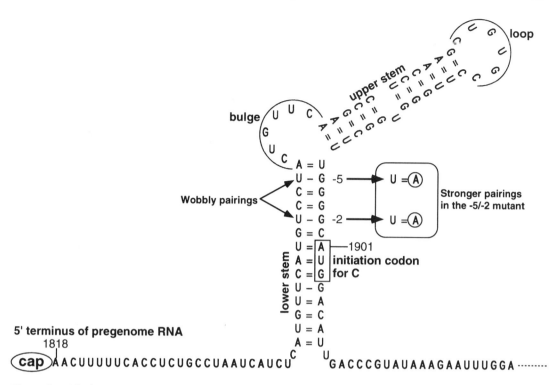

Figure 6-7. *The hepatitis B virus (HBV) pregenome encapsidation signal ε.* The conformational stability of this important structure is enhanced by the G to A mutations at both the -5 and -2 nucleotide positions.

cytes, are already activated and perform their functions continuously and effectively. So if a mutant with a high replicative efficacy evolves and begins growing in a hepatocyte at a certain time during a persistent infection, the hepatocyte will soon be recognized and destroyed by the CTLs. In contrast, in persons for whom the infection was the first encounter with HBV, there would be a substantial interval until the responsive CTLs show up, and during this time the virus can grow and infect a greater number of hepatocytes that will later be ravaged by CTLs. Thus, more massive degeneration of liver will occur in such an acute case compared with a chronic case. In this situation, viral factors become more important than host factors. The faster the replication of the virus in the first hepatocyte(s) that are infected, the greater the number of hepatocytes elsewhere in the liver that would become infected within a given period. Thus, if the time lag before activation of CTLs is constant, a replication-efficient mutant, for example, the -5/-2 G to A mutant, would infect a larger volume of the liver than a wild-type HBV. Together with the absence of the immunosuppressive e antigen, this replication

advantage can explain why the precore-defective mutants are more frequently the cause of fulminant hepatitis than are wild-type HBVs.

As a side-note, although the two daughters of the parents in this case had been infected with HBV (they were positive for hepatitis B antibodies at the time of their father's illness), fortunately, they did not contract fulminant hepatitis. Terazawa et al. (1991) detected precore-defective HBV mutants in two infants with fulminant hepatitis who were born to mothers seropositive for anti-HBe and who are harboring the same HBV mutants. Why did the same events not occur in the present case? It must be a matter of the timing of transmission. Vertical transmission of HBV occurs most frequently at the time of delivery. The younger child of the wife of the patient had been born 8 years before her father died of fulminant hepatitis. According to Okamoto et al. (1990), the precore-defective HBV mutants prevail in persistently infected hosts over time. Most likely, at the time of the delivery of the two daughters, the precore-defective mutants of HBV had not yet evolved in the mother.

In conclusion, this case illustrates several important aspects of HBV infection: (1) sexual transmission as an important route for horizontal spread of the virus; (2) genetic drift of HBV from wild-type (e-plus phenotype) to precore-defective type (e-minus phenotype) or to more replication-competent mutants during persistent infection; and (3) the potential of such mutants to cause fulminant hepatitis in acutely infected individuals.

THERAPY

Because fulminant hepatitis leads to multiple organ failure (i.e., dysfunction of multiple organs, such as liver, kidney, lung, and others, as is occasionally observed in patients with severe infectious diseases), patients should be removed as soon as possible after diagnosis to the intensive care unit and be treated by a team of experienced personnel.

Hepatic coma is one of the most prominent features of fulminant hepatitis, although the mechanisms are not yet fully appreciated. Antibiotics are given *per os* and *per anum* to eliminate the possible toxic substances generated by microorganisms in the gastrointestinal tract. Plasma exchange therapy can be employed to remove toxins and to supply the necessary components (coagulation factors, for example) that are decreased as a result of insufficient biosynthesis in the liver. The therapeutic use of amino acid solutions enriched in the branched chain amino acids, as in the present case, is now regarded as rather controversial. The use of sedativa is contraindicated. Because cerebral edema is observed in 70 to 80% of patients with fulminant hepatitis and often causes herniation of brainstem, intravenous infusion of mannitol is recommended to reduce the intracranial pressure.

Acute renal failure develops in more than 50% of patients with fulminant hepatitis. This renal insufficiency is mostly functional and is probably due to an imbalance of vasoactive substances. Hemodialysis is the first choice of treatment, combined in most instances with plasma exchange. In the early phase of renal dysfunction, hypokalemia and hyponatremia develop. Because hypokalemia is often followed by metabolic alkalosis, potassium chloride supplements are recommended at this stage.

Symptoms that resemble adult respiratory distress syndrome (i.e., dyspnea in adults with acute infiltrative lung lesions characterized by a prominent arterial hypoxemia) are often associated with fulminant hepatitis. Infections and hemorrhage will worsen the situation. Thus, if respiratory failure is suspected, the patient should be placed immediately under respiratory control and pulmonary functions carefully monitored. Measures to control infections and bleeding are also required.

Patients with fulminant hepatitis are particularly susceptible to bacterial infections caused by the decreased function of reticuloendothelial cells, such as Kupffer cells in the liver. Blood, sputum, urine, and other body fluids should be frequently examined for pathogenic bacteria during the course of the disease to select appropriate antibiotics. Administration of antibiotics for prophylactic purposes only is not recommended because antibiotics in general are hepatotoxic.

A bleeding tendency is often associated with fulminant hepatitis; it arises from the impaired production of coagulation factors by the liver as well as from an increased consumption of these factors because of other complications, such as disseminated intravascular coagulopathy. Clinically, bleeding from the gastrointestinal tract is most frequently seen, and the prophylactic use of H_2-receptor antagonists such as cimetidine (800 mg/day) is recommended. Supplementing clotting factors by transfusing fresh-frozen plasma and platelets is also recommended. Use of an antithrombin III preparation is another therapeutic option.

An "artificial liver support system" is used to some cases to remove toxic substances of various molecular sizes and to maintain patients until spontaneous recovery of their liver functions. It is more or less a combination of plasma exchange, molecular-sieving hemofiltration, charcoal-affinity hemoperfusion, and hemodialysis and has been reported to have some temporary beneficial effects.

Liver transplantation has become one of the major treatments of fulminant hepatitis in western countries. The survival rate of fulminant hepatitis patients with liver transplantation is reported to be 65%, much higher than that for those who do not undergo this procedure (roughly 20%).

QUESTIONS

1. What are the clinical features that characterize fulminant hepatitis?

2. What laboratory findings are of particular importance to the diagnosis of fulminant hepatitis?
3. What viruses should be considered the cause of fulminant hepatitis, and what laboratory tests should be done for the differential diagnosis?
4. Why are the precore-defective HBV mutants regarded as more virulent than wild-type HBVs?
5. Why are the clinical courses different for chronically infected and acutely infected persons, even when both were infected with an identical genotype of HBV?

REFERENCES

Junker-Niepmann M, Bartenschlager R, Schaller H: A short *cis*-acting sequence is required for hepatitis B virus pregenome encapsidation and sufficient for packaging of foreign RNA. *EMBO J* **9**:3389–3396, 1990.

Kosaka Y, Takase K, Kojima M, et al.: Fulminant hepatitis B: induction by hepatitis B virus mutants defective in the precore region and incapable of encoding e antigen. *Gastroenterology* **100**:1087–1094, 1991.

Liang TJ, Hasegawa K, Rimon N, Wands JR, Ben-Porath E: A hepatitis B virus mutant associated with an epidemic of fulminant hepatitis. *N Engl J Med* **324**:1705–1709, 1991.

Okamoto H, Yotsumoto S, Akahane Y, et al.: Hepatitis B viruses with precore region defects prevail in persistently infected hosts along with seroconversion to the antibody against e antigen. *J Virol* **64**:1298–1303, 1990.

Omata M, Ehata T, Yokosuka O, Hosoda K, Ohto M: Mutations in the precore region of hepatitis B virus DNA in patients with fulminant and severe hepatitis. *N Engl J Med* **324**:1699–1704, 1991.

Terazawa S, Kojima M, Yamanaka T, et al.: Hepatitis B virus mutants with precore-region defects in two babies with fulminant hepatitis and their mothers positive for antibody to hepatitis B e antigen. *Pediatr Res* **29**:5–9, 1991.

Tong S-P, Li J-S, Vitvitski L, Kay A, Trépo C: Base pairing in the pregenome encapsidation signal of HBV: A clue for the prevalence of naturally occurring HBe-Ag-minus precore mutations, *in* Nishioka K, Suzuki H, Mishiro S, Oda T (eds): *Viral Hepatitis and Liver Disease.* Tokyo, Springer-Verlag, 1994, pp 269–272.

Yotsumoto S, Kojima M, Shoji I, Yamamoto K, Okamoto H, Mishiro S: Fulminant hepatitis related to transmission of hepatitis B variants with precore mutations between spouses. *Hepatology* **16**:31–35, 1992.

7

Sickle Cell Anemia

SAMUEL CHARACHE AND AJOVI B. SCOTT-EMUAKPOR

CASE REPORT

The patient, a 25-year-old black man with sickle cell anemia, had been hospitalized for vaso-occlusive crises 10 times, mostly in late childhood and early adolescence.[1] He had been in good health for the past 6 to 8 years, during which time his minor aches and pains could be managed at home with oral analgesics. Four to 5 days before he came to the emergency department, he noted the gradual onset of moderately severe flank and back pain. On admission, he was found to be afebrile and was treated with intravenous fluids and analgesics, with some improvement. The total serum bilirubin value was 5.1 mg/dL (normal, 0.3–1.2 mg/dL), the white blood cell (WBC) count was 18,000/mm³ (normal for black adults, 2400–10,800 cells/mm³), and the hematocrit was 27% (normal adult black man, 37.2–50.2%). He was sent home with a prescription for oxymorphone (a morphine derivative) for pain. However, when his pain became generalized and he developed fever and sweats, he returned to the emergency department, whereupon he was found to have pleuritic chest pain and mild *dyspnea* (shortness of breath).

His blood pressure was 135/70 mm Hg, pulse 88 beats per minute, respirations 18 per minute, and oral temperature 38.3°C. He was an acutely ill, thin, jaundiced man complaining of severe pain. There was poor inspiratory effort, and a few rales were

heard at the base of both lungs. The liver was palpable one finger's breadth below the right costal margin.

The hematocrit was 26%, but his WBC had risen to 26,000/mm³. The total bilirubin was 9.1 mg/dL and the serum electrolytes were sodium, 138 mEq/L (normal, 135–147); potassium, 5.9 mEq/L (normal, 3.5–5.0); chloride, 109 mEq/L (normal, 95–105); HCO_3^-, 26 mEq/L (normal, 22–28). His arterial pH was 7.40 (normal, pH 7.35–7.45) with a P_{O_2} of 86 torr) and P_{CO_2} of 37 torr (normal, 35–45 torr) while breathing room air.

The chest roentgenogram showed a slightly enlarged heart, fluid in the right minor fissure of the lung, and nonvisualization of the posterior diaphragm, consistent with a pleural effusion. There was also a suggestion of an infiltrate at the right lung base. An electrocardiogram showed sinus tachycardia with a pattern of left ventricular enlargement.

Blood, throat, and urine cultures were obtained, and he was treated with cefotaxime (an antibiotic), oxygen, and meperidine (a narcotic analgesic). He spent a difficult night and developed a temperature of 39.3°C within 12 hours. He developed *tachypnea* (respiratory rate 40 per minute), a loud left pleural friction rub was heard, and an arterial blood sample showed a P_{O_2} of 41 torr. Despite the administration of 40% oxygen by facemask, the arterial P_{O_2} remained at 43 torr. The oxygen content of the inspired gas was increased to 100%, and the patient was transferred to the medical intensive care unit (ICU). A repeat chest roentgenogram showed consolidation and *atelectasis* (collapse) in both lungs

[1]This patient's case history was initially presented on April 7, 1984, at medical grand rounds. Johns Hopkins Hospital, by Dr. Phillip C. Buescher.

and bilateral pleural effusions. Blood, throat, urine, and the pleural effusions were cultured. Gram's stains of the pleural fluid and the scant sputum were negative, as was a fluorescent-antibody stain for *Legionella* organisms.

Urinalysis showed specific gravity of 1.005 (dilute urine; normal, 1.015–1.025), pH 8.0 (normal fasting, 5.5–6.5), with trace blood, trace protein, and large amounts of urobilinogen. Antibiotics were changed to ampicillin, gentamicin, and trimethoprim-sulfamethoxazole (Bactrim), because pneumonia could not be ruled out and the patient was dangerously ill.

His condition continued to deteriorate for several days. His temperature stayed above 39°C and his WBC count increased to 46,000/mm³. On the 4th hospital day the patient's P_{O_2} again fell to 50 torr despite the administration of 100% oxygen ($P_{O_2} \sim$ 700 torr) by facemask. An endotracheal tube was inserted in an effort to force oxygen into his lungs with positive pressure and so that the P_{O_2} in the inspired gas mixture could be lowered in an attempt to avoid oxygen-induced lung damage. This maneuver was successful because it was possible to maintain Pa_{O_2} above 70 torr despite a decreased P_{O_2} in the inspired gas. He was given an exchange transfusion with 5 U of packed red blood cells over the next 2 days, bringing the percentage of hemoglobin (Hb) A to 70%. Thereafter, he received transfusions as necessary to keep his hematocrit above 35%.

By the 9th day in the ICU, his temperature had returned to normal; after gradual weaning off the ventilator, the endotracheal tube was removed. None of the cultures obtained earlier provided evidence of an infectious cause of his illness. Antibiotics were discontinued, and the patient was transferred to a general medical ward on the 13th hospital day, where he received a mixture of oxygen and room air by nasal cannula. At the time of discharge, on his 22nd hospital day, a roentgenogram showed no infiltrates or effusions, and the Pa_{O_2} (while breathing room air) was 88 torr. The discharge diagnosis was adult respiratory distress syndrome complicating sickle cell vaso-occlusive crisis.

DIAGNOSIS

A definitive diagnosis of sickle cell disease is routinely made by electrophoretic analysis of lysed red cells. This information revealed the presence of hemoglobin S early in the course of the patient's illness.

The properties of a molecule that influence its electrophoretic mobility are its net electric charge and frictional coefficient. In the case of proteins, the former is the sum of the positive and negative charges on exposed amino acid side chains and the amino and carboxyl ends, whereas the latter is a result of the size and shape of the molecule. The sickle cell mutation causes the loss of two negative charges in the Hb tetramer at pH 8.6 because of the substitution in the β subunits of nonpolar valine for glutamic acid. The glutamic acid side chain is negatively charged at this pH. Thus, Hb A migrates more rapidly toward the *anode* (positive pole) than Hb S on a cellulose acetate strip at pH 8.6 (Fig. 7-1, lane 5).

Electrophoretic analysis for the presence of hemoglobin S in cord blood is complicated by the presence of large amounts of fetal Hb (F), which may obscure Hb A and Hb S. To avoid this, electrophoresis is also carried out in citrate agar at pH 6.0, where Hb S migrates completely free of Hb F (Fig. 7-1, lane 8).

MOLECULAR PERSPECTIVES

The early history of sickle cell anemia has been elegantly described by Conley (1980), and much of what follows is taken from that description. In 1910, Herrick noticed that some of the red cells on the blood smear of a West Indian student had "peculiar elongate forms," and that the student was anemic. In 1922 Mason noted the falciform (sickle) shape of some of the red cells on the smear of a patient with severe anemia and an ankle ulcer and named the disease *sickle cell anemia*. Emmel (1950) had shown earlier that although only occasional red cells were deformed on blood smears from a similar patient, all of the red cells assumed a bizarre shape in a sealed wet preparation. Further, he noted that the red cells of the patient's father behaved similarly, although the father was apparently normal in other respects. More cases were reported, but there was considerable confusion between the "active" and "latent" forms of the disease:

The active form was represented by the patient and the "latent" form was represented by the pa-

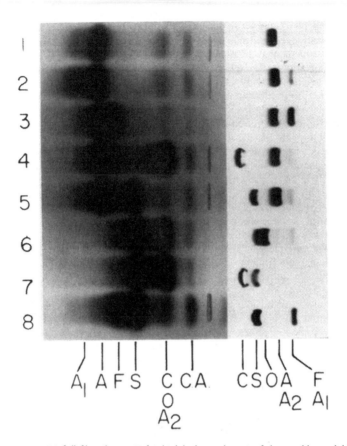

Figure 7-1. Cellulose acetate pH 8.6 (left) and agar pH 6.0 (right) electrophoresis of abnormal hemoglobins, stained for protein. The anode is to the left, and band C.A. is erythrocyte carbonic anhydrase. Lanes are as follows: (1) normal (AA$_2$); (2) a diabetic with increased glycosylated hemoglobin (A$_1$, A, A$_2$); (3) umbilical cord (AF A$_2$); (4) hemoglobin C trait (AC); (5) sickle cell trait (AS A$_2$); (6) hemoglobin S-O$_{Arab}$ disease (SO); (7) hemoglobin SC disease (SC); (8) sickle cell anemia (SF A$_2$). Hemoglobin O$_{Arab}$ migrates with Hb C on cellulose acetate, but between A and S on agar: glycosylated hemoglobin (A$_1$) migrates faster than A on cellulose acetate, but with F on agar.

tient's father. Red cells from all cases changed shape (*sickled*) when sealed in wet preparations. Whereas the active form had intermittent serious clinical problems (*crises*), the latent form was not associated with any significant clinical manifestations. In between crises, the active form behaved like the latent form, and it was not clear what factors caused this shift. Those early reports stressed the presence of severe anemia and ankle ulcers but made little of the recurrent attacks of abdominal, joint, and bone pain that dominate contemporary descriptions of the disease.

In 1927 Hahn and Gillespie showed that it was deoxygenation that caused cells in sealed preparations to sickle. The "peculiar elongated forms" seen on oxygenated blood smears were irreversible sickle cells (ISC), which are now recognized as having an acquired membrane defect causing them to retain an abnormal shape even after the Hb is oxygenated. Some years after discovery of the role of deoxygenation in inducing sickling, a conversation on an overnight train led Pauline et al., (1949) to subject the Hb of a patient with sickle cell anemia to electrophoresis. The patient's Hb (Hb S) migrated differently from normal Hb (Hb A), and relatives with latent disease had two Hb peaks, one normal and one not. For the first time, a genetic disorder had been traced directly to an abnormal protein; it soon became clear that active patients were homozygotes, and latent patients heterozygotes. Since that initial demonstration, Hb electrophoresis has become a simple clinical laboratory procedure (Fig. 7-1). To date more than 300 abnormal Hbs have been described, most of which are produced by single amino acid substitutions in either the α- or β-globin chains.

Following identification of sickle cell Hb, studies of the sickling process took two directions. The structural abnormality of the mutant Hb molecule was shown to be replacement of hydrophilic, or acidic, glutamic acid in position 6 of the β chain by hydrophobic, nonpolar valine, and it was deduced that sickling was caused by a polymerization process involving that site. After Perutz and coworkers (1960) defined the three-dimensional arrangement of normal α and β chains with respect to each other (*tertiary structure*), Wishner et al. in 1975 solved the structure of the basic unit of the Hb S polymer. When deoxygenated, the abnormal Hb tetramers formed paired linear filaments in which the hydrophobic side chain of valine fit nicely into a similarly hydrophobic acceptor area of an adjacent Hb molecule.

Studies of "supramolecular" structure demonstrated that filaments associate to form into larger fibers. Early on, Harris (1950) showed that deoxygenated Hb S solutions contained "tactoids," which, by analogy to tobacco mosaic virus, appeared to be composed of bundles of linear polymers. Murayama confirmed that suggestion in a series of ingenious studies and proposed a model for bundle or fiber formation. Electron-micrographic (Fig. 7-2) and radiographic diffraction studies eventually led to what is widely accepted as the model of supramolecular Hb structure: The paired filaments described by Wishner and co-workers (1975) aggregate into 14-stranded fibers that then aggregate, side to side, to form tactoids. It is these fibers of deoxygenated Hb molecules that not only deform red cells into the characteristic sickled shape but render them stiff and inflexible as well. The clinical effects of stiff sickle cells, described in 1940 by Ham and Castle, are discussed as follows.

Twenty to thirty percent of West Africans are carriers of the β^S gene. This high prevalence, confined to West Africa and other areas of the Mediterranean Basin, raises a question as to the mechanism of evolution and establishment of this gene.

Almost certainly, the occurrence in one population of significant numbers of β^A and β^S genes (a *polymorphism*) is not a consequence of recurrent mutation. Restriction endonuclease cleavage site polymorphisms around the β-globin gene suggest that the change in codon β^6 occurred several but not hundreds of times (Kan and Dozy, 1980). Thus, the large number of carriers of Hb S in numerous parts of the world is probably a consequence of "balanced" polymorphism. Sickle cell trait conveys a survival advantage to young children in areas where *falciparum* malaria is endemic. Typically, parasitized red cells leave the circulation and are sequestered in relatively hypoxic areas of the liver and spleen; if these cells can sickle, they may be destroyed by reticuloendothelial cells, and the loss of K^+ ion that accompanies sickling may kill *trophozoites* (the motile feeding stage of the parasite). The protection is not complete, but parasite density may be kept low enough so that heterozygote children have a significantly increased chance to survive long enough to develop partial immunity to infection and to reproduce, thereby increasing the numbers of β^S genes in the gene pool.

The β^A *homozygotes* (normal persons) do not have a similar protection against malaria. Malaria infection is often lethal for these homozygotes, and they do not live long enough to reproduce, causing loss of two β^A genes from the pool. On the other hand, homozygosity for the β^S gene (*sickle cell anemia*) leads to severe clinical consequences. A large number of β^S homozygotes do not reach reproductive age, which leads to the increased loss of two β^S genes from the pool. Thus, we have a situation in which the heterozygote is genetically fitter than both homozygotes. This is selection balanced by selection and is referred to as *balanced polymorphism*. By this mechanism, the incidence of the sickle cell trait increases until the loss of β^S genes is balanced by the gain of the gene through increased survival of the heterozygotes. With eradication of malaria, or movement of heterozygotes to areas free of malaria, all the advantage and much of the disadvantage of sickle trait is lost, and gene frequency is expected to remain nearly constant, apart from effects of societal factors such as racial admixture and birth control.

The "central dogma" of the Hb aficionado is that a single base-pair substitution in the DNA of both copies of chromosome 11 is responsible for all the clinical manifestations of sickle cell disease. In the case report described at the beginning of this chapter, little defense of the dogma is necessary; in oth-

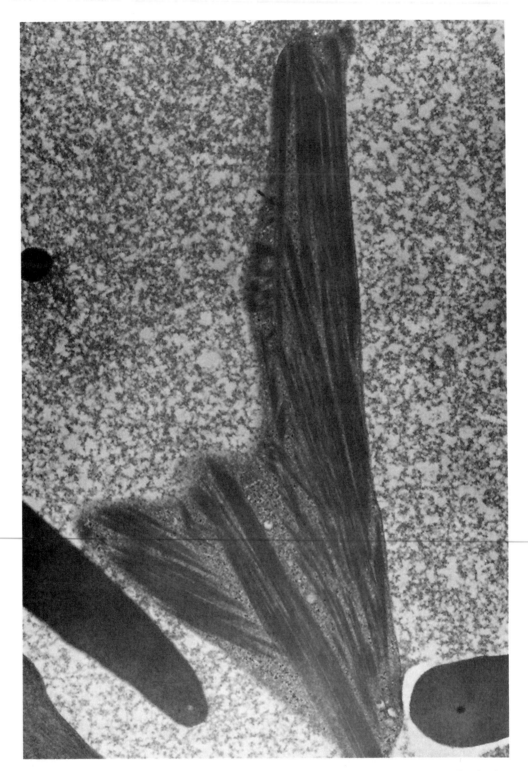

Figure 7-2. Electron micrograph of a sickled cell, showing fibers of polymerized deoxyhemoglobin S. Reproduced with permission of Dr. Isabelle Telez-Nagel.

ers, more faith is required. Substitution of a T-A base pair for an A-T base pair in that portion of the β gene that codes for the sixth amino acid of the β chain leads to a substitution of valine for glutamic acid. The presence of valine permits formation of the relatively weak intermolecular bonds that lead to polymerization of Hb. Such bonds can form only when Hb molecules are in the deoxygenated conformation, when their concentration is high and when they happen to collide at just the appropriate angle. Those conditions were apparently satisfied in the patient 3 days before he first came to the emergency room: His Hb polymerized and he developed a painful or vaso-occlusive sickle cell crisis.

Polymerization leads to hemolytic anemia as well as decreased deformability of red cells. The pathogenesis of *accelerated* red cell destruction is poorly understood; it involves membrane damage, cation loss, Hb denaturation, and fragmentation of cells. Although the same process alters both deformability and red cell survival, exacerbations of one abnormality are not usually associated with worsening of the other process. Typically, the patient described here was no more anemic than usual, even at a time of significant vaso-occlusive disease.

Ham and Castle's original description (1940) of the "vicious cycle of sickling" reported measurement of blood viscosity, and the belief that blood viscosity is abnormally high in patients with sickle cell anemia persists today. Actually, viscosity is not high, as all but the most unusual of patients are so anemic that their red cells do not interact sufficiently to alter blood flow. Intracellular viscosity is increased, and it is the increased rigidity of individual cells that prevents them from passing through narrow channels in the microvasculature. If enough microvascular channels are occluded, the tissue they supply becomes ischemic; if all collaterals are occluded, the tissue becomes infarcted. The mild pains experienced by many patients from day to day are probably ischemic episodes; those that bring them to the emergency department are infarctions, and those that produce fever and leukocytosis are large infarctions.

Sickling occurs when red cells are deoxygenated—but how much deoxygenation does it take? Sickling of SS (homozygous) red cells begins at P_{O_2} values as high as 80 torr, and nearly all cells are sickled at P_{O_2} values of ≤60 torr. Cells of heterozygotes (AS) do not begin to sickle until the P_{O_2} falls below ~20 torr,

and those of compound heterozygotes (SC, or S/β⁺ thalassemia) sickle at intermediate P_{O_2} values. Whether cells will sickle at usually encountered P_{O_2} values determines the relative severity of these conditions (SS SC AS) and accounts for the effects of lowered ambient P_{O_2} values on clinical manifestations. Stated another way, many red cells are exposed to P_{O_2} values of 60 torr, but few spend any time in tissues with P_{O_2} values of 20 torr; as a result, many SS cells sickle, but few AS cells do so.

Clearly, one can anticipate that clinical situations that lower P_{O_2} are likely to provoke increased polymerization of Hb and, hence, clinical symptoms. Cyanotic heart disease, chronic lung disease, and exposure to high altitude can produce shortening of red cell survival or vaso-occlusive lesions in normally asymptomatic persons with sickle cell trait (Diggs, 1984).

The dramatic course of events that followed the initial attack of pain in the patient described herein may be reconstructed as follows. His original pain probably represented bone marrow infarction: P_{O_2} is low in the marrow cavity, and blood flow is sluggish, permitting cells to deoxygenate and sickle within the sinusoids. The infarction was relatively large, for the patient developed fever and increased leukocytosis. Then some of the necrotic marrow, or perhaps an aggregate of sickled cells, became dislodged from the medullary cavity, entered the venous side of the circulation, and lodged in the next small vessel it encountered, producing a pulmonary infarct. In retrospect, the "suggestive infiltrate" seen on his chest roentgenogram was probably quite significant; unfortunately, there were probably multiple episodes of embolization, each small, but in aggregate enough to lower his Pa_{O_2} to the point where cells began to sickle everywhere, thereby impairing microvascular perfusion. At a Pa_{O_2} of 43 torr, sickling would be expected in *all* blood vessels; for unclear reasons, the primary target organ was the patient's lung.

If the liver happened to be the major organ affected in the sickle cell patient, high levels of serum bilirubin might occur because of accelerated red cell destruction and a so-called *hepatic crisis*. Bilirubin is a normal product of Hb catabolism. It is made more water-soluble by the attachment of glucuronic acid residues in the liver and then excreted in the bile. In persons with normal liver function, serum bilirubin may rise if the increased amount of bilirubin exceeds the glucuronidating capacity of the liver (*hemolytic jaundice*). If the capacity to attach glucuronic acid to bilirubin is also decreased by injury to the liver (e.g., infarction due to vaso-occlusion by sickled cells), the result may be a spectacular degree of jaundice.

In the kidney, one might expect acute renal failure, hematuria, or even papillary necrosis. The kidneys are usually mildly affected in all sickle cell cases. The microvasculature of the kidney is sensitive to the hypoxia that results from the sickling of erythrocytes. Thus, the entire length of the nephron is affected, from the glomerulus to the papillary tip. Three primary abnormalities are recognized in sickle cell nephropathy: (1) an inability to concentrate urine, leading to hyposthenuria; (2) some degree of distal renal tubular acidosis; and (3) impaired potassium metabolism. In the patient described here, a urine-specific gravity of 1.005 in a patient who is obviously dehydrated indicates the marked inability of the kidney to concentrate urine. This inability to concentrate urine has been shown to be due to the loss of deep juxtamedullary nephrons that are required for maximal concentration of urine. The urine pH of the patient was 8.0, indicating that the urine was inadequately acidified.

The process of acidification of the urine is a combination of events, including reabsorption of bicarbonate, tubular ammonia production, and excretion of hydrogen ions and titratable acid. In sickle cell disease, aside from being unable to perform these functions adequately, the distal tubules and collecting ducts have an altered ability to maintain the hydrogen ion gradient necessary for the acidification of urine. The patient described here also had slightly elevated serum potassium ($K^+ = 5.9$ mEq/dL). Defective potassium excretion by the kidneys leading to hyperkalemia, has been well described in sickle cell disease (De Fronzo et al., 1979).

In the intestinal tract, there is a peculiar abdominal syndrome that may represent mesenteric occlusion, but in small vessels, not arteries. In the spleen, at least in young children, massive sequestration of sickle cells, or infarction, occurs and in the lung, the respiratory distress syndrome, which is uncommon in adults but a major problem for pediatricians, who frequently see severe pulmonary malfunction complicating bacterial pneumonia in sickle cell disease.

THERAPY

Treatment

The first and still the only fairly reliable method for prevention of crises in sickle cell anemia is partial-exchange transfusion. If patients receive such exchanges and are maintained with a significant number of normal red cells in their veins, crises at least become less frequent and less severe. In acute emergencies, such as a fall in P_{O_2} to 43 torr despite administration of oxygen, an exchange transfusion can be lifesaving, as it may have been in this patient.

Studies of microvascular perfusion and of tissue obtained on biopsy or at autopsy make it clear that sickled cells cannot be "flushed out" of occluded vessels and that necrotic tissue that typifies sickle cell crises cannot be revivified by transfusion of normal red cells (or hyperbaric oxygenation or chemotherapeutic agents that decrease the likelihood that cells will sickle). Transfused red cells prevent new occlusions during intercritical periods as well as in desperate situations such as that described here. Attempts to prevent recurrent crises or strokes or to restore splenic function suggest that the proportion of sickle cells must be reduced to 30 to 50% if transfusions are to be effective. The mechanism of action of transfusions is unclear; it does not involve alterations of Hb concentration or of blood viscosity, but it may decrease the likelihood of two sickled cells arriving in the same microvascular junction at the same time.

It must be emphasized that there has never been a controlled study of the efficacy of transfusion in the acute or chronic care of patients with sickle cell anemia. Despite the lack of that highly desirable evidence, the inescapable effects of low P_{O_2}, low pH, and fever on deoxygenation, and hence sickling, have prompted use of transfusions in situations like that in the patient described herein, in addition to vigorous efforts to maintain normal P_{O_2}, pH, and temperature.

Sickle cell anemia and residence at high altitudes have much in common because the adaptation to chronic tissue hypoxia permits patients or highlanders to carry out their daily activities with surprising ease. Anemia in sickle cell patients is not a cause for transfusion unless either cardiopulmonary compensation or erythropoiesis falters, as in heart disease, lung disease, or bone marrow failure. Patients now live long enough to develop angina pectoris from coronary artery disease; overzealous transfusion and hyperviscosity must be avoided, but patients have less chest pain if their Hb concentrations are kept 7 g/dL. Fetal oxygenation is a potential problem when a severely anemic woman becomes pregnant; a cooperative study may eventually tell us whether transfusions can prevent spontaneous abortion and intrauterine growth retardation in such patients.

Other Forms of Treatment

Two other main forms of treatment have been attempted with some success in sickle cell disease. One of them is bone marrow transplantation (BMT), the rationale for which is the repopulation of a patient's bone marrow with that of a normal donor (Vermylen et al., 1988). This method requires finding appropriately human leukocyte antigen (HLA)-matched bone marrow donors, and it involves the use of preparatory regimens that include high-dose cytotoxic drugs or total body irradiation to obliterate the patient's own marrow. Thus, BMT can lead to severe clinical consequences (i.e., prolonged morbidity and even death) because of the occurrence of severe graft-versus-host disease, the potential for secondary malignancies (Witherspoon et al., 1992), and growth retardation (Wingard et al., 1992). These problems have combined to make BMT a less attractive an option for treating patients with sickle cell disease.

The second approach evolved through the study of patients with sickle cell disease who demonstrate mild clinical course (Noguchi et al., 1988). Through these studies, we now know that red blood cells containing both Hb F and Hb S survive longer than those containing only Hb S. This knowledge has stimulated interest in finding methods for inducing fetal Hb synthesis in patients with sickle cell disease and other β-chain hemoglobinopathies. Early in this effort, 5-azacytidine was successfully used because it was capable of inducing fetal Hb synthesis in anemic baboons (DeSimone et al., 1982). This drug, which is a cytotoxic drug and a carcinogen, can have considerable toxicity in addition to causing profound myelosuppression. It was therefore not widely used. More recently, another cytoxic drug, hydroxyurea, has gained more acceptance because it is much less

toxic and capable of inducing fetal hemoglobin production (Charache et al., 1992, 1995). In spite of its promise, hydroxyurea has not gained widespread use because its long-term carcinogenic and mutagenic effects cannot be predicted.

The search for a safe compound capable of inducing fetal Hb production led to the discovery of butyrate derivations. It was found that infants of diabetic mothers who develop in the presence of high maternal plasma α-amino-*n*-butyric acid do not switch off their F globin genes at the expected 28 to 32 weeks of gestation (Perrine et al., 1985). Derivatives of butyric acid have been tested in patients with sickle cell disease in several small studies, with some success. In addition, butyric acid derivatives appear to be safe, as they have been used for a long time without adverse effects as a cancer-differentiating agent and in treating patients with inborn errors of urea metabolism. The mechanism by which these drugs induce fetal hemoglobin synthesis is not fully understood.

Prevention

At present, the only way to prevent sickle cell anemia is to prevent the birth of persons homozygous for the β^S gene. We saw earlier in this chapter how carriers could be identified by analysis of hemolysates using a simple electrophoretic procedure (Fig. 7-1). Using this technique, it is possible to screen all members of a population carrying the β^S gene and explain to the carriers who are detected how sickle cell disease is inherited. Responsible, sensitive, and effective genetic counseling requires skill, patience, and lots of time, prerequisites that often are not met. Additionally, it is sometimes difficult to explain the risks of sickle cell anemia to prospective parents, especially because the disease is highly variable in its clinical severity and because the counselor must describe a spectrum of illness that in most cases is not nearly as severe as the case reported here.

It is generally much easier to counsel couples who have already decided that they do not want an affected (or, frequently, another affected) child, but who do want more children. Prenatal diagnosis of the presence of the β^S gene can be accomplished biochemically by determining the type of β-globin chains synthesized by a small sample of fetal blood (Alter, 1981); however, this approach involves a sophisticated surgical procedure and depends on a biochemical assay that must be used late in the second trimester when β-globin synthesis is high enough to be detected in the fetal blood sample.

Since 1980 our ability to detect the β^S gene has advanced dramatically, largely because of developments in molecular biology that permit the direct analysis of DNA structure. The technique may be used for prenatal diagnosis with little risk to the fetus or the mother because it requires only a small sample of fetal tissue. Thus, amniocentesis in the second trimester can provide sufficient fetal DNA for the identification of the β-globin genotype by the 20th week of gestation. In fact, the technique is so sensitive that a single chorionic villus, which represents extraembryonic fetal tissue, contains enough DNA to permit diagnosis during the later half of the first trimester (Williamson et al., 1981).

Recent advances in chorionic villus sampling have led to safe and efficient acquisition of fetal tissue much earlier in pregnancy, permitting early *in utero* diagnosis of sickle cell disease. Because elective abortion in the first trimester is safer and often more acceptable socially than the same procedure done later in pregnancy, early chorionic villus sampling has become the diagnostic method of choice for intrauterine diagnosis β-globin structure and synthesis.

The technique that made possible the direct analysis of DNA structure grew out of the discovery of a family of enzymes called *restriction endonucleases* (Roberts, 1979). To date, more than 200 restriction endonucleases have been identified. Each restriction endonuclease binds to double-stranded DNA at a specific sequence and cleaves one phosphodiester bond in each strand; An enzyme will not cleave a sequence that differs from its recognition sequence by as little as a single base pair.

The locations of restriction endonuclease cleavage sites within or next to a gene are determined by a systematic characterization of the number and size of fragments carrying the gene in endonuclease digests of DNA. The rationale of this approach is summarized in Figure 7-3. First, the DNA fragments in a digest are separated according to size by electrophoresis through an agarose gel. The hundreds of thousands of fragments generated by digestion causes the genomic DNA to be distributed nearly continuously from the top to the bottom of the gel. Because of the sieving action of the gel, small fragments migrate fast and are found near the anode (+). Large fragments migrate slowly and are found nearest the origin.

Nucleic acid hydridization is used to detect fragments in the gel that carry DNA sequences present in the gene of interest. Two circumstances must prevail if this is to be successfully accomplished. A radiolabeled molecular probe specific for the DNA sequences in the gene must be available, and the DNA must be removed from the agarose gel and rendered

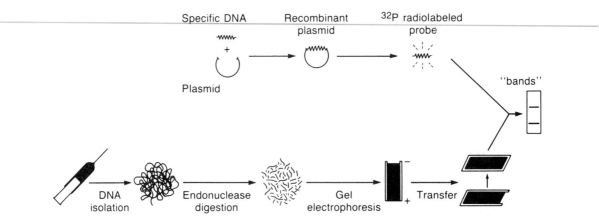

Figure 7-3. Steps in restriction endonuclease analysis of DNA. The upper portion illustrates the preparation of the radioactive probe. The specific DNA must first be inserted into the plasmid and amplified by replication in a bacterial host to produce a large amount of probe. Recombinant plasmid DNA is then isolated from the host, and the specific fragment is removed from the plasmid and radiolabeled with ^{32}P. See text for a description of the lower portion of the figure. Reproduced with permission from Antonarakis et al. (1982).

accessible to the probe. The technique is often referred to as *Southern blot hybridization* after its originator, Dr. Southern.

Most frequently the molecular probe is available as a recombinant plasmid that contains part of the gene. Bacterial cells carrying the recombinant plasmid provide a ready source of this DNA. Radiolabeling and denaturing this DNA result in a single-stranded DNA preparation with sequences complementary to the gene.

The genomic DNA fragments in the agarose gel are denatured by treatment of the gel with mild alkali. The denatured fragments are made accessible to the probe by capillary blotting onto a nitrocellulose membrane. The strong bonds that form between the denatured DNA and membrane preserve the spatial relationship between DNA fragments of different size that was present in the gel. Newer nylon membranes are finding increasing use because of

their greater mechanical strength and DNA-binding capacity.

After exposure of the membrane to the probe under conditions where it will only bind (*hybridize*) to complementary DNA sequences, the membrane is placed in contact with photographic film. Specifically bound radiolabeled probe will be indicated by a band of exposed film at a position corresponding to the location of genomic DNA fragments in the agarose gel that carry gene sequences. The size of these fragments is determined by comparison of the position of the band with DNA size standards included in a separate lane of the gel.

Every gene contains a unique distribution of restriction endonuclease cleavage sites along its length. Thus, the sizes of fragments in an endonuclease digest are characteristic of each gene. For example, if a gene does not contain a cleavage site for an endonuclease and is present in one copy per haploid

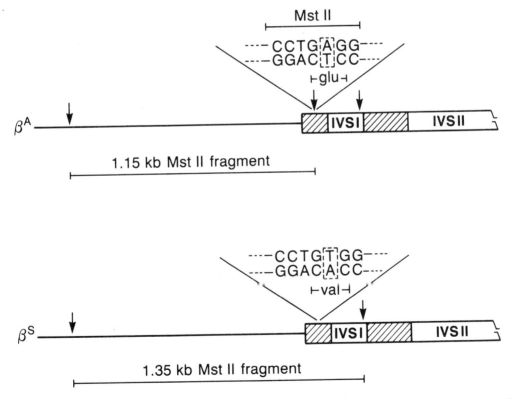

Figure 7-4. Diagram of the flanking region and the 5′ portion of the β-globin gene. Arrows indicate the *Mst*II cleavage sites. The DNA sequences illustrate the base pair change that destroys a *MST*II cleavage site and causes the amino acid substitution in the β-globin protein. Using the ^{32}P-labeled 1.15-kb *Mst*II fragment indicated in the diagram as a molecular probe, the 1.15-kb fragment was detected in digests of normal DNA, and the 1.35-kb fragment in DNA from a patient with sickle cell disease. IVS denotes intervening sequences. Reproduced in modified form with permission from Chang and Kan (1982).

genome, then it will be found on one size of fragment in the endonuclease digest. The fragment will appear as a single band whose location on the film (autoradiogram) is a function of the distance between the endonuclease cleavage sites nearest each end of the gene. If additional endonuclease cleavage sites are also present within the sequence detected by the radiolabeled probe for the gene, more than one band will appear on the autoradiogram.

The mutation that causes sickle cell disease may be directly detected by this powerful new technique because it coincidently destroys an *Mst*II restriction endonuclease cleavage site that overlaps the β^6-glutamic acid codon in the β-globin gene, resulting in an increase in the size of fragment that carries the 5' end of the β-globin gene in *Mst*II digests of human DNA. The 1.15 kilobase pair (kb) fragment from the β^A gene is increased to 1.35 kb in the β^S gene because of the addition of 200 base pairs of adjoining sequence (Fig. 7-4).

Chang and Kan (1982) and Orkin and co-workers (1982) demonstrated that this difference offers a practical prenatal test for the presence of the β^S gene. They analyzed *Mst*II digests of DNA from members of several families expecting a child at risk for sickle cell disease. The radiolabeled molecular hybridization probe used in both analyses was the 1.15-kb *Mst*II fragment carrying DNA sequence from the 5' end of the β^A gene (see Fig. 7-4). Therefore, only the 1.15- and 1.35-kb fragments were detected in the autoradiograms. Figure 7-5 presents an autoradiogram for one of the families that has a normal child. Remember that the expected child was at risk for sickle cell disease because the parents were known carriers of the β^S gene. Amniocytes were used as the source of fetal DNA. Because only a single 1.35-kb fragment was detected in the *Mst*II digest of fetal DNA (lane 4, SS) the analysis unambiguously demonstrated that the fetus was homozygous for the β^S gene. Furthermore, the data confirmed the previous diagnosis because of the presence of both fragments in digests of parental DNA (lanes 1 and 2: AS, AS) and the 1.15-kb fragment in a digest of the previous child's DNA (lane 3, AA).

Even though there are an increasing number of inherited diseases caused by mutations that also alter DNA fragment sizes in endonuclease digests (Antonarakis et al., 1982), the prospects are low for direct detection of most defective genes. Coincident

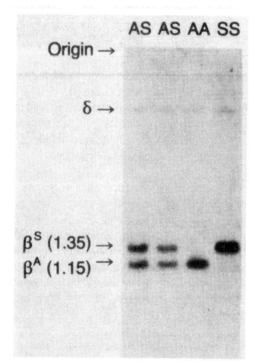

Figure 7-5. Blot hybridization analysis of *Mst*II-digested DNA from parents (AS, AS), a previous child (AA), and cultured amniotic fluid cells. The faint 6-kb band ($\beta \rightarrow$) seen in some samples is due to cross-hybridization of the molecular probe with the β-globin gene sequence. Reproduced with permission from Chang and Kan (1982).

loss of function and alteration of endonuclease cleavage of a gene is likely to be an infrequent event. Furthermore, molecular probes are not available for most genes. Because restriction endonuclease cleavage site polymorphisms appear to be quite abundant in the human population, however, genetic linkage between polymorphic sites and defective genes is finding increasing application in tracking these genes in families (Boehm et al., 1983). The potential for widespread use of this approach is great because nothing needs to be known about the structure of a defective gene or the activity of its product.

QUESTIONS

1. Hemoglobin C disease is caused by a mutation leading to a Glu $\rightarrow$ Lys substitution in the sixth amino acid of the β-globin protein.
   (a) Describe the chemical basis for the different electrophoretic mobilities of Hb A, Hb S, and Hb C on cellulose acetate at pH 8.6.

(b) Discuss whether the Hb C mutation can be detected by the blot hybridization method described in this chapter.

2. Before a biochemical test can be brought into general use in diagnosis, the frequency and causes of false-positive and false-negative results must be evaluated. Two circumstances lead to false results: failure of the biochemical test or the absence of a 100% association between the biochemical condition (correctly identified by the biochemical test) and the illness for which a diagnosis is being sought. The advantage of the restriction endonuclease and blot hybridization methods described in this chapter is that a null result is neither positive nor negative; failure of this biochemical test is quite unlikely to produce misleading results; however, one must consider whether the β^A gene always contains one MstII cleavage site that is never present in the β^S gene. Given the fact that the sequence of the fifth, sixth, and seventh positions (from the amino end) of all β^A proteins has been shown to be Pro-Glu-Glu, discuss the potential causes of false-positive or -negative results and describe how a DNA analysis should be conducted to address this uncertainty (hint: codon degeneracy).

3. Considerable interest has developed in synthesizing nontoxic compounds that block aggregation of Hb S because of their potential use in preventing clinical manifestations of the disease. Discuss the effect, if any, that widespread use of this kind of drug will have on the frequency of the β^S gene in the human population.

4. Suppose a family with one child with sickle cell disease (SS) informed you that they were happily planning to have another child or two because they would certainly not be affected. How would you respond to their belief?

5. A woman with sickle cell trait is 4 months pregnant and knows that her fetus is homozygous for the β^S gene. She wants to visit her mother in Denver but worries whether the decreased P_{O_2} there will cause the fetus to have a sickle cell crisis. What do you tell her?

6. Why would Hb F ameliorate the phenomenon of sickling? Consider O_2 dissociation curves of Hb F and Hb A in your answer.

7. In the patient described in the case report, suppose his arterial blood gases showed a pH of 7.30. How would you explain the mechanism of metabolic acidosis in this patient?

REFERENCES

Alter BP: Prenatal diagnosis of hemoglobinopathies: A status report. *Lancet* **2**:1152–1154, 1981.

Antonarakis SE, Phillips JA III, Kazazian HH: Genetic diseases: Diagnosis by restriction endonuclease analysis. *J Pediatr* **100**:845–856, 1982.

Boehm CD, Antonarakis SE, Phillips JA, et al.: Prenatal diagnosis using DNA polymorphism: Report on 95 pregnancies at risk for sickle-cell disease of β-thalassemia. *N Engl J Med* **308**:1054–1058, 1983.

Chang JC, Kan YW: A sensitive new prenatal test for sickle-cell anemia. *N Engl J Med* **307**:30–32, 1982.

Charache S: Treatment of sickle cell anemia. *Annu Rev Med* **32**:195–206, 1981.

Charache S, Dover GH, Moore BD, et al.. Hydroxyurea. Effects on hemoglobin F production in patients with sickle cell anemia. *Blood* **78**:212–216, 1992.

Charache S, Terrin ML, Moore RF, et al.: Effects of hydroxyurea on the frequency of painful crises in sickle cell anemia. *N Engl J Med* **332**:1317–1322, 1995.

Conley CL: Sickle-cell anemia—the first molecular disease, *in* Wintrobe MM (ed): *Blood, Pure and Eloquent.* New York, McGraw-Hill, 1980, pp 319–371.

De Fronzo RA, Taufield PA, Black H, et al.: Impaired renal tubular potassium secretion in sickle cell disease. *Ann Intern Med* **90**:310–316, 1979.

DeSimone J, Heller P, Hall L, Zwiers D: 5-Azacytidine stimulates fetal hemoglobin synthesis in anemic baboons. *Proc Natl Acad Sci USA* **79**:4428–4431, 1982.

Diggs LW: The sickle cell trait in relation to the training and assignment of duties in the Armed Forces. *Aviat Space Environ Med* **55**:180–185, 271–276, 358–364, 1984.

Emmel VE: A study of erythrocytes in a case of severe anemia with elongated and sickle-shaped red blood corpuscles. *Arch Intern Med* **20**:197–201, 1950.

Friedman MJ, Trager W: The biochemistry of resistance to malaria. *Sci Am* **244**:154–164, 1981.

Hahn EV, Gillespie EB: Sickle cell anemia: report of a case greatly improved by splenectomy; experimental study of sickle cell formation. *Arch Intern Med* **39**:233–254, 1927.

Ham TH, Castle WB: Relation of increased hypotonic fragility and of erythrostasis to the mechanisms of hemolysis in certain anemias. *Trans Assoc Am Physicians* **55**:127–135, 1940.

Harris JW: Studies on the destruction of red blood cells. VIII. Molecular orientation of sickle cell hemoglobin solutions. *Proc Soc Exp Biol Med* **75**:197–201, 1950.

Herrick JB: Peculiar elongated and sickle shaped red blood corpuscles in a case of severe anemia. *Arch Intern Med* **6**:517–521, 1910.

Kan YW, Dozy AM: Evolution of the hemoglobin S and C genes in world populations. *Science* **209**:388–390, 1980.

Mason VR: Sickle Cell Anemia. *JAMA* **79**:1318–1320, 1922.

Noguchi CT, Rodgers GP, Sergeant G, Schecter AN: Levels of fetal hemoglobin necessary for treatment of sickle cell disease. *N Engl J Med* **318**:96–99, 1988.

Orkin SH, Little PFR, Kazazian HH, et al.: Improved detection of the sickle mutation by DNA analysis. *N Engl J Med* **307**:32–36, 1982.

Pauline L, Itano HA, Singer SJ, et al.: Sickle cell anemia, a molecular disease. *Science* **100**:543–548, 1949.

Perrine SP, Greene MF, Faller DV: Delay in the fetal globin switch in infants of diabetic mothers *N Engl J Med* **312**:224–228, 1985.

Perutz MF, Rossman MG, Cullis AF, et al.: Structure of haemoglobin. A three-dimensional Fourier synthesis at 5.5 resolution, obtained by x-ray analysis. *Nature* **185**:416–422, 1960.

Roberts RJ: Directory of restriction endonuclease. *Meth Enzymol* **68**:27, 1979.

Vermylen C, Niname J, Fernandez-Robles E, et al.: Bone marrow transplantation in five children with sickle cell anemia. *Lancet* **1**:1427–1428, 1988.

Williamson R, Eskdale J, Coleman DV, et al.: Direct gene analysis of chorionic villi: A possible technique for first trimester antenatal diagnosis of hemoglobinopathies. *Lancet* **2**:1125–1127, 1981.

Wingard JR, Plotnick LP, Freemer CS, et al.: Growth in children after bone marrow transplantation; busulfan plus cyclophosphamide versus cyclophosphamide plus total body irradiation. *Blood* **79**:1068–1073, 1992.

Witherspoon RP, Storb R, Pepe, M, et al.: Cumulative incidence of secondary solid malignant tumors in aplastic anemia patients given marrow grafts after conditioning with chemotherapy alone. *Blood* **79**:289–290, 1992.

Wishner BC, Ward KB, Lattman EE, et al.: Crystal structure of sickle-cell deoxyhemoglobin at 5 Å resolution. *J Mol Biol* **98**:179–194, 1975.

Part II

Metabolism and Energetics

8

Glucose 6-Phosphate Dehydrogenase Deficiency

ERNEST BEUTLER AND KEVIN LAUBSCHER

CASE REPORTS

Case 1

A.R., a 26-year-old black male had been in good general health until 1 week before admission to the hospital, when he developed signs of a respiratory infection and a low-grade fever. Self-medication with an over-the-counter cold preparation failed to alleviate his symptoms, and one day before admission he began to experience chills and a hacking cough. When his temperature rose to 40.6°C (normal, 36–37°C) his mother brought him to the emergency department. He was noted to be acutely ill, *dyspneic,* (labored breathing), and coughing and was admitted to the hospital.

Physical examination revealed slight *icterus* (yellowing of the sclera), bronchial breathing over the left lower lung fields with scattered rales (suggesting consolidation seen in pneumonia), a temperature of 40°C, pulse 120 beats per minute (normal, 60–90 beats per minute), and a moderate degree of dyspnea.

Laboratory findings included a hemoglobin of 8.4 g/dL (normal, >14.0 g/dL), white cell count of 18,000/μL (normal, 5,000–10,000/μL) with 80% polymorphonuclear leukocytes and a bilirubin of 3.2 mg/dL (normal, 0.1–0.5 mg/dL). The reticulocyte count was 1.2% Gram-positive diplococci were found in the sputum. Sputum and blood cultures were obtained, and the patient started on therapy with penicillin. The next day his condition had already considerably improved, and cultures confirmed the presence of pneumococci in both the sputum and blood. His maximum temperature was 38.2°C and his dyspnea less pronounced. Over the next few days, the fever abated completely. The hemoglobin, however, fell to a nadir of 7.2 g/dL. The reticulocyte count rose rapidly so that seven days after admission, it had reached 12% (normal, <1%). One month after the episode of pneumococcus pneumonia, the hemoglobin was nearly normal at 13.8 g/dL, and the patient felt quite well. He was warned never again to take aspirin, counsel he received with considerable skepticism because he had previously taken this drug without untoward effect. He was also supplied with a long list of drugs (Table 8-1), none of which were familiar to him, and advised never to take any of them. Observed intermittently over the next several years, the patient experienced no further hemolytic episode.

Case 2

When D.M. was 1 day old, his bilirubin was 14 mg/dL (normal, 0.4–4.0 mg/dL). He was treated with ultraviolet light, and during the 2nd day of life his bilirubin level climbed to 17 mg/dL. Preparations for exchange transfusion were made but abandoned when subsequent bilirubin readings were lower, and the level gradually declined over the next few days. The hemoglobin level of the blood fell to 13 g/dL, and the reticulocyte count (normal 3.2 ± 1.4%) was recorded at levels ranging from 5 to 10%. Family history revealed that an older brother experienced anemia and darkening of the urine on two occasions, once during a respiratory infection and again when a urinary tract infection was treated with a sulfonamide of unknown type. The parents were both well, but a maternal uncle had a history of intermittent jaundice and anemia.

The child developed normally with a steady-state hemoglobin of 10.5 g/dL and a reticulocyte count of about 10%. At age 6 years, he developed dark urine in the course of a respiratory infection, and his hemoglobin had declined to 5.4 g/dL. He had a transfusion of 1 U of packed red cells, subsequently, the hemoglobin concentration of his blood rose to the level that was usual for him. In the following year, a splenectomy was performed because a diagnosis of hereditary spherocytosis had been made erroneously. There was no change in the steady-state hemoglobin level of the blood, although now the peripheral blood contained nucleated red cells and red cells with nuclear fragments (Howell-Jolly bodies), and the platelet count was elevated to 700×10^9/L (normal $= 150–300 \times 10^9$/L).

When D.M. was aged 14 years, his anemia was reevaluated; his red cells were profoundly deficient in glucose 6-phosphate dehydrogenase (G6PD) activity. He has continued to get along quite well clinically. At times he is mildly jaundiced. When he has infections he sometimes experiences a hemolytic episode with a fall in the hemoglobin concentration of the blood and darkening of the urine. He has been cautioned to seek medical attention promptly for these symptoms but also patients who have undergone splenectomy are more likely to succumb to overwhelming sepsis in a relatively short time. Up to now, however, D.M. has dealt well with infections.

DIAGNOSIS

G6PD deficiency should be considered in the differential diagnosis of any patient with hemolytic anemia (Beutler, 1978; Luzzato and Mehta, 1996). This enzyme catalyzes the following reaction:

$$\text{Glucose 6-phosphate} + \text{NADP}^+ \rightarrow$$
$$\text{6-phosphogluconolactone} + \text{NADPH} + \text{H}^+$$

6-Phosphogluconolactone, which is a product of the reaction, hydrolyzes spontaneously and through the catalytic effect of 6-phosphogluconolactonase is converted to 6-phosphogluconic acid. The latter serves as substrate for a second NADPH-yielding reaction.

$$\text{6-phosphogluconate} + \text{NADP}^+ \rightarrow \text{ribulose-5-P} + \text{NADPH}$$
$$+ \text{H}^+ + \text{CO}_2$$

The demonstration of G6PD activity depends on the measurement of NADPH generation from NADP^+ when glucose 6-phosphate is supplied as a substrate. NADPH formation can be detected by a variety of methods. It can be quantitated spectrophotometrically by measuring light absorbance of NADPH at 340 nm, fluorometrically by estimating light emission when NADPH is exposed to ultraviolet light in this range, or by coupling to a dye, such as brilliant cresyl blue, methylene blue, or a tetrazolium compound. Numerous screening tests that can rapidly detect G6PD deficiency in blood samples are available, and in most instances a screening test is perfectly adequate for the diagnosis of this disorder.

Difficulties may arise, however, in two circumstances. Because G6PD deficiency is a sex-linked disorder, the blood of female heterozygotes contains varying proportions of G6PD-deficient and normal erythrocytes. In patients in whom the proportion of G6PD-normal red cells is fairly high, the enzyme activity of the mixed red cells approaches normal levels. Several histochemical methods have been introduced to increase the accuracy of diagnosis of enzyme deficiency in heterozygous females. In these methods the activity of individual red cells is measured so that even a relatively small proportion of enzyme-deficient erythrocytes can be detected.

A second problem in diagnosis arises because the G6PD activity in some of the milder variants, such as G6PD A-, is nearly normal in reticulocytes. Thus, a patient who has recently undergone hemolysis and who has a reticulocytosis may have normal or near-normal enzyme activity. This difficulty may be overcome by waiting for a few days until the newly produced red cells have an opportunity to age; centrifuging blood samples and examining the most dense, reticulocyte-poor fraction; or carrying out quantitative G6PD assay and adjusting for red cell age by concurrent assay of another enzyme.

The most powerful method of diagnosis is identification of the mutations that cause G6PD. Genetic analysis of DNA from circulating leukocytes can identify carriers and establish a diagnosis in the context of hemolysis or mild enzyme deficiency. DNA has further advantages in being more stable than enzymes for shipping or storage, and with today's amplification techniques little DNA is needed.

MOLECULAR PERSPECTIVES

Mammalian tissues must phosphorylate glucose to extract energy from it. Under ordinary circumstances, most of the glucose 6-phosphate formed in the phosphorylation of glucose by ATP is metabolized to pyruvate and lactate in the Embden-Myerhof pathway. Another pathway exists, however, for the direct nonmitochondrial oxidation of glucose 6-phosphate: the hexose monophosphate pathway. Glucose 6-phosphate dehydrogenase is the first enzyme of this alternative route of glucose metabolism.

G6PD normally exists as a dimer with a subunit molecular weight of approximately 55,000 d. It catalyzes the oxidation of glucose 6-phosphate to 6-phosphogluconolactone, reducing NADP$^+$ to NADPH in the process (Luzzatto and Battistuzzi, 1985). Under steady-state circumstances, almost all of this pyridine nucleotide is in the reduced state; there is very little NADP$^+$ in the erythrocyte. G6PD activity is profoundly regulated by the NADP$^+$/NADPH ratio. If NADPH is oxidized through the glutathione reductase (GR) reaction, which reduces oxidized glutathione (GSSG) to reduced glutathione (GSH), G6PD is activated:

$$\text{GSSG} + \text{NADPH} + \text{H}^+ \xrightarrow{\text{GR}} 2 \text{ GSH} + \text{NADP}^+$$

As with many other enzymes, only a small fraction of the potential maximum G6PD activity of erythrocytes is used under normal circumstances. Thus, even a relatively severe deficiency of this enzyme is well tolerated except when the enzyme is called on to reduce large amounts of NADP$^+$. Such circumstances arise when certain drugs are administered and during the course of some infections. Such stresses result in hemolytic anemia.

The mechanism by which stresses such as drug administration result in shortening of the life span of G6PD-deficient cells appears to involve, as a common pathway, oxidation of important red cell components. The principal function of erythrocytes is to carry a large load of oxygen. In the course of the normal loading and unloading of this cargo, highly reactive oxygen species, such as hydrogen peroxide and the superoxide anion, are continually being created. Hemolytic drugs increase the rate at which active oxygen species are formed and thus call into play the defense mechanisms of the cell. The erythrocyte is richly endowed with superoxide dismutase,

which catalyzes the decomposition of the superoxide anion into the somewhat less reactive hydrogen peroxide moiety. Catalase, which is also present in red cells, breaks down hydrogen peroxide; but the most important pathway is probably the glutathione peroxidase reaction, which uses reduced glutathione as a substrate for the detoxification of low levels of hydrogen peroxide:

$$2 \text{ GSH} + \text{H}_2\text{O}_2 \rightarrow 2 \text{ H}_2\text{O} + \text{GSSG}$$

It is likely that when the capacity of red cells to maintain glutathione in the reduced form is impaired in G6PD deficiency, the accumulation of hydrogen peroxide produces damage to erythrocytes, which shortens their life-span. The nature of such damage is complex, but it does not usually involve outright lysis of the erythrocyte. Rather, cross-linking of membrane proteins, denaturation of hemoglobin, and peroxidation of membrane lipids all may change the physical characteristics of the red cell in such a way that it is removed from the circulation by a perceptive reticuloendothelial system.

Collectively, more than 400 G6PD variants have been described and differentiated biochemically (Yoshida and Beutler, 1983). The mutations involving G6PD have been divided into five classes. Class I variants are so severe that they produce hemolysis even in the absence of stress, resulting in a clinical syndrome called *hereditary nonspherocytic hemolytic anemia*. Case 2 represents an example of such a variant. Class I variants may appear to have more G6PD activity than do class II variants, those that are severely deficient but in which a stress is required to precipitate hemolysis. The reason for this apparent discrepancy is that the enzyme is ordinarily assayed under optimal conditions with saturating substrate concentrations and in the absence of significant concentrations of inhibitors. Under physiologic conditions, in the red blood cell, the enzyme must work under much less advantageous circumstances. As a result, its capability to perform its function *in vivo* may be much less than indicated by *in vitro* assay values. One of the factors that may be important in this respect is inhibition of the enzyme by NADPH. A number of variants associated with hereditary nonspherocytic hemolytic anemia are extraordinarily sensitive to NADPH inhibition. Class III variants are mildly deficient and are associated with self-limiting hemolysis under conditions of stress. Class IV variants are not deficient at all but may be of great interest as genetic markers, and class V variants have increased activity compared to normals.

In the common forms of G6PD deficiency (i.e., class II and III variants), hemolysis occurs only when the patient is subjected to certain stresses. Case I was a typical example of G6PD A⁻, a common class III variant found in 11% of black men. In this case, the stress precipitating hemolysis was infection. Other stresses that cause hemolysis include exposures to certain "oxidizing" drugs and to fava beans. Table 8-1 provides a list of drugs that have been shown to induce hemolysis in some G6PD-deficient individuals. This is the same list that was given to A.R. in case report 1. Table 8-2 is a list of drugs that can probably be ingested safely by G6PD-deficient individuals, even though many of these drugs have, at one time or another, been considered hemolytic.

GENETICS

Because G6PD is on the X chromosome, inheritance is sex-linked; father-to-son inheritance is not ob-

Table 8-1. Drugs and Chemicals That Should be Avoided by Persons with G6PD Deficiency

Acetanilid	Phenylhydrazine
Furazolidone (Furoxone)	Primaquine
Methylene Blue	Sulfacetamide
Nalidixic acid (NeGram)	Sulfamethoxazole (Gantanol)
Naphthalene	Sulfanilamide
Niridazole (Ambilhar)	Thiazolesulfone
Naphthalene	Toluidine blue
Nitrofurantoin (Furadantin)	Trinitrotoluene (TNT)
Phenazopyridine (Pyridium)	Urate oxidase

G6PD, glucose 6-phosphate dehydrogenase deficiency.

served. The G6PD gene is situated among a cluster of genes, including hemophilia A, color vision, fragile X, and dyskeratosis congenita. G6PD on the inactive X chromosome of women is associated with methylation of certain upstream CpG islands. Expression of G6PD deficiency, like that of other sex-linked traits, varies greatly in female heterozygotes. Their red cells represent a mosaic of G6PD-deficient and normal erythrocytes. As noted earlier, because the proportion of normal and deficient cells may vary widely,

Table 8-2. Drugs That Can Probably Safely Be Given in Normal Therapeutic Doses to G6PD-Deficient Subjects Without Hereditary Nonspherocytic Hemolytic Anemia

Acetaminophen (paracetamol, Tylenol, Tralgon, hydroxyacetanilide)	p-Aminobenzoic acid
	Phenylbutazone
Acetophenetidin (phenacetin)	Phenytoin
Acetylsalicylic acid (aspirin)	Probenecid (Benemid)
Amiopyrine (Pyramidon, Aminopyrine)	Procain amide hydrochloride (Pronestyl)
Actazoline (Antistine)	
Antipyrine	Pyrimethamine (Daraprim)
Ascorbic acid (vitamin C)	Quinidine
Benzhexol (Artane)	Quinine
Chloramphenicol	Streptomycin
Chlorguanidine (Proguanil, Paludrine)	Sulfacytine
Chloroquine	Sulfadiazine
Colchicine	Sulfaguanidine
Diphenhydramine (Benadryl)	Sulfamerazine
Isoniazid	Sulfamethoxypyridazine (Kynex)
L-Dopa	Sulfisoxazole (Gantrisin)
Menadione sodium bisulfite (Hykinone)	Tiaprofenic acid
	Trimethoprim
Menapthone Vitamin K	Tripelennamine HCl (Pyribenzamine)

G6PD, glucose 6-phosphate dehydrogenase deficiency.

there are difficulties in diagnosing the heterozygous state.

More than 60 mutations or combinations of mutations have been identified at the DNA level. Most mutations are in the coding region, with one splice-site mutation identified but no promotor region abnormalities. Distribution of mutations in the gene is not random among four classes of this disease. Class I disease has mutations clustered around the glucose 6-phosphate and putative $NADP^+$/NADPH binding domains, whereas the mutations that cause class II, III, and IV deficiencies are distributed throughout the gene. Class V mutations have not been identified. G6PD mutations are found in all populations, but occurrence is highest in Mediterranean, African, and Southeast Asian peoples (Table 8-3). Certain mutations in G6PD deficiency are specific to populations or geographic regions. For example African populations usually carry the mutation designated A^-. In the Mediterranean region, the common mutations include G6PD Mediterranean[563T] and G6PD Seattle[844C], which are common in many countries along this sea. One exception to this rule is the Union[1306T] mutation, which has been detected in distant corners of the globe. Currently, it is unknown whether this mutation arose in many populations independently or spread with ancient human migrations.

DNA analysis provides accurate results in patients without symptoms and those undergoing hemolysis, and it can be used to identify heterozygotes accurately. Molecular techniques, such as the polymerase chain reaction amplification and restriction enzyme digestion, make mutation detection simple and cost-effective for diagnosis.

THERAPY

G6PD-deficient patients should avoid the drugs listed in Table 8-1. It is important, however, that they not be overwhelmed by uncritical lists of proscribed medications, such as aspirin and acetaminophen, which have not lived up to their reputation of inducing clinically significant hemolytic episodes. When hemolysis does occur in such G6PD-deficient persons, either as a result of infection or inadvertent administration of the hemolytic drug or fava beans, therapeutic intervention is rarely necessary. In very severe cases, blood transfusion may be required.

The use of vitamin E has been advocated as a possible treatment for chronic hemolysis in G6PD deficiency, but its role has not been firmly established and its effect is at best modest. It has been suggested that administration of the iron-chelating drug desferroxamine may ameliorate hemolysis.

Splenectomy is occasionally useful in lessening hemolysis in patients with G6PD deficiency and nonspherocytic hemolytic anemia, but more often than not it is unsuccessful.

Genetic counseling is useful only in families in whom type I variants occur. DNA analysis is the best method for identifying these patients and carriers. Fortunately, G6PD deficiency, even in the case of class I variants, is rarely so severe as to pose a major

Table 8-3. Some Properties of Common G6PD Variants

Designation	Geographic Distribution	Biochemical Properties	Nt Substitution (cDNA#)	Amino Acid Substitution
A	Africa, Southern Europe	N Activity & Kinetics. Elect fast	376 A→G	126 Asn→Asp
A^-	Africa, Southern Europe	Activity ↓. N Kinetics. Elect fast	202 G→A 376 A→G	68 Val→Met 126 Asn→Asp
Mediterranean	Southern Europe, Middle East, Indian subcontinent	Activity ↓↓. K_m G6P and $NADP^+$. Elect N	563 C→T	188 Ser→Phe
Seattle	Southern Europe, Canary Islands	Activity ↓. K_m G6P and $NADP^+$. Elect slow	844 G→C	282 Asp→His
Union	Europe, Hawaii, Phillipines, China, southwest Pacific	Activity ↓↓. K_m G6P ↓ $NADP^+$ N. Elect N	1360 C→T	454 Arg→Cys

G6PD, glucose 6-phosphate dehydrogenase deficiency; K_m, Michaelis constant; N, Normal; ↓, moderately decreased, ↓↓, severely decreased; Elect, electrophoretic mobility.

health problem. Thus, genetic counseling is not frequently a pressing consideration.

QUESTIONS

1. What enzyme-catalyzed reactions in liver and macrophages use NADPH as a substrate?
2. Why is the level of G6PD activity lower in old red blood cells compared with that in young red blood cells?
3. What might some of the abnormal properties be of the different variants of G6PD deficiency?
4. What complications of G6PD deficiency make DNA analysis best for identification of carriers and patient diagnosis?

Acknowledgment: This work was supported by the National Institute of Health grant HL 2555 and the Walker Foundation.

REFERENCES

Beutler E: *Hemolytic Anemia in Disorders of Red Cell Metabolism.* New York, Plenum Publishing 1978.

Luzzato L, Mehta A: Glucose 6-Phosphate Dehydrogenase Deficiency, *in* Scriver C, A Beaudet, Sly W, Valle D (eds): *The Metabolic and Molecular Basis of Inherited Disease,* 7th ed. New York, McGraw-Hill, 1996, p 3367–3398.

Luzzatto L, Battistuzzi G: Glucose 6-Phosphate Dehydrogenase, *in* Harris H, Hirschhorn K, (eds): *Advances in Human Genetics,* Ch 4. New York, Plenum Publishing 1985, pp 217–329.

Yoshida A, Beutler E: G-6-PD variants: Another up-date. *Ann Hum Genet* **47:**25–38, 1983.

9

Neonatal Hypoglycemia and the Importance of Gluconeogenesis

IAN R. HOLZMAN AND J. ROSS MILLEY

CASE REPORT

Female infant L. weighed 3.980 kg at birth to a 29-year-old mother after a 35-week pregnancy. Mrs. L. was an insulin-requiring diabetic who had had diabetes since she was 15 years old and had not yet shown signs of vascular disease (class C, White classification). Her pregnancy had been complicated by multiple episodes of *hyperglycemia* (excess sugar in the blood) and *glycosuria* (presence of abnormal amounts of sugar in the urine). Her prenatal care was only episodic because her husband had been part of a layoff at work, and the family was without health insurance. On the day of delivery, Mrs. L. had a routine nonstress test because she noticed that her fetus had decreased movement over the preceding 2 days. The nonstress test showed a flat baseline heart rate without any variation, a finding suggesting that the fetus was at risk for *asphyxia* (lack of oxygen). Following the rupture of membranes, a blood sample taken from the fetal scalp revealed an acidotic pH of 6.9 (normal, >7.3). Because these findings were clear evidence of fetal distress, an immediate cesarean section was performed.

The infant's Apgar scores (scale 0–10, with 10 being best) of two at 1 minute and six at 5 minutes suggested depression of neurological and cardiopulmonary function. The physicians present resuscitated the infant, who was then taken to the neonatal intensive care unit. She had a normal pulse, respiratory rate, and rectal temperature. The infant's head circumference and length were both normal for this gestational age; however, she was clearly *macrosomic* (large body and organs) and *plethoric* (ruddy with an increased red blood cell mass) and had a protuberant, firm abdomen. The liver edge was 4 to 5 cm below the right costal margin; the kidneys were large bilaterally but of normal shape and position, and the initial cardiac examination revealed no abnormalities. The pulses were symmetric but difficult to feel in all extremities. There were no other congenital anomalies.

When the infant was aged 30 minutes, the hematocrit was 0.63 (normal, 0.45–0.62) and the serum glucose 2.5 mmol/L (normal, 2.8–3.3). An intravenous (i.v.) line was established. The initial i.v. fluid was 10% dextrose in water and was administered at a rate of 10 ml/h or a total of 60 mL/kg/day (4 mg/kg/min of glucose). Several minutes later, the infant's blood glucose concentration was 1.2 mmol/L, and 10 mL of 25% dextrose in water was given via the i.v. catheter over a 5-minute period (125 mg/kg/min). The first arterial blood gas determination at 45 minutes of life revealed a pH of 7.18 (normal, 7.30–7.35), a P_{O_2} of 6.3 kPa (normal, 6.7–9.3 kPa), a P_{CO_2} of 6.1 kPa (normal, 4.7–6.0 kPa), and a bicarbonate concentration of 17 mmol/L (normal, 18–21 mmol/L), with a base excess (anion gap, see Chapter 12), of -11 mmol/L. A chest radiograph film showed that the lungs were clear and the heart was large. One hour and 10 minutes after birth, the infant's blood sugar was

21.0 mmol/L (after infusion of 10 ml of 25% dextrose noted above). About 45 minutes later, the blood sugar was 1.8 mmol/L, and 8 ml of 10% dextrose was given through the i.v. catheter over 5 minutes (40 mg/kg/min). The i.v. infusion was changed to 12.5% dextrose in water at a rate of 13 mL/h (78 mL/kg/day or 6.8 mg/kg/min of glucose). Within 10 to 15 minutes, the serum glucose level had fallen to between zero and 1.4 mmol/L, and an additional 4 ml of 12.5% dextrose was given via the i.v. catheter. A catheter was then inserted into the umbilical vein to lie in the lower part of the right atrium, and an infusion of 15% dextrose was begun. By 5 hours of age, this infant was receiving glucose at a rate of 13.5 mg/kg/min. The blood glucose concentration continued to be <1.1 mmol/L, and the infant was given 15 mg of hydrocortisone every 6 hours. Echocardiography showed decreased left ventricular contractility and hypertrophy of the ventricular septum but no other structural abnormalities. These findings were consistent with the cardiomyopathy often seen in infants of diabetic mothers.

By 12 hours of age, the infant had seizure activity that included rhythmic movement of both upper extremities, hiccuping, and repetitive chewing movements. An electroencephalogram was grossly abnormal, showing paroxysmal bursts of activity (*seizures*) and periods of suppression. Phenobarbital was given to alleviate the seizure activity.

Eventually, the infant's need for hydrocortisone began to decrease so that by the 9th day of life she no longer required steroids, and she maintained serum glucose concentrations >2.8 mmol/L with a glucose infusion of <7 mg/kg per minute. Subsequently, glucose control was no longer difficult, and no further medications were given for this problem.

Sonar examination of this infant's head at one week of age showed an infarction of the right parietooccipital area and hemorrhage within the right ventricle. This brain damage was manifested clinically: Infant L. had great difficulty with sucking and swallowing. She was also diffusely *hypotonic* (decreased muscle tone), with fewer movements of the lower extremities than of the upper extremities. Hearing tests revealed severe bilateral central hearing loss. At age 1 month, the infant was discharged to a transitional care center, where she could receive developmental stimulation and the parents could be educated as to how to feed her.

DIAGNOSIS

This case exemplifies many of the problems classically associated with infants born to diabetic mothers (Cowett, 1991a and 1991b). Inadequate maternal glucose control during pregnancy generates potential metabolic difficulties in the infant (see below). Meticulous attention to diabetic control during pregnancy has markedly improved the outlook for these infants, in terms of both morbidity and mortality. Indeed, in many high-risk centers, the outlook for a diabetes-associated pregnancy is indistinguishable from that of a normal pregnancy. The size of this infant at birth (nearly 4 kg in a preterm infant), however, categorizes her as large for gestational age, a finding characteristic of affected infants of diabetic mothers. This infant is therefore likely to have the other manifestations associated with this pathophysiology. Indeed, many characteristics of this infant are typical for a child born to a mother with diabetes mellitus. Specifically, the *macrosomia* (large organs), round facies, plethora, and overall weight, length, and head circumference are all consistent with poorly controlled maternal diabetes mellitus that has significantly affected fetal growth and metabolism.

As the end of gestation approaches, the fetus of a diabetic mother is more likely to be poorly oxygenated *in utero*. The markedly decreased scalp pH and low Apgar scores are convincing evidence that this infant's supply of oxygen was insufficient to meet its needs. The etiology of the hypoxemia is not always apparent at the time of birth. Any mechanical disruption of the fetal-placental circulation (e.g., abruption or separation, placenta previa or placenta located over the cervical os, and cord accidents) could compromise fetal oxygen supply, as could a fetal infection. In the present case, however, there was no evidence of such problems. Consequently, it seems more likely that the fetus exhibited the chronic oxygen deficit that occurs in infants of diabetic mothers and becomes more severe as the pregnancy progresses.

Hypoglycemia, beginning soon after birth, is typical for infants of diabetic mothers. Indeed, the physicians caring for this child should have expected this problem because the infant was so conspicuously affected. Fortunately, the severity of the present case, including the need for glucocorticoids, has become rare since the advent of more sophisticated maternal care during pregnancy. Seizures are an unfortunate and serious complication of hypoglycemia, but it is not possible to determine whether the lack of oxygen during prenatal life, the hypoglycemia, or a combination of both is responsible for the infant's brain damage.

MOLECULAR PERSPECTIVES

To understand the etiology of hypoglycemia in the newborn, it is first necessary to know the principles of fetal metabolism that form the basis for newborn physiology and pathology. A unique characteristic of the fetus is the need for the continual provision of substrates across the maternal and placental circulations for growth and energy. A second unique characteristic of the fetus is its biochemical development so that it no longer needs this constant substrate supply (i.e., is capable of independent existence) at birth.

The primary metabolic substrates the fetus receives from the mother are glucose, lactate, amino acids, essential fats, free fatty acids (primarily stored and not oxidized) and oxygen. Each of these is required for three ongoing processes: energy metabolism, growth, and preparation for extrauterine life. The provision of glucose is especially important because of its central role in fetal brain metabolism; cerebral glucose utilization is obligatory at a rate of ~ 5 mg/min/0.1 kg of tissue. The brain of the term human fetus weighs approximately 0.4 kg and thus would require ~ 20 mg/kg per minute of glucose for brain use alone. Most of this glucose is needed for cerebral oxidative metabolism, but there is a further requirement for the synthesis of macromolecules. Other fetal tissues are less dependent on glucose as an oxidative fuel but still require glucose for growth. In addition, tissues such as liver, lung, heart, and skeletal muscle use glucose to form glycogen, and adipocytes distributed throughout the fetus convert glucose into lipid (triglycerides). To provide glucose for all these purposes, the fetus must receive glucose at a rate of 7 to 8 mg/kg per minute.

What system is in place to ensure that the fetus receives this constant supply of glucose? The transport of glucose from the maternal to the fetal circulation occurs by facilitated diffusion across the pla-

cental chorionic membrane (i.e., it occurs by carrier-mediated transport). This system equilibrates glucose concentrations across the membrane but will not move sugar against a concentration gradient; therefore, the amount of glucose received by the fetus depends on the concentration gradient between the fetus and mother. Consequently, under circumstances of increased maternal glucose concentration, the fetomaternal glucose concentration gradient will increase and more glucose will be delivered to the fetus. Conversely, if the maternal glucose concentration falls, the fetomaternal glucose concentration gradient will decrease and the fetus will receive less glucose.

The maternal glucose concentration is extremely critical in determining fetal glucose supply, and a normal fetal endocrine environment is important in modulating the way the fetus uses this supply of glucose. The endocrine milieu of the fetus provides an anabolic environment within which the fetus can produce complex macromolecules from simpler precursors. Although the placenta is essentially impermeable to maternal insulin, the fetal pancreas releases insulin in response to increases in fetal blood glucose concentration. The pattern of insulin effects on the fetus makes sense if one knows which tissues have receptors to insulin and realizes that effects of activation of these receptors differ in various tissues. Because the fetus in late gestation contains insulin-sensitive glucose transporters (GLUT4) in only fat and muscle, a major effect of fetal insulin is to regulate the use of glucose by these two tissues. Thus, in muscles, both skeletal and cardiac, higher insulin concentrations promote increased glucose uptake and oxidation as well as the storage of glucose in the form of glycogen. In adipose tissue, insulin promotes lipogenesis. In addition, there are numerous effects of insulin, generally anabolic, not mediated through its well-known effects on glucose transport. For example, in muscle, insulin decreases glycogenolysis, proteolysis, and gluconeogenesis. Lipolysis is inhibited by insulin in adipocytes. The effect of insulin on hepatic tissue is to promote increased glycogen production and protein synthesis and to inhibit glycogenolysis, proteolysis, lipolysis, and gluconeogenesis (Fig. 9-1). Other hormones, notably glucagon and epinephrine, are important counterregulators of the action of insulin in postnatal life; however, both fetal glucagon and epinephrine

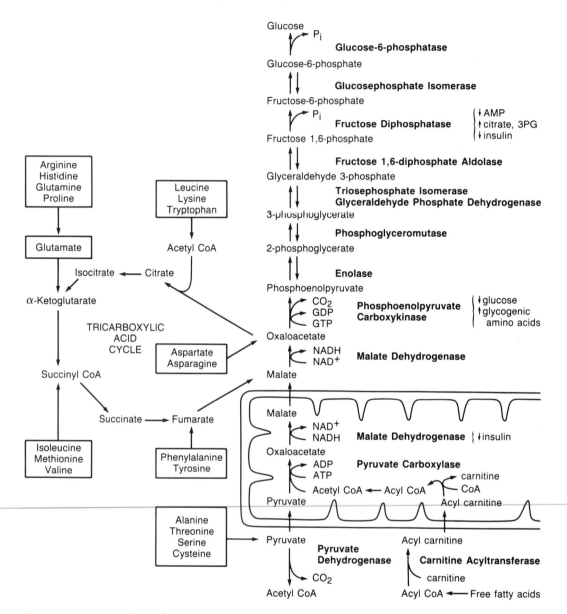

Figure 9-1. Enzymatic pathways for glucose synthesis from amino acids or pyruvate in mammalian liver. Enclosed in the boxes are the glucogenic amino acids with arrows indicating the points where carbon skeletons from these amino acids enter the pathways of gluconeogenesis or the tricarboxylic acid cycle. Free fatty acids provide intramitochondrial acetyl coenzyme A (CoA) needed to convert pyruvate to oxaloacetate but cannot be used as the sole source of carbon skeletons for gluconeogenesis. Bracketed next to the rate-controlling enzymes for gluconeogenesis are some of the substances that increase (⇑) or decrease (⇓) the activity of these enzymes. P_i, inorganic phosphate; 3PG, 3-phosphoglycerate; AMP, adenosine monophosphate; ADP, adenosine diphosphate; ATP, adenosine triphosphate; GDP, guanosine diphosphate; GTP, guanosine triphosphate; NAD^+ and NADH, nicotinamide adenine dinucleotide, oxidized and reduced forms, respectively.

concentrations are normally quite low through fetal life until birth. Thus, as the action of insulin is predominant, the endocrine milieu of fetal life is uniquely anabolic.

The most obvious perinatal event is the loss of the constant supply of nutrients to the infant. At birth the serum glucose concentration of a normal infant is approximately 4.2 mmol/L and the serum volume 45 mL/kg. Therefore, the total amount of available circulating glucose is 0.19 mmol/kg. At a utilization rate of 0.03 mmol/kg/min, the fetus receives enough glucose to support 7 minutes of normal metabolism. Obviously, continued existence depends on the ability of the infant to produce glucose or alternative fuels from endogenous sources. This is especially crucial for human brain cells, which have been shown to require some glucose constantly as a source of energy. Glucose transport into human brain cells is not regulated by insulin; rather, it occurs by facilitated transport. Therefore, unlike muscle and fat cells, in which high insulin concentrations can continue to maintain glucose entry in the face of hypoglycemia, in brain cells, the lower the serum concentration of glucose, the less glucose the brain cells receive. Consequently, prolonged periods without glucose produce irrevocable brain damage.

The consequences of severe hypoglycemia to the newly born infant are significant; therefore, late fetal and early neonatal metabolism is specifically adapted to alleviate these effects. Initially, there is a precipitous decline of blood glucose in the newborn infant (Fig 9-2). When the blood glucose pool is abruptly depleted, the initial source for replacement is from hepatic glycogen. The liver of the newborn infant contains about 0.012 kg of glycogen (Fig. 9-3), representing sufficient glucose for about 12 hours of normal glucose use. Mobilization of these stores is dependent on a rapid change in the neonatal hormonal environment (Girard and Narkewicz, 1992; Jones, 1991). Over the first hours, there is a marked decline in the fetal insulin concentration and a striking rise in fetal glucagon concentration (Fig. 9-4). Other counterregulatory hormones are also affected by birth. Plasma epinephrine and norepinephrine concentrations increase markedly, as does the cortisol concentration. These rapid changes in hormone levels set in motion a cascade of enzymatic reactions that generate active phosphorylase, which in turn catalyzes the degradation of glycogen to glucose

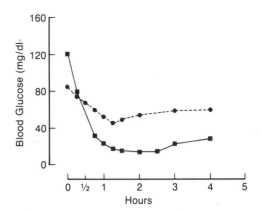

Figure 9-2. The decline of blood glucose after birth in healthy full-term infants (● - - - ●) and infants of diabetic mothers (■ —— ■). The latter group, if untreated, will achieve much lower blood glucose concentrations within the first hour of life and sustain a lower blood glucose level for an extended period. Reproduced with permission from Mc-Cann ML, Chen CH, Katigbak EB, et al.: Effects of fructose on hypoglycemia in infants of diabetic mothers. *N Engl J Med* **275:**1–7, 1966.

6-phosphate. These same hormonal changes are likely also responsible for the remarkable postnatal induction of glucose 6-phosphatase, the enzyme responsible for the further metabolism of glucose 6-phosphate to glucose. Because infants normally do not receive an adequate supply of exogenous glucose (from feeding) for the first weeks of life, however, hepatic glycogen stores are soon exhausted (see Fig. 9-3), and the glucose pool must be replenished from other endogenous sources (e.g., gluconeogenesis).

The only other endogenous source for glucose production is the generation of glucose from gluconeogenic amino acids. By late fetal life, all the enzymes needed for gluconeogenesis are present; however, because there is an easily obtainable source of glucose (i.e., across the placenta) and the fetal endocrine environment is not suitable for gluconeogenesis, the pathways for the production of newly formed glucose are not used. Shortly after birth, the fall of the blood glucose concentration and the rise in glucagon concentrations, catecholamines, and possibly the corticosteroid hormones serve as strong stimulants for the initiation of gluconeogenesis. These factors increase the synthesis and activity of cytosolic phosphoenolpyruvate carboxykinase, an enzyme that is directly related to hepatic gluconeogenic capacity. This activity of this enzyme,

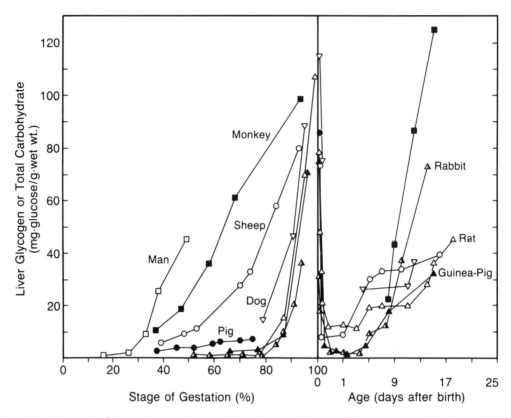

Figure 9-3. The quantity of hepatic glycogen (shown on the ordinate as milligrams of glucose per gram of wet liver weight) in a number of mammalian species throughout gestation (left panel). The increase in humans (□ —— □) occurs earlier in gestation than in some other mammals. The precipitous decline of hepatic glycogen is shown on the right panel for all species studied. Replenishment occurs after many days of a normal neonatal diet. Reproduced with permission from Shelley HJ: *Br Med Bull* **17:**137–143, 1961.

which is minimal in the near-term fetus, rises remarkably postnatally (Fig. 9-5). That gluconeogenesis is an important mode of glucose production during the first weeks of life has now been shown unequivocally using radioactive tracer techniques. Amino acids derived from protein breakdown in skeletal muscle provide the most important source of gluconeogenic precursors. This source of glucose allows the newborn to maintain normal blood glucose concentrations during the period before the onset of adequate feeding (and adequate exogenous carbohydrates). In addition, hepatic fatty acid oxidation is also required to sustain gluconeogenesis. These fatty acids may be obtained from exogenous feeding or metabolism of fatty acids released from endogenous lipid stores. Beta-oxidation of fatty acids provides the acetyl-coenzyme A needed to activate mitochondrial pyruvate carboxylase and the NADH

used as the substrate in the reaction catalyzed by glyceraldehyde 3-phosphate dehydrogenase in the direction of gluconeogenesis (see Fig. 9-1).

Although glycogenolysis and gluconeogenesis represent the only pathways that the newborn can call on to produce glucose from endogenous sources, glucose usage could be minimized, and thus the blood glucose level maintained, if other substrates were to supply the metabolic needs of tissues. The newborn has a potential source of energy in the lipid stores present primarily in white adipose tissue (Girard et al., 1992). Indeed, among species, the human is unique in having a body fat content of about 16% of body weight. These stores are present almost entirely in the form of triacylglycerols that contain significant amounts of palmitic and oleic acid. Mobilization of these stores in adipose tissue is controlled by a lipase that is regulated by the hormonal envi

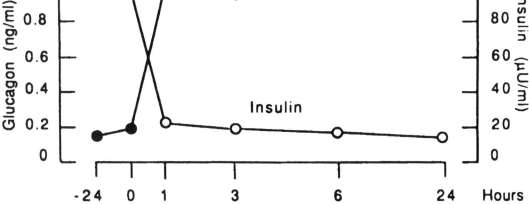

Figure 9-4. Postnatal changes in newborn rat plasma insulin and glucagon concentrations. Reprinted with permission from Girard et al. (1992).

ronment. Insulin is probably the most important inhibitor of lipolysis. In contrast to adults, in whom catecholamines represent the most important stimulators of lipolysis, thyrotropin (TSH) is the most important stimulator of lipolysis in the newborn. Plasma-free fatty acid concentrations rise markedly in the first hours after birth in response to a marked increase in the TSH concentration and a fall in the insulin concentration. The fatty acids released from lipid stores are oxidized by some extrahepatic tissues (e.g., heart and skeletal muscle, kidney, intestine, and lung). Because the *respiratory quotient* (the ratio of carbon dioxide production to oxygen use) falls from a value of 1.0 (showing that carbohydrate oxidation is the primary source of energy) to a value of 0.8 to 0.9 (showing increasing oxidation of pro-

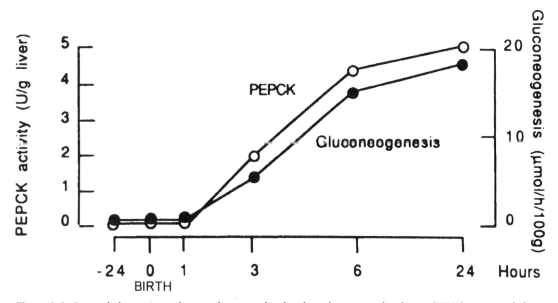

Figure 9-5. Postnatal changes in newborn rat liver cytosolic phosphoenolpyruvate carboxykinase (PEPCK) activity and gluconeogenic rate *in vivo* from [14C-lactate]. Reprinted with permission from Girard et al. (1992).

tein or fatty acids) at 2 to 12 hours of age, and at a time when protein catabolism is usually insignificant, fatty acid oxidation must represent a significant energy source in the early postnatal period.

Fatty acids are metabolized differently in the liver than they are in other tissues (Fig. 9-6). Only a small portion of the fatty acids are oxidized totally to the level of CO_2 and water in liver. Hepatic tissues convert most of the fatty acids they oxidize to ketone bodies, which are released into the bloodstream and carried to peripheral tissues, most notably the brain, where they are used as metabolic fuels. Because

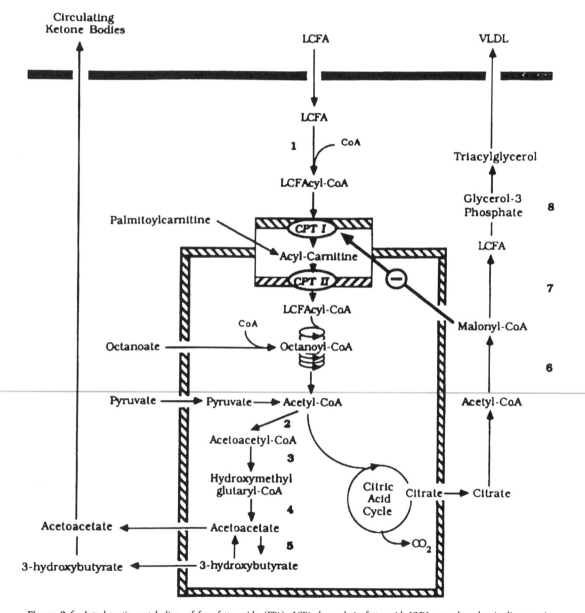

Figure 9-6. Intrahepatic metabolism of free fatty acids (FFA). LCFA, long-chain fatty acid; VLDL, very low-density lipoprotein; CPT I, CPT II, carnitine palmitoyltransferase I, II. 1, long-chain acylcoenzyme A (CoA) synthase; 2, acetoacetyl-CoA thiolase; 3, hydroxymethylglutaryl-CoA synthase; 4, hydroxymethylglutaryl-CoA lyase; 5, 3-hydroxybutyrate dehydrogenase; 6, acetyl-CoA carboxylase; 7, fatty acid synthase; 8, glycerolphosphate acyltransferase. Reprinted with permission from Girard et al. (1992).

glucagon stimulates ketogenesis and insulin inhibits ketogenesis, the hormonal changes that occur at birth would be expected to promote ketone body formation; however, blood ketone bodies remain quite low during the first hours after birth, reaching a maximal value only after 1 to 2 days. The reason for this delay in ketone body formation may be the low liver concentrations of carnitine in the human newborn liver. Carnitine is needed to transfer long-chain fatty acids into the mitochondrion, where beta-oxidation occurs (Fig. 9-6). Because newborn infants have a limited capacity for carnitine synthesis, exogenous carnitine must be supplied through the diet before ketogenesis can proceed optimally. Thus, although cerebral oxidation of ketone bodies, occurs shortly after birth and spares some of the cerebral glucose requirement, there still is a major need for glucose as an energy source in the brain.

With the above discussion in mind, it is possible to predict the consequences to the fetus and newborn of an elevated maternal blood glucose concentration, such as occurs in diabetes mellitus (Cornblath and Schwartz, 1991). As the maternal blood glucose level rises, the gradient between fetal and maternal blood glucose concentrations increases, causing more glucose to be transported to the fetus. With the consequent rise in the fetal blood glucose concentration, the fetal pancreas releases more insulin (fetal hyperinsulinism). Fetal skeletal and cardiac muscles now become exposed to higher blood concentrations of both glucose and insulin. In response to the consequent increase in the rate of glucose transport, muscles metabolize more glucose and store more of it as glycogen. The fetal liver, too, has a higher than usual glycogen content. In addition, the activities of the key gluconeogenic enzymes (see Fig. 9-1), phosphoenolpyruvate carboxykinase in particular, are depressed. The hyperinsulinemia stimulates fat cells throughout the body, including subcutaneous adipocytes to deposit lipid at a maximal rate, causing the fetus to weigh more than would be expected based on its length or head circumference.

In addition, the metabolic effects of insulin ultimately increase fetal oxygen consumption. The circulation of the fetus is unique; specifically, because blood in the fetal descending aorta contains a portion of venous return after tissue perfusion, the increased rate of consumption of oxygen by fetal tissues decreases the arterial oxygen concentration of

the fetus. The fetal tissues supplied by this circulation (which include most of the mass of the fetus) are then at risk for inadequate tissue oxygenation. There are two consequences of such tissue hypoxia. First, as renal oxygenation becomes inadequate, the fetal kidney produces erythropoietin, which in turn stimulates the production of new erythrocytes. This response leads to an increased hematocrit and an increase in the oxygen-carrying capacity of the blood of the fetus. Second, normal fetal metabolism may be altered if the supply of oxygen to the fetus becomes marginal. Generally, the normal fetus receives about twice as much oxygen across the placenta as needed for normal metabolism. For any fetus, labor increases the likelihood of decreased oxygen supply as uterine contractions interfere with blood flow to the intervillous space of the placenta. The fetus of the diabetic mother, even if it receives a normal oxygen supply, has, as already noted, an accelerated rate of oxidative metabolism. The fetus of a diabetic mother is therefore at greater risk for hypoxic damage, as illustrated by the present case.

When the fetus lacks an adequate oxygen supply, it must satisfy its energy needs through anaerobic pathways (e.g., glycolysis); however, the glycolytic pathway of glucose utilization, while generating adenosine triphosphate (ATP), produces lactic acid (by reducing pyruvate) (see Fig. 9-1). A fall in the blood pH is indicative of anaerobic metabolism. The use of glycolysis for energy production is an inefficient process that yields only two molecules of ATP per molecule of glucose metabolized, compared with the 38 ATP molecules produced by the combined action of glycolysis, the citric acid cycle, and oxidative phosphorylation. Indeed, anaerobic glycolysis is too inefficient to provide the energy the fetus needs to survive for more than a few hours or days. The finding of a pH of 6.9 in the infant described in the present case report was evidence of significant anaerobic metabolism and impending fetal death. It was imperative that the physicians caring for this patient remove the fetus from the hostile intrauterine environment so that effective oxygenation and aerobic metabolism could proceed.

Once one understands the normal metabolic adaption to extrauterine life, it is easy to see why the infant whose mother has diabetes is also likely to have problems maintaining neonatal glucose homeostasis. Before birth, infants of diabetic mothers whose placentas have functioned normally will receive a constant oversupply of glucose, which will induce high insulin levels and low concentrations of the principal counterregulatory hormones: glucagon and the catecholamines. Glucose utilization can be increased to rates as high as 10 mg/kg per minute in some infants of diabetic mothers. Even with the fetal blood glucose concentration (because of the maternal diabetes) as high as 8.3 mmol/L (representing a glucose pool of 0.45 mmol at birth), this source of glucose will be exhausted within 8 minutes. Therefore, the infant of a diabetic mother, like a normal infant, must generate endogenous glucose to maintain the metabolism of tissues, such as brain, that are constantly dependent on this metabolic substrate. Such infants have, as mentioned, abundant liver glycogen stores. Over the first hours of life, however, such infants persist in having higher than normal insulin concentrations and lower than normal glu-

cagon concentrations (Fig. 9-7). In addition, the concentrations of other counterregulatory hormones, such as catecholamines, remain low. This particular hormonal milieu will seriously inhibit glycogenolysis, thereby decreasing the rate of glucose release from the liver.

Unfortunately, the endocrine environment of the infant whose mother is diabetic also suppresses the production of glucose from its only other major potential source namely, amino acids. High insulin levels in both fetal and neonatal life inhibit protein breakdown, thereby decreasing the availability of amino acids from endogenous sources for potential use as gluconeogenic substrates. In addition, the marked increase that normally occurs in the activities of two important rate-controlling gluconeogenic enzymes, cytosolic phosphoenolpyruvate carboxykinase and glucose 6-phosphatase, is markedly sup-

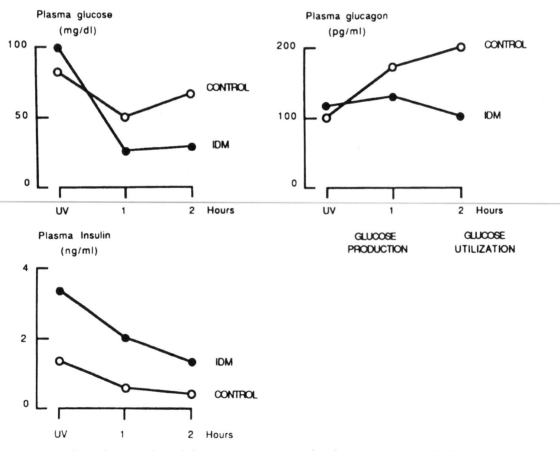

Figure 9-7. Plasma glucose, insulin, and glucagon concentrations in infants from diabetic mothers (IDM). UV, umbilical vein. Reprinted with permission from Girard et al. (1992).

pressed owing to the higher insulin and lower counterregulatory hormone concentrations of infants born to diabetic mothers. The combined effect of the decreased capacity for glycogenolysis and gluconeogenesis in infants of diabetic mothers is a marked decrease in the ability of the newborn to release glucose from the liver into the blood.

Such a decrease in glucose production would have less impact if other metabolic fuels could be mobilized and used. As noted, the fetus whose mother has diabetes has greatly increased fat stores. In these infants, the amount of fat present is theoretically sufficient to supply adequate metabolic substrate for weeks, but the high insulin concentrations markedly inhibits lipolysis. As a consequence, tissues like heart and skeletal muscle, which are otherwise capable of using fatty acids to satisfy metabolic needs are compelled to continue oxidizing glucose. The infant of a diabetic mother, therefore, in the face of impaired glucose production, has a higher than normal rate of glucose consumption. This circumstance precipitates a marked fall in the blood glucose concentration of the neonate.

The cerebral requirement for oxidative substrate can be met by only two substrates: glucose and ketone bodies. Unfortunately, the endocrine milieu of the infant of the diabetic mother inhibits both *lipolysis* (i.e., the mobilization of fatty acid stores) and hepatic *ketogenesis* (formation of ketone bodies). Consequently, the brain is left with no alternative to glucose as a metabolic substrate, and the use of glucose to support normal metabolism becomes obligatory. Unless steps are taken to supply exogenous glucose or to alter the endocrine environment so endogenous stores can be mobilized, the infant of a diabetic mother will be at great risk for brain injury.

The present case presentation and discussion of the consequences of maternal hyperglycemia presume that placental function is sufficiently preserved to allow maternal hyperglycemia to be reflected in fetal hyperglycemia. Some diabetic mothers whose disease is sufficiently long-standing or advanced to cause renal or retinal vascular disease will also have vascular disease that adversely affects the placenta and compromises its ability to transport substrates to the fetus. In such cases, the infants are affected by a chronic undersupply of both oxygen and other critical metabolic substrates, including glucose. Because the infants have received subnormal quantities of glucose, they have low insulin levels and higher than normal concentrations of counterregulatory hormones. Consequently, both their glycogen and lipid stores are minimal. Such an undersupply of fuel reserves results in an infant that is notably smaller than would be expected for its gestational age.

Despite the small size of the infant at birth, an obligate need for glucose ($\sim$4 mg/kg/min) still exists. Thus, an infant born with a subnormal serum glucose concentration of 3.3 mmol/L will have used up the entire circulating glucose pool within about 8 minutes. With such a rapid depletion of serum glucose, the infant must reply on glycogenolysis to replenish blood glucose. Although the endocrine environment of such infants, specifically one in which there are low insulin levels and higher than normal concentrations of counterregulatory hormones, favors glycogenolysis, complete depletion of glycogen reserves will occur in about 4 hours, which is much faster than normal. These infants must then resort to another source of endogenous glucose production, namely, gluconeogenesis. The endocrine environment of such infants, like that of the macrosomic infants, is conducive to both mobilization of amino acids from protein breakdown and induction of the hepatic enzymes needed for gluconeogenesis. Nonetheless, gluconeogenesis remains deficient as a result of the lack of free fatty acid from lipolysis, which diminishes intramitochondrial acetyl-coenzyme A and compromises hepatic gluconeogenesis. Other potential substrates such as fat are not available to provide metabolic substrate because lipolysis, although favored by the endocrine milieu, is limited by a lack of adipose triglyceride. Therefore, infants born to diabetic mothers, in whom placental function has been compromised, lack the endogenous sources of glucose and are also at risk for hypoglycemia; however, the etiology is one of decreased substrate stores rather than an inappropriate endocrine environment.

THERAPY

Because all the myriad consequences to the infant of a diabetic mother arise from maternal hyperglycemia, the therapy of hypoglycemia for the infant should begin before birth. Careful management of the maternal diabetes to prevent both hypoglycemia and hyperglycemia will lessen the likelihood of fetal death or neonatal hypoglycemia. In the present case, economic hardship (the husband's layoff and loss of health insurance) prevented Mrs. L. from obtaining adequate prenatal care. The resultant neonatal complications can be traced directly to this problem.

There are circumstances that preclude the preventive measures outlined above. In such cases, there are two main methods of relieving the hypoglycemia: provision of exogenous substrate or alteration of the infant's endocrine status. After delivery, assuming the infant is otherwise healthy, the early provision of calories by milk feedings can provide adequate exogenous sources of glucose to prevent hypoglycemia. In some infants, however, either because of other illnesses or because of the severity of the hypoglycemia, it is necessary to provide i.v. glucose. Although this was done in the present case, the provision of glucose at only 4 mg/kg per minute was inadequate to ensure a sufficient quantity of glucose for use by the brain. The initial i.v. therapy should provide at least 6 mg/kg per minute.

When hypoglycemia does occur, it is imperative for the physician to respond rapidly and appropriately. Exogenous glucose delivered directly into a vein is the treatment of choice; but caution must be exercised because the rapid injection of quantities of glucose far in excess of requirements will lead to a sudden increase of blood glucose to hyperglycemic levels. For infants of diabetic mothers, this further stimulates insulin release, which then rapidly produces rebound hypoglycemia, as we saw in the present case. The use of 10 ml of 25% dextrose produced a blood glucose concentration of nearly 22.2 mmol/L, followed by a rapid decrease. It is more prudent and efficacious to administer 1 to 2 mL/kg of 10% dextrose over approximately 5 minutes and then begin a continuous i.v. infusion calculated to supply 6 to 8 mL/kg of glucose per minute. In an emergency, when an i.v. site cannot be rapidly obtained, the endocrine environment of the infant can be made more conducive to glucose release by use of intramuscular or subcutaneous injection of glucagon (0.3 mg/kg per dose) to produce a short-lived (<30 min) increase in blood glucose while an i.v. catheter is being inserted. Infants whose glycogen is depleted (i.e., growth-retarded neonates) cannot be expected to respond as effectively to glucagon as can an infant of a diabetic mother. If possible, milk feeding should also be instituted to stimulate the secretion of many glucoregulatory gut hormones and

to supply an additional source of glucose and gluconeogenic precursors.

In a few infants, massive quantities of i.v. glucose fail to prevent repeated episodes of hypoglycemia, and manipulation of the neonatal endocrine status is required to minimize glucose use and maximize glucose production. The use of a brief course of glucocorticoids, one of the counterregulatory hormones, as in the present case, can effectively treat the hypoglycemia. The mechanisms of action are threefold: (1) glucocorticoids counteract the effect of insulin on peripheral muscle glucose uptake, thereby "sparing" glucose for brain use and raising the blood glucose concentration; (2) glucocorticoids stimulate hepatic glycogenesis and gluconeogenesis; and (3) glucocorticoids increase proteolysis in peripheral tissues, thereby increasing the availability of gluconeogenic substrates. The effectiveness of this therapy was clearly shown in the present case.

It is not surprising that infant L. suffered a diffuse *encephalopathy* (brain disorder), a cerebral infarction, and seizures during the neonatal period. Both asphyxia and hypoglycemia are injurious to the brain. The treatment for seizures consists of providing normal metabolic substrates (e.g., glucose) and appropriate anticonvulsant therapy (phenobarbital), as was done in the present case. The long-term treatment for the child's developmental disabilities is complex and involves the skills of many members of the health-care team. The prognosis of infant L. is uncertain. Asymptomatic hypoglycemia in an infant of a diabetic mother is usually less injurious than those episodes associated with central nervous symptoms. Obviously, in the present case, although the child had symptoms of seizures and an abnormal neurological examination, it is not possible to differentiate these symptoms from those that might have resulted from the chronic inadequacy of cerebral oxygenation *in utero*. Nevertheless, the prognosis for an asphyxiated child with an abnormal electroencephalogram, a cerebral infarction, and persistent abnormalities on neurological examination is guarded at best. The bilateral hearing loss and the inability to swallow and feed adequately at the time of discharge are strong evidence of some degree of severe neurological disability in the future. Predictions about specific motor and mental potentials are impossible to make in the early neonatal period.

Generally, the prognosis for infants born to diabetic mothers is good; however, severe symptomatic hypoglycemia can lead to lifelong problems. Infants whose hypoglycemia reflects a long-term lack of adequate nutrition and oxygenation *in utero* (such as severe growth-retarded infants) are at even greater risk for developmental disabilities. In both cases the additional burden of birth asphyxia will increase the likelihood of long-term problems. Obviously, the severity of illness in the infant herein described and the ominous signs of cerebral disturbance at the time of discharge bode poorly for the child's future development.

QUESTIONS

1. Compare the hormonal changes that occur at birth and their effects on carbohydrate homeostasis with those that occur in adults during starvation.
2. What was the primary medical cause of infant L's problems? Why was appropriate therapy not initiated in the present case?
3. What substance is an important circulating oxidative substrate in fetal life but uncommon postnatally? What common metabolic substrate of postneonatal life is relatively less important during fetal life?
4. Can free fatty acids serve as a direct source of glucose (i.e., can fatty acids be converted into glucose)? Why or why not?
5. Would glucagon or glucocorticoids be as effective a therapy for hypoglycemia in the growth-retarded infant of a diabetic mother as in newborns who are large for gestational age?

REFERENCES

Cornblath M, Schwartz R: *Disorders of Carbohydrate Metabolism in Infancy.* Boston, Blackwell Scientific Publications, 1991.

Cowett RM: Neonatal glucose metabolism, *in* Cowett RM (ed): *Principles of Perinatal-Neonatal Metabolism.* New York, Springer-Verlag, 1991a, pp. 356–389.

Cowett RM: Infant of the diabetic mother, *in* Cowett RM (ed): *Principles of Perinatal-Neonatal Metabolism.* New York, Springer-Verlag, 1991b, pp. 678–698.

Girard J, Ferré P, Pégorier J-P, et al.: Adaptations of glucose and fatty acid metabolism during the perinatal period and suckling-weaning transition. *Physiol Rev* **72:**507–562, 1992.

Girard J, Narkewicz M: Role of glucoregulatory hormones on hepatic glucose metabolism during the perinatal period, *in* Polin RA, Fox WW (eds): *Fetal and Neonatal Physiology.* Philadelphia, WB Saunders Company, 1992, pp 390–401.

Jones CT: Control of glucose metabolism in the perinatal period. *J Dev Physiol* **15:**81–89, 1991.

10

Jaundice and Gallstone Diseases

SUSUMU TAZUMA AND GORO KAJIYAMA

CASE REPORT

A 37-year-old woman visited her physician because of pain in the right upper abdominal quadrant associated with nausea and vomiting. The pain, which radiated to the back, occurred three hours after enjoying a heavy dinner in a restaurant. It lasted overnight, and early in the morning of the next day she noted the gradual onset of moderate chills and sweating and darkening of the color of the urine. She had experienced a similar episode 1 month before; however, it resolved within 6 hours. Review of systems was completely normal. She was sent to the emergency department and hospitalized.

On physical examination, the patient appeared well developed and well nourished (52 kg, 157 cm). Her blood pressure was 132/66 mm Hg and her heart rate 96 beats per minute and regular. Her respiration rate was 20 per minute and her temperature 38.3°C. She was *icteric* (jaundiced), and her skin was warm and moist. The cardiopulmonary examination was unremarkable. There was deep tenderness in the upper right abdominal quadrant with no organomegaly or *ascites* (fluid accumulation in the abdominal cavity). The neurological examination was unremarkable.

Urinalysis demonstrated 2+ urobilinogen; however, the urine was negative for bilirubin. The hematocrit was 38% (normal range, 35–40), but the white blood cell (WBC) count had risen from 4800/mm³ (normal, 4000–8000) to 10,300/mm³ (neutrophils 70%, lymphocytes 17%, monocytes 11%, eosinophils 1%, and basophils 1%). The total serum bilirubin concentration was 2.9 mg/dL (normal, <1.0) and direct-reacting bilirubin was 1.5 mg/dL (normal, <0.2). The activity level of serum aspartate aminotransferase (AST) was 185 IU/L (normal, <41), alanine aminotransferase (ALT) 69 IU/L (normal, <41), γ-glutamyl transpeptidase 148 IU/L (normal, 8–45), alkaline phosphatase 189 IU/L (normal, <120), and leucine aminopeptidase 421 IU/L (normal, 70–200). Her serum total cholesterol and triglyceride levels were within normal ranges. Serum cholinesterase, lactic acid dehydrogenase, creatine phosphokinase, amylase, blood glucose, total protein, protein fractions (albumin, 56.0–72.0%; α1-globulin, 1.6–3.5%; α2-globulin, 6.4–11.0%; β-globlin, 6.2–10.5%; γ-globulin, 9.5–21.4%), and electrolytes were within normal ranges (Na, 137–149 mEq/L; K, 3.7–5.0 mEq/L; Cl, 98–109 mEq/L). The level of C-reactive protein was 6.9 mg/dL (normal, <0.4) and erythrocyte sedimentation was elevated to 32 mm per hour (normal, <15). Hepatitis B surface antigen and hepatitis C virus antibody were negative. The tests for autoantibodies against nuclei, smooth muscle, microsomes, and mitochondria were negative.

Abdominal ultrasound revealed a single stone (diameter, 18 mm) in the gallbladder, thickening of the gallbladder wall, and slight dilatation of the common bile duct (internal diameter, 9 mm); but the images of liver, pancreas, spleen, and kidneys were normal. The abdominal roentgenogram was normal.

A diagnosis of acute cholecystitis resulting from stasis of the gallbladder or cystic duct obstruction by gallstones was made. For further examination of common bile duct dilatation evidenced by abdominal ultrasound, *endoscopic retrograde cholangiopancreatography* (a diagnostic method for identifying biliary and pancreatic ductal abnormalities by injecting contrast materials through an indwelling catheter endoscopically) was performed and the presence of 5-mm-diameter stones, in the common duct was confirmed. Common duct stones were removed nonsurgically by a basket through an endoscope after *endoscopic sphincterotomy* (an endoscopic technique that enlarges the papillary orifice by cutting the sphincter of Oddi with a papillotome). After successful removal of common bile duct stones, laboratory parameters returned to normal values in a week.

Finally, laparoscopic *cholecystectomy* (surgical removal of the gallbladder) was performed. Infrared spectrophotometry revealed that the gallstones consisted of cholesterol (88%) and calcium salts (12%). The removed gallbladder showed signs of mild acute inflammation with edema and cellular infiltration, but no perforation was evident. Bile sterilely obtained at surgery was subjected to lipid analysis, including the fatty acid composition of the lecithin and bile acid composition by simultaneous microanalyses using capillary gas chromatography. These data revealed that the bile was supersaturated with cholesterol; the cholesterol saturation index was 1.8 as calculated by *Carey's table* (a relative value of cholesterol concentration to maximal cholesterol solubility calculated from the molar ratio of cholesterol, phospholipids, and bile acids). Furthermore, the *nucleation time* (the interval required for the first detection of cholesterol monohydrate crystals by polarizing microscopy) was 3 days. The concentration of high molecular weight glycoprotein in bile, as determined by gel chromatography, was 5.5 mg/mL (normal, 0.9–3.5). After no leakage of bile was determined by intravenous cholangiography, the patient was discharged.

DIAGNOSIS

Causes of Hyperbilirubinemia

In general, the serum level of bilirubin reflects a state of dynamic equilibrium between its rate of production and rate of clearance (Tazuma and Holzbach, 1987). Hyperbilirubinemia is caused by either an increase in bilirubin production or a decrease in its clearance, or some combination of the two (Table 10-1). In most cases, the cause of jaundice can be diagnosed from the clinical history, physical examination, routine laboratory tests, and especially the increased serum level of bilirubin (unconjugated bilirubin or its conjugates).

Because bilirubin conjugates are structurally unstable and undergo oxidation, their analysis is performed using two dipyrrolic derivatives formed by the reaction of bilirubin with a diazo reagent. Conjugated bilirubin reacts with sulfanilic acid diazo reagent to form azodipyrrols; unconjugated bilirubin reacts with such an agent only in the presence of accelerator substances, such as methanol or caffeine. The first type of reaction is called *direct;* the second *indirect.* The unconjugated bilirubin is called indirect-reacting bilirubin, and the conjugated bilirubin is called direct-reacting bilirubin.

Increased Bilirubin Production

Common causes of bilirubin overproduction are hemolysis and transfusion of stored blood. Chronic hemolysis usually results in mild unconjugated hyperbilirubinemia and a serum bilirubin concentration below 4 mg/dL. A bilirubin value exceeding the 4.0 mg/dL level indicates the additional presence of hepatic dysfunction. In contrast, acute hemolysis leads to a striking elevation of the serum unconjugated bilirubin concentration (also called indirect-reacting bilirubin), as the bilirubin production rate exceeds the hepatic bilirubin clearance capacity in such circumstances. Another major cause of jaundice is blood transfusion because a fraction of stored blood tends to hemolyse immediately after transfusion. Ineffective erythropoiesis (e.g., megaloblastic anemia, polycythemia, thalassemia) is another cause of jaundice.

Table 10-1. Causes of Hyperbilirubinemia

Increased bilirubin production
  Hemolysis, transfusions

Decreased bilirubin clearance
  Hereditary defects in hepatic bilirubin clearance
  Cholestasis
    Hepatocellular diseases
    Biliary tract obstruction

Decreased Bilirubin Clearance

Hereditary Hyperbilirubinemia Caused by Defects of Hepatic Clearance. Hyperbilirubinemias are caused by defects of hepatic bilirubin clearance. Hereditary defects of hepatic uridine diphosphate (UDP)-glucuronyl transferase activity results in unconjugated hyperbilirubinemias (e.g., Gilbert's syndrome and Crigler-Najjar syndrome types I and II). In contrast, impairment of hepatic excretion of conjugated bilirubin (also called direct-reacting bilirubin) into bile causes conjugated hyperbilirubinemias (e.g., Dubin-Johnson syndrome). The identified defects in bilirubin metabolism in Gilbert's syndrome are decreases in glucuronyl transferase activity and hepatic uptake of bilirubin. The activity of glucuronyl transferase is absent in Crigler-Najjar syndrome type I and markedly decreased or absent in Crigler-Najjar syndrome type II. In contrast, the presumed defect in bilirubin metabolism of Dubin-Johnson syndrome is impaired biliary excretion of conjugated organic anions.

Cholestasis. Cholestasis can be subdivided into intrahepatic and extrahepatic causes. Various hepatic parenchymal diseases cause intrahepatic cholestasis, in which hepatocytes are unable to excrete bile; these include viral hepatitis, alcoholic hepatitis, and drug- or toxin-induced liver injury. In contrast, biliary obstruction, commonly caused by a neoplasm or gallstones, is the cause of extrahepatic cholestasis. In most cases, conjugated hyperbilirubinemia is caused by a reflux of conjugated bilirubin into serum.

Clinical Diagnosis of Patients with Jaundice

The diagnosis of jaundice can usually be made from the clinical history, the physical examination, and laboratory data. Outline of a clinical approach to jaundiced patients is shown in Figure 10-1. Among the various causes of jaundice, extrahepatic cholestasis resulting from biliary obstruction requires more extensive examinations to image the biliary

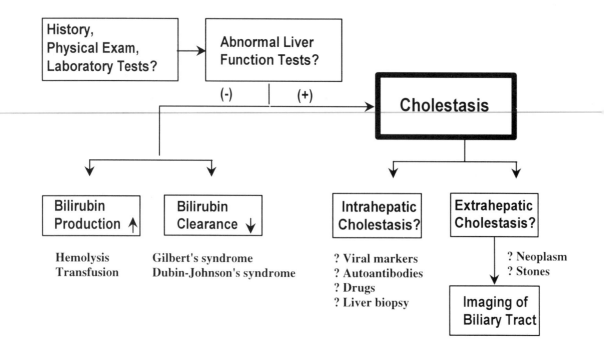

Figure 10-1. Clinical approach to jaundiced patients. Imaging of the biliary tract includes ultrasonography and computed tomography. In cases where biliary obstruction is suspected or evidenced by noninvasive imaging, direct visualization, endoscopic retrograde or percutaneous transhepatic cholangiography must be performed.

tree for definitive or palliative treatment. The differential diagnosis of causes of extrahepatic biliary obstruction is of clinical importance, because it will determine the treatment that the patient will receive.

In the present case, the patient's history and physical examination provided important diagnostic clues. Collectively, the presence of postprandial abdominal pain with nausea and vomiting, fever, dark urine, and abdominal tenderness all pointed to biliary disease. Furthermore, routine laboratory data revealed conjugated hyperbilirubinemia with hepatic dysfunction, indicating the presence of extrahepatic obstruction with inflammation. Noninvasive imaging of the biliary tree by ultrasound revealed the presence of a gallbladder stone with cholecystitis and mild dilatation of the common bile duct. Finally, direct imaging of the bile duct by endoscopic retrograde cholangiography confirmed the presence of common bile duct stones (Fig. 10-2). Thus, the present case was diagnosed to be jaundice caused by

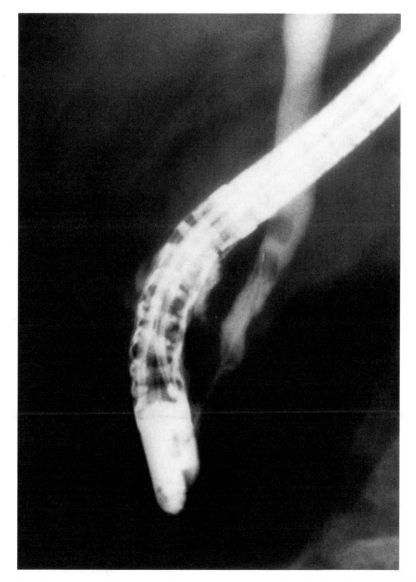

Figure 10-2. Endoscopic retrograde cholangiograph. Two ductal stones are seen. The dilatation of the common bile duct is mild. Stones were removed after endoscopic sphincterotomy.

cholecystitis owing to gallstones in the gallbladder and common bile duct.

MOLECULAR PERSPECTIVES

Bilirubin Metabolism

Catabolism of Heme to Bilirubin Glucuronides

Bilirubin is derived mainly from hemoglobin liberated from the destruction of senescent erythrocytes by the reticuloendothelial-macrophage system (e.g., liver, spleen, bone marrow). Heme dissociates from the globin apoprotein as a complex of iron with protoporphyrin IX; the selective cleavage of the porphyrin ring at the α-methene bridge to form biliverdin is catalyzed by the combined activity of the microsomal enzymes NADPH-cytochrome *c*-reductase and heme oxygenase (Fig. 10-3). Subsequently, conversion of biliverdin to bilirubin is catalyzed by the cytosolic enzyme biliverdin reductase. Because bilirubin is toxic and hydrophobic, conjugation of bilirubin with glucuronide moieties is catalyzed by the microsomal UDP-glucuronyl transferase before excretion.

Hepatic Uptake, Transport, Metabolism, and Biliary Secretion of Bilirubin

A schematic summary of hepatic uptake, intracellular transport and metabolism, and biliary secretion of bilirubin is shown in Figure 10-4. Bilirubin is transported in the plasma primarily bound to albumin and is efficiently taken up by the liver through a carrier-mediated process. After uptake from plasma, unconjugated bilirubin binds to cytosolic binding proteins (also called ligandins) and then transported to its intracellular metabolic site (e.g., the endoplasmic reticulum). Conjugation of bilirubin with glucuronide moieties occurs when bilirubin is presented to the microsomal UDP-glucuronyl transferase. Bilirubin glucuronides (e.g., bilirubin diglucuronide, bilirubin monoglucuronide) are transported to the canalicular membrane mainly by cytosolic binding proteins (ligandins). Bilirubin bound to ligandin (e.g., glutathione S-transferase) can also be stored in the liver. Another route for bilirubin transport is the vesicle pathway, the physiological role of which still needs further clarification. Canalicular

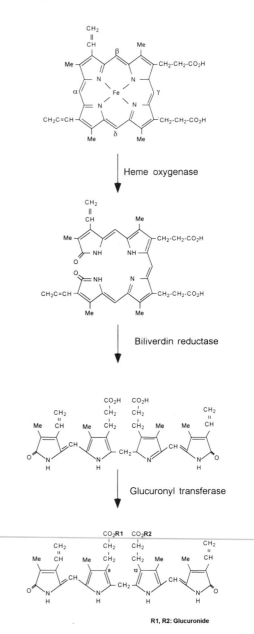

Figure 10-3. Catabolism of heme to bilirubin glucuronides. Heme is a complex of iron with protoporphyrin IX and is degraded by microsomal heme oxygenase to biliverdin. Biliverdin is converted to bilirubin by a cytosolic enzyme, biliverdin reductase. Bilirubin is conjugated with one or two glucuronic acids by glucuronyl transferase.

secretion of bilirubin is the rate-limiting step, mediated by the multispecific organic anion transporter (Coleman, 1987).

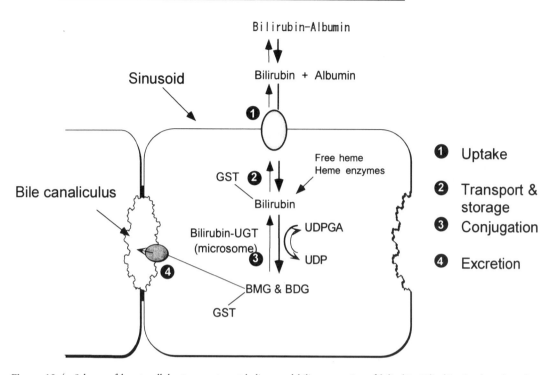

Figure 10-4. Scheme of hepatocellular transport, metabolism, and biliary excretion of bilirubin. Bilirubin circulates bound to albumin. Despite high-affinity binding to albumin, bilirubin is rapidly transferred from plasma into the liver by a carrier-mediated process. After uptake from plasma, bilirubin binds to cytosolic binding proteins (i.e., glutathione S-transferase [GST]) and then is transported by these soluble proteins to intracellular sites of metabolism. Conjugation of bilirubin with glucuronic acids is catalyzed by a family of microsomal enzymes, uridine-diphosphoglucuronoside glucuronosyltransferase (UGT). Bilirubin-UGT catalyzes the transfer of the glucurosyl moiety of UDP-glucuronic acid (UDPGA) to bilirubin. Bilirubin conjugates are either secreted into bile or stored in the liver bound to GST. Biliary excretion of bilirubin conjugates are mediated by a canalicular membrane protein.

Gallstone Formation

No conclusive evidence concerning the origin of common bile duct stones is available, but most (95%) patients with common bile duct stones also have gallbladder stones. Conversely, 15% of gallbladder stone patients also have stones in the common duct. Thus, most ductal stones appear to originate in the gallbladder.

Types of Gallstones

The classification of gallstones is based on the major components that constitute them (Table 10-2). With rare exception, human gallstones are classified into two major categories: cholesterol stones (Admirand and Small, 1978) and pigment gallstones (Ostrow,

1984). These two major groups are subdivided further. In the cholesterol gallstone group, pure radiate cholesterol stones are generally less common; are usually round or oval; are pale whitish yellow; and

Table 10-2. Types of Gallstones (Components, Location)

Cholesterol stones; >70% cholesterol, commonly in the gallbladder
  Pure radiate cholesterol stones: >90% cholesterol
  Mixed stones: cholesterol and calcium bilirubinate
  Combination stones: radiate cholesterol stone as a center with an outer layer shell structurally similar to mixed stones

Pigment stones: >50% calcium bilirubinate, gallbladder and bile ducts
  Black stones: insoluble bilirubin polymer, gallbladder
  Brown stones: calcium bilirubinate, gallbladder and bile ducts

Other rare stones

often solitary. The more common mixed cholesterol stones are also yellow but usually occur as multiple stones. The diameter of mixed stones ranges from 5 to 25 mm, which is smaller than that of pure cholesterol stones. Gallstones with a radiate cholesterol nucleus with an outer shell the structure of which is similar to that of laminated mixed stones are designated *combination stones.*

Pigment stones are subdivided into two categories: black stones and brown stones. Black stones contain considerably more of a polymerized form of an oxidized bilirubin degradation product, coloring them black. This bilirubin polymer is combined with calcium bilirubinate and other calcium salts. Brown stones are composed primarily of calcium bilirubinate and calcium soaps of long-chain fatty acids. Black stones are located in the gallbladder, whereas brown stones may occur in the gallbladder and bile ducts.

Pathogenesis of Cholesterol Gallstones

Cholesterol gallstone disease can be subdivided into five stages as proposed by Small (1980) (Table 10-3). Either biliary cholesterol hypersecretion or biliary bile salt hyposecretion or a combination of the two (the *genetic-metabolic stage*) results in bile cholesterol supersaturation (the *chemical stage*). Because of the limitation of the cholesterol-solubilizing capacity of biliary cholesterol carriers (e.g., bile salt-micelles, lecithin-cholesterol vesicles), cholesterol nucleates and precipitates under an excessive cholesterol supersaturation state (the *physical stage*) (Holan et al., 1979; Groen et al., 1991). Nucleated and precipitated cholesterol crystals grow into macroscopic stones (the *growth stage*), and then biliary obstruction by stones leads to clinical symptoms (the *clinical stage*) (Holzbach, 1990).

Defects in Biliary Lipid Secretion. Bile becomes supersaturated with cholesterol as a result of the two metabolic defects in biliary lipid secretion: cholesterol hypersecretion and biliary bile acid hyposecretion (Admirand and Small, 1978). Excessive cholesterol secretion is related to increased cholesterol synthesis. One sees increased cholesterol biosynthesis in obesity, aging, oral contraceptive use, pregnancy, familial hyperlipoproteinemias IV and IIb, and with hypolipidemic agents (e.g., clofibrate).

In contrast, a decrease in the rate of bile acid secretion is caused by an abnormally hypersensitive bile acid feedback mechanism, impaired bile acid synthesis, or abnormal intestinal bile acid loss. A combination of these two defects, along with impaired gallbladder function, results in bile cholesterol supersaturation.

The primary human bile acids, cholic acid and chenodeoxycholic acid, are synthesized by saturation and hydroxilation of cholesterol with oxidative cleavage of its side chain (Fig. 10-5). Thus, cholesterol is a precursor of primary bile acids, and bile acid biosynthesis plays a role in cholesterol homeostasis. Also, the activity of microsomal cholesterol 7α-hydroxylase, the rate-limiting enzyme in the main pathway for bile acid synthesis, is reduced by the more hydrophobic bile acids (e.g., chenodeoxycholic acid, deoxycholic acid, and lithocholic acid). Because secondary bile acids, which are produced by the exposure of primary bile acids to intestinal bacteria (Fig. 10-6) are hydrophobic, the enterohepatic circulation of bile acids plays a role in regulating hepatic bile acid biosynthesis.

Cholesterol Crystal Nucleation in Bile. Nucleation of cholesterol monohydrate crystals is an initial and essential step in the process of cholesterol gallstone formation (Carey, 1978). It is generally agreed that nucleation occurs rapidly in the gallbladder bile of cholesterol gallstone patients, whereas it does so only slowly in the gallbladder bile from stone-free subjects. Thus, determination of the *nucleation time,* which is the interval needed for the first detection of cholesterol monohydrate crystals by polarizing microscopy, permits a clear delineation of normal bile from abnormal bile. Recent reports demonstrate that the difference in nucleation time between metastable bile from cholesterol gallstone patients and from stone-free subjects is based on the balance between pronucleating factors and antinucleating factors. The principal pronucleating factor, which promotes the nucleation of cholesterol monohydrate crystals, is mucin secreted by the gallbladder mucosa. Based on data demonstrating that mucin accelerates the nucleation of cholesterol monohydrate crystals in supersaturated model bile solution and native bile, mucin is considered to play a role as a pronucleating factor. Mucin has hydrophobic domains, a binding site for hydrophobic molecules (e.g., cholesterol, lecithin, bilirubin), and hy-

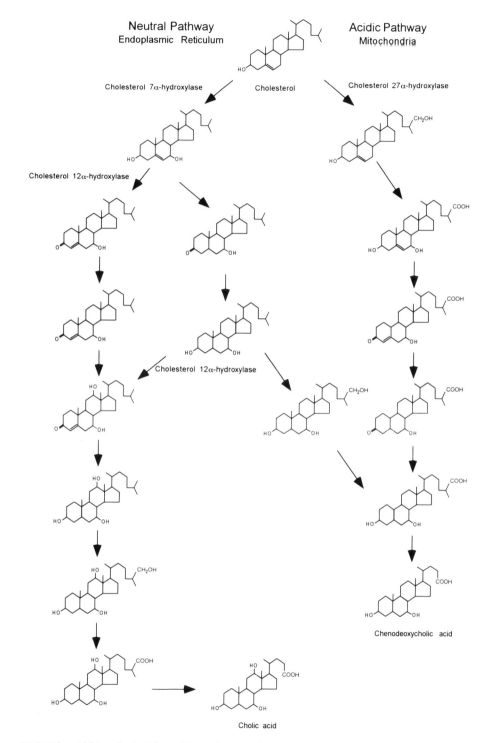

Figure 10-5. Bile acid biosynthesis. Bile acid biosynthesis involves two pathways: The main pathway (the 'neutral pathway') accomplishes the conversion of cholesterol to cholic acid or chenodeoxycholic acid, which is catalyzed by the microsomal enzymes, cholesterol 7α-hydroxylase, and 12α-hydroxylase. In contrast, another pathway (the 'acidic pathway') involves oxidative cleavage of the side chain of cholesterol, which is catalyzed by the mitochondrial enzyme, 27α-hydroxylase.

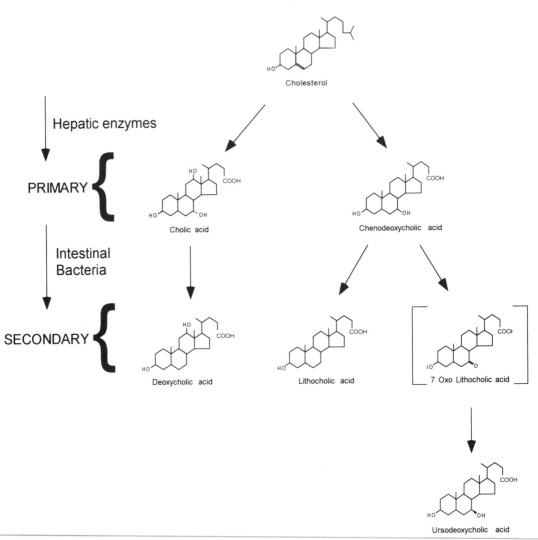

Figure 10-6. Structures of major bile acids in human bile. Primary bile acids are converted to secondary bile acids by bacterial 7-dehydroxylation, which occurs in the intestine.

drophilic domains to which water-soluble molecules (e.g., calcium ions) in bile can bind. Furthermore, mucin serves as a protective layer over the gallbladder mucosa. A thick viscous mucin gel forms as the unstirred water layer over the gallbladder surface. The nucleation of cholesterol crystals occurs in the mucin gel. Thus, the mucin gel serves as a site for nucleation. In contrast, potential antinucleating factors, which have been demonstrated to retard the nucleation of cholesterol monohydrate crystals, are apolipoproteins A-I and A-II, which are the principal constituents of human high-density lipoprotein. These apolipoproteins are also present in human bile, where they prolong the nucleation of cholesterol monohydrate crystals. The proposed mechanism whereby apolipoproteins A-I and A-II inhibit cholesterol crystal nucleation is stabilization of nonmicellar cholesterol through formation of lipid-protein complexes.

Lecithin-cholesterol vesicles are metastable, whereas bile acid micelles are stable (Hatsushika et al., 1993). Cholesterol-rich vesicles with a molar ratio of cholesterol to lecithin greater than 1.0 are unstable; they preferentially aggregate and fuse to form larger muiltilamellar vesicles which release cholesterol, thereby resulting in cholesterol nucleation. In contrast, lecithin-rich vesicles with a molar ratio of cholesterol to lecithin of less than 1.0 are stable and hold their cholesterol tightly. Thus, the vesicle is thought to be the site where cholesterol monohydrate crystals nucleate. Such a vesicle transformation process is enhanced by mucin that has a hydrophobic domain to which lipids in bile can bind. In contrast, apolipoproteins A-1 and A-2 stabilize vesicles by forming lipid-protein complexed particles similar to lipoproteins in the serum and thereby inhibit cholesterol crystal nucleation.

Cholesterol-packing density in lipid bilayers of biliary vesicles is regulated by the hydrophobicity of lecithin. Hydrophobic lecithin binds tightly to cholesterol to form stable vesicles, whereas hydrophilic lecithin binds less tightly to cholesterol to form unstable vesicles (Hatsushika et al., 1993; Tao et al., 1993). Lecithin hydrophobicity relates to the degree of fatty acyl chain saturation. Because lecithin species are subject to dietary manipulations, the bile cholesterol metastability is determined in part by the fatty acid composition of dietary fat.

Gallbladder Function and Cholesterol Gallstone Formation. The gallbladder plays a crucial role in the process of cholesterol crystal growth to macroscopic stones. A significant proportion of patients with gallstones have a hypofunctioning gallbladder. Impaired gallbladder emptying leads to the stasis of bile, and this provides the time needed for cholesterol crystal nucleation and precipitation to occur within a mucin gel on the surface of the gallbladder.

Prolonged exposure of the gallbladder epithelium to bile with a high degree of cholesterol saturation (termed *lithogenic bile*) and a high proportion of arachidonoyl or linoleoyl lecithin is thought to result in mucin hypersecretion by the gallbladder wall. Free polyunsaturated fatty acids and lysolecithin produced by phospholipase A_2 present in the bile or on the surface of the gallbladder mucosa stimulate mucin secretion by the gallbladder epithelium.

Long-term parenteral *hyperalimentation* (intravenous nutrition without oral intake for patients with inflammatory bowel diseases or those after gastrointestinal surgery) causes gallbladder stasis and also frequently causes the formation of biliary sludge, which is an amorphous material. When sludge is examined microscopically, both cholesterol monohydrate crystals and insoluble calcium bilirubinate granules (presumably bilirubin polymers) embedded in a mucin gel can be seen. The gallbladder mucosa shows glandular hyperplasia, and hyper secretion of epithelial mucin into the gallbladder bile is evident. Thus, gallbladder stasis leads to the formation of a thick viscous mucin gel that provides a site for the formation of biliary sludge. Other causes of gallbladder stasis include pregnancy and use of oral contraceptives. Under these situations, the rate of emptying of the gallbladder decreases progressively with the duration of gestation, thereby increasing the fasting gallbladder volume and the residual volume after contraction.

Pathogenesis of Pigment Gallstones

The mechanism(s) whereby pigment gallstones form remains conjectural, although stone composition, clinical associations, and natural history are well documented (Ostrow, 1984).

Black Stones

Black stones form in the gallbladder. Their major components are mucin glycoproteins and insoluble unconjugated bilirubin polymers. Pathogenic factors include: (1) a high concentration of insoluble unconjugated bilirubin; (2) a decrease in the quantity of bile acid available to solubilize bilirubin; (3) an excess of mucin glycoproteins secreted from the gallbladder epithelium; and (4) an increased concentration of ionized calcium. These factors support the following mechanistic hypothesis: (1) that increased excretion of free bilirubin or nonbacterial hydrolysis of conjugated bilirubin leads to an excess amount of unconjugated bilirubin; (2) that a relative deficiency of bile salts results in an increase in ionized calcium and a decrease in the solubility of unconjugated bilirubin, which together, result in precipitation of unconjugated bilirubin; and, finally, (3) that an excess of mucin glycoprotein secreted by the gallbladder enhances precipitation of bilirubin.

Brown Stones

The clinical correlations of brown stones are biliary stasis and bacterial infection. Bacteria and an injured biliary epithelium release β-glucuronidase and phospholipase into bile. These enzymes hydrolyze conjugated bilirubin and lecithin to produce unconjugated bilirubin and free fatty acids, respectively.

Thus, the major components in brown stones (i.e., calcium bilirubinate and calcium soaps of fatty acids) are formed as a result of the action of these enzymes.

THERAPY

Dissolution Therapy with Bile Acids (Adjuvant Bile Acid Therapy)

One well-established nonsurgical treatment of cholesterol gallstones involves dissolution therapy with chenodeoxycholic acid (CDCA) and ursodeoxycholic acid (UDCA). The ideal candidate for bile acid therapy is a mildly symptomatic patient with uncalcified small stones with a diameter of <15 mm in a functioning gallbladder. UDCA dissolves cholesterol stones through liquid crystal formation, whereas CDCA does so by forming micelles with cholesterol and lecithin. UDCA alone or in combination with CDCA is used preferably for dissolution therapy because CDCA has the side effect of being hepatotoxic.

Direct Dissolution Therapy

Direct dissolution therapy with the organic solvent methyl *tert*-butyl ether can be performed via *percutaneous transhepatic catheterization* (indwelling a catheter into the bile duct through the liver and skin) or *endoscopic transpapillary catheterization* (indwelling a catheter into the bile duct through the papilla of Vater using an endoscopy). In general, this strategy is still considered a supplementary option.

Extracorporeal Shock Wave Lithotripsy (ESWL)

Fragmentation of stones by extracorporeal shock waves is highly effective in eliminating a solitary cholesterol gallstone if its diameter is <30 mm. A combination of ESWL and adjuvant bile acid therapy is performed for patients with a larger cholesterol stone in a functioning gallbladder. Fragmentation of gallstones into small particles can aid in overcoming problems of large stones by increasing the surface area/volume ratio and disrupting localized area of calcium salts. Thus, stone dissolution by bile acids (i.e., UDCA, CDCA) is accelerated after fragmentation by ESWL. Fragments with a diameter <3 mm can be cleared by gallbladder emptying in a few weeks.

Endoscopic Lithotripy

Based on a number of clinical investigations, endoscopic extraction is to be initially attempted for the treatment of *choledocholithiasis* (stones located in the common bile duct). Most stones that occur in bile ducts are successfully extracted by endoscopic lithotripsy alone. A combination of endoscopic sphincterotomy and ESWL is occasionally effective for the treatment of large stones with a diameter >30 mm. The present case was subjected to endoscopic extraction of stones in the common bile duct.

Cholecystectomy

Symptomatic gallstone patients who cannot be successfully treated with nonsurgical approaches and those who have stones in both of the gallbladder and bile ducts are candidates for laparoscopic or open cholecystectomy. The present case was subjected to laparoscopic cholecystectomy after successful extraction of ductal stones by endoscopic lithotripsy.

QUESTIONS

1. What is the mechanism(s) whereby substances influencing cholesterol crystal nucleation modulate bile cholesterol metastability?
2. What is the mechanism(s) by which the ratio of calcium bilirubinate to black pigment polymers in pigment gallstones is regulated?
3. What is the major disadvantage of cholecystectomy? Do any defects occur in the enterohepatic circulation of bile acids and lipids after cholecystectomy?
4. What is the difference in the pathogenesis of pure cholesterol gallstone formation and mixed gallstone formation?

REFERENCES

Admirand WH, Small DM: The physicochemical basis of cholesterol gallstone formation in man. *J Clin Invest* **61**:998–1026, 1978.

Carey MC: Critical tables for calculating the cholesterol saturation of native bile. *J Lipid Res* **19**:945–955, 1978.

Coleman R: Biochemistry of bile secretion. *Biochem J* **244**:249–261, 1987.

Groen AK, Noordam C, Drapers JAG, et al.: Isolation of a potent cholesterol nucleation-promoting activity from human gallbladder bile: role in the pathogenesis of gallstone disease. *Hepatology* **11**:525–533, 1991.

Hatsushika S, Tazuma, S, Kajiyama G: Nucleation time and fatty acid composition of lecithin in human gallbladder bile. *Scand J Gastroenterol* **28**:131–136, 1993.

Holan KR, Holzbach RT, Hermann RE, et al.: Nucleation time: a key factor in the pathogenesis of cholesterol gallstone disease. *Gastroenterology* **77:**611–617, 1979.

Holzbach RT: Nucleation of cholesterol crystals in native bile. *Hepatology* **12:**155s–161s, 1990.

Ostrow JD: The etiology of pigment gallstones. *Hepatology* **4:**215S–222S, 1984.

Small DM: Cholesterol nucleation and growth in gallstone formation. *N Engl J Med* **302:**1305–1307, 1980.

Tao S, Tazuma S, Kajiyama G: Fatty acid composition of lecithin is a key factor in bile metastability in supersaturated model bile systems. *Biochim Biophys Acta* **1167:**142–146, 1993.

Tazuma S, Holzbach RT: Transport of conjugated bilirubin and other organic anions in bile: relation to biliary lipid structures. *Proc Natl Acad Sci USA* **84:**2052–2056, 1987.

11

Pernicious Anemia

DOROTHY J. VANDERJAGT AND DENIS M. McCARTHY

CASE REPORT

The patient, a 52-year-old man, made an appointment with his primary care physician because he was concerned about his progressive loss of energy. He complained of numbness and tingling in his toes and feet and a loss of balance on several occasions, most noticeably when walking in the dark. He also complained of a sore tongue, which made it difficult to eat. The patient was 5 ft 10 in (178 cm) tall and weighed 146 lbs (66.4 kg). He reported having lost 10 lbs (4.5 kg) over the last 6 months. The physical examination was normal except for pale skin and mucous membranes and a bald, pale atrophic tongue. His blood pressure was 128/72 mm Hg (normal, 120/80 mm Hg). His pulse rate was 86 beats per minute (normal, 72 beats per minute) and his respiration rate was 18 per minute (normal, 12 per minute). The physical examination revealed that the patient had difficulty keeping his balance and knowing the position of his fingers and toes when his eyes were closed. He also exhibited a loss of vibrational sense at the ankles and wrists.

Based on the finding of pale mucous membranes during the physical examination and the report of fatigue by the patient, a preliminary diagnosis of anemia was made. A complete blood count with differential white blood cell count was ordered as well as determinations of serum iron and total iron binding capacity, serum vitamin B_{12}, and serum and red blood cell folate concentrations. The hemoglobin concentration (10 g/dL) and hematocrit (38%) were below the normal limits for the patient's age and sex

(14–18 g/dL and 42–53%, respectively). The white blood cell count was 6100/mm³ (normal, 5000–11,000/mm³), and the platelet count was 110,000/mm³ (normal, 150,000–400,000/mm³). A peripheral blood smear (Fig. 11-1) showed the presence of *macro-ovalocytes* (large, egg-shaped red cells) and an increase in hypersegmented neutrophils (Fig. 11-2, polymorphs with five or more lobes in the nucleus). The mean corpuscular volume was 115 fL (normal, 80–94 fL), with a mean cell hemoglobin of 26 pg (normal, 25–32 pg) and a mean cell hemoglobin concentration of 26.3 g/L (normal, 31.5–36.5 g/L). The serum iron was 34 μmol/L (normal, 14–32 μmol/L) and the total iron binding capacity was 45 μmol/L (normal, 45–82 μmol/L), with a 77% saturation of transferrin (normal, 30–35%). The serum folate concentration was 32 nmol/L (normal, 4–22 nmol/L), whereas the red blood cell folate concentration was depressed at 317 nmol/L (normal, 550–2200 nmol/L). The serum vitamin B_{12} was 48 pmol/L (normal, 150–750 pmol/L).

A diagnosis of vitamin B_{12} deficiency was made on the basis of clinical findings and laboratory data. The patient was administered cyanocobalamin (1000 μg intramuscularly) and injections of 1000 μg per day thereafter for 10 days while his reticulocyte count was monitored. Three weeks after the initiation of vitamin B_{12} therapy, the Schilling test was performed (see Diagnosis section). The amount of radio-labelled aqueous vitamin B_{12} excreted over 24 hours was <1% of the administered dose (normal, ≥10%). When the test was repeated with exogenous intrinsic factor (IF) added to the oral dose of radio-

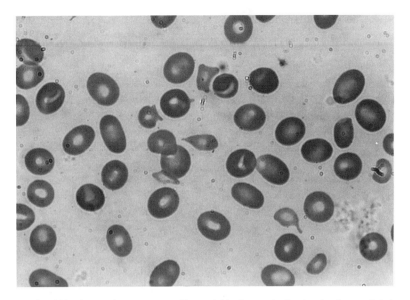

Figure 11-1. A peripheral blood smear from a patient with megaloblastic anemia showing the characteristic large oval red blood cells (>8 μm in diameter) referred to as *macro-ovalocytes.*

labelled aqueous vitamin B_{12}, the patient excreted 13% of the total labelled B_{12} dose. His serum contained high titers of antibodies both to IF and to gastric parietal cells. Together, these findings confirm the diagnosis of pernicious anemia (PA). The patient was then started on monthly injections of 1000 μg vitamin B_{12}.

Follow-up hematological tests were repeated after the patient had been receiving vitamin B_{12} therapy for 3 months. A peripheral blood smear showed an absence of macrocytes and hypersegmented neutrophils. The mean corpuscular volume decreased to 92 fL, and the hemoglobin and hematocrit levels increased to 16 g/dL and 46.8%, respectively. The

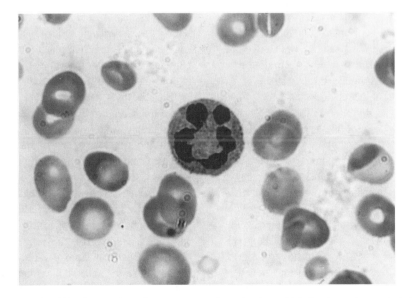

Figure 11-2. A peripheral blood smear from the same patient shown in Figure 11-1 showing a characteristic hypersegmented neutrophil (>5 nuclear lobes) observed in macrocytic anemia due to vitamin B_{12} or folate deficiency.

plasma folate concentration was 20 nmol/L, the red blood cell folate concentration 530 nmol/L. The serum vitamin B_{12} concentration increased to 155 pmol/L. The patient also stated that he had more energy and that the tingling in his extremities had decreased greatly. In addition, he had gained 3 lbs (1.4 kg) since his first clinic visit. Vitamin B_{12} injection therapy will be continued for the lifetime of the patient because of his confirmed inability to produce IF. The patient will be monitored on a regular basis to determine the optimal frequency and amount of intramuscular B_{12} necessary to maintain acceptable hematological indices over the long term.

ETIOLOGY AND PATHOGENESIS

Megaloblastic anemia is characterized by the presence of megaloblasts (unusually large stem cells) in the bone marrow that mature into unusually large erythrocytes (*macrocytes*) in the circulation. Although the hemoglobin content in the red cells is normal, the nucleus is disproportionately small in relation to the size of the bone marrow cell as the result of defective DNA synthesis.

Pernicious anemia is a megaloblastic anemia that occurs after prolonged deficiency of vitamin B_{12}. It arises from a failure of secretion of IF, a vitamin B_{12} binding protein that is required for the intestinal absorption of the vitamin. Decreased secretion of IF is a consequence of atrophy of the glands of the fundus and body of the stomach, which secrete HCl and pepsin and is thought to be caused by complement-fixing autoantibodies directed against parietal cells (Burman et al., 1989; Karlsson et al., 1988). The region of the tubulovesicular membrane where the enzyme H^+/K^+ ATPase (the "proton pump") is located is a specific target of antiparietal cell autoantibodies. Gastric H^+/K^+-ATPase, which mediates the secretion of protons across the apical membrane of parietal cells, consists of a catalytic α-subunit and a β-subunit whose functions are unknown (Gleeson and Toh, 1991; Song et al., 1994).

Pernicious anemia is the most common cause of vitamin B_{12} deficiency in Western populations, although achlorhydria, gastric surgical procedures, abnormal colonization of the small intestine, ileal disease or resection, and certain parasitic infestations may also cause it (Cooper and Zittoun, 1989).

It is more common in blacks and in persons of northern European descent and less common in Orientals and those of southern European descent. The incidence of the disease increases with age: It is estimated that one in 100 people over the age of 65 has the disease. Except for congenital or juvenile PA, which manifests at about 2 years of age, it is rare in people aged under 30 years. Juvenile PA is not due to immune-mediated gastric injury but results from secretion of an abnormal, biologically ineffective IF by an otherwise normal mucosa.

DIAGNOSIS

The symptoms associated with PA are primarily those characteristic of vitamin B_{12} deficiency and include a variety of hematological, neurological, and gastrointestinal symptoms. The principal hematological sign of vitamin B_{12} deficiency is anemia, accompanied by findings of an elevated mean corpuscular volume and hypersegmentation of neutrophils in the bone marrow and peripheral blood. The red cells usually vary in size so that the mean corpuscular volume in patients with severe megaloblastic anemia ranges from 110 to 140 fL (normal, <100 fL). The size of the red cell is usually proportional to the severity of disease.

The neurological symptoms of PA include weakness, *paresthesiae* (numbness and tingling) of the extremities, ataxia, forgetfulness, and in the more severe cases, dementia, which occurs late in the course of the disease. Neurological problems or cognitive impairment may present even in the absence of obvious anemia, but this is exceptional.

When the disease is advanced, epithelial cell turnover and differentiation are abnormal throughout the gastrointestinal tract, resulting in a variety of minor nonspecific symptoms. Lack of acid peptic activity results in an inefficient release of protein bound B_{12} in food. Because of achlorhydria, gastric antral D-cells, which secrete somatostatin in response to luminal H^+ concentration, are unstimulated, resulting in unopposed release of gastrin by antral G-cells and consequent hypergastrinemia. Gastrin is trophic to the enterochromaffin-like (ECL) cells of gastric fundic mucosa, and with prolonged hypergastrinemia these cells proliferate and form multiple small benign carcinoid tumors in the stomachs of patients with PA. These tumors regress following excision of the gastric antrum. Although most are benign, these tumors do have a low malignant potential; 1 to 2% of PA patients also develop hyperplastic gastric polyps and rarely gastric adenocarcinomas.

Laboratory tests for PA include a complete blood count and the determination of serum vitamin B_{12} concentrations, measured using either microbiological or radioimmunoassay procedures. Microbiological assays use microorganisms that have a specific requirement for vitamin B_{12} for growth. The microorganisms used most frequently for vitamin B_{12} determinations are *Lactobacillus leichmanni, Euglena gracilis,* and *Ochromonas malhamensis.* In the microbiological assay, an aliquot of diluted serum is added to medium containing all of the necessary nutrients required by the microorganism except vitamin B_{12}. Growth of the culture is monitored by changes in the turbidity of the culture medium. Because the test microorganisms cannot use nonfunctional analogues of vitamin B_{12}, this assay reliably measures the biologically active form of vitamin B_{12}. Because microbiological assays are time consuming and subject to interference by antibiotics, antimetabolites, or tranquilizers present in the blood, most laboratories now use radioimmunoassay methods to measure vitamin B_{12} concentrations in serum.

The radioimmunoassay for serum vitamin B_{12} is a competitive binding assay that uses radiolabelled vitamin B_{12} (^{58}Co or ^{57}Co) and a specific B_{12} binding protein, such as IF, which is added to the assay mixture in limiting amounts. The unlabeled B_{12} from the serum competes with labelled vitamin B_{12} for the binding sites on the protein, thus reducing the amount of isotope that is bound. Separation of the bound and free vitamin B_{12} is accomplished by the addition of activated charcoal to the reaction mixture to absorb the free vitamin B_{12} molecules. Following centrifugation to pellet the charcoal, the amount of radioactivity remaining in the supernatant is measured. The amount of bound radiolabelled cobalamin remaining in the supernatant fraction is inversely proportional to the amount of vitamin B_{12} present in the original sample. Procedures that employ purified IF provide the best estimate of "true" cobalamin concentration because the high degree of specificity of the IF for cobalamin eliminates any interference from nonfunctional vitamin B_{12} analogues that may be present in the specimen being analyzed. In pernicious anemia, serum concentrations of vitamin B_{12} are usually below 74 pmol/L (normal 150–750 pmol/L) by the time anemia is present.

Macrocytic anemia caused by vitamin B_{12} deficiency is indistinguishable by hematological methods from anemia caused by folic acid deficiency. Therefore, serum and red blood cell folate should also be measured in patients suspected of having PA (Allen et al., 1993). In macrocytic anemia resulting from folic acid deficiency, both serum and red blood cell folate concentrations are abnormally low, whereas in vitamin B_{12} deficiency with adequate folic acid, the red blood cell folate concentration is usually diminished with a slight elevation of 5-methyl-folate in serum. Serum and urinary homocysteine concentrations are elevated in both vitamin B_{12} and folate deficiency, with similar elevations of serum and urinary methylmalonic acid in B_{12} deficiency but not in folate deficiency. Elevations of serum and urinary homocysteine and methylmalonic acid are not specific to vitamin B_{12} deficiency but are sensitive indicators of its existence in patients.

Folates exist in food as polyglutamates that contain a chain of two to seven glutamic acid residues long linked to the *p*-aminobenzoic acid portion of the folate molecule. Before intestinal absorption, the polyglutamate forms of folate are converted to the monoglutamate form by pteroylpolyglutamate hydrolase located on the brush borders of cells of the proximal small intestine. After the monoglutamate form of folate is absorbed, it is transported to the liver and peripheral tissues, where the polyglutamate form is resynthesized. In vitamin B_{12} deficiency, the unconjugated methyl-folate is not converted to the forms of folate required for DNA synthesis (see Molecular Perspectives section). In experimental animals, 5-methyl-folate is a poor substrate for the conjugating enzyme that forms the polyglutamated derivative of folic acid; therefore, 5-methyl-folate that remains unconjugated slowly leaks from the cells, resulting in decreased cellular and elevated serum concentrations.

Once vitamin B_{12} deficiency has been confirmed by measurement of serum vitamin B_{12}, the diagnosis of PA is made by means of the Schilling test (Schilling, 1995) and measurement of gastric autoantibodies. In the Schilling test, which measures vitamin B_{12} absorption, the patient is administered a parenteral injection of "cold" aqueous vitamin B_{12} to saturate all the B_{12} binding sites in the liver and on transcobalamin (TCII, vitamin B_{12} transport protein) in the blood to ensure that any radiolabelled B_{12} that is absorbed will remain unbound and be excreted in the urine. The patient is then given an oral dose of radioactively labelled aqueous B_{12} (^{57}Co or ^{58}Co cyanocobalamin) (Part I of the Schilling test). The total amount of radiolabelled vitamin B_{12} excreted in the urine over a 24-hour period is then determined. Healthy adults without PA will excrete more than 10% of the labelled dose, whereas a patient with PA will excrete less (usually 1–4%). To prove that the vitamin B_{12} absorption problem is due to a lack of IF, the test is then repeated using the same dose of labelled B_{12} combined with exogenous IF (Part II of the Schilling test). If the vitamin B_{12} deficiency is the result of insufficient secretion of endogenous IF, the Part II Schilling test should yield a normal result (>10% of the labelled dose will be absorbed). This will not be the case if the patient has bacterial overgrowth, parasitic infestation, or pancreatic insufficiency, however. The Schilling test should be postponed until the patient has been treated for B_{12} deficiency for several weeks because many patients have intestinal mucosal abnormalities due to B_{12} deficiency, which interferes with vitamin B_{12} absorption. All gastric antisecretory drugs, such as H_2-receptor antagonists or proton pump inhibitors, should be stopped one week before the test.

Anti-intrinsic factor (anti-IF) antibody is present in the serum of 60 to 90% of patients with PA. Because false-positive results are extremely uncommon, the presence of anti-IF antibody in the serum is a useful marker for PA; thus, it can be assumed with a high degree of certainty that a cobalamin-deficient patient who has anti-IF antibody has PA; however, the absence of anti-IF antibody does not exclude the diagnosis. Antiparietal cell microsomal antibodies are also usually present in the serum of patients with PA; however, because these antibodies also occur in about 50% of patients with gastric atrophy without apparent PA, their presence is not specific to PA. In addition, the serum gastrin concentration should be determined; although it is not diagnostic of PA, patients who have very high serum gastrin concentrations are at increased risk of carcinoid tumor development. In the absence of circulating antigastric antibodies and in the presence of vitamin B_{12} malabsorption that does not correct with IF administration,

other causes of vitamin B_{12} deficiency should be sought. Deficiency should be treated with vitamin B_{12} injections in all cases for life.

In some elderly patients or in those with acquired immunodeficiency syndrome (AIDS), serum B_{12} concentrations may be low without evident hematologic or neurologic abnormalities. In such patients exposure to nitrous oxide anaesthesia may precipitate neurological deterioration. Nitrous oxide irreversibly oxidizes the cobalt atom in the corrin ring of vitamin B_{12}, resulting the the excretion of inactive vitamin B_{12} in the urine (see Molecular Perspectives section).

MOLECULAR PERSPECTIVES

The structure of vitamin B_{12} (cobalamin) and its role in human metabolism were revealed largely through the study of PA. Although PA was described as long ago as 1870, it was not until 1926 that George Minot and William Murphy (Minot and Murphy, 1926) demonstrated that the symptoms of this once fatal disease could be alleviated by nutritional intervention, specifically by the ingestion of large amounts of liver. It was also recognized in the 1920s that PA is associated with significant atrophy of the gastric mucosa. These observations led William Castle in 1928 to hypothesize that the stomach produces a substance (intrinsic factor) that acts with some dietary substance (extrinsic factor) to prevent PA. The extrinsic factor, later named vitamin B_{12}, was obtained in crystalline form in 1948. Its final structure was determined by Dorothy Hodgkins using X-ray crystallography, an accomplishment for which she was awarded the Nobel Prize in chemistry in 1964.

The structure of vitamin B_{12} is shown in Figure 11-3. It is composed of a planar corrin ring that contains a single cobalt atom at the center. The corrin ring system, which resembles the porphyrin rings of heme, is composed of four reduced pyrrole rings linked by three methylene bridges and a single saturated bond between the third and fourth rings. The cobalt atom is coordinated to each of the nitrogen atoms of the four pyrrole rings, a dimethylbenzimidazole group, and a sixth ligand, which may be a cyanide, hydroxyl, methyl, or adenosyl moiety.

Because the vitamin B_{12} that occurs in nature is produced almost entirely by bacterial synthesis (Bat-

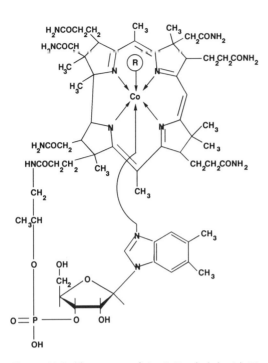

Figure 11-3. The structure of vitamin B_{12} (cobalamin). Vitamin B_{12} is composed of a planar corrin ring containing a cobalt atom at the center. The corrin ring system is composed of four pyrrole rings and is similar to porphyrin in heme. The cobalt atom is coordinated to the nitrogens of each pyrrole ring and to a dimethylbenzimidazole group. The R group attached to the sixth coordination site of the cobalt atom in vitamin B_{12} can be a -CN, -OH, $-CH_3$, or adenosyl group.

tersby, 1994), humans must obtain the vitamin from the diet. The richest dietary sources of vitamin B_{12} are organ meats, such as liver and kidney. Lesser amounts are present in shellfish, chicken, fish, muscle meats, and dairy products. Plants contain no vitamin B_{12} unless they are contaminated by bacteria, and foods that contain microorganisms often provide the only source of B_{12} for strict vegetarians, such as the vegans of southern India.

The two active coenzyme forms in human metabolism are 5'-adenosylcobalamin and methyl-cobalamin. Adenosylcobalamin is the primary form of vitamin B_{12} in tissues. Cyanocobalamin, the therapeutic form of vitamin B_{12}, is produced by the cleavage of the unstable linkage between the 5'-deoxyadenosyl group and the cobalt ion in adenosylcobalamin during its isolation from liver. The adenosyl group is replaced by a molecule of cyanide that is leached from the charcoal columns used in the purification

procedure. Cyanocobalamin, which is not physiologically active, is readily hydrolyzed in tissues to hydroxycobalamin. As shown in Figure 11-4, hydroxycobalamin is then converted to adenosylcobalamin by the successive reactions of two flavoprotein-dependent reductases, which reduce Co^{3+} to Co^{1+}, a powerful nucleophile. The Co^{1+} then attacks the 5'-carbon of adenosine triphosphate (ATP), expelling a triphosphate anion and resulting in the synthesis of 5'-adenosylcobalamin.

Absorption and Transport of Vitamin B_{12}

In the diet, vitamin B_{12} occurs bound to proteins. Some release of protein-bound vitamin B_{12} in food begins in the mouth, but most of the release occurs in the stomach on exposure of food to gastric acid (HCl) and the proteolytic enzyme pepsin. For this reason, either *hypochlorhydria* (abnormally low concentration of HCl in the gastric fluid) or *achlorhydria* (the absence of HCl in gastric fluid) may decrease the availability of dietary vitamin B_{12} for absorption by preventing the activation of pepsinogen to pepsin, the enzyme responsible for proteolysis in the stomach. Achlorhydric patients with adequate production of IF may have low serum vitamin B_{12} concentrations, even though the absorption of labelled aqueous B_{12} (Schilling test) may be normal.

The receptor-mediated intestinal absorption of vitamin B_{12} and the delivery of the vitamin to remote sites require a series of carrier proteins for vitamin B_{12} (Fig. 11-5) (Schjonsby, 1989). The two major classes of vitamin B_{12} binding proteins present in the stomach are IF and R proteins (also referred to as haptocorrin) (Neale, 1990). The *R proteins* consist of a family of glycoproteins that can be fractionated on the basis of their sialic acid content. *Sialic acid* is a nine-carbon acidic sugar. R proteins are synthesized primarily in granulocytes but are also present in saliva, plasma, bile, tears, and milk. They were designated R proteins on the basis of their more *rapid* migration relative to IF during electrophoresis. The affinity of R proteins for vitamin B_{12} at pH 2 is about 50 times that of IF. In addition, the R protein-B_{12} complex is resistant to proteolytic degradation by pepsin at this low pH. Therefore, most vitamin B_{12} becomes bound to R protein during transit through

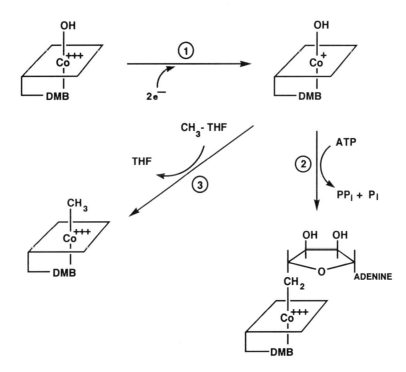

Figure 11-4. The conversion of hydroxycobalamin to methyl- and adenosylcobalamin. The cobalt atom in vitamin B_{12} that is released into the cytosol following lysosomal degradation of the TCII-cobalamin complex is in the trivalent state (Co^{+3}). After reduction of the cobalt atom to Co^{+1} by flavoprotein reductases in the cytosol ①, the cobalamin enters the mitochondria and is converted to adenosylcobalamin by adenosyl transferase ②. Alternatively, the cobalamin can remain in the cytosol, where it is methylated and bound to the enzyme methionine synthetase ③. DMB, dimethylbenzimidazole; ATP, adenosine triphosphate; THF, tetrahydrofolate; CH_3-THF, 5-methyltetrahydrofolate.

the stomach, thereby protecting the vitamin B_{12} moiety from hydrolysis.

Intrinsic factor is a 60,000-Da glycoprotein that is synthesized and secreted by gastric parietal cells. The secretion of IF is stimulated by several endogenous agents, including insulin, gastrin, histamine, and acetylcholine. Although the release of IF parallels that of gastric acid, each is secreted by distinct mechanisms. Whereas the secretion of both gastric acid and IF is decreased by atropine or by vagotomy, other agents, such as secretin and omeprazole, a H^+/K^+-ATPase antagonist drug, inhibit secretion of HCl but not of IF. The average concentration of IF in gastric fluid is 1 μg/mL, and it is secreted in amounts that are approximately 50 times greater than the estimated physiological need.

When the gastric contents reach the duodenum and the pH of the chyme is raised to neutrality, the R proteins become susceptible to degradation by pancreatic proteolytic enzymes (e.g., trypsin), causing vitamin B_{12} to be released: The free vitamin B_{12} is then immediately bound to IF. In the presence of pancreatic disease, the lack of proteolytic enzymes may result in malabsorption of B_{12} bound to R proteins, which do not bind to the receptors on ileal cells, resulting in the loss of B_{12} into the colon, where it cannot be absorbed. Intrinsic factor has two binding sites, one for vitamin B_{12} and one for the ileal receptor, which recognizes the IF-vitamin B_{12} complex (Tang et al., 1992). IF is highly specific for vitamin B_{12} and does not bind nonfunctional cobalamin analogues ingested in food or excreted in the bile.

In the duodenum, gastric contents are also mixed with bile, which contains approximately 0.5 nmol/L cobalamins. Intrinsic factor is thus available in duodenal contents to bind not only recently ingested vitamin B_{12} but also any cobalamin that has been

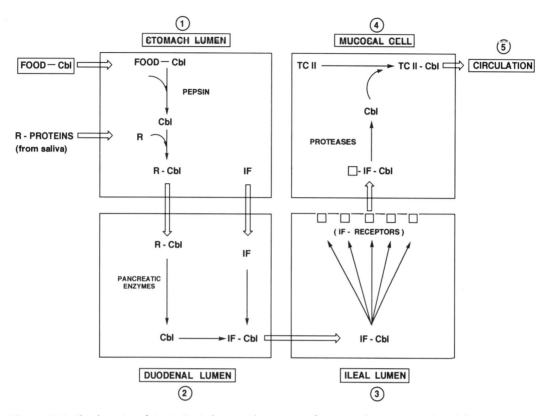

Figure 11-5. The absorption of vitamin B_{12} in humans. The sequence of transitions between protein-bound dietary vitamin B_{12} and circulating B_{12} bound to TCII. Cbl, cobalamin, vitamin B_{12}; R, R proteins; vitamin B_{12} binding proteins; IF, intrinsic factor; TCII, transcobalamin.

secreted in bile. In this way, about 90% of the vitamin B_{12} excreted in the bile is reabsorbed. This enterohepatic recirculation provides for efficient conservation of vitamin B_{12} and, together with the fact that large amounts are stored in the liver, accounts for the fact that vitamin B_{12} deficiency does not occur rapidly even in the prolonged absence of vitamin B_{12} intake. Anemia usually develops 5 to 7 years after the onset of reduced vitamin B_{12} intake or absorption whether due to dietary or other causes.

In the ileum, the IF-B_{12} complex binds to specific receptors on ileal cells for IF, resulting in absorption of the IF-B_{12} complex by receptor-mediated endocytosis. Vitamin B_{12} bound to defective forms of IF is not absorbed. Once inside the cell, the vitamin combines with an intracellular receptor before its release across the basolateral membrane into the bloodstream, where it becomes bound to transcobalamin (TCII). TCII is a β-globulin with a molecular weight of 50,000 Da, which is synthesized by a variety of tissues (primarily the liver) and is the B_{12} transport protein for recently absorbed vitamin B_{12}. Normal serum contains 0.7 to 1.5 nmol/L of TCII, which is capable of binding 600 to 1300 ng of vitamin B_{12}; however, only 10 to 20% of its binding capacity is used at any one time. Unlike TCI and TCIII, the other serum transport proteins for vitamin B_{12}, TCII is not a glycoprotein. The TCII-B_{12} complex is recognized by specific high-affinity plasma membrane receptors present on cells. After internalization, the complex is transferred to lysosomes, where TCII is rapidly degraded and the vitamin B_{12} is released. About 20% of plasma vitamin B_{12} is bound to TCII; the remainder of vitamin B_{12} in plasma is transported by TCI and TCIII, primarily in the form of 5-methylcobalamin. The specific functions of TCI and TCIII have not been determined; however, they are believed to transport potentially toxic vitamin B_{12} analogues to the liver for excretion in the bile. Vitamin B_{12} present in plasma in excess of the binding capacity of the transport proteins is excreted in the urine. Radiolabelled vitamin B_{12} is sometimes used for the determination of glomerular filtration rate in humans.

In the early stages of vitamin B_{12} deficiency, the amount of vitamin B_{12} bound to TCII decreases without any decrease in the total serum B_{12} level. The total vitamin B_{12} concentration begins to decline only when the saturation of TCII falls below 5%. Reduced saturation of TCII is one of the earliest indicators of vitamin B_{12} deficiency and may be a diagnostic feature of vitamin B_{12} deficiency in advance of developing clinical disease. Elevated serum and urine concentrations of methylmalonic acid may serve a similar purpose.

The total body pool of vitamin B_{12} in humans ranges from 2 to 5 mg, most of which is stored in the liver. The total serum B_{12} concentration reflects body stores of B_{12} only when liver concentrations fall below 0.6 μg/g wet weight (normal, 0.6–1.5 μg/g wet weight). Moderately low serum vitamin B_{12} concentrations (110–148 pmol/L) may not be specific for vitamin B_{12} deficiency; however, serum vitamin B_{12} concentrations below 74 pmol/L are almost always associated with B_{12} deficiency. Daily losses of vitamin B_{12} are usually 1 to 3 μg/day, or approximately 0.1% of total body stores. These losses occur primarily through excretion of vitamin B_{12} in bile and through sloughing of gastrointestinal epithelium. Although a dietary intake of 1 μg/day is probably sufficient to meet the needs of most adults, the recommended dietary allowance is 2 μg/day to allow for individual variability and to ensure maintenance of body stores (Herbert, 1987). The average American diet contains 5 to 30 μg/day of vitamin B_{12}. Elderly achlorhydric patients with normal IF but low serum vitamin B_{12} are usually treated with a multivitamin complex containing 10 μg of aqueous cyanocobalamin.

Metabolic Functions of Vitamin B_{12}

Vitamin B_{12} is required by only two mammalian enzymes, methionine synthetase and L-methylmalonyl-coenzyme A (CoA) mutase. Methionine synthetase has an absolute requirement for methylcobalamin and catalyzes the conversion of homocysteine to methionine (Fig. 11-6.) Methyltetrahydrofolate, which is formed by an irreversible reaction catalyzed by

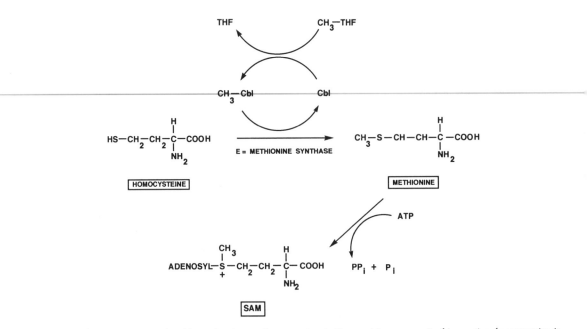

Figure 11-6. The reaction catalyzed by methionine synthetase, a vitamin B_{12} requiring enzyme. In this reaction, homocysteine is converted to methionine, with the simultaneous production of tetrahydrofolate (THF) from 5-CH_3- THF. Methionine can then be converted to S-adenosylmethionine (SAM), the universal methyl-group donor.

methylene-THF-reductase, is simultaneously converted to tetrahydrofolate in this reaction. This vitamin B_{12}-catalyzed reaction is the only means by which THF can be regenerated from 5-methyl-THF in humans. Therefore, in vitamin B_{12} deficiency, folic acid can become "trapped" in the 5-methyl-folate form, and THF is then unavailable for conversion to other coenzyme forms required for purine, pyrimidine, and amino acid synthesis. All folate-dependent reactions are impaired in vitamin B_{12} deficiency, resulting in indistinguishable hematologic abnormalities in both folate and B_{12} deficiencies.

The catabolism of certain amino acids (e.g., valine, isoleucine, methionine) and odd-chain fatty acids produces propionyl-CoA. Propionyl-CoA enters the TCA cycle following conversion to succinyl-CoA, as shown in Figure 11-7. Propionyl-CoA is first carboxylated to produce D-methylmalonyl-CoA, which in turn is then racemized to L-methylmalonyl-CoA, which is then converted to succinyl-CoA in an intra-

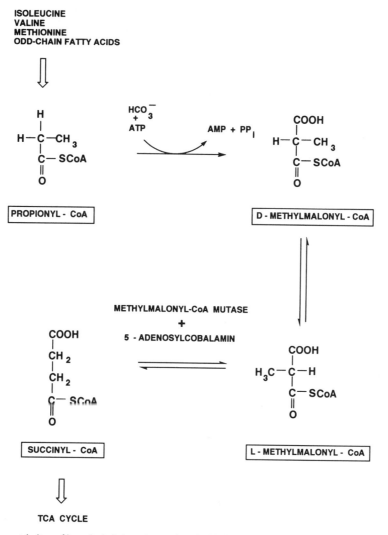

Figure 11-7. The metabolism of branched-chain amino acids and odd-chain fatty acids via propionyl-CoA. Propionyl-coenzyme A (CoA) is converted to D-methylmalonyl-CoA by propionyl-CoA carboxylase. D,L-methylmalonyl-CoA racemase catalyzes the conversion of D-methylmalonyl-CoA to L-methylmalonyl-CoA. L-methylmalonyl-CoA mutase, an adenosylcobalamin-requiring enzyme, converts L-methylmalonyl-CoA to succinyl-CoA. TCA cycle: citric acid cycle, Kreb's cycle.

molecular rearrangement reaction catalyzed by L-methylmalonyl-CoA mutase, a vitamin B_{12}-requiring enzyme. As a consequence of vitamin B_{12} deficiency, cellular levels of both propionyl-CoA and methylmalonyl-CoA increase. Propionyl-CoA can then substitute for acetyl-CoA in fatty acid synthesis, leading to the production of fatty acids comprised of an odd number of carbon atoms. Similarly, methylmalonyl-CoA can substitute for malonyl-CoA in fatty acid synthesis, resulting in the synthesis of branched chain fatty acids. Myelination is essential to the normal function of sensory neurons. Because the synthesis of normal myelin is dependent on the availability of specific fatty acids, the inclusion of abnormal fatty acids (e.g., odd-chain, branched-chain fatty acids) in myelin may alter neural function or cause premature demyelination. This hypothesis has been put forth to explain the neurological impairment observed in vitamin B_{12} deficiency (Shevell and Rosenblatt, 1992).

Methionine, through subsequent conversion to S-adenosylmethionine (see Fig. 11-6), is also required for the synthesis of choline and choline-containing phospholipids and for the methylation of myelin basic protein. Although the mechanism responsible for the development of neurological impairment resulting from vitamin B_{12} deficiency has not been precisely defined, defective methionine metabolism may also contribute to neurological complications in vitamin B_{12}-deficient patients.

THERAPY

Treatment of PA is accomplished by vitamin B_{12} replacement therapy. Because the defect is one of absorption, the vitamin B_{12} must be administered parenterally, usually by intramuscular injection of cyanocobalamin. Initial therapy usually consists of four alternate-day injections of vitamin B_{12} intramuscularly or intravenously and an additional injection 2 weeks later. Subsequently, injections of 1000 μg of vitamin B_{12} every 4 weeks should be continued for life. The response to replacement therapy is usually rapid, with changes noted in the first days after treatment. The morphology of the bone marrow cells begins to return to normal a few hours after administration of the vitamin. In clinical practice, approximately 4 to 5 days after initiation of therapy, an increasing reticulocytosis is observed, which

peaks at 15 to 20% on approximately day 7. The painful tongue improves in several days and serum folate levels decrease, indicating increased use of folate by cells. There are no known toxic effects of cobalamin.

An important point to recognize in patient management is that patients with megaloblastic anemia should never be treated with folic acid until their serum vitamin B_{12} concentrations have been measured and any vitamin B_{12} deficiency corrected. Administration of folic acid to vitamin B_{12} deficient patients may promote B_{12} use by bone marrow, which could cause an already low serum B_{12} concentration to fall precipitously, resulting in severe and sometimes irreversible deterioration in the patient's neurological status. Similar deterioration can follow anesthesia with nitrous oxide (Metz, 1992). Once the vitamin B_{12} and folate deficiencies have been corrected, anemia caused by other deficiencies (e.g., iron and copper) may be unmasked and also require specific correction.

QUESTIONS

1. What metabolites in serum and urine can be used to differentiate between a vitamin B_{12} deficiency and a folic acid deficiency?
2. In the presence of adequate intake of vitamin B_{12} and normal secretion of intrinsic factor, how can pancreatic insufficiency contribute to the development of vitamin B_{12} deficiency?
3. In addition to the absence of intrinsic factor, what other types of metabolic abnormalities could cause symptoms characteristic of megaloblastic anemia?
4. What are the metabolic and clinical consequences of treating a vitamin B_{12} deficiency with folic acid?
5. How does a vitamin B_{12} deficiency result in a decreased hemoglobin level and hematocrit?

REFERENCES

Allen RH, Stabler SP, Savage DG, Lindenbaum J: Metabolic abnormalities in cobalamin (vitamin B_{12}) and folate deficiency. *FASEB J* 7:1344–1353, 1993.

Battersby AR: How nature builds the pigments of life: The conquest of vitamin B_{12}. *Science* **264**:1551–1557, 1994.

Burman P, Mardh S, Norberg, Karlsson FA, Parietal cell antibodies in pernicious anemia inhibit H, K-adenosine triphosphatase, the proton pump of the stomach. *Gastroenterology* **96**:1434–1438, 1989.

Cooper BA, Zittoun J (eds.): *Folates and Cobalamins,* New York, Springer Verlag, 1989, pp. 71–84.

Gleeson PA, Toh B-H: Molecular targets in pernicious anemia. *Immunology Today* **12:**233–238, 1991.

Herbert V: Recommended dietary intake (RDI) of vitamin B_{12} in humans. *Am J Clin Nutr* **45:**671–678, 1987.

Karlsson FA, Burman P, Loof L, Mardh S: The major parietal cell antigen in autoimmune gastritis with pernicious anemia is the acid-producing H,K-ATPase of the stomach. *J Clin Invest* **81:**475–479, 1988.

Metz J: Cobalamin deficiency and the pathogenesis of nervous system disease. *Annu Rev Nutr* **12:**59–79, 1992.

Minot, GR, Murphy, WP: Treatment of pernicious anemia by special diet. *J Am Med Assoc* **87:**470–476, 1926.

Neale G: B_{12} binding proteins. *Gut* **31:**59–63, 1990.

Schilling RF: Vitamin B_{12} deficiency: Underdiagnosed, overtreated? *Hosp Pract* **30:**47–54, 1995.

Schjonsby H: Vitamin B_{12} absorption and malabsorption. *Gut* **30:**1686–1691, 1989.

Shevell MI, Rosenblatt DS: The neurology of cobalamin. *Can J Neurol Sci* **19:**472–486, 1992.

Song Y-H, Ma J-Y, Mardh S, et al.: Localization of a pernicious anemia autoantibody epitope on the α-subunit of human H,K-adenosine triphosphate. *Scand J Gastroenterol* **29:**122–127, 1994.

Tang L-H, Chokshi H, Hu C-B, et al.: The intrinsic factor (IF)-cobalamin receptor binding site is located in the amino-terminal portion of IF. *J Biol Chem* **267:**22982–22986, 1992.

12

Pyruvate Dehydrogenase Complex Deficiency

DAVID W. JACKSON AND WILLIAM S. HAYS

CASE REPORT

Pyruvate dehydrogenase complex (PDHC) deficiency is a heterogeneous metabolic disease, the presentation of which ranges from fulminant neonatal lactic acidosis to developmental abnormalities that appear gradually during childhood. Therefore, no two patients with this disease will present exactly alike. The following is a description of the first reported case of pyruvate decarboxylase (E_1 component of PDHC) deficiency described by John P. Blass and colleagues in 1970 (Blass et al., 1970; Blass et al., 1971).

A 9-year-old boy arrived in the clinic accompanied by his parents. His mother complained that the child was, once again, "acting strange, walking and talking like he were drunk." She stated that since he was 16 months old, the child had experienced similar problems intermittently. These episodes often occurred after a febrile illness, fatigue, or other stressors and lasted anywhere from a few hours to as long as 3 weeks. The attacks occurred two to six times per year. Associated symptoms included "erratic, writhing movements," weakness, *tachypnea* (rapid breathing), and a fine *papular rash* (superficial raised areas of skin) over the child's nose and cheeks, although not all symptoms were always present. The symptoms and their severity varied greatly with each attack. During the least severe episodes, the child was able to attend school; however, the most severe attacks reduced the child to crawling and bed rest.

There was no prenatal history of drug, alcohol, or tobacco abuse. The mother (gravida 3, para 2) experienced adequate weight gain and nutrition during the pregnancy and no *pica* (eating of dirt, stones, etc.) was noted. Neither sexually transmitted disease nor exposure to toxins was identified. The *vertex* (head first) delivery and perinatal period were unremarkable. There was no history of *dysmorphic* (abnormal) features, head injury, anoxia, seizures, or perinatal infections. The child reached developmental milestones in gross motor, language, and personal function on schedule, with a slight delay in fine motor function that became more apparent after age 16 months. There was no family history of consanguinity or movement disorders.

Except for acute exacerbations of the disease, the child's life was normal. He enjoyed riding his bicycle and playing the piano. He attended school regularly, and, despite particularly poor handwriting, kept up with his peers academically and physically.

On admission to the hospital, the child did not complain of any head injury, hearing difficulty, nasal discharge, mouth or throat soreness, heart problems, nausea, vomiting, diarrhea, abdominal pain, or *dysuria* (painful urination). He did complain of *diplopia* (double vision), muscle weakness, incoordination, and a facial rash. His mother also stated that he was tachypneic.

The child was 1.37 m tall (4 ft 6 in, 48th percentile) and weighed 32 kg (72 lbs, 67th percentile). He was afebrile, tachypneic, and *tachycardic* (rapid heart rate). The patient walked to the examining table unsteadily, using a wide-based gait. No head trauma was noted. His eye movements were irregular and interfered with fixation but did not exhibit true *nystagmus* (an involuntary, rapid movement of the eye). His pupils were dilated and slowly reactive to light. *Coloboma* (a developmental defect) of the right optic disk was noted. There was no *clubbing* (obliteration of the normal angle between the nail and digit), *cyanosis* (bluish discoloration of the skin), or *edema* (swelling) of the extremities. His lungs were clear to auscultation bilaterally and exhibited good air movement. *Leukoderma* (white patches of skin due to loss of skin pigment) was present on the right trunk. His heart beat had a regular rate and rhythm, and no murmurs were heard. Neurological examination revealed a bilateral generalized weakness of the extremities, *hypotonia* (reduced muscle tension), *choreiform movements* (jerky, involuntary movements) of the arms and hands, a slight intention tremor, and decreased vibratory sense in the toes. The deep tendon reflexes and remaining cranial nerves were normal on examination.

Extensive medical evaluation and laboratory studies revealed elevated levels of blood lactate (3.8 mM; normal range, 0.5–2.2 mM) and blood pyruvate (0.36 mM; normal, 0.03–0.08 mM), but a normal serum lactate/pyruvate ratio of 10/1. Alanine (852 μM; normal 338–472 μM) was the only serum amino acid whose concentration was elevated. The blood glucose, plasma insulin levels, ketones, and serum osmolality were normal. In addition, the glucose tolerance test and fasting blood glucose levels were normal. The blood pH was 7.30 (normal, 7.35–7.45), the P_{CO2} was 30 mm Hg (normal, 33–38 mm Hg), and the bicarbonate concentration was 18 mM (normal, 22–30 mM). The anion gap (serum $[Na^+]$ - $[Cl^-]$ - $[HCO_3^-]$) was 16 (normal, 10–14). Urine pyruvate was elevated at 0.21–0.32 mmol/day (normal, 0.04–0.08 mmol/day), as was urinary alanine excretion at 1,496–1,568 μmols/day (normal, 60–500 μmol/day). No other amino acids or organic acids were abnormal in the serum or the urine. A skeletal muscle biopsy revealed an increase in lipid droplets, but no ragged red fibers (characteristic of certain mitochondrial DNA mutations) were observed. Finally, analysis of cerebrospinal fluid revealed elevated levels of lactate (3.4 mM, normal <2.2 mM) and pyruvate (0.35 mM, normal <0.15 mM) with a normal lactate/pyruvate ratio of 10. No other cerebrospinal fluid abnormalities were observed.

DIAGNOSIS

The clinical diagnosis of PDHC deficiency requires rigorous exclusion of alternative diagnoses. It should be considered when neurological abnormalities, an unexplained high anion gap, and lactic acidosis or selective elevation of cerebrospinal fluid lactate are present. Ultimately, PDHC deficiency is confirmed by assaying cultured skin fibroblasts, lymphocytes, or tissues for PDHC activity (Robinson, 1995). DNA analysis is employed to identify the specific defect and to demonstrate a genetic defect in the face of ambiguous activity levels, which are often the result of *lyonization* (random inactivation of one X chromosome in somatic cells). It is instructive to review the differential diagnosis of metabolic acidosis, which ultimately leads to the diagnosis of PDHC deficiency, before focusing on the specific diagnosis of this enzymatic deficiency.

A careful history, physical examination, and the appropriate laboratory studies are necessary for a correct diagnosis. Clinically, several syndromes can present initially as a metabolic acidosis with central nervous system (CNS) sequelae. *Ketoacidosis* (decreased serum pH caused by increased levels of ketones) as a result of diabetes, starvation, or acute ethanol ingestion is an unlikely diagnosis for the present patient because neither blood glucose nor ketones were elevated, and there was no history of ethanol intake. The chronic nature of the disease virtually eliminates methanol, ethylene glycol, or salicylate intoxication. Septicemia, shock, and profound tissue hypoxemia are also unlikely candidates for similar reasons. Thus, in this child's case, the chronic nature of the disease is a significant clue in helping to narrow the etiology of the lactic acidemia.

Having ruled out diabetes and consumption of exogenous agents (i.e., methanol, ethylene glycol, and others), an enzymatic disorder producing a primary lactic acidosis appears likely. Several enzymatic deficiencies can produce elevated serum lactate and a high anion gap acidosis: (1) defects in the metabolism of organic acids or in the oxidation of fatty acids; (2) mutations in the mitochondrial DNA or in the enzymes of oxidative phosphorylation; (3) deficiencies of pyruvate carboxylase or other enzymes of gluconeogenesis; and (4) defects in the pyruvate dehydrogenase complex. In this case, the normal fasting glucose levels and the lack of a pathognomonic organic aciduria indicate that deficiencies in the metabolism of fatty acids or organic acids are unlikely. The absence of ragged red fibers on skeletal muscle biopsy rules out mutations in mitochondrial DNA, and the normal serum ketone profile makes deficiency in oxidative phosphorylation improbable. A key diagnostic feature is the normal ratio of lactate to pyruvate: Balanced elevations of lactate and pyruvate are characteristic of deficiencies of pyruvate carboxylase, the enzymes of gluconeogenesis, and of PDHC. A functional deficiency of PDHC can also be caused by mutations in PDHC phosphatase, a regulatory enzyme that activates PDHC. Disorders in the gluconeogenic enzymes glucose 6-phosphatase, fructose-1,6-bisphosphatase, and phosphoenolpyruvate carboxykinase are distinguished by fasting hypoglycemia and hepatomegaly. Additionally, deficiencies in pyruvate carboxylase can lead to elevated serum levels of proline and other amino acids in addition to alanine. Thus, the enzymatic disorders most consistent with the clinical and laboratory data in this case are defects in either PDHC or PDHC phosphatase. Enzymatic defects of gluconeogenesis and pyruvate carboxylase are less likely.

To establish the diagnosis, skin fibroblasts should be isolated, cultured, and assayed for the suspected enzymatic defects. Using this approach, the patient's mean pyruvate dehydrogenase complex activity was found to be <4% of the mean control values: $1.93 \pm 1.28 \times 10^{-7}$ μmol pyruvate converted per minute per 10^4 cells for the patient versus $53.3 \pm 6.42 \times 10^{-7}$ μmol per min per 10^4 cells for the controls. This result demonstrated unequivocally the enzymatic deficiency of pyruvate dehydrogenase.

Imaging of the brain by computed tomography or magnetic resonance imaging often shows developmental and degenerative abnormalities, the awareness of which can be helpful in the diagnosis of PDHC deficiency (De Meirleir et al., 1993). *Agenesis* (total absence) of the corpus callosum or medullary pyramids and abnormal inferior olives are seen occasionally, as are cerebral atrophy, ventricular dilatation, and symmetrical cystic lesions of the basal ganglia and brain stem characterized by *gliosis* (an excess of astrocytes in damaged areas of the CNS) and capillary proliferation. None of these findings, however, are pathognomonic for PDHC deficiency.

MOLECULAR PERSPECTIVES

To understand the neurological and metabolic consequences of PDHC deficiency, it is necessary to appreciate: (1) the metabolism of pyruvate in humans; (2) the central role of the pyruvate dehydrogenase complex in carbohydrate, fat, and amino acid metabolism (Fig. 12-1); and (3) the dependence of the CNS on glucose and aerobic energy production.

Pyruvate is derived either from glycolysis or from the catabolism of amino acids (Fig. 12-1). Pyruvate derived from glycolysis is converted into acetyl-coenzyme A (CoA) in the mitochondria via the PDHC (Fig. 12-2). In general, this pathway operates when the intracellular levels of acetyl-CoA, ATP, and NADH are low. Acetyl-CoA generated by the PDHC is responsible for much of the ATP generated by the electron transport chain. Pyruvate, derived from the carbon skeletons of amino acids, is carboxylated by the mitochondrial enzyme pyruvate carboxylase, yielding oxaloacetate (see Fig. 12-1). This is the first step in gluconeogenesis, which occurs exclusively in the liver and kidney. Gluconeogenesis is supported by the β-oxidation of fatty acids. Acetyl-CoA derived from β-oxidation enters the mitochondrial TCA cycle (tricarboxylic acid/Krebs cycle) and generates ATP, thus sparing glucose, derived primarily from gluconeogenesis, for use by the CNS during the fasting state. Additionally, pyruvate may be enzymatically and reversibly converted to either lactate (by lactate dehydrogenase) or to alanine by transamination.

A deficiency in the enzymatic activity of the PDHC severely limits the amount of acetyl-CoA available for entry into the TCA cycle, reducing the amount of NADH and $FADH_2$ generated by the TCA cycle, which in turn reduces the amount of ATP generated by electron transport chain-dependent oxidative phosphorylation. The brain has a constant demand for ATP that is met largely by aerobic metabolism via the TCA cycle and oxidative phosphorylation. In addition, the CNS depends exclusively on glucose, through glycolysis and the PDHC, to supply acetyl-CoA for the TCA cycle (fatty acids derived from adipocytes do not cross the blood–brain barrier). In contrast, the peripheral tissues can use a variety of substrates as fuel for the TCA cycle in lieu of glucose (i.e., fatty acids, ketones). With extended starvation, the brain can adapt to use ketones for a significant

METABOLIC FATES OF PYRUVATE

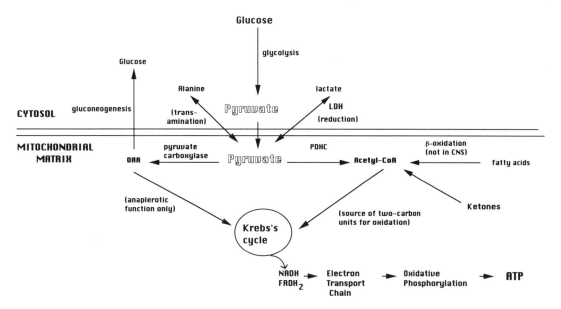

Figure 12-1. The relationship of pyruvate to lipid, carbohydrate, and alanine metabolism. OAA, oxaloacetate; ATP, adenosine triphosphate; PDHC, pyruvate dehydrogenase complex; LDH, lactate dehydrogenase.

fraction of its energy requirements. However, in well-nourished children with PDHC deficiency the major fuel source remains glucose. (Lactate accumulation, not ketone production, is responsible for the metabolic acidosis seen in PDHC deficiency.) This dependence on glucose is the basis for the effects of PDHC deficiency on the CNS. In a PDHC-deficient person, pyruvate is produced by glycolysis, but it accumulates because of its inability to enter the TCA cycle. The CNS becomes starved for substrate for the TCA cycle. The situation is further complicated by peripheral homeostatic mechanisms that maintain normal glucose levels. For example, the catabolism of liver glycogen by glycogen phosphorylase is directly stimulated by a drop in serum glucose levels. Thus, ketogenesis is inhibited, and the brain is deprived of an alternative substrate (ketones) that can provide acetyl-CoA for the TCA cycle. Without an adequate energy supply to the brain, CNS dysfunction becomes apparent in the form of choreiform movements, intention tremors, and other abnormalities. Some of the accumulated pyruvate is either reduced to lactate or transaminated to alanine. Thus, the levels of lac-

tate, pyruvate, and alanine increase in bodily fluids (Fig. 12-3). The high anion gap acidosis results from lactate accumulation.

The PDHC is the principal source of two-carbon compounds entering the TCA cycle when glucose is plentiful. Its activity is regulated by both product inhibition and by changes in its phosphorylation state (Fig. 12-4). The products of the reaction catalyzed by the PDHC (acetyl-CoA and NADH) inhibit their further production, whereas the substrates (pyruvate, NAD^+, and CoA) all activate the complex (Behal et al., 1993). As the NAD^+/NADH or CoA/acetyl-CoA ratio increases, the activity of PDHC also increases. The PDHC is inactive when phosphorylated and active when dephosphorylated. High levels of NAD^+, CoA, and pyruvate inactivate PDHC kinase and prevent PDHC phosphorylation. Ca^{2+} and Mg^{2+} activate the PDHC phosphatase, which in turn activates the PDHC. In general, the PDHC is active when glucose is being used for ATP production and is inhibited during the β-oxidation of fatty acids when mitochondrial NADH and acetyl-CoA are elevated. Finally, insulin and catecholamines (e.g., epi-

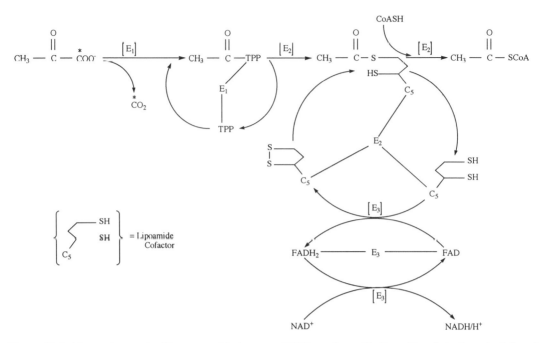

Figure 12-2. The reactions catalyzed by pyruvate dehydrogenase (PDHC) are shown. The lipoamide cofactor is covalently bound to the E_2 subunit, whereas thiamine pyrophosphate (TPP) and FAD/FADH$_2$ are noncovalently but tightly bound to the $E_1\alpha$ and E_3 subunits, respectively. The enzyme subunits responsible for catalysis of each step are indicated in brackets (e.g., $[E_1]$). E_1 catalyzes the oxidative decarboxylation of pyruvate and is the rate-limiting step in the overall reaction catalyzed by the PDHC. The irreversibility of the reaction catalyzed by the PDHC is the main reason why fat cannot be converted into glucose.

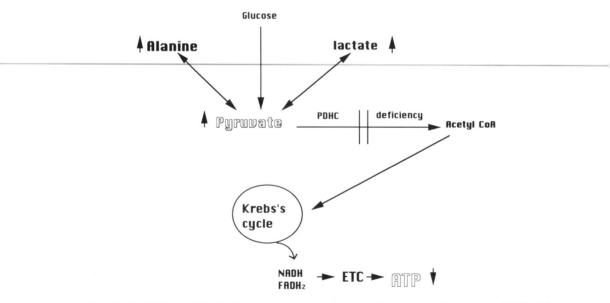

Figure 12-3. Bodily fluid levels of alanine, lactate, and pyruvate are increased in pyruvate dehydrogenase (PDHC) deficiency, which deprives the central nervous system of its main source of two carbon units (acetyl-coenzyme A) for the entry into the Kreb's cycle, resulting in decreased adenosine triphosphate (ATP) production and consequent neurological sequelae.

Regulatory Mechanisms for Pyruvate Dehydrogenase

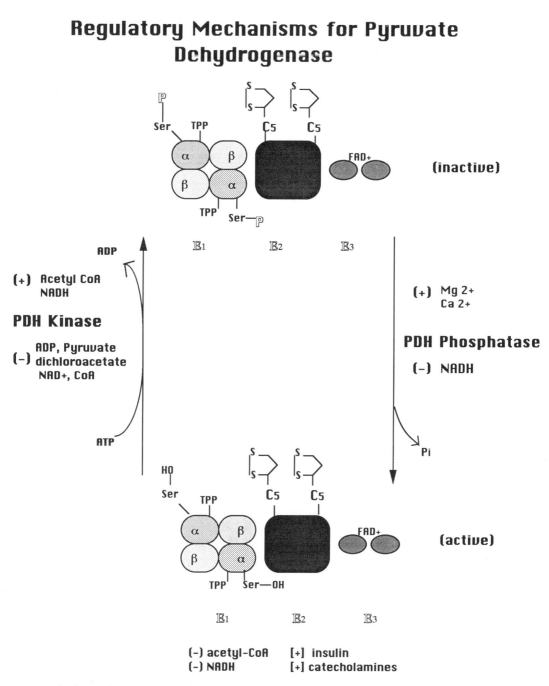

Figure 12-4. The regulatory mechanisms for pyruvate dehydrogenase. The dephosphorylated pyruvate dehydrogenase (PDH) complex is active. E_1 is the enzyme pyruvate dehydrogenase (pyruvate decarboxylase) attached to the cofactor thiamine pyrophosphate, (TPP). E_2 is the enzyme dihydrolipoyl transacetylase with two molecules of the cofactor lipoamide attached. E_3 is the enzyme dihydrolipoyl dehydrogenase with its cofactor NAD^+. α and β subunits of E_1 form dimers that coalesce to form the active E_1 tetramer. Ser, serine residue on α subunit of E_1; P, = phosphate group.

nephrine) activate the PDHC in adipose and cardiac muscle, respectively. The mechanisms of these hormonal actions are not well understood.

The PDHC consists of multiple copies of the four enzyme subunits involved in the conversion of pyruvate to acetyl-CoA, along with multiple copies each of PDHC kinase and PDHC phosphatase (Fig. 12-2). The subunits involved are E_1 (pyruvate dehydrogenase, also called pyruvate decarboxylase), E_2 (dihydrolipoyl transacetylase), and E_3 (dihydrolipoyl dehydrogenase). The E_1 component uses thiamine pyrophosphate (TPP) as a prosthetic group and catalyzes the oxidative decarboxylation of pyruvate. E_2 has two lipoamide chains as cofactors and catalyzes the transfer of the acetyl group to CoA, whereas E_3 uses FAD as a prosthetic group to catalyze the oxidative regeneration of lipoamide. Protein X, a recently described component of the PDHC, performs an acyl transfer function and is involved in the binding of E_3 to the PDHC.

Molecular genetics has shown defects in the E_1 component to be the most prevalent cause of PDHC deficiency (more than 200 described cases). The E_1 component is a tetramer composed of two identical $\alpha\beta$ dimers. Most mutations occur in the α gene, which is located on the X chromosome at p22.1-22.2 (Robinson, 1995). The critical role of the PDHC in CNS metabolism explains both the dominance of mutant $E_1\alpha$ alleles and the different patterns of mutations seen in males and females. Mutations that result in a complete loss of function are fatal; so the mutations seen in males (who have only a single allele) show significant residual function. These mutations are typically located near the 3' end of the coding sequence. The presence of two X chromosomes in females, however, allows the expression of a normal allele to compensate in part for a mutant allele (Brown et al., 1994). Thus, whereas mutations are dominant in females, the range of specific molecular defects is greater than in males, including mutations that completely inactivate the gene. These observations help to explain why severe neonatal lactic acidosis predominates in males, and the chronic neurological form of PDHC deficiency is more common in females. In addition to insertions and deletions, defects that alter the TPP binding site (resulting in an increased Michaelis constant, K_m, for TPP) and the regulatory phosphorylation sites in the $E_1\alpha$ protein have been described. In contrast to the heterogeneity in $E_1\alpha$ mutations, no defects have

been described in the $E_1\beta$ gene, which suggests that mutations at this locus are invariably fatal.

In addition to the E1α gene, mutations have been reported in the E_2, E_3, and protein X genes. The E_3 gene is unique among these three in that it is shared by the other α-keto acid dehydrogenases, namely, the α-ketoglutarate dehydrogenase complex of the TCA cycle and the α-keto acid dehydrogenase responsible for the catabolism of the branched chain amino acids valine, leucine, and isoleucine. As a result, the few patients who have been described with E_3 deficiency also have elevated serum levels of α-ketoglutarate and branched chain amino acids in addition to elevated levels of lactate and pyruvate. Deficiencies in PDHC phosphatase have also been described but are rare.

THERAPY

Several therapies are available for treating PDHC deficiency. Administration of dichloroacetate increases the activity of the PDHC complex by inhibiting PDHC kinase (Robinson, 1995). (Fig. 12-3), which results in dephosphorylation and activation of PDHC. In theory, a high-fat, low-carbohydrate "ketogenic" diet decreases carbohydrate availability and increases the supply of acetyl-CoA for entry into the TCA cycle via fatty acid β-oxidation while increasing ketone production. A high-fat, low-carbohydrate diet decreases carbohydrate intake, lowering serum glucose levels, which activates gluconeogenesis. Gluconeogenesis diminishes the supply of oxaloacetate, which is necessary for the entry of acetyl-CoA into the TCA cycle. Thus, acetyl-CoA accumulates, and the liver produces ketone bodies. The fatty acids in the diet are a rich source of acetyl-CoA, which is used both as a fuel molecule in the TCA cycle and as the precursor to ketone bodies. In addition, some patients respond to thiamine and carnitine loading, which necessitates a combined trial of each for each patient. Thiamine is useful in thiamine-deficient patients or in those whose $E_1\alpha$ PDHC subunits have an abnormally high K_m (low affinity) for TPP (Brown et al., 1994); carnitine is essential for the transport of long-chain fatty acids into mitochondria. The objective of thiamine therapy is to increase the activity of the PDHC, and that of carnitine therapy in this setting is to increase the total liver output of ketones. Because many CNS abnormalities are present before birth, therapy rarely influences the course of PDHC deficiency. The poor correlation between the levels of residual PDHC activity and phenotype confounds prognosis; in general, the more severe the lactic acidosis, the more severe the disease. Finally, prenatal diagnosis by means of assay for PDHC activity in cultured chorionic villus cell remains the best way of detecting PDHC deficiency before birth, although lyonization can make diagnosis difficult in female fetuses.

QUESTIONS

1. Name the five cofactors necessary for the pyruvate dehydrogenase complex to catalyze the conversion of pyruvate into acetyl-CoA. What function does each serve?
2. Why is CNS tissue so dependent on glycolysis and the TCA cycle for energy production?
3. What are the key laboratory values that suggest PDHC deficiency? Why are they abnormal in this disease?
4. Why would stress, such as an infection, cause an exacerbation of PDHC deficiency?
5. What is the rationale behind the different therapies for treating PDHC deficiency, and why are they not successful?
6. What is the main fuel supply for the brain, skeletal muscle, and the liver in the fed and unfed states? How might feeding the patient a high-fat, low-carbohydrate diet influence this energy supply?
7. Why is PDHC deficiency such a heterogeneous disease?
8. Most cases of deficiency in the $E_1\alpha$ subunit of PDHC appear to arise from *de novo* mutations, rather than by inheritance from either parent. What might explain this pattern of occurrence?
9. Review the differential diagnosis of lactic acidemia. Defects in oxidative phosphorylation are associated with an increase in the ratio of 3-hydroxybutyrate to acetoacetate. What might explain this defect? Why would a defect in pyruvate carboxylase lead to an increased serum concentration of proline?

REFERENCES

Behal RH, Buxton DB, Robertson JG, Olson MS: Regulation of the pyruvate dehydrogenase multienzyme complex. *Annu Rev Nutr* **13:**497–520, 1993.

Blass JP, Avigan J, Uhlendorf BW: A defect in pyruvate decarboxylase in a child with an intermittent movement disorder. *J Clin Inves* **49:**423–432, 1970.

Blass JP, Kark RAP, Engel WK: Clinical studies of a patient with pyruvate decarboxylase deficiency. *Arch Neurol* **25:**449–460, 1971.

Brown GK, Otero LJ, Legris M, Brown RM: Pyruvate dehydrogenase deficiency. *J Med Genet* **31:**875–879, 1994.

De Meirleir L, Lissens W, Denis R, Waynberg JL, et al. Pyruvate dehydrogenase deficiency: Clinical and biochemical diagnosis. *Ped Neurol* **9:**216–220, 1993.

Robinson BH: Lactic acidemia (disorders of pyruvate carboxylase, pyruvate dehydrogenase), *in The Metabolic and Molecular Basis of Inherited Diseases,* 5th ed. 1995, pp 1479–1499.

13

Biotin and Multiple Carboxylase Deficiency

KRISHNAMURTI DAKSHINAMURTI AND BARBARA TRIGGS-RAINE

CASE REPORT

Case 1

Patient P1 was born at 41 weeks of gestation following an uncomplicated pregnancy, labor, and delivery (Roth et al., 1976). The parents were not consanguineous. A previous male child had died soon after birth. On admission at 46 hours of age, the female infant was *cyanotic* (a bluish discoloration due to deficient oxygenation of the blood) and in severe respiratory distress. Laboratory data indicated severe metabolic acidosis. Arterial blood lactate and pyruvate levels were elevated, and the lactate to pyruvate ratio was 40:1. The blood ammonia concentration was 10 times normal. Gas chromatographic analysis of urine indicated the presence of propionic acid. A multivitamin preparation containing biotin was administered intravenously. Although there was initial improvement, the infant died at 4 days of age.

Case 2

A subsequent pregnancy in the family of patient P1 came to our attention when the mother was in the 34th gestational week. Prenatal diagnosis was not attempted because of the late stage of pregnancy. Because of the previous family history, it was decided to start prenatal therapy by oral administration of biotin (10 mg/day) to the mother. Clinically normal twins were delivered. The results of organic acid analysis by gas chromatography of cord blood and urine were normal during the first 7 days of life for both infants, and they were discharged. Patient P2 was normal until 3 months of age. During the week prior to admission the parents noted irritability, fussy feeding along with development of a skin rash and the odor of "cat's urine" emanating from soiled diapers. Physical examination revealed a moribund, ashen male infant with marked *tachypnea* (increased respiration rate) (80/min) and chest wall retractions. His rectal temperature was 34°C and blood pressure 45/20. The physical examination was unremarkable except for a generalized erythematous exfoliative dermatitis. Laboratory data on admission were as follows: arterial blood, pH 6.99; P_{CO2} 14 mm Hg (torr); base deficit, 38 mmol; serum Na^+, 142 mmol/L; K^+, 44 mmol/L; Cl^-, 118 mmol/L; total CO_2, 2 mmol; blood urea nitrogen, 7.2 mmol/L; glucose, 9.0 mmol/L; hemoglobin, 108 g/L; white blood cells, (WBC), 10.9 × 10^9/L; platelets, 220 × 10^6/L; cerebrospinal fluid (CSF) protein, 4.94 g/L; glucose, 5.2 mmol/L; and CSF cell count, unremarkable. Urinalysis indicated marked *ketonuria* (ketones in urine). Serum lactate concentration was 8.42 mmol/L, pyruvate 0.368 mmol/L, acetoacetate 3.6 mmol/L and β-hydroxybutyrate 2.44 mmol/L. The infant was treated with fluids containing sodium bicarbonate intravenously and biotin 2.5 mg every 6 hours via a nasogastric tube. Cultures of blood, CSF, and urine were sterile. After 24 hours of sodium bicarbonate and biotin treatment his respiration rate had decreased from 80/min to 40/min. He was alert and vigorously taking oral feeding. There was dramatic improvement in acid-base values. Feeding was cautiously advanced to a standard proprietary formula, which he tolerated. He was discharged receiving biotin 2.5 mg four times a day. Six months after discharge, he was thriving and developing normally on biotin 10 mg per day (Roth et al., 1980). In the years since, the child has been completely normal, like his unaffected twin sibling.

Cultured fibroblasts were grown from the patient's foreskin obtained at circumcision. Assay of biotin-dependent carboxylases in fibroblasts after growth in biotin-containing or biotin-deficient culture medium was carried out. Genetic complementation experiments were performed with fibroblasts from affected patients.

The mother reported no untoward effects of biotin therapy during gestation. Gas chromatographic analysis of the mother's urinary organic acid excretion pattern revealed no abnormalities. Assays of biotin carboxylases in fibroblasts from the affected twin B (patient P2), the unaffected twin A, and normal controls were compared under biotin-rich and biotin-depleted cell growth conditions. As shown in Table 13-1, in biotin-depleted medium the cells of twin B (patient P2) showed virtually complete deficiencies of all three carboxylases: propionyl-CoA carboxylase, β-methyl-crotonyl-coenzyme A (CoA) carboxylase and pyruvate carboxylase. The cells of the unaffected twin A had activity levels comparable to those of control cells. In biotin-rich medium, the carboxylase activities of the cells of twin B (patient P2) were comparable to those of control cells. On the basis of complementation studies, twin B could be assigned to the biocomplementation group.

DIAGNOSIS

Arriving at a diagnosis based on the presentation is an exigency. When one sees a very ill infant in the newborn nursery, the first impression is that of an infant with sepsis, hence the workup for culture of body fluids. A positive blood culture could even be confusing. A workup for metabolic diseases should be considered in view of the prevalence of inborn errors of metabolism, particularly if there is a family history of a sibling death, even if the cause of death was not established.

In the present case, the family history suggested the possibility of a mitochondrial carboxylase deficiency and prompted the decision to attempt a prenatal therapy even in the absence of a confirmed prenatal diagnosis. Subsequent findings have confirmed the wisdom of this approach. Since this first attempt at prenatal therapy, similar treatment of other such patients has proved successful. Analysis of samples of body fluids and tissues obtained immediately before initiation of therapy and those obtained after therapy could confirm the diagnosis.

Respiratory distress and metabolic acidosis indicate the need to identify the organic acid(s) responsible for the anion gap. Laboratory data on the presence in serum and excretion in urine of abnormal organic acids provide valuable information, which, along with the nature of the response to biotin therapy, permit determination of whether the condition is associated with a single or multiple carboxylase deficiency (MCD). Single carboxylase deficiencies have all been unresponsive to biotin therapy.

Table 13-1. Biotin-dependent Carboxylase Activity of Cultured Fibroblasts

Cell Line	Propionyl-CoA Carboxylase[a]		β-Methyl-crotonyl-CoA Carboxylase[a]		Pyruvate Carboxylase[a,b]	
	+Biotin	−Biotin	+Biotin	−Biotin	+Biotin	−Biotin
Control 1	1.02	0.70	0.50	0.24	2.56	1.24
Control 2	0.82	0.56	0.39	0.25	0.56	0.26
Control 3	0.86	0.42	0.33	0.10	0.38	0.23
Twin A	1.11	0.63	0.49	0.16	2.46	1.15
Twin B	1.19	0.01	0.37	<0.01	1.16	0.05

CoA, Coenzyme A

[a] Values represent the means of duplicate determinations; specific activities are expressed as nmole/min/mg protein.

[b] Pyruvate carboxylase activities are strain-specific.

Data from: *Pediatr Res* **16**:126, 1982.

The clinical symptoms of the holocarboxylase synthetase (HCS)-deficient and the biotinidase-deficient variants of MCD are similar. Both disorders are characterized by deficient activities of biotin carboxylases in peripheral blood leukocytes before therapy with biotin. Age of onset was thought to be useful in discriminating between the two disorders, but it is not necessarily so. The differential diagnosis would depend on the following information: (1) Serum biotin concentrations are usually in the normal range in patients with the HCS-deficient variant, whereas biotin concentrations are low in the biotinidase-deficient variant of MCD; (2) Differences between the biotin carboxylase activities in extracts of fibroblasts cultured in biotin-depleted medium can be used to distinguish between the variants. Fibroblasts of patients with the HCS-deficient variant have low levels of biotin carboxylase activities, whereas fibroblasts from patients with the biotinidase variant have normal levels of biotin carboxylase activities; and (3) Serum biotinidase activity is normal in the HCS-deficient variant, whereas it is decreased or absent in the biotinidase-deficient variant of MCD. Based on the data from fibroblast culture studies, patient P2 was diagnosed as having the HCS-deficient variant of the MCD syndrome. This conclusion was confirmed by genetic complementation experiments.

MOLECULAR PERSPECTIVES

Biotin is a water-soluble vitamin; its formal chemical name is cis-hexahydro-2-oxo-14-thieno [3,4] imidazole-4-valeric acid, (Dakshinamurti and Bhagavan, 1985; Dakshinamurti and Chauhan, 1989). Only the (+) stereoisomer has significant biological activity. Various biotin derivatives, analogues, and antagonists are known. Desthiobiotin, a sulphur-free analogue of biotin, is the direct precursor of biotin in microorganisms, algae, and plants which synthesize biotin and are the food sources for animals. It was generally believed that the enteric synthesis of biotin by bacteria is a source of biotin for humans, based on the observation that the total excretion of biotin in urine and the feces exceeds the dietary intake. Dietary biotin absorbed in excess of requirement and storage capacity of tissues, along with its metabolites, such as bisnorbiotin and biotin sulfoxide, is excreted in urine. Unabsorbed biotin and

biotin synthesized by bacteria, essentially in the large intestines, are excreted in feces. The absorption of biotin is higher in the jejunum than in the ileum and minimal in the colon. These observations indicate that enterically synthesized biotin is less important for the nutrition of the human host than previously thought. There is no specific recommendation regarding dietary allowance for biotin because no definitive studies on human requirements have been done. In adults receiving total parenteral nutrition, daily administration of 60 μg biotin prevents the appearance of signs of biotin deficiency. Lacking information about the bioavailability of biotin in foods, a daily intake of 100 μg has been recommended for adults. Based on the biotin content of human milk, which is all in the free form, and assuming a daily milk consumption of 750 mL by an infant, the daily biotin intake of breast-fed infants would be in the range of 2 to 15 μg per day. For formula-fed infants, an intake of 10 to 15 μg biotin per day is recommended during the first year of life. Recommended intakes for children and adolescents are gradually increased to adult levels by 11 years of age.

Nonprosthetic Group Functions of Biotin

Various reports indicate a requirement for biotin for cells in culture. The addition of biotin to the culture medium of cells enhances protein synthesis, DNA synthesis, and cell growth. These capabilities are reduced when cells are grown in a medium deficient in biotin. The nonprosthetic group functions of biotin are analogous to those of insulin inasmuch as both positively regulate the transcription of glucokinase (EC 2.7.1.2) and negatively regulate the transcription of phosphoenolpyruvate carboxykinase (EC 4.1.1.32) (Chauhan and Dakshinamurti, 1991). We have also shown that biotin influences palatal development of mouse embryos in organ culture.

Prosthetic Group Functions of Biotin

The best understood role of biotin is as the prosthetic group of biotin-containing enzymes, although information on the nonprosthetic group functions of biotin is increasing. There are only four biotin-containing enzymes in mammalian tissues; they include acetyl-coenzyme A carboxylase (ACC), propionyl-coenzyme A carboxylase (PCC), β-methyl-crotonyl-coenzyme A carboxylase (MCC), and pyruvate carboxylase (PC). Each of the biotin-containing carboxylases catalyzes an adenosine triphosphate (ATP)-dependent CO_2 fixation reaction. Biotin functions as a CO_2 carrier on the surface of the enzyme. The role of biotin enzymes in intermediary metabolism shown in Figure 13-1 emphasizes its obligatory requirement in carbohydrate and lipid metabolism and in the further metabolism of certain amino acids after they have been deaminated.

ACC (EC 6.4.1.2) catalyzes the ATP-dependent carboxylation of acetyl-CoA in the first step of fatty acid synthesis, leading to lipogenesis. The key enzyme in the catabolic pathway of isoleucine, threonine, methionine, and valine and also of odd-chain fatty acids is PCC (EC 6.4.1.3). It catalyzes the conversion of propionyl-CoA to methylmalonyl-CoA, which is converted to succinyl-CoA (by a vitamin B_{12}-dependent enzyme) before its entry into the tricarboxylic acid cycle. The conversion of β-methyl-crotonyl-CoA to β-methylglutaconyl-CoA, a key step in the degradative pathway of leucine, is catalyzed by MCC (EC 6.4.1.4), and PC (EC 6.4.1.1) is a key regulatory enzyme of gluconeogenesis. It catalyzes the formation of oxaloacetate from pyruvate, the first step in the gluconeogenic pathway. Pyruvate carboxylase is present in lipogenic tissues and participates in fatty acid synthesis by transporting acetyl groups through citrate and reducing groups through malate, from mitochondria to cytosol. In all tissues

PC has an anaplerotic role in the formation of oxaloacetate.

Biotin Holocarboxylase Synthetase

Biotin carboxylases are synthesized in the form of apoproteins that undergo posttranslational covalent modification by the addition of biotin, the prosthetic group, to the ε-amino group of lysine. This covalent attachment of biotin is catalyzed by biotin HCS in a two-step reaction:

$$\text{Biotin} + \text{ATP} \rightarrow 5'\text{-adenylate-biotin} + \text{PP}_i \quad \text{(Step 1)}$$

$$5'\text{-adenylate-biotin} + \text{apoenzyme} \rightarrow \text{holoenzyme} + \text{AMP} \quad \text{(Step 2)}$$

Holocarboxylase synthetase is responsible for the formation of the holoforms of ACC, PCC, MCC, and PC.

HCS cDNA clones have been isolated using two independent approaches; both cDNA sequences predicted a polypeptide of 726 amino acids with a molecular mass of 80,759 Da. Suzuki et al. (1994) employed degenerate oligonucleotide primers predicted from the amino acid sequence of purified bovine liver HCS to isolate a fragment of the bovine HCS cDNA. This was used to design oligonucleotide primers to amplify a segment of the human HCS cDNA ultimately used as a hybridization probe to isolate the human cDNA from a library. Leon-Del-Rio

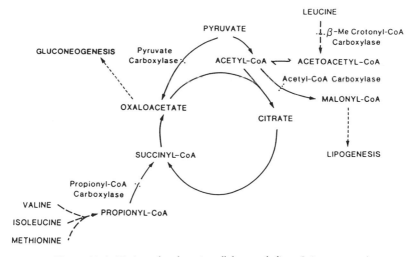

Figure 13-1. Biotin carboxylases in cellular metabolism. CoA, coenzyme A.

et al. (1995) used a unique approach, the complementation of an *Escherichia coli* mutant deficient in biotin-ligase (*birA*), to achieve the same outcome. Given the requirement of sequence or functional conservation for the success of these approaches, it is not surprising that the human HCS protein sequence is strikingly similar to the *E. coli/birA* protein in the biotin-binding region as well as in a potential ATP-binding site. Homology with avian avidin is also evident in a short region (47 amino acids) of HCS thought to bind biotin. A genomic clone containing the human HCS gene was isolated from a cosmid library and shown to map to human chromosome 21q22.1 using fluorescent *in situ* hybridization.

The HCS cDNA has provided the tool to begin the analysis of the structure and expression of HCS. In the various tissue mRNA samples examined by Northern blot analysis, a 5.7 kb mRNA was detected; an additional 8.3-kb mRNA was detected in some tissues. The isolation of cDNA clones of differing sequences has provided evidence for alternative splicing, but the significance of these various mRNA species is unknown. Because the predicted protein sequence reveals no classic mitochondrial targeting sequence, the mechanism by which HCS enters the mitochondria to biotinylate mitochondrial apoenzymes remains obscure. Perhaps an as yet undetected sequence could be introduced by alternative splicing to provide a signal for mitochondrial import.

Biotinidase

Acid hydrolysis of biotin proteins releases free biotin, whereas proteolytic hydrolysis results in the formation of biotin peptides, the smallest among these being biocytin (N-ϵ-(d-biotinyl)-L-lysine). Biotinidase (biotin-amide aminohydrolase, EC 3.5.1.12) releases biotin from the proteolytic degradation product of carboxylases or biocytin so that biotin can be reutilized (Fig. 13-2) (Chauhan and Dakshinamurti, 1986; Cole et al., 1994a). This enzyme has been detected in many mammalian tissues, and it has been purified to homogeneity from human serum. The purified enzyme, which is a glycoprotein, is a single polypeptide with a molecular mass of 68,000 Da. We isolated a biotinidase clone of 1.25 kb from a human liver λgt_{11} library in 1988. The poly (A+) RNA corresponding to the clone is 1.8 kb, which was sequenced by the dideoxy-chain termination method. Although the predicted amino acid sequence determined from the biotinidase clone did not share extensive homology with avidin or strepavidin, there was conservation of sequence around tryptophan residues, which have been shown to be critical for biotin binding in both avidin and strepavidin.

Biotin binding studies performed with purified biotinidase as well as with biotinidase in human serum indicate that biotinidase is the biotin-carrier protein in blood (Chauhan and Dakshinamurti, 1988; Cole et al., 1994a). There are two classes of biotin binding sites, one of high (Ka, 0.5 nM) and one of low (Ka, 50 nM) affinity. The requirement of tryptophan and cysteine residues for binding is shown by the complete inhibition of biotin binding activity of biotinidase by treatment of the enzyme with the tryptophan and cysteine reagents N-bromosuccinimide and p-chloromercuribenzoate, respectively. The decreased level of plasma biotin in biotinidase-deficient patients underscores the role of

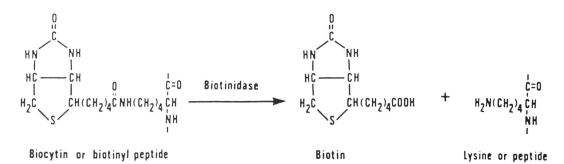

Figure 13-2. Hydrolysis of biocytin or biotinyl peptides by biotinidase.

biotinidase in biotin transport. It is well-known that epileptic patients on long-term therapy with anticonvulsants have a low level of plasma biotin. We have shown that all the anticonvulsants compete with biotin for the biotin binding activity of biotinidase, providing an explanation for the low serum biotin levels in anticonvulsant drug-treated epileptics.

We have reported that the uptake of biotin by various human cell lines occurs by a saturable transport process. Based on the binding of avidin and avidin-biotin complex to rat liver plasma membranes, it was suggested that avidin might be mimicking a natural biotin-carrier involved in biotin transport. This idea was corroborated by subsequent studies. We have also shown that the uptake of biotin and biocytin by rat jejunal segments is biphasic. Based on studies with fractionated solubilized brush-border membranes from rat intestines, we showed that biotinidase is the only protein in brush-border membranes that binds biotin. We suggested that when the biotin concentration in the gut is below 50 nM (as is the case under normal physiological conditions) the saturable uptake mechanism operates. Such a biphasic uptake would be advantageous in the context of fluctuating amounts of biotin in the diet. It is thought that in the late-onset multiple carboxylase syndrome, patients lack the transport system for absorbing biotin when it is present in the lower nanomolar concentration range. The responses of these patients to pharmacological doses of biotin indicate that only the saturable portion of the biotin transport system is defective in these patients. These studies highlight the dual function of biotinidase. As an enzyme releasing biotin from biocytin, it is responsible for the intracellular recycling of biotin and for the absorption of dietary protein-bound biotin in the gastrointestinal tract. As a biotin-binding protein, it has a role in biotin transport.

Biotinidase-encoding cDNAs have been isolated using two independent approaches. We first isolated a partial cDNA clone from a human liver library with an antibody prepared against human serum biotinidase. Using degenerate oligonucleotide primers predicted from amino acid sequence generated from the purified serum protein, Cole et al. (1994a) isolated a full-length biotinidase cDNA clone by polymerase chain reaction (PCR) amplification. We were also able to extend our partial biotinidase cDNA clone to full-length using a PCR-based approach. Our cDNA sequence is in complete agreement with

that of Cole et al. (1994a) with the exception of a C1413T substitution, which does not alter the amino acid at this position. The 543-residue polypeptide predicted by both cDNA sequences is identical, starting with a 41 amino acid signal sequence which is predicted to be cleaved to produce a mature protein of 502 amino acids and a molecular mass of 56,771 Da.

We localized the biotinidase gene, *BTD*, in the human genome by PCR amplification of DNA from somatic cell hybrids using primers specific for human *BTD* that do not amplify rodent DNA. The sequence of the forward PCR primer (5′GAGAATGAC-CACTATTTCCTGAGG-3′) was specified from the sequence near the 3′ end of the coding region, and the reverse primer (5′AGCCTGTGGAAGTGCAAG-GCTGT-3′) was specified from sequence in the 3′ untranslated region of the cDNA. The size of the PCR product resulting from these primers was 156 bp. Only DNA from somatic cell hybrids (Bios Corporation, New Haven, CT) containing human chromosome 3 yielded an amplification product. *BTD* was further localized between 3pter and 3q21 of chromosome 3 using DNA from hybrids containing differing regions of chromosome 3. Fluorescent *in situ* hybridization (FISH) with the biotinidase cDNA refined the position of the gene to 3p25, which is consistent with the FISH mapping described by Cole et al. (1994b) using a fragment of genomic DNA containing *BTD*.

Northern blot analysis of fibroblast mRNA from normal and biotinidase-deficient subjects revealed an mRNA of approximately 2.3 kb in all samples. This finding agrees with the analysis of Cole et al. (1994a) who observed a 2.0-kb biotinidase mRNA in several human tissues. Interestingly, the mRNA in all three biotinidase-deficient cell lines that we examined were normal in size and abundance. Although these cell lines were not available for mutation analysis, the presence of a substantial level of mRNA suggested that the mutations in these probands affect the level of activity of the biotinidase protein and not the synthesis or stability of the mRNA.

Multiple Carboxylase Deficiency Syndrome

Since 1976 the incidence in infants with various organic acidemias has been investigated using molecular biology techniques. Many of these disorders have been characterized as occurring in association with the lack of one or more of the biotin carboxylases. Inherited disorders of individual carboxylases are distinct from the biotin-responsive MCD inasmuch as patients with inherited disorders of individual carboxylases do not respond even to pharmacologic doses of biotin. In MCD, all three mitochondrial carboxylases are deficient. The abnormal metabolites due to deficiency of individual carboxylases are shown in Figure 13-3. Two distinct types of MCD have been recognized based on the nature of the clinical presentation and also on the serum biotin concentration of the patient. The neonatal form is recognized during the first week of life by vomiting, lethargy, and hypotonia. Metabolic ketoacidosis in the infant is associated with excretion of metabolites characteristic of MCD (Fig. 13-3). The infant could die in an overwhelming acidotic episode before development of cutaneous eruptions, although skin lesions usually are a component of the clinical picture. Carboxylase activities of blood leukocytes are low before treatment with biotin but return to normal levels after biotin administration. Nevertheless, serum biotin concentration and urinary excretion of biotin by the untreated infant are normal. When skin fibroblasts from the patient are cultured in a medium containing physiologic concentrations of biotin, the carboxylase activities are below normal levels. When the fibroblasts are cultured in a medium containing a high concentration of biotin, however, the carboxylase activities increase to normal levels. A deficiency of biotin holocarboxylase synthetase, the enzyme that covalently adds the biotin prosthetic group to the apobiotin carboxylase, is the primary biochemical lesion in the neonatal type of MCD. The beneficial response of the affected infant to pharmacologic doses of biotin administered prenatally suggests a defective holocarboxylase synthetase with a Michaelis constant (K_m) for biotin that is about 60 times greater than the normal K_m (8 μM) (Roth et al., 1982). The mode of inheritance of this disorder is autosomal recessive.

Biotinidase deficiency is the underlying defect in patients with the late-onset type of MCD. It is also an autosomal recessively inherited disorder. There is significant phenotypic variation in this syndrome. It was generally assumed that children with biotinidase deficiency developed clinical symptoms only by about 3 to 4 months of age. In view of the ease of biochemical diagnosis, there has been a spate of

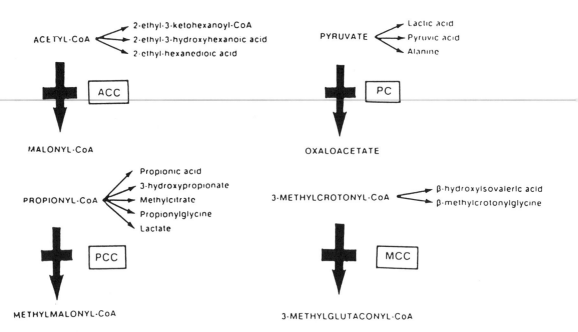

Figure 13-3. Accumulation of intermediary metabolites in individual carboxylase deficiency. Accumulated metabolites are shown with multiple arrows. ACC, acetyl coenzyme A carboxylase; PC, pyruvate carboxylase; PCC, propionyl coenzyme A carboxylase; MCC, β-methylcrotonyl coenzyme A carboxylase.

reports of biotinidase deficient patients presenting from as early as two weeks of age to adolescence. Patients who develop clinical symptoms in late childhood are distinct compared with the classic phenotype described for infants with complete biotinidase deficiency. Clinical features seen in infants commonly include seizures, hypotonia, ataxia, and breathing problems. If treatment is delayed, optic atrophy and neurosensory hearing loss may result. Alopecia, skin rashes, developmental delay, and recurrent infections are also reported in patients who have not been diagnosed and treated early.

Analysis of urine for abnormal organic acids (Fig. 13-3) is a useful screening technique. Excretion of organic acids (such as β-hydroxyisovaleric acid, β-methylcrotonylglycine, or methyl citrate) is seen in classic presentations of this syndrome. Increased serum lactate and hyperammonemia are also common findings, although a determination of serum biotinidase activity must be done for positive diagnosis of biotinidase deficiency. These values could range from virtually undetectable levels to less than 5% of normal values in profoundly biotinidase-deficient patients.

Serum biotinidase levels of parents of affected children are in the heterozygous range, intermediate between those of affected children and normal adult controls. In the group with partial biotinidase deficiency, the serum enzyme activity could be 10 to 30% of normal values. It should be noted that newborns with the partial biotinidase deficiency phenotype have been identified only by serum enzyme determinations and have shown no clinical manifestations to suggest that partial biotinidase deficiency is harmless. It is possible that their biotinidase has normal catalytic properties but the amount synthesized is low. The other possibility is that in this phenotype the tissues have adequate enzyme with normal catalytic activity, but the enzyme is not secreted. The situation may not be entirely benign, however, as there are reports that some, if untreated, become symptomatic with eczema and alopecia. Some patients with complete serum biotinidase deficiency have not shown any urinary excretion of abnormal organic acids or any clinical manifestations of MDC. This result could be due to early identification and treatment with biotin, particularly as an elevation of blood ammonia was noted in these patients during a lapse in their treatment. Clinical symptoms at presentation have varied considerably.

Whereas infants identified through neonatal screening could be symptom free, older patients could be severely ill with neurological abnormalities.

Abnormal function of the central nervous system is more common in MCD patients with biotinidase deficiency than in those with HCS deficiency, possibly because of the more acute illness associated with HCS deficiency, which is fatal if not treated with biotin. An analysis of MCD symptomatic children with profound biotinidase deficiency indicates that more than 55% have clinically apparent seizures, usually in combination with other clinical features. Electroencephalographic findings are abnormal in patients with seizures. Computed tomography scan shows hypodensity of white matter. The selective vulnerability of the central nervous system in biotinidase deficiency could be due to the lower stores of biotin in the brain than in peripheral tissues and the consequent accumulation of abnormal organic acids, such as β-hydroxyisovaleric acid, in the MCD patient. The fact that cerebrospinal fluid/plasma ratios of lactate and β-hydroxyisovaleric acid in patients with biotinidase deficiency are high supports the above contention. The role of biotinidase in the uptake and transport of biotin is in keeping with the above observations. The suggestion that the accumulation of biocytin in the brain could contribute to the toxicity of biotinidase deficiency is only a speculation.

The molecular basis of the multiple carboxylase deficiency resulting from mutations in the HCS gene is being explored. Suzuki et al. (1994) identified two mutations: delG1067, which generates a premature stop codon, and T997C, which results in a Leu237Pro substitution. In an analysis of five Japanese patients with HCS deficiency, these mutations were found to account for seven of eight alleles. A cDNA harbouring the Leu237Pro mutation did not complement HCS deficiency when expressed in patient fibroblasts, whereas the corresponding wild-type cDNA clone did, confirming the disease-causing nature of the Leu237Pro mutation. This result provides strong evidence that the Leu237Pro mutation can result in HCS deficiency.

The isolation of a biotinidase cDNA also allows characterization of the molecular basis of multiple carboxylase deficiency caused by mutation in the biotinidase-encoding genes. A 7-bp deletion accompanied by a 3-bp insertion on 50% of the alleles of symptomatic children with biotinidase deficiency has been reported. In our examination of DNA from French-Canadian probands, identified through newborn screening programs to have partial biotinidase deficiency, we identified a G1330C (Asp444His) mutation on at least one allele of each proband. The capacity of this mutation to cause biotinidase deficiency is under investigation. Further characterization of the mutations underlying biotinidase deficiency should facilitate the diagnosis of this disorder and allow genotype/phenotype correlations to be made.

THERAPY

The two biotin-responsive disorders, referred to collectively as multiple carboxylase deficiency syndrome, have different biochemical etiologies. One variant, referred to as the *early onset* type, is due to a deficiency of HCS, leading to a deficiency of tissue biotin-dependent carboxylases. The other variant, referred to as the *late onset* type, is due to a deficiency of biotinidase, which is involved in intracellular biotin recycling as well as biotin uptake and transport. Biotinidase deficiency also results in a deficiency of tissue biotin-dependent carboxylases. Holocarboxylase synthetase deficiency is a clinically severe form in the neonate and is fatal if untreated. In view of the insidious nature of biotinidase-deficient MCD, clinical symptoms might appear later. Biotinidase deficiency is more prevalent than HCS deficiency. The incidence of biotinidase deficiency (profound as well as partial) is 1 in 60,000 (1 in 50,000 to 1 in 73,000, 95% confidence limits) with an estimated 1 in 123 persons being heterozygous. Both variants of MCD respond to biotin treatment (10 mg daily). Early treatment is crucial for significant recovery. It has been shown that biotin treatment can arrest progressive deterioration of visual, motor, and mental deficits. When diagnosis and treatment are delayed, the outcome, although remarkable, has residual deficiency in regard to development.

As the treatment itself is so simple, specific early diagnosis through neonatal screening or even prenatal diagnosis is an important factor in the successful outcome of therapy. Neonatal screening for biotinidase deficiency is currently done in 14 countries. Biotinidase activity can be measured in both amnionitic fluid and cultured amniotic cells obtained by amniocentesis of normal pregnancies. A recent report of transcervical chorionic villus biopsy at the 11th week of gestation and assay of sonicated chorionic villi for biotinidase indicates that prenatal diagnosis for biotinidase deficiency can be easily performed during the first trimester of pregnancy. Prenatal diagnosis of HCS deficiency is made by demonstrating decreased biotin carboxylase activities in cultured amniocytes. The enzyme activities increase toward normal values after the cells have been incubated in the presence of a large concentration of biotin. The presence of increased amounts of β-hydroxyisovaleric acid and methyl citrate in amniotic fluid is a rapid method of prenatal diagnosis of the early onset type of MCD.

Neonates with HCS deficiency are acutely ill with keto-lacticacidosis, hyperammonemia, and respiratory distress. Treatment with biotin (10 mg daily) would be appropriate even before a diagnosis of HCS deficiency is confirmed. In cases of a pregnancy at risk, indicated by neonatal death of a previous child with any of the symptoms of MCD, prenatal treatment consisting of a biotin supplement (10 mg daily) to the mother during the last trimester of pregnancy is indicated in view of the demonstrated success of prenatal treatment of early-onset MCD.

The late-onset type patient may not present with the classical symptoms of MCD. Biotinidase deficiency should be considered in the differential diagnosis of infantile spasms regardless of the age of the patient. Infants with seizures who are unresponsive to the usual anticonvulsants should be tested for their responsiveness to biotin. Even when the patient responds favorably to treatment with corticotropin (an ACTH preparation), a meticulous search for other symptoms, such as dermatitis and alopecia, should be made. Because in some infants muscle jerks may be the only symptom in early infancy, biotinidase activity in serum should be assayed in these patients. Extracts of fibroblasts and peripheral leukocytes of normal subjects have a low but detectable activity of biotinidase. Similar extracts from patients with biotinidase deficiency have 1% of the mean normal activity for these cells and should be useful in confirming diagnosis. The question of whether to treat patients who do not have clinical symptoms but have only a biochemically determined deficiency of biotinidase can be answered with reasonable confidence. Clinical and experimental data indicate that biotin administration in pharmacological doses over time is essentially innocuous. There is no substantiation for the suggestion that sensorineural deafness and optic atrophy might be exaggerated by treatment with pharmacological doses of biotin. It appears that despite reversal of dermatological and psychomotor abnormalities, patients are likely to have residual auditory or visual handicaps if diagnosis and treatment are delayed beyond the first year of life. The watchword would therefore be to treat and not wait.

QUESTIONS

1. What are the clinical variants of the multiple carboxylase deficiency syndrome? Indicate the nature of the biochemical lesion in each.
2. In as much as both variants of multiple carboxylase deficiency respond to biotin therapy, can the blood level of biotin in a patient be used to identify either of these variants?
3. You are consulted on an infant in the newborn nursery who has intermittent seizures unresponsive to valproic acid. How would you proceed further? Indicate the rationale.
4. You have successfully treated a 3-month-old child with biotin for the biotinidase-deficient variant of MCD. It comes to your attention later that the mother of that child is in the 30th week of gestation. What would be your recommendation?

REFERENCES

Chauhan J, Dakshinamurti K: Purification and characterization of human serum biotinidase. *J Biol Chem* **261**:4268–4275, 1986.

Chauhan J, Dakshinamurti K: Role of human serum biotinidase as biotin-binding protein. *Biochem J* **256**:265–270, 1988.

Chauhan J, Dakshinamurti K: Transcriptional regulation of glucokinase gene by biotin in starved rats. *J Biol Chem* **266**:10035–10100, 1991.

Cole H, Reynolds TR, Lockyer JM, Buck GA, Denson T, Spence JE, Hymes J, Wolf B: Human serum biotinidase. *J Biol Chem* **269**:6566–6570, 1994a.

Cole H, Weremowicz S, Morton CC, Wolf B: Localization of serum biotinidase (BTD) to human chromosome 3 in band p25. *Genomics* **22**:662–663, 1994b.

Dakshinamurti K, Bhagavan HN, (eds.): Biotin. *Ann NY Acad Sci* **447**:1–447, 1985.

Dakshinamurti K, Chauhan J: Biotin. *Vitamins and Hormones* **45**:337–384, 1989.

Leon-Del-Rio A, Leclerc D, Akerman B, Wakamatsu N, Gravel RA: Isolation of a cDNA encoding human holocarboxylase synthetase by functional complementation of a biotin auxotroph of *Escherichia coli. Proc Natl Acad Sci USA* **92**:4626–4630, 1995.

Roth K, Cohn R, Yandrasitz J, Preti G, Dodd P, Segal S: Beta-methylcrotonic aciduria associated with lactic acidosis. *J Pediatr* **88**:229–235, 1976.

Roth KS, Yang W, Foremann JW, Rothman R, Segal S: Holocarboxylase synthetase deficiency: a biotin-responsive organic acidemia. *J Pediatr* **96**:845–849, 1980.

Roth KS, Yang W, Allan L, Saunders M, Gravel RA, Dakshinamurti K: Prenatal administration of biotin in biotin responsive multiple carboxylase deficiency. *Pediatr Res* **16**:126–129, 1982.

Suzuki Y, Aoki Y, Ishida Y, Chiba Y, Iwamatsu A, Kishino T, Niikawa N, Matsubara Y, Narisawa K: Isolation and characterization of mutations in the human holocarboxylase synthetase cDNA. *Nat Genet* **8**:122–128, 1994.

14

Lactose Intolerance

BEULAH M. WOODFIN AND SANJEEV ARORA

CASE REPORT

A 54-year-old Hispanic woman presented with complaints of abdominal distension and bloating after meals, with increased flatulence and episodic diarrhea of about 1 year's duration. These symptoms occur 30 minutes to 4 hours after meals. She knows of no aggravating factors and feels best early in the morning before she eats. Fasting for 8 hours results in complete relief of all symptoms. She has had no nausea or vomiting. She described mild suprapubic cramping and urgency before bowel movements; this discomfort was promptly relieved by defecating.

There is no history of diabetes, previous gastrointestinal surgery, foreign travel, skin rash, or previous radiation exposure. Her past history was significant for low back pain; she had sustained a pathological compression fracture of the lumbar spine 15 months ago. At that time, she had been diagnosed as having osteoporosis and was advised to increase her dietary calcium intake. She estimated her average milk consumption for the last 6 months to be about 3 cups (24 oz) per day. Her physical examination was normal and the stool was negative for occult blood. Flexible sigmoidoscopy was performed and was normal.

DIAGNOSIS

Laboratory Tests

The symptoms of lactose intolerance are nonspecific, and numerous other serious gastrointestinal disorders can cause similar symptoms. The following laboratory tests were performed: hemoglobin, 15 g/dL (normal, 14–16 g/dL); hematocrit, 46% (normal, 44–50%); serum albumin, 4.5 g/dL (normal, 3.8–4.8 g/dL); serum cholesterol, 210 mg/dL (normal, <200 mg/dL); serum β-carotene, 35.7 μg/dL (normal, 20–60 μg/dL); stool ova and parasites, negative for Giardia and amoeba; fecal leukocytes, negative; and thyroid stimulating hormone (TSH), 1 μIU/mL (normal, 0.6–4.6 μIU/mL).

Normal hemoglobin, hematocrit, albumin, cholesterol, and β-carotene levels indicate that malabsorption of iron, amino acids, and fat is not occurring. In celiac disease, for example, one would expect iron deficiency and anemia and low levels of serum cholesterol and β-carotene.

A stool test for ova and parasites allows exclusion of infectious etiologies, such as giardiasis and amebiasis, which often present with similar symptoms. A negative test for fecal leucocytes indicates the absence of an inflammatory mucosal disease, such as ulcerative colitis or Crohn's disease. Patients with hypothyroidism or hyperthyroidism can present with gastrointestinal complaints; a normal TSH level indicates a *euthyroid* (normally functioning thyroid) state.

Fecal occult blood testing and a flexible sigmoidoscopy are performed as screening tests for colonic polyps and cancer. The patient's symptoms of suprapubic cramping, urgency, and relief with defecation could also be produced by a cancer or polyp in the rectum or sigmoid colon.

Diagnostic Tests

The first diagnostic test should be a trial of lactose withdrawal. If this does not result in complete relief of symptoms, the following tests should be performed. The following are the most useful clinical tests:

Breath Hydrogen Test

The breath hydrogen test is a sensitive test based on the metabolism of undigested lactose by colonic bacteria. Bacterial fermentation releases a large quantity of hydrogen (H_2), which is absorbed in the colon and exhaled in the lungs. After an overnight fast, the patient exhales into a breath analyzer (i.e., gas chromatograph) and the concentration of H_2 is determined in parts per million (ppm). A water solution of 50 g of lactose (equivalent to 32 oz of milk) is then ingested.

The dose of lactose administered in this test is greater than that commonly consumed by the population at large. Although this is a useful test to diagnose lactose deficiency, its results cannot be extrapolated to indicate that a patient will necessarily be symptomatic when lesser, more physiologic quantities of lactose are consumed in the diet.

Oral Lactose Tolerance Test

This test measures the serum glucose profile after ingestion of 50 g of lactose. The serum glucose is measured in the fasting state and then every 30 minutes thereafter for 2 hours following lactose ingestion. As with the breath hydrogen test, the results should be interpreted with caution. Neither of these tests can distinguish between primary and secondary lactase deficiency.

Quantitation of Small Bowel Lactase Activity

This test can be performed on a tissue sample obtained from the distal duodenum by endoscopy or jejunal biopsy. Although useful for research purposes, because of its invasive nature, this test is seldom used clinically to make the diagnosis of lactase deficiency.

Case Discussion

Lactose intolerance is a prevalent clinical problem. It is estimated that 50 million Americans may experience some discomfort after consuming lactose-rich products. The prevalence of this condition varies greatly between different races and populations, from less than 30% in Europeans to nearly 100% in some Asian populations. In North America, the prevalence varies according to ethnic origin (see section on Ethnic Distribution).

It is important to distinguish between *lactase deficiency,* or *hypolactasia* (a marked diminution in lactose-phlorizin hydrolase), and *lactose intolerance* (a clinical syndrome of milk intolerance). Symptoms of lactose intolerance develop in only a subset of patients with hypolactasia and include *meteorism* (abnormal distension resulting from the presence of gas or air in the intestine or in the peritoneal cavity), *borborygmi* (rumbling noises caused by propulsion of gas through the intestines), flatulence, distension, dyspepsia, fullness, colicky pains, loose stools, and diarrhea. Patients often are unable to make the connection between the consumption of milk products and their symptoms because they have tolerated milk products in the past (Aurusicchio and Pitchumoni, 1994). An increasing number of patients with hypolactasia develop symptoms as soon as the quantity of lactose ingested is increased. Other variables that can influence development of lactose intolerance are gastric-emptying time and small intestinal transit time.

Patients with rapid gastric emptying are more susceptible to symptoms of lactose intolerance because a large amount of lactose is delivered rapidly into the small intestine, overwhelming its capacity to digest lactose. Consuming milk products as a part of a meal reduces symptoms by slowing the rate of delivery of lactose to the small intestine. Patients with irritable bowel syndrome and inflammatory bowel disease (ulcerative colitis, Crohn's disease) are more sensitive to intestinal distension and therefore are more symptomatic if lactase deficiency is present (Fig. 14-1). Gastric surgery, such as *vagotomy* (surgical division of the vagus nerve) and *pyloroplasty* (an operation on the pylorus), can bring on symptoms of previously subclinical lactase deficiency by enhancing gastric emptying.

Most adult patients with lactase deficiency can

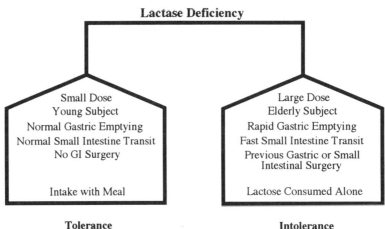

Figure 14-1. Characteristics of different presentations of lactose deficiency.

tolerate a modest intake of lactose, for example, the amount contained in a cup of milk (12 g). Lactase deficiency presents in three distinct clinical syndromes:

1. *Congenital:* This is a very rare inborn error of metabolism transmitted in an autosomal recessive pattern (*alactasia*).
2. *Primary,* adult lactase deficiency, isolated: This is the common type discussed in detail as the subject of this chapter (*hypolactasia*).
3. *Secondary:* This type is caused by a decrease in lactase activity in the small intestine as a result of disease or damage to the small intestine villous structure or its function (Table 14-1).

The patient developed symptoms characteristic of lactose intolerance soon after she modified her diet. Attempts to increase dietary calcium led her to consume increased quantities of milk products containing lactose, which unmasked her underlying lactase deficiency. When taking the history and physical, it is important to exclude other causes of gastrointestinal symptoms, such as infectious enteropathy, inflammatory bowel disease, diabetic autonomic neuropathy with gastrointestinal symptoms, celiac disease, and gastrointestinal malignancy. An absence of weight loss and normal hemoglobin, hematocrit, serum albumin, and cholesterol levels make a generalized malabsorption disorder unlikely. Causes of second-

Table 14-1. Causes of Secondary Lactase Deficiency

Celiac disease	Acute enteritis
Tropical sprue	Viral
Cystic fibrosis	Bacterial
Protein calorie malnutrition	Parasite infection Giardia
Blind loop syndrome	AIDS enteropathy Whipple's disease
Short gut syndrome (small bowel resection)	Radiation enteropathy
Zollinger Ellison syndrome	

AIDS, acquired immunodeficiency syndrome.

ary lactose deficiency should also be considered and excluded by using appropriate tests, if indicated.

MOLECULAR PERSPECTIVES

History

Two thousand years ago Galen reported that milk had a cathartic effect and could produce other gastrointestinal symptoms. It was not until the late nineteenth century, however, that it was shown in dogs that milk sugar (*lactose*) was the responsible agent, causing an osmotic diarrhea due to lack of lactase activity. The lactose-splitting enzyme activity could be demonstrated in the intestines of a wide variety of young animals but rarely in adult animals. The observation was extended to humans in the mid-twentieth century (Sahi, 1994a). Lactase activity was associated with the mucosa of the small intestine, being highest in the jejunum and decreasing with progression toward the ileum. Although some studies reported finding lactase activity in the intestinal juice, by the late 1950s it was generally accepted that lactase activity is localized to the brush border of the small intestine.

Early studies were conducted on adults of Northern European origin. The results of these studies led to the conclusion that high lactase activity throughout life was normal. Subsequent studies, however, showed that many healthy adults with a normal small intestinal mucosa were almost completely devoid of lactase activity. Recent data indicate that lactase expression correlates directly with the concentration of lactase mRNA. Sequencing of the lactase cDNA from adults with high and low lactase activities showed no differences, suggesting that activity is directly related to the level of transcription.

The observation that lactase activity persisted after weaning in some individuals gave rise to the theory that lactase activity could be induced by dietary lactose. A series of animal studies in the early twentieth century and others in mid-century, however, led to the conclusion that adaptation to dietary lactose does not occur (Sahi, 1994b). Studies in the 1960s using more accurate assay methods showed some increase in lactase activity in adult animals and humans when fed lactose, but the increase was insignificant compared with the postweaning loss in activity. Continued feeding of lactose after weaning, however, might delay the decline in activity (Johnson, et al., 1993).

Incidence

Lactose intolerance is usually a disease of adults and is most often associated with an inadequate amount of the enzyme *lactase* in the small intestine (Fig. 14-2) (Auricchio and Maiuri, 1994). The term *milk intolerance* is frequently used interchangeably with lactose intolerance, but the latter can also be caused by milk factors other than lactose. Transient lactose intolerance is observed secondary to enteritis, in celiac disease, and in protein-calorie malnutrition. Lactase activity returns following healing of the intestine. Because of the immaturity of the villi, lactose intolerance is also usually observed in preterm infants.

As noted earlier, the common reduction in lactase activity observed in most adults is referred to as *hypolactasia*, or *lactase deficiency*. The term *alactasia* refers to a total lack of lactase activity. The line between hypolactasia and the higher activity observed in *lactase persistence* is arbitrary, but lactase

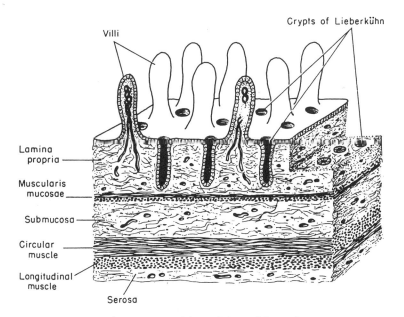

Figure 14-2. Structure of the epithelium of the small intestine.

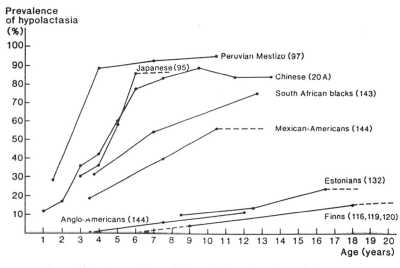

Figure 14-3. The prevalence of lactase deficiency in various ethnic groups.

activities observed in adults show a bimodal distribution. This terminology implies that low lactase activity in adults represents an abnormality, but it has been shown to be the most common situation when many different populations are examined.

Lactase-phlorizin hydrolase (LPH) is a brush-border enzyme with two active sites and three catalytic activities. One active site expresses lactase (EC 3.2.1.23) activity and catalyzes the hydrolysis of lactose to D-glucose and D-galactose; the other site is

extremely low level in adults, reaching a minimum of about 10% of the infant level at about 20 years of age (hypolactasia) (Montgomery et al., 1991). In some ethnic groups, however, lactase activity continues throughout life (*lactase persistence*) (Flatz, 1987) (Fig. 14-3).

Metabolism of Lactose

Lactase catalyzes the following reaction in the intestinal lumen:

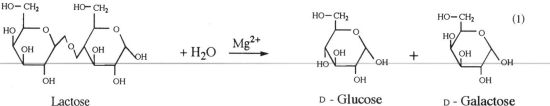

responsible for both phlorizin hydrolase (EC 3.2.1.62) activity (aryl glycosidase) and β-glucosylceramidase (EC 3.2.1.45-46) activity. The lactase activity of LPH is responsible for the hydrolysis of dietary lactose (Greenberger and Isselbacher, 1994).

During human development, lactase activity appears in the fetus late in gestation, continues at a high level until weaning, and then declines to an

The monosaccharide products are actively transported from the lumen and transferred to the portal circulation by the cells of the intestinal epithelium (Brooks et al., 1980). In the liver, glucose is phosphorylated at C_6 by glucokinase and stored as glycogen or metabolized. Galactose, however, is phosphorylated at the C_1 position by a specific enzyme, namely galactokinase:

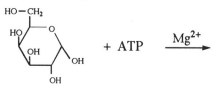

D - Galactose

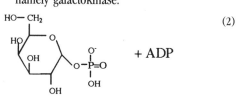

D - Galactose 1-phosphate

The galactose 1-phosphate is then transferred to uridylic acid (UMP) in a reversible reaction by galactose 1-phosphate uridyltransferase:

(3)

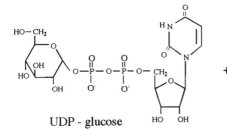 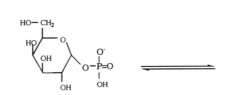

UDP - glucose   D - Galactose 1-phosphate

UDP - galactose   D - Glucose 1-phosphate

The interconversion of UDP-galactose and UDP-glucose is catalyzed by the enzyme UDP-galactose-4-epimerase, historically called *galactowaldenase* because it accomplishes a Walden inversion on C_4. NAD^+ acts as a true coenzyme in this reaction. The C_4 is oxidized to a carbonyl and subsequently reduced back to the alcohol; the configuration of the hydroxyl group is randomized, and the NAD^+ is regenerated.

$+ NADH + H^+$ (4)

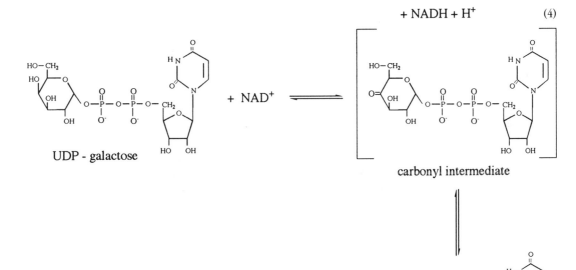

UDP - galactose

$+ NAD^+$

carbonyl intermediate

UDP - glucose

The net of these last 3 reactions is

$$\text{D-Galactose} + \text{ATP} \rightarrow \text{D-glucose 1-phosphate} + \text{ADP} \quad (5)$$

The glucose moiety of glucose 1-phosphate can be directly incorporated into glycogen; alternatively, glucose 1-phosphate can be isomerized to glucose 6-phosphate. Glucose 6-phosphate, in turn, can be metabolized through glycolysis or the pentose phosphate pathway, or it can be hydrolyzed to free glucose, which can enter the blood circulation for transport to other tissues. The hydrolysis of glucose 6-phosphate to produce free glucose occurs only in the liver.

The inability to convert galactose to glucose leads to an accumulation of galactose (*galactosemia*), which can cause mental retardation and even death.

Ethnic Distribution

The persistence of lactase activity is greatest in those geographic areas where adults consume milk and milk products. As shown in Table 14-2, less than ¼ of the white population of the United States exhibit hypolactasia, and among those of Northern European descent, this group falls to less than 10%. Low lactase levels are observed in much larger proportions of Native Americans and blacks and universally among Asian-Americans. Among Europeans, Scandinavians are far less likely to suffer from hypolactasia than are people from the Mediterranean countries (Table 14-3) (also Rao et al., 1994).

A recent study relates lactase persistence to the decline in female fertility above 30 years of age (Cramer et al., 1994). Populations in whom the incidence of hypolactasia is low and consumption of dairy products is considerable have a high level of exposure to dietary galactose, which has been shown to be toxic to ovarian germ cells. A positive correlation is reported between the decline in fertility at older ages and per capita milk consumption.

Table 14-2. Lactase Phenotypes in the United States by Ethnicity

Ethnic Group	% Lactase Deficient
Vietnamese	100
Native American	95
Black	65
White	22
Northern European	7

Table 14-3. Lactase Phenotypes in European Populations

Nationality	% Lactase Deficient
Italian	
Southern	72
Northern	50
French	
Total	32
Southern	44
Austrian	20
Swedish	1
Dutch	0

Diagnostic Tests

Enzyme Assay

The most accurate, but also the most invasive, method for determining lactase activity is from a jejunal biopsy, which is not necessarily diagnostic of lactose intolerance per se; normal lactase activity can be present in more distal areas of the small intestine (Arola, 1994).

The activity can be assayed at pH 7.0 by either of two colorimetric methods:

1. *Direct,* using p-NO_2-phenyl-β-D-galactoside as substrate: the reaction is stopped by adjusting the pH to 9.0, at which the product p-NO_2-phenylate anion produces a strong yellow color.

2. *Indirect,* by coupling to the glucose oxidase/peroxidase reactions.

$$\text{Lactose} + H_2O \rightarrow \text{D-Galactose} + \text{D-Glucose}$$

$$\text{D-Glucose} + O_2 \rightarrow \text{D-Gluconic acid} + H_2O_2$$

$$H_2O_2 + \text{o-Dianisidine} \rightarrow \text{oxidized o-Dianisidine (brown)}$$

A variation of this test, which is faster but less accurate, measures the glucose product using a glucose test strip designed for urine glucose testing. Chemicals in the test strip react with glucose to produce a visible color, the intensity of which is compared with a color key to estimate glucose concentration.

Lactose Tolerance Tests

Breath Hydrogen Test. This test, often referred to as the "gold standard," is based on the determination of H_2 in expired air after an oral lactose dose. H_2 is produced in the colon by colonic flora and 15 to 20% is exhaled through the lungs. Usually, end-expiratory samples are taken at 30-minute intervals after ingestion of 50 g of lactose (equivalent to 32 oz of milk) and compared with the zero-time level. The quantity of H_2 is determined by gas chromatography. An increase in the amount of breath H_2 in excess of 20 ppm above the zero-time level supports the diagnosis of lactase deficiency (Rumessen et al., 1994).

In some cases, colonic flora do not metabolize lactose, especially in infants. Reduced pH and active diarrhea can also produce false-negative results. In addition, the presence of methane-producing bacteria (which consume H_2) has been noted in a number of cases; simultaneous determination of CH_4 has been recommended to interpret H_2 breath-test data accurately.

Blood Tests.

1. The Oral Lactose Load Test: This test is most widely used and is based on the measurement of increased blood glucose after oral administration of lactose. Blood samples are taken at intervals at zero time and at 30-minute intervals and analyzed for glucose. A rise in blood glucose of less than 1.1 mmol/L (20 mg/dL) is indicative of hypolactasia, whereas a rise greater than 1.7 mmol/L (30 mg/dL) is indicative of lactose persistence. An incremental rise of 1.1 to 1.7 mmol/L is inconclusive. Symptoms after the test are recorded and used to help evaluate equivocal situations (Greenberger and Isselbacher, 1994).
2. The Lactose-Ethanol Load Test: This test measures blood galactose and is a more specific test for lactase activity. Because of the rapid conversion of galactose to glucose by the liver, there is no significant increase in blood galactose after oral administration of lactose. Administration of ethanol just before lactose ingestion inhibits galactose metabolism. Metabolism of ethanol by the liver transiently depletes intracellular NAD^+, preventing the epimerization reaction (see section entitled Metabolism of Lactose). In the simplest method reported, ethanol (300 mg/kg) is administered 15 minutes before lactose, and a single blood sample is taken 40 minutes after lactose ingestion. Hypolactasia is indicated by a blood galactose level of less than 0.3 mmol/L (5 mg/dL). This test is used widely in Europe but not in the United States.

THERAPY

Dietary management is the mainstay of treatment of lactose intolerance. Patients should be educated with regard to which foods contain lactose and how much they contain. Patients are advised to read labels carefully to identify sources of lactose. When lactose is consumed, it is preferable to divide it into several meals and to combine it with other solid food, such as fats or dietary fiber, to slow the rate of gastric emptying (Billako and Maaroos, 1994).

It is advisable to start with complete lactose restriction to confirm that all the symptoms are indeed related to the lactose intolerance. For the long term, the degree of lactose restriction required depends on individual tolerance (Tamm, 1994). Calcium supplementation may be needed in patients requiring severe lactose restriction. Table 14-4 lists common foods with a high lactose content.

It is noteworthy that hard cheeses (e.g., cheddar, swiss) are low in lactose and are often well tolerated. Although yogurt contains more lactose per serving than milk, it is better tolerated by patients with lactose deficiency. It is hypothesized that the live bacteria in yogurt release lactases when the bacteria are digested by stomach acid and proteolytic enzymes. These lactases then assist in digestion of the lactose (Kolars et al., 1984). Milk containing *Lac-*

Table 14-4. Lactose Content of Common Milk Products

Food	Serving Size	Approximate Lactose Content (g)
Milk		
Whole (3.3%)	8 oz	11.0
Lowfat (1% and 2%)	8 oz	12.0
Nonfat, skim	8 oz	12.0
Cheeses		
American, pasteurized process	1 oz	0.5
Cheddar	1 oz	0.4
Mozzarella, part skim	1 oz	0.8
Swiss	1 cu in.	0.6
Soft cheeses		
Cream cheese	1 oz	0.8
Cottage cheese lowfat (1%)	4 oz	3.0
Yogurt		
Plain, skim with solids	8 oz	17.0
Vanilla ice cream	1 cup	10.0

From Aurusicchio LN, Pitchumoni CS (1994).

tobacillus acidophilus does not appear to have the same effect.

A large number of prescription and over-the-counter medicines contain lactose as a filler or drug carrier. A list is available from the Food and Drug Administration. Commercially available products to relieve the symptoms of lactase deficiency are sold under the tradenames Lact-Aid, Dairy-Ease, and Lactrase.

QUESTIONS

1. What are the reactions that enable galactose to be metabolized by the glycolytic pathway?
2. Suggest a mechanism for the reaction catalyzed by galactose 1-phosphate uridyltransferase.
3. The incidence of adult hypolactasia is high in countries such as Afghanistan (83%), Egypt (73%), Jordan (75%), and Singapore (93%); it is low in Australia (6%), Denmark (4%), New Zealand (9%), and the United Kingdom (5%). The following are the corresponding declines in fertility after age 30 years for each population: Afghanistan, 31%; Egypt, 34%; Jordan, 23%; Singapore, 70%; Australia, 83%; Denmark, 87%; New Zealand, 84%; the United Kingdom, 84%. Cramer, et al. (1994) suggest that these data are the result of exposure to different levels of galactose in adult females. Can you suggest another explanation?
4. What results can be expected from a breath hydrogen test (lactose breath test) and an oral lactose tolerance test in a patient with untreated celiac disease?
5. What effect would eating a beefsteak along with a glass of milk have on symptoms of lactose intolerance in a patient with lactose intolerance?
6. Which of the following statements are true of the patient in this chapter?
   a. Visual appearance of the duodenal and jejunal mucosa on endoscopy is normal.
   b. On light microscopy of jejunal biopsies, the villi in the jejunum are blunted.
   c. Measurement of fecal fat for 72 hours reveals steatorrhea.

REFERENCES

Arola H: Diagnosis of hypolactasia and lactose malabsorption. *Scand J Gastroenterol* 29(suppl) 202:26–35, 1994.

Auricchio S, Maiuri L: Cellular basis of adult-type hypolactasia. *Acta Paediatr* 395:14–17, 1994.

Aurusicchio LN, Pitchumoni CS: Lactose intolerance: Recognizing the link between diet and discomfort. *Postgrad Med* 95:113–120, 1994.

Billako K, Maaroos H: Clinical picture of hypolactasia and lactose intolerance. *Scand J Gastroenterol* 29(suppl) 202:36–54, 1994.

Brooks SM, Paynton-Brooks N: *The Human Body. Structure and Function in Health and Disease.* St. Louis, MO, CV Mosby Company, 1980, p. 313.

Cramer DW, Xu H, Sahi T: Adult hypolactasia, milk consumption, and age-specific fertility. *Am J Epidemiol* 139:282–289, 1994.

Flatz G: Genetics of lactose digestion in humans, *in* Harris H, Hirschhorn H (eds): *Advances in Human Genetics,* New York, Plenum, 1987, pp 1–77.

Greenberger NJ, Isselbacher KJ: Disorders of absorption/disaccharidase deficiency syndromes, *in* KJ Isselbacher et al., (eds): *Harrison's Principles of Internal Medicine, 13th edition,* New York, McGraw Hill, 1994, pp 1399–1401.

Johnson AO, Semenya JG, et al. Adaptation of lactose maldigesters to continued milk intake. *Am J Clin Nutrition* 58:879–881, 1993.

Kolars JC, Levitt MD, et al. Yogurt: an autodigesting source of lactase. *N Eng J Med* 310:1–3, 1984.

Montgomery RK, Büller HA, et al.: Lactose intolerance and the genetic regulation of intestinal lactase-phlorizin hydrolase. *FASEB J* 5:2824–2832, 1991.

Rao DR, Bello H, Warren AP, Brown GE: Prevalence of lactose maldigestion: Influence and interaction of age, race, and sex. *Dig Dis Sci* 39:1519–1524, 1994.

Rumessen JJ, Nordgaard-Andersen I, Gudmand-Høyer E: Carbohydrate malabsorption: Quantification by methane and hydrogen breath tests. *Scand J Gastroenterol* 29:826–832, 1994.

Sahi T: Hypolactasia and lactase persistence. *Scand J Gastroenterol* 29(suppl) 202:1–6, 1994a.

Sahi T: Genetics and epidemiology of adult-type hypolactasia. *Scand J Gastroenterol* 29(suppl) 202:7–20, 1994b.

Tamm A: Management of lactose intolerance. *Scand J Gastroenterol* 29(suppl) 202:55–63, 1994.

15

Systemic Carnitine Deficiency:
A Treatable Disorder

HARBHAJAN S. PAUL AND GAIL SEKAS

CASE REPORT

This 3½-year-old boy was born to nonconsanguineous parents from Chihuahua, Mexico, after an uncomplicated pregnancy and delivery. A brother had died at 3 months of age of a "liver problem" after an unexplained coma. The parents and three siblings are well.

At 3 months of age, the patient was in a coma and admitted to a community hospital, where he suffered a cardiac arrest. Examination revealed hepatomegaly and cardiomegaly and a blood glucose concentration of 15 mg/dL (normal, 60–100 mg/dL). Hepatomegaly and hypotonia were noted on admission. On day 3, he became lethargic and generalized seizure activity and cardiac arrest developed, but he was successfully resuscitated. The patient eventually recovered and the hepatomegaly resolved. At six months of age, he developed congestive heart failure after an upper respiratory tract infection and was brought to the medical center of the University of California, Los Angeles. Hepatomegaly and hypotonia were noted on admission. On day 3, he became lethargic and generalized seizure activity and cardiac arrest developed. Laboratory studies at the time of the arrest revealed a blood glucose level of 15 mg/dL without associated acidosis or ketosis; mild elevation of serum aspartate aminotransferase (SGOT) (337 IU/L; normal, 6–36 IU/L) and alanine aminotransferase (SGPT) (179 IU/L; normal = 10 to 45 IU/L); and hyperammonemia (300 μg/dL; normal,

<69 μg/dL). Delayed milestones (developmental quotient 66; normal, 100), proximal-muscle weakness, and growth retardation (weight and height below the third percentile) were noted after recovery. Metabolic studies showed normal glucose, galactose, and fructose tolerance and a normal 10-hour fasting blood glucose level, with no increase in lactate, pyruvate, or ketone bodies. The electroencephalogram, brain scan, and chromosomal studies were unremarkable. Also normal were the plasma levels of electrolytes, calcium, phosphorus, magnesium, bilirubin, thyroxine, thyroid-stimulating hormone, and growth hormone. Results of total serum protein determination, serum electrophoresis, cerebrospinal fluid studies, and studies of immune function were also normal. Between acute episodes, blood glucose levels, ammonia, SGOT, SGPT, and creatine phosphokinase were all normal.

The patient was again admitted with cardiorespiratory arrest after upper respiratory tract infections at the ages of 20, 24, and 33 months. The episodes were associated with liver enlargement, elevations of transaminases to >2000 IU/L, and of creatine phosphokinase from 1500 to 33,000 IU/L. Maintenance glucose requirements varied from normal (3 mg/kg of body weight per min) to slightly elevated (5–7 mg/kg/min).

A muscle biopsy contained large amounts of neutral lipids, and a liver biopsy also showed severe but nonspecific fatty changes. Also evident were abnormal mitochondrial structure, many electron-dense lysosome-like bodies, and dense, laminate, rounded lipofuscin-like particles.

A 32-hour fasting study was performed. During the fasting period, the patient had no nausea, cramps, or pigmenturia; however, at 32 hours he suddenly had a cardiorespiratory arrest characterized by an absence of cardiac electrical activity. He was successfully resuscitated and intravenous glucose was administered.

At the start of the fast, his blood glucose was 91 mg/dL, but by 24 hours it had fallen to 66 mg/dL. Plasma triglyceride levels rose from 66 to 126 mg/dL and free fatty acids increased from 0.1 to 2.0 mEq/L. Serum SGOT rose from 36 to 1450 IU/L, but there was no increase in creatine phosphokinase or aldolase. Ammonia increased from 40 to 134 μg/dL. The most significant finding, however, was the lack of production of measurable ketone bodies.

During the 11th admission, the diagnosis of carnitine deficiency was considered because of fatty changes in the liver and the lack of production of ketone bodies after 24 hours of fasting. At that time the patient's height and weight were normal, but his developmental quotient was 40, and he had a variety of neuromuscular abnormalities. A computerized axial tomography (CT) scan of the brain revealed marked enlargement of both lateral ventricles and of the sulci between the cerebral gyri.

DIAGNOSIS

The diagnosis of carnitine deficiency requires determination of carnitine levels in tissues (Broquist, 1982; Bieber, 1988). The syndrome of carnitine deficiency can be classified as myopathic (Waber et al., 1982) or systemic (Chapoy et al., 1980), depending on which tissues are involved. The syndrome is considered *myopathic* when carnitine deficiency is limited to muscle. If several tissues and plasma are involved, the syndrome is called *systemic*.

Myopathic

1. Only muscle tissue involved
2. Carnitine levels reduced only in muscle
3. Plasma carnitine levels often normal
4. Elevated serum enzymes of muscle origin
5. Fatty infiltration in muscle
6. Able to produce ketone bodies

7. Usually not associated with hepatic and central nervous system dysfunctions
8. Less responsive to carnitine therapy

Systemic

1. Several tissues involved
2. Carnitine levels reduced in several tissues
3. Plasma carnitine levels either normal or decreased
4. Elevated serum enzymes of muscle and liver origin
5. Fatty infiltration in muscle, liver, and other tissues
6. Unable to produce ketone bodies
7. Often associated with hepatic and central nervous system dysfunctions
8. Often responsive to carnitine therapy

Failure to produce ketone bodies on fasting and the accumulation of lipids in tissues are suggestive of carnitine deficiency; however, a key feature in establishing the diagnosis is the determination of carnitine levels in tissues. Decreased carnitine levels concomitant with lipid accumulation in tissues are more reliable criteria for the diagnosis of systemic carnitine deficiency than serum carnitine levels alone. As shown in Table 15-1, before therapy there was a marked deficiency of carnitine in muscle, liver, serum, and urine of this patient, indicating that the patient suffers from systemic carnitine deficiency.

To establish a firm diagnosis, it is essential to rule out any defect in carnitine acyltransferase I and II (CAT-I, CAT-II) and the enzymes of the β-oxidation pathway. Carnitine is present in tissues in free and esterified forms; together, these constitute *total carnitine*. For diagnostic purposes it is essential to measure total carnitine.

Two other disorders that could be easily confused with systemic carnitine deficiency are urea cycle enzymopathies (Chapter 24) and Reye syndrome, in which liver dysfunction, hyperammonemia, and central nervous system involvement are observed. None however, of these disorders, is associated with carnitine deficiency, and patients with a defective urea cycle enzyme or Reye syndrome often have either normal or only slightly depressed plasma and tissue carnitine levels. Furthermore, unlike patients with urea cycle disorders, patients with systemic carnitine deficiency do not exhibit protein intolerance and

Table 15-1. Carnitine Levels in Muscle, Liver, Serum, and Urine

Tissue	No. of Samples	Controls	Patient Before Therapy	Patient After Therapy
Muscle				
Total Carnitine (nmol/mg noncollagen protein)	9	13.4 ± 2.6[a]	0.19	
Total Carnitine (mmol/g wet weight)	9	1.2 ± 0.3	0.02	0.5
Liver				
Total Carnitine (nmol/mg noncollagen protein)	10	6.8 ± 0.7	0.37	
Total Carnitine (mmol/g wet weight)	1	1.2	0.04	5.0
Serum (mmol/L)	10	35.5 ± 5.6	4.82	18.5
Urine (mmol/24 h)	1	231	47	1660

From Chapoy et al., (1980).

[a] Mean ± SD

have normal plasma and urinary levels of citrulline, argininosuccinate, and arginine. Reye syndrome can also be distinguished from carnitine deficiency on the basis of the case history in that the former is often preceded by a viral illness.

In general, the following steps should be taken to establish a diagnosis of carnitine deficiency:

1. Case history: frequency of illness, symptomology
2. Familial history: death of any sibling and the cause of that death
3. Physical examination: muscle weakness
4. Biochemical analysis: serum enzymes, blood levels of glucose, carnitine, ammonia, free fatty acids
5. Dietary studies: response to fasting, ability to produce ketone bodies, improvement with fat-restricted diet
6. Tissue biopsy: lipid accumulation and tissue levels of carnitine.

MOLECULAR PERSPECTIVES

L-Carnitine is required in humans for the oxidation of long-chain fatty acids (Engel, 1980). It is synthesized endogenously from the essential amino acid lysine, with terminal methyl groups donated by S-adenosylmethionine according to the scheme outlined in Fig. 15-1. Methylation of the lysine side chain occurs when this amino acid is in proteins. In humans the final reaction in the pathway, catalyzed by a cytosolic hydroxylase, occurs in the liver, kidney, and other tissues but not in cardiac or skeletal muscle (Bieber, 1988; Broquist, 1982). The carnitine requirement of these tissues is met by carnitine transported to them via the plasma from sites of biosynthesis (Paul et al., 1992). Failure of cardiac and skeletal muscles to obtain sufficient carnitine results in cardiomyopathy and muscular weakness, respectively.

In addition to endogenous synthesis, a significant amount of carnitine is usually provided by dietary sources. Meat products, particularly red meats, and dairy products are important dietary sources of carnitine. Because the human body can usually synthesize adequate amounts of carnitine, it is not considered an essential nutrient. Many infant formulas, particularly those based on soy protein, are low in carnitine; so infants receiving a significant part of their nutrition from such formulas may be susceptible to carnitine deficiency.

Long-chain fatty acids cannot penetrate the inner membrane of mitochondria. The primary function of carnitine is to transfer long-chain fatty acids from the cytosol into mitochondria for oxidation. In contrast to long-chain fatty acids, the transport of medium-chain fatty acids (C_6 to C_{10}) into mitochondria does not depend on carnitine. Free fatty acids enter the cell and are activated to their coenzyme A (CoA) esters in the reaction catalyzed by fatty acyl-coenzyme A synthetase:

$$\text{Fatty acid} + \text{ATP} + \text{CoASH} \rightarrow \text{fatty acyl-CoA} + \text{AMP} + \text{PP}_i$$

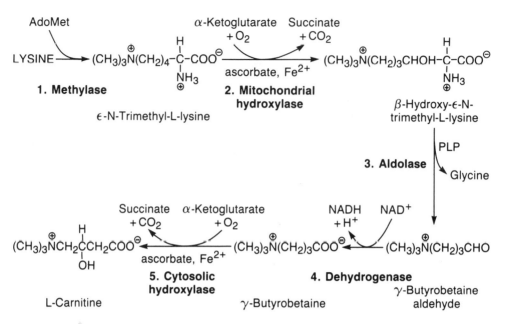

Figure 15-1. Carnitine biosynthetic pathway. AdoMet, S-adenosylmethionine. *From* Broquist (1982).

The mitochondrial inner membrane is impermeable to fatty acyl-CoA. To be transported into mitochondria, fatty acyl-CoA must first be converted to fatty acylcarnitine, which can readily cross the mitochondrial inner membrane. This reaction is catalyzed by CAT-I localized on the outer surface of the mitochondrial inner membrane:

Fatty acyl-CoA + carnitine ⇔ fatty acylcarnitine + CoASH

Once inside the mitochondria, another enzyme, CAT-II, located on the matrix side of the mitochondrial inner membrane, catalyzes the reconversion of fatty acylcarnitine to fatty acyl-CoA. Intramitochondrial fatty acyl-CoA then undergoes β-oxidation, and the carnitine molecule returns to the cytosolic compartment. These reactions are shown schematically in Figure 15-2. Failure of this transport mechanism because of a carnitine deficiency or abnormalities of one or both of the carnitine acyltransferases blocks fatty acid oxidation. Most ketone bodies are synthesized from acetyl-CoA units derived from the oxidation of fatty acids in liver; therefore, any defect in fatty acid oxidation will necessarily also impair ketogenesis. Another consequence of impaired fatty acid oxidation is lipid accumulation in tissues (e.g., muscle).

Besides mitochondria, peroxisomes are also active in the oxidation of fatty acids, particularly the very-long-chain fatty acids ($>C_{18}$), and require the participation of carnitine. Unlike the oxidation of fatty acids in mitochondria, the oxidation of fatty acids in peroxisomes is not complete but terminates at acyl-CoA residues of medium-chain length. These acyl-CoA residues, as well as acetyl-CoA produced by β-oxidation, are then transported out of peroxisomes as acylcarnitines for further metabolism. Formation of acylcarnitines is catalyzed by carnitine acyltransferases, enzymes that are located in peroxisomes and that use carnitine as a substrate. Therefore, peroxisomal metabolism of fatty acids requires a substantial amount of carnitine. The source of carnitine for peroxisomal metabolism had not been known; however, a recent study demonstrated that hepatic peroxisomes contain γ-butyrobetaine hydroxylase, an enzyme that catalyzes the crucial final step in the biosynthesis of carnitine, and indeed are capable of synthesizing carnitine (Paul et al., 1992). The implication of this observation is that persons with genetic disorders of peroxisomes may be at risk for developing carnitine deficiency.

Clinically, the myopathic form of carnitine deficiency is characterized by progressive muscle weakness, lipid accumulation in muscle, and elevated serum enzymes of muscle origin (e.g., aldolase, SGPT) (Rebouche and Engel, 1983). Onset may occur early in life, or it may be delayed until middle

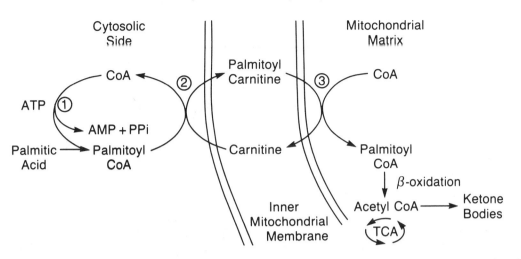

Figure 15-2. Transport of long-chain fatty acids into mitochondria. Palmitoyl-CoA synthetase; "outer" carnitine palmitoyltransferase; "inner" carnitine palmitoyltransferase CoA, coenzyme A; ATP, adenosine triphosphate; AMP, adenosine monophosphate; TCA, tricarboxylic acid; PP_i. *From* Broquist (1982).

age. Carnitine levels in the muscles of such patients are markedly reduced, whereas levels in liver and serum are usually normal. Many of these patients also develop cardiomyopathy. It is believed that diminished ATP resulting from impaired fatty acid oxidation is the contributing factor to the skeletal and cardiac muscle dysfunctions. It is postulated that patients with the myopathic disease have normal carnitine biosynthesis, but carnitine transport into muscle is defective.

The manifestations of the systemic form of carnitine deficiency are usually expressed early in life. Systemic carnitine deficiency is associated with hepatic dysfunction and central nervous system symptoms, including repeated episodes of acute encephalopathy and vomiting, followed by deepening stupor, confusion, and coma. Other symptoms and signs include hypoglycemia, hyperammonemia, and elevated levels of liver and muscle enzymes in serum. The patient's plasma free fatty acid levels are usually elevated but cannot produce ketone bodies. A mild to pronounced increase of neutral lipids in both liver and muscle is found. The patients have low levels of carnitine in the liver and in skeletal muscle and variable levels in serum. Cardiomyopathy accompanied by reduced carnitine levels in the heart is also a prominent feature of many cases of systemic carnitine deficiency.

The recurrent crises in systemic carnitine deficiency appear to be provoked by caloric deprivation. This situation calls for increased use of fatty acids and increased gluconeogenesis. Effective use of fatty acids, however, is limited by the carnitine deficiency. Gluconeogenesis, which occurs mostly in the liver, requires large amounts of ATP, the generation of which depends largely on the oxidation of fatty acids. Consequently, the patient who cannot oxidize long-chain fatty acids is unable to make adequate amounts of glucose and becomes hypoglycemic. Another reason for the hypoglycemia is that most peripheral tissues, which normally use fatty acids, become glucose dependent. Failure of hepatic ATP production also impairs urea cycle functions, leading to elevated blood ammonia levels (the synthesis of one molecule of urea requires the equivalent of four high-energy phosphoanhydride bonds). It is postulated that systemic carnitine deficiency represents a defect in carnitine biosynthesis.

Cases of carnitine deficiency as a result of genetic disorders, such as the present case, are classified as primary deficiency of carnitine. Cases of secondary deficiency of carnitine have also been described. Such cases are due to disorders of organic acid metabolism or therapy with certain drugs. In such cases, acyl-CoA intermediates accumulate in the tissues, which, by reacting with carnitine, results in the formation of acylcarnitines followed by their urinary excretion (Nishida et al., 1987; Chalmers et al., 1984; Sekas and Paul, 1993). Excretion of large amounts of acylcarnitines depletes the body pool of carnitine, resulting in secondary deficiency. Carnitine supplementation is beneficial and is recommended for these patients.

THERAPY

In a patient with carnitine deficiency, several therapeutic options are available. First, the patient can be treated with either oral or intravenous carnitine. Second, because carnitine deficiency results in lipid accumulation, patients can be maintained on a lipid-restricted and carbohydrate-rich diet. Third, because carnitine is essential for the oxidation of long-chain fatty acids but not medium-chain fatty acids, patients can be given medium-chain triglycerides as a source of dietary fat. Finally, patients with myopathic forms of carnitine deficiency can be treated with glucocorticoids. The beneficial effect of glucocorticoids appears to be due to their ability to enhance the uptake of carnitine by muscle.

In the present case, as soon as the diagnosis of carnitine deficiency was considered, the patient was given a high-carbohydrate, low-fat diet containing 20% of the calories as protein. In addition, the patient was given a total of 2.0 g of carnitine per day administered in three equal doses. Carnitine therapy resulted in dramatic clinical and biochemical changes.

After 3 months of therapy (see Table 15-1), the muscle carnitine levels approached the lower limit of normal and increased nearly 20-fold over pretreatment levels. Carnitine levels in the liver increased nearly three times normal. Serum levels of carnitine, although still lower than controls, increased markedly from the pretherapy levels. Similar increases occurred in urinary carnitine.

In addition to the biochemical changes, dramatic clinical improvements occurred. Hepatomegaly was no longer evident after 2 weeks, and his SGPT level returned to normal. Neurological disturbances, including hyperreflexia of lower extremities, bilateral Babinski responses, and walking disability from weakness and ataxia disappeared after 2 weeks of therapy. His muscle strength increased from 2/5 to 4/5, and he could run for the first time in his life. Sensory-nerve conduction in the left peroneal nerve, virtually unmeasurable before therapy, was normal. Somatosensory-evoked potentials, strikingly abnormal before therapy, showed marked improvement

after 3 months of treatment. The cardiomyopathy was largely resolved.

After establishing the diagnosis and instituting carnitine therapy, the prognosis in such cases is generally quite favorable. Cases of carnitine deficiency have been reported only since the mid-1970s. Therefore, the outcome for patients on a long-term basis is not yet known. Because systemic carnitine deficiency is due to a defect in carnitine biosynthesis, carnitine administration must be lifelong.

QUESTIONS

1. What are the reasons for lipid accumulation in the liver?
2. Why was the patient unable to produce ketone bodies after 24 hours of fasting before carnitine therapy?
3. How can you differentiate whether the carnitine deficiency is systemic or myopathic?
4. What is the cause of hypoglycemia observed in the patient described in this case report?
5. What is "secondary" carnitine deficiency?
6. How can the secondary carnitine deficiency be diagnosed?

REFERENCES

Bieber LL: Carnitine. *Annu Rev Biochem* **57**:261–283, 1988.

Broquist HP: Carnitine biosynthesis and function. *Fed Proc* **41**:2840–2842, 1982.

Chalmers RA, Roe CR, Stacey TE, Hoppel CL: Urinary excretion of L-carnitine and acylcarnitines by patients with disorders of organic acid metabolism: Evidence for secondary insufficiency of L-carnitine. *Pediatr Res* **18**:1325–1328, 1984.

Chapoy PR, Angelini C, Brown WJ, Stiff JE, Shug AL, Cederbaum SD: Systemic carnitine deficiency—A treatable inherited lipid-storage disease presenting as Reye's syndrome. *N Engl J Med* **303**:1389–1394, 1980.

Engel AG: Possible causes and effects of carnitine deficiency in man, *in* Frenkel RA, McGarry JD (eds): *Carnitine Biosynthesis, Metabolism, and Functions.* New York, Academic Press, 1980, pp. 271–284.

Nishida N, Sugimoto T, Araki A, Woo M, Sakane Y, Kobayashi Y: Carnitine metabolism in valproate-treated rats: The effect of L-carnitine supplementation. *Pediatr Res* **22**:500–503, 1987.

Paul HS, Sekas G, Adibi SA: Carnitine synthesis in hepatic peroxisomes. Demonstration of γ-butyrobetaine hydroxylase activity. *Eur J Biochem* **203**:599–605, 1992.

Rebouche CJ, Engel AG: Carnitine metabolism and deficiency syndromes. *Mayo Clin Proc* **58**:533–540, 1983.

Sekas G, Paul HS: Hyperammonemia and carnitine deficiency in a patient receiving sulfadiazine and pyrimethamine. *Am J Med* **95**:112–113, 1993.

Waber LJ, Valle D, Neill C, DiMauro S, Shug A: Carnitine deficiency presenting as familial cardiomyopathy: A treatable defect in carnitine transport. *J Pediatr* **101**:700–705, 1982.

16

Diabetes Mellitus

ABBAS E. KITABCHI AND JOSEPH N. FISHER

CASE REPORT

A 47-year-old white man was brought by his family to the emergency department; he was in a semi-comatose state. His general health was said to have been good, and he had been on no medication. A few weeks before admission he began to complain of excessive thirst. At that time his wife noted that he had started to awaken at night and go to the bathroom, first once, and more recently, several times nightly. Despite having what was described as a good, if not excessive, appetite he had begun to lose weight. Although he was able to continue his work as a draftsman, he complained of visual blurring, which he ascribed to excessive work on a large set of plans he was drawing. On the day before admission, his wife noted that he drank a 2-L bottle of soft drink before noon. His office was in his home, and after lunch he went to take a nap complaining of excessive fatigue. Several hours later his wife found him still in bed and had difficulty arousing him. She noted that he was breathing very deeply and had a "fruity" odor to his breath. Their son helped her get him out of bed and into the car for transportation to the local emergency department.

On examination there he was somnolent but could be aroused and would respond to his name. His pulse was 112 (normal, 60–100), blood pressure 130/70 (normal, 120/80), respiration 28 (normal, 16–20) and very deep, temperature 97.8°F (normal, 98.6). His skin turgor was poor and his eyes appeared sunken. There was no *lipemia retinalis* (lipid deposition in the retina). His lungs were

clear to auscultation and his heart rate was regular with no murmurs, S3 or S4. The abdomen was soft and nontender and the genitalia were those of a normal male. The extremities were free of edema, and pulses were good. On neurological exam there were no focal neurological findings. The laboratory data were as follows: sodium, 128 mEq/L (normal, 135–148); potassium, 0.9 mEq/L (normal, 3.5–5.3); chloride 88 mEq/L (normal, 96–106); bicarbonate 5 mEq/L (normal, 21–28); glucose, 967 mg/dL (normal, 75–115); blood urea nitrogen, 30 mg/dL (normal, 7–18); creatinine, 2.2 mg/dL (normal, 0.9–1.5); complete blood count hematocrit, 48% (normal, 42–50); white blood cells (WBC), 12,300 with 47 neutrophils, no bands, 41 lymphs, 4 basophils, 7 monos, 1 eosinophil; urinalysis 4+ glucose, heavy ketone, protein negative, 2–4 WBC and no red blood cells.

The diagnosis of diabetic ketoacidosis was made, and the patient was started on appropriate therapy. Within 24 hours he was alert, eating, and back to his "normal" self.

DIAGNOSIS

Classification of Diabetes

In the past, there were no uniform criteria for the diagnosis of diabetes mellitus (DM) and its various types. New terminology, classifications, and diagnostic criteria were developed in 1979 by an international workshop, the National Diabetes Data Group, sponsored by the National Institutes of Health and endorsed by the American Diabetes Association and other major diabetes associations. Table 16-1 lists the present classifications of diabetes and other categories of glucose intolerance together with the "statistical-risk classes" (persons who have a high risk of developing diabetes) that may be part of the natural history of diabetes.

Type I Diabetes

Insulin-dependent diabetes mellitus (IDDM), formerly referred to as juvenile-onset diabetes mellitus, is a severe form of diabetes that often involves ketosis. Because of the destruction of beta cells, there is eventually a near total absence of insulin. The loss of beta cells is the result of an autoimmune process, which in some patients may involve other organs, such as the thyroid, in addition to the endocrine pancreas. Both environmental (viral infection or exposure to toxins) and genetic factors (specific major histocompatibility complex [MHC] linkage) are re-

sponsible for the beta cell damage. There is a strong association with human leukocyte antigens (HLA), with predominance in *DR*3 and *DR*4 genes (in 95% of white patients with IDDM versus only 45% of non-IDDM controls). The DQ locus (*DQW 3.2*) has been identified as the susceptibility gene for IDDM. Without insulin, the insulin-sensitive tissues (muscle, fat, liver) cannot metabolize glucose efficiently. In uncontrolled diabetes, excess counterregulatory hormones (catecholamines, glucagon, cortisol, and growth hormone) cause proteolysis of muscle with the release of amino acids, lipolysis of fat with release of free fatty acids, and glycogenolysis in the liver with the release of glucose. All this in turn is associated with an increase in glucose production from noncarbohydrate precursors (*gluconeogenesis*) and ketone body synthesis (*ketogenesis*), both in the liver. A severe metabolic decompensation, diabetic ketoacidosis, may ensue which, without prompt and appropriate treatment, will lead to stupor, coma, and death.

Table 16-1. Types of Diabetes Mellitus and Other Categories of Glucose Intolerance

Disease Classifications	*Distinguishing Characteristics*
Clinical Classes	
Diabetes mellitus (DM)	Patients may be of any age, are usually thin, and have
Type I: insulin-dependent diabetes mellitus (IDDM)	abrupt onset of signs and symptoms before age 40. These patients have ketonemia and are dependent on insulin to sustain life.
Type II: non-insulin-dependent diabetes mellitus (NIDDM) (obese or nonobese)	Patients usually are older than 40 years at diagnosis, are obese, and have a family history of diabetes. Although not dependent on exogenous insulin on discovery, they may require it to sustain euglycemia.
Other types of diabetes mellitus or glucose intolerance	Pancreatic disease: endocrinopathies (Cushing's, acromegaly, pheochromocytoma): drug-induced glucose intolerance
Impaired glucose tolerance (IGT) (obese or nonobese)	Patients with IGT have plasma glucose levels that are higher than normal but not diagnostic for diabetes mellitus.
Gestational diabetes mellitus (GDM)	Patients with GDM have onset or discovery of glucose intolerance during pregnancy.
Statistical Risk Classes[a]	
Previous abnormality of glucose tolerance (PrevAGT)	Persons in this category have normal glucose tolerance but a history of transient diabetes mellitus or impaired glucose tolerance.
Potential abnormality of glucose tolerance (PotAGT)	Persons in this catetory have never experienced abnormal glucose tolerance but have a greater than normal risk for developing diabetes mellitus or impaired glucose tolerance.

Adapted from National Diabetes Data Group (1979) and *Medical Management of Non-Insulin-Dependent* (1994).

[a]Used for epidemiological and research purposes.

Type II Diabetes

Non insulin dependent diabetes mellitus (NID-DM), previously called maturity-onset diabetes, is a heterogeneous form of diabetes that usually has onset in persons over the age of 40 years. The familial incidence of NIDDM is greater than in IDDM (concordance in identical twins is >90% for NIDDM versus 25 to 50% for IDDM). It is characterized by insulin resistance, manifested by impaired glucose uptake and a compensatory increase in insulin secretion. In some patients, this may be accompanied by hypertension and *dyslipidemia* (abnormalities in blood lipoproteins). About 85% of NIDDM patients are obese. The pathogenesis remains uncertain, but it may be the result of both a relative decrease in insulin secretion and action. Most NIDDM patients eventually require insulin for the control of diabetes, in which case they become "insulin-requiring" as opposed to "insulin-dependent"; that is they are *not* reclassified as type I diabetics. Various distinguishing characteristics of these two classes are summarized in Table 16-2. Table 16-3 provide criteria for diagnosis of diabetes in adults and children as well as gestational diabetes, together with criteria for impaired glucose tolerance (IGT).

Diabetic Ketoacidosis and Hyperglycemic, Hyperosmolar Nonketotic State

Diabetic ketoacidosis (DKA) and hyperglycemia, hyperosmolar nonketotic state (HHNS) are two of the most frequently encountered metabolic endocrine emergencies (Kitabchi and Fisher, 1981; Kitabchi et al., 1994; Kitabchi and Wall, 1995). Table 16-4 provides the diagnostic criteria of DKA versus HHNS.

It must be emphasized that because about 70% of the "ketone bodies" are usually present as β-hydroxybutyrate, which gives a negative nitroprusside reaction (Acetest, Ketostix), DKA may still be present when this test is negative. To differentiate DKA from lactic acidosis, serum β-hydroxybutyrate and lactate concentrations must be determined. Increased plasma triglyceride levels, a frequent concomitant of DKA, can cause spuriously low estimates of serum sodium and other electrolytes but do not interfere

Table 16-2. Characteristics for Types I and II Diabetes Mellitus

Features	Types I (IDDM) Ketosis Prone	Type II (NIDDM) Ketosis Resistant
Age at onset (yr)	Usually <20	Usually >40
Proportion of all diabetes	<10%	About 90%
Seasonal trend	Fall and winter	None
Appearance of symptoms	Acute or subacute	Slow
Metabolic ketoacidosis	Frequent	Rare
Obesity at onset	Uncommon	Common
β-Cells	Decreased	Variable
Insulin	Decreased	Variable
Concordance in identical twins	30–50%	90 to 95%
Inflammatory cells in islets	Present initially	Absent
Family history of diabetes	Uncommon	Common
HLA association	Yes	No
Insulin autoantibodies (IAA)	Yes	No
Antibody to islet cells (ICA)	Yes	No
"64K" GAD antibodies	Yes	No
Treatment	Diet and insulin	Diet, oral hypoglycemic agents, or insulin

GAD, Glutamic acid decarboxylase; IDDM, insulin dependent diabetes mellitus; NIDDM, non-insulin-dependent diabetes mellitus; HLA, human lymphocyte antigen.

Table 16-3. Diagnostic Criteria for Diabetes Mellitus (DM), Impaired Glucose Tolerance
(IGT), and Gestational Diabetes Mellitus (GDM)

Nonpregnant Adults

DM Criteria: at least one of the following:
1. Random plasma glucose level of ≥200 mg/dL plus classic DM signs and symptoms,
   including polydipsia, polyuria, polyphagia, and weight loss
2. Fasting plasma glucose level of ≥140 mg/dL on at least two occasions
3. Fasting plasma glucose level of <140 mg/dL plus sustained elevated plasma glucose levels
   during an oral glucose tolerance test. The 2-hr sample and at least one other between 0
   and 2 h after the 75-g glucose dose should be ≥200 mg/dL. Oral glucose tolerance
   testing is not necessary if criteria 1 or 2 have been met.

IGT Criteria: all the following:
1. Fasting plasma glucose <140 mg/dL
2. Two-hour oral glucose tolerance test plasma glucose level between 140 and 199 mg/dL
3. An intervening oral glucose tolerance test plasma glucose value of ≥200 mg/dL

Pregnant Women

GDM Criteria: Following an oral glucose load of 100 g, two plasma glucose values equal or
exceed the following: fasting, 105 mg/dL; 1 h. 190 mg/dL; 2 h. 165 mg/dL; 3 h. 145 mg/dL.

Children

DM Criteria: one of the following:
1. Random plasma glucose level of ≥200 mg/dL plus classic DM signs and symptoms,
   including polyuria, polydipsia, ketonuria, and rapid weight loss
2. Fasting plasma glucose level of ≥140 mg/dL on at least two occasions and sustained
   elevated plasma glucose levels during an oral glucose tolerance test. Both the 2-h plasma
   glucose and at least one other between 0 and 2 h after the glucose dose (1.75 g/kg ideal
   body weight up to 75 g) should be ≥200 mg/dL.

Adapted from National Diabetes Data Group (1979) and *Medical Management of Non-Insulin-Dependent* (1994).

Table 16-4. Criteria for Diagnosis of Diabetic
Ketoacidosis (DKA) and Hyperglycemic,
Hyperosmolar Nonketotic Coma (HHNC)

Parameter	DKA	HHNC
Blood glucose (mg/dL)	>300	>500
Blood pH	<7.3	>7.3
Serum HCO_3^- (mEq/L)	<15	>15
Ketonemia	>1:2 dilution	Negative
Serum osmolarity	Variable	>330 mOsm/kg H_2O
Mental obtundation	Variable	Always present

Adapted from Kitabchi et al., (1994).

with blood gas determination. Although the ratio of
lactate to pyruvate is >20 in most DKA patients,
<20% of these patients have lactate levels >3 mM.

Figure 16-1 depicts causes of hyperglycemia (DM,
HHNC, IGT, and stress hyperglycemia), metabolic acidotic states (lactic acidosis, hyperchloremic acidosis, drug-induced acidosis), and other ketotic
states (ketotic hyperglycemia and alcoholic ketosis).
Table 16-5 lists the most common precipitating fac-

tors for DKA, of which the most frequent omission of
insulin, infection, and undiagnosed diabetes.

MOLECULAR PERSPECTIVES

Diabetes mellitus is a chronic disorder characterized
by fasting hyperglycemia or plasma glucose levels
that are above defined limits during oral glucose
tolerance testing (Kitabchi and Fisher, 1991; National Diabetes Data Group, 1979). It is a genetically
determined, heterogeneous group of clinical disorders with abnormalities in the metabolism of carbohydrates, proteins, and fat that result primarily
from deficiency in the synthesis, secretion, or function of insulin. The disease is associated with microvascular, macrovascular, and metabolic complications.

It was estimated recently that as many as 14 million Americans suffer from DM, although only about
half of this group have been diagnosed (Harris et al.,
1987; National Diabetes Data Group, 1995). About

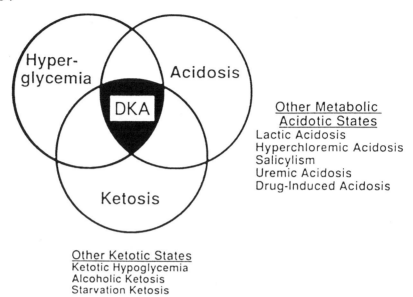

Other Hyperglycemic States
Diabetes Mellitus
Non-Ketotic Hyperosmolar Coma
Impaired Glucose Tolerance
Stress Hyperglycemia

Hyper-
glycemia

Acidosis

DKA

Other Metabolic
Acidotic States
Lactic Acidosis
Hyperchloremic Acidosis
Salicylism
Uremic Acidosis
Drug-Induced Acidosis

Ketosis

Other Ketotic States
Ketotic Hypoglycemia
Alcoholic Ketosis
Starvation Ketosis

Figure 16-1. Other conditions in which the components of the diagnostic triad for diabetic ketoacidosis (DKA) (hyperglycemia, ketosis, and acidosis) may be found. Adapted from Kitabchi AE, Fisher JN: Diabetes mellitus. *In* Glew RA, Peters SP (eds): *Clinical Studies in Medical Biochemistry.* New York, Oxford University Press, 1987, pp 102–117; with permission.

Table 16-5. Common Precipitating Factors Involved in the Development of Diabetic Ketoacidosis or Hyperglycemic, Hyperosmolar Nonketotic Coma[a]

Undiagnosed or untreated diabetes mellitus
Failure to take insulin
Emotional stress
Acute myocardial infarction
Infection
Treatment with steroids or thiazide diuretics
Thromboembolic episodes
Hypertensive crisis
Vomiting

[a]Adapted from Kitabchi et al., (1994).

600,000 new cases of diabetes are diagnosed each year, and nearly 40,000 deaths per year are attributable to the disease. Although no segment of the population is spared, some ethnic groups are at elevated risk. The Pima Indians in Arizona have an incidence in adult age groups near 50%, whereas adult Hispanics have an incidence of about 12%, and blacks 5%, compared with 2.5% for the population in general. The duration and quality of life of persons with diabetes may be considerably lessened. Compared with nondiabetics, persons with diabetes in North America and Western Europe are 25 times more likely to develop blindness (diabetes causes 15% of all blindness), 17 times more prone to kidney disease (diabetes causes 20% of all kidney failure), five times more susceptible to gangrene (diabetes is the cause of 50% of all amputations of the foot and leg among adults), and twice as likely to have heart disease and stroke (diabetes is one of the four major risk factors for cardiovascular disease).

Physiology of Pancreatic Hormone Secretions

The adult pancreas contains about one million islets, with the largest concentration in the tail. The islets are highly vascularized and innervated by the autonomic nervous system, the parasympathetic (vagus) nerve and the sympathetic (middle splanchnic) nerve. There are at least four major cell types in the islets of Langerhans: α-cells responsible for production of glucagon, β-cells responsible for production of insulin, D cells responsible for production of somatostatin, and F cells responsible for production of pancreatic polypeptide.

Insulin

Insulin biosynthesis occurs in rough endoplasmic reticulum from a single-chain precursor, preproinsulin, with a molecular weight of 11,500 and containing 109 amino acids (Kitabchi et al., 1990). This molecule consists of proinsulin with an additional hydrophobic extension of 23 amino acids (preregion) on the N terminus. This hydrophobic region is rapidly removed *in vivo* before the peptide chain is completed. Human proinsulin is a single polypeptide chain of 86 amino acids with a molecular weight of 9000. It has A and B chains, as does insulin, but the A chain is linked to the B chain by a connecting peptide of 35 amino acids that connects the C terminus of the B chain to the N terminus of the A chain

(Fig. 16-2). Proinsulin has only 5% of the biological effect of insulin.

C-peptide, consisting of 31 amino acids, is the connecting peptide minus one dibasic amino acid from each end. The connecting peptide is produced in an equimolar ratio to insulin during insulin secretion. C-peptide has no biological activity, but because of its common antigenic determinant with proinsulin, it cross-reacts with proinsulin, but not with insulin in their specific radioimmunoassays (RIAs). Hence, the assay of C-peptide in blood under conditions when endogenous insulin cannot be measured may be a clinically useful method of assessing pancreatic insulin reserve. For example, patients who receive exogenous insulin treatment quickly develop antibodies directed against that "foreign" protein. Although these antibodies usually do not significantly influence the biological effect of the injected insulin, they do interfere with the RIA for insulin. In that situation, measurement of C-peptide will provide an estimate of the patient's own remaining insulin-secretory capacity.

Human insulin is a 6000-Da protein made up of 51 amino acids, arranged as two polypeptide chains. The A chain has 21 amino acids and is linked to the

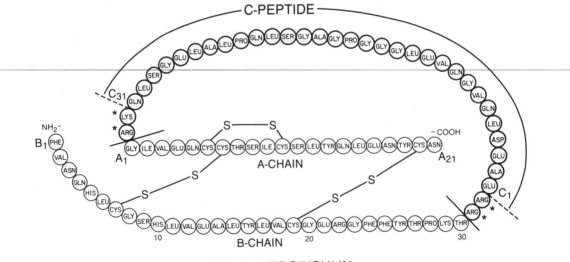

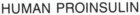

Figure 16-2. Structure of human insulin. The connecting segment (C-peptide) is shown at the top, enclosed by the curved line. The loss of four basic amino acids during conversion of proinsulin to insulin (indicated with asterisks) results in formation of equimolar concentrations of C peptide and insulin. The numbering of the proinsulin molecule for each component of the molecule is designated by A for the A chain, B for the B chain, and C for the C peptide. Reproduced with permission from Kitabchi et al., (1990).

B chain by two disulfide bridges. There is a single intrachain disulfide bridge on the A chain.

The insulin concentration in blood is about 10^{-10} M. It is stored in the B granules in the form of hexamers that contain two atoms of zinc per hexamer. The insulin B chain has a helical region, whereas the A chain contains two α-helical regions that lie within the hydrophobic cleft formed by the B chain. Residues B[23-26] are part of the active site (Gly-Phe-Phe-Tyr) of insulin. Substitution of the Phe residue by other amino acids may result in a reduction of insulin activity. Pork insulin differs from human insulin in only one amino acid (B[30] consists of Ala in pork in place of Thr in human); beef insulin varies by three amino acids (A[8], A[10] and B[30]) from human insulin and is therefore more immunogenic than pork insulin in humans.

With the introduction of the appropriate stimulatory agent, a rapid depolarization of the plasma membrane of β-cells occurs as a result of a reduction in its permeability to K^+, which opens voltage-dependent calcium channels in the membrane and permits a rapid accumulation of Ca^{2+} within the cytoplasm of β-cells. Thus, the cytosolic Ca^{2+} concentration increases from 10^{-7} to 10^{-5} M, resulting in increased insulin secretion. This is the first or rapid phase of insulin secretion, which lasts only a few minutes; it is stimulated by compounds such as glucose and amino acids, in which Ca^{2+} plays an important role. Thus, Ca^{2+}, like sulfonylureas (a class of so-called *oral hypoglycemic agents* used in the treatment of type II DM that has effects on insulin secretion as well as extrapancreative actions) stimulates insulin secretion but not synthesis. The second phase of insulin secretion, which is delayed and lasts longer, appears to be mediated through cyclic adenosine monophosphate (cAMP). The release of insulin involves two processes: (1) a microtubular system (*margination*) for the transport of granules from the cytoplasm toward the plasma membrane; and (2) a microfilamentous system for final delivery of the granule to the membrane (*exocytosis*). In addition to glucose, there are other stimuli for insulin secretion.

Thus, the β-cell response to insulin secretagogues is biphasic. An initial rapid burst occurs within the first 5 minutes that releases preformed insulin from a rapidly mobilizable pool. This phase usually responds to glucose, amino acids, sulfonylurea, glucagon, and gastrointestinal hormones.

The second phase, which occurs after about 20 minutes and continues for as long as an hour, is stimulated by glucose and amino acids and involves the release of preformed insulin, newly synthesized insulin, and proinsulin. The gastrointestinal hormones (e.g., gastric inhibitory polypeptide, gastrin, secretin, and enteroglucagon) are modulating agents for the alimentary phase of insulin secretion. Thus, a greater insulin response occurs following an oral glucose compared with an intravenous glucose challenge. Additional agents that stimulate or inhibit insulin secretion are listed in Table 16-6. An adult human secretes about 40 to 50 U (depending on the purity of the preparation, 1 mg is equal to approximately 26–30 U) of insulin per day, of which about 40% is unstimulated or "basal" (preprandial) and the remaining is secreted as pulses in response to food ingestion.

Insulin Action

Insulin is essential for survival; its lack leads to rapid wasting and death. Insulin has major effects on lipid,

Table 16-6. Stimulators and Inhibitors of Insulin Release

Stimulators	Inhibitors
Carbohydrates	Carbohydrates
Glucose	2-Deoxyglucose
Fructose	D-Mannoheptulose
Mannose	
	Hormones
Polypeptide hormones	Epinephrine
Glucagon	Norepinephrine
ACTH (not in human)	Somatostatin
Growth hormone	
	Miscellaneous
Amino acids	Starvation
Fatty acids	Diazoxide
Enteric hormones	Hypoxia
Secretion	Hypothermia
Pancreozymin	Vagotomy
Gastrin	
Gut glucagon	
Miscellaneous	
Cyclic 3', 5'-AMP	
Glucocorticoids	
Ketones	
Potassium	
Calcium	
Sulfonylurea	
Vagal stimulation	
Methylxanthines	

ACTH, adrenocorticotropin; AMP, adenosine monophosphate.

protein, and carbohydrate metabolism in insulin-sensitive tissues (e.g., fat, muscle, liver) where its action is exerted at physiological concentrations of the hormone ($\sim 10^{-10}\ M$). The actions of insulin may be classified as immediate, intermediate, or long-term, as indicated in Table 16-7. Insulin, in general, is an anabolic hormone that stimulates protein, glycogen, and lipid synthesis and prevents lipolysis and gluconeogenesis.

Although the molecular basis of insulin action has been the subject of intensive investigation, and numerous low and higher molecular weight compounds have been proposed as putative mediators of insulin action on certain enzymes, to date the identity of these "second messengers" has remained elusive. Table 16-8 summarizes the effect of insulin on various enzymes.

Glucagon

The second hormone produced by the islets of Langerhans is glucagon, a 3485-Da single-chain, poly-peptide hormone comprising 29 amino acids. It is synthesized in and released from the α-cell from proglucagon, a higher molecular weight (~ 9000) precursor. Whereas insulin and C-peptide have species specificity, the glucagon structure appears to be identical in all mammalian species. The concentration of glucagon in blood is normally 10^{-10}M and occurs as a monomer. Table 16-9 summarizes the stimulators and inhibitors of glucagon secretion. Unlike insulin secretion, which is biphasic in normal individuals, the glucagon response to a standard meal containing carbohydrate, fat, and protein involves a gradual, modest increase in the rate of secretion. In insulin-dependent diabetics however, glucagon levels rise abruptly to a peak after 30 minutes. Conventional insulin therapy significantly reduces the glucagon response in diabetics, but usually levels are still above those found in normal subjects. The major action of glucagon is in the liver, where it stimulates glycogen breakdown (*glycogenolysis*), glucose production (*gluconeogenesis*), and ketone production (*ketogenesis*). Table 16-10 summarizes the effects of glucagon on intermediary metabolism. At the molecular level, production of cAMP is the dominant mechanism for physiological action of glucagon.

Somatostatin

A third hormone of the endocrine pancreas is *somatostatin,* a cyclic tetradecapeptide secreted by D cells of the islets of Langerhans. Somatostatin is derived from a larger precursor called *prosomatostatin.* Between the outer rim of the α-cell and the β-cell core are scattered somatostatin-containing D cells, which constitute about 10% of the total cells. All three cell types are in intimate contact with each other through gap junctions. Glucagon is a potent stimulant of insulin and somatostatin secretion. On the other hand, somatostatin inhibits both insulin and glucagon secretion. Somatostatin, in conjunction with insulin, inhibits glucagon secretion and diminishes postprandial hyperglycemia by about 50%. Table 16-11 summarizes the biological activities of somatostatin.

Fed and Fasting States

Feeding

To understand the interrelationships of fuel metabolism under feeding and fasting situations, these con-

Table 16-7. Effects of Insulin on Target Tissues

Effect	Tissue
Rapid	
Membrane transport of glucose	Muscle, adipose
Membrane transport of amino acids	Muscle, adipose, liver
Intermediate	
Carbohydrate metabolism	
↑ Glycogen synthesis	Muscle, liver
↓ Glycogenolysis	Muscle, liver
↓ Glucoeneogenesis	Liver
Lipid metabolism	
↑ Lipogenesis	Liver adipose
↑ Esterification	Liver, adipose
↓ Lipolysis	Adipose
↑ Cholesterol synthesis	Liver
↓ Ketogenesis	Liver
↑ Utilization of dietary lipid	Liver, adipose
↓ Fatty acid oxidation	Liver, adipose
Protein metabolism	
↑ Protein synthesis	Liver, muscle, adipose
↓ Proteolysis	Liver, muscle
Long-term	
Promotion of cell growth	
Promotion of cell division	
Promotion of DNA synthesis	
Promotion of RNA synthesis	

Adapted from Montague, (1983).

Table 16-8. Effects of Insulin on Enzyme Activity

Enzyme	Effect of Insulin on Activity	Molecular Basis of Activity Change
Carbohydrate metabolism		
Glycogen	↑	DPh
Phosphorylase	↓	DPh
Phosphorylase kinase	↓	DPh
Pyruvate dehydrogenase	↑	DPh
Pyruvate kinase	↑	DPh
Fructose-6-phosphate-2-kinase	↑	DPh
Phosphoprotein phosphatase inhibitor 1	↓	DPh
Lipid metabolism		
Triacylglycerol lipase	↓	DPh
Hydroxymethylglutaryl-CoA reductase	↑	DPh
Hydroxymethylglutaryl-CoA reductase kinase	↓	DPh
Acetyl-CoA carboxylase	↑	Ph
ATP-Citrate lyase	?	Ph
Glycerol phosphate acyltransferase	↑	DPh
Diacylglycerol acyltransferase	↑	DPh
Phosphoprotein phosphatase and protein kinase enzymes		
Glycogen synthase phosphatase	↑	PF
Pyruvate dehydrogenase phosphatase	↑	PF
AMP-independent protein kinase	↑	?
AMP-dependent protein kinase	↓	PF
Membrane enzymes		
Na/K-ATPase	↑	Ph
Low K_m AMP phosphodiesterase	↑	Ph
Ca-ATPase	↓	DPh?

Adapted from Montague, (1983).

DPh, Dephosphorylation; PF, peptide factor; Ph, phosphorylation; CoA, coenzyme A; ATP, adenosine triphosphate; AMP, adenosine monophosphate.

Table 16-9. Stimulators and Inhibitors of Glucagon Release

Stimulators	Inhibitors
Pancreozymin	Glucose
Amino acids	Glucagon
Starvation	Secretin
Hypoglycemia	Somatostatin
Exercise	Serotonin
D-Mannoheptulose	Fatty acids
Gastrin	
Catecholamines	
Gastric inhibitory polypeptide	
Vasoactive intestinal polypeptide	

ditions are described in some detail. Figure 16-3 depicts the sources and metabolic fates of glucose and shows how glucose homeostasis is maintained through a variety of processes. Note that muscle glycogen cannot directly contribute to blood glucose because of a lack of glucose 6-phosphatase in muscle. Muscle glycogen must therefore be converted to various intermediates before it can be used as a source of energy. The ingestion of a meal increases insulin secretion immediately. This rise in serum insulin is proportional to the rise in serum glucose for a short time and promotes the assimilation of glucose, amino acids, and fatty acids into energy stores. For each 100 g of glucose ingested, about 60 g is taken up by the liver for glycogen synthesis, 25 g by non-insulin-dependent tissues, and 15 g by insulin-dependent tissues, especially muscle and fat. The dominant hormone of the fed state is insulin. Insulin is the major metabolic hormone that stimulates transport of glucose into insulin-dependent tissues, such as the liver, muscle, and fat, and it increases protein and fat synthesis while inhibiting lipolysis and proteolysis. During this period of food

Table 16-10. Effects of Glucagon
on Intermediary Metabolism

Effect	Tissue
Carbohydrate metabolism	
Stimulation of glycogenolysis	Liver
Inhibition of glycogen synthesis	Liver
Stimulation of gluconeogenesis	Liver, kidney cortex
Inhibition of glycolysis	Liver
Lipid metabolism	
Stimulation of lipolysis	Adipose
Stimulation of ketogenesis	Liver
Inhibition of triglyceride synthesis	Liver
Protein metabolism	
Stimulation of proteolysis	Liver, muscle

Adapted from Montague, (1983).

intake, there is a reduced requirement for fatty acids for fuel; in fact, lipolysis of triglycerides to glycerol and free fatty acid (FFA) is inhibited by insulin. Carbohydrate ingestion is a signal for reduced secretion of the catabolic hormone glucagon. Thus, eating a meal usually reduces the need for glucagon-mediated fuel mobilization. These interrelationships are depicted in Figure 16-4.

Fasting

When ingestion of food is delayed, the prevailing condition is that of the nonabsorptive or fasted state; the blood insulin concentration falls to a level that prevents significant transfer of glucose to muscle and adipose tissue while still permitting glucose uptake by non-insulin-dependent tissues such as the brain, WBC, and RBC. Thus, of the total amount of glucose produced by the liver as a result of glycogenolysis and gluconeogenesis, about 60% of the glucose is used by the brain, 20% by WBC, and 20% by RBC,

with negligible amounts going to adipose tissue or muscle. Glucagon favors hepatic use of amino acids, especially alanine, to produce glucose (*gluconeogenesis*), and the glycogenolytic action of glucagon augments hepatic glucose output. Fatty acids are used not only by muscle for energy; they also serve as substrates for ketogenesis. Thus, the hormones of starvation are: (1) glucagon, which stimulates gluconeogenesis and ketogenesis; and (2) catecholamines, which in humans serve as the major lipolytic hormones, facilitating breakdown of triglycerides to FFA and glycerol. Glycerol serves as a major carbon skeleton for gluconeogenesis, whereas the oxidation of fatty acids provides reducing equivalents for the gluconeogenic pathway. Excess FFA, as a result of increased lipolysis, serve as substrate for triglyceride production and ketogenesis in the liver as well as substrate for cardiac and skeletal muscle. These interrelating mechanisms are depicted in Figure 16-5.

Pathogenesis of Diabetes Mellitus

Type I Diabetes

Multifactorial inheritance and poorly understood environmental factors are involved in the pathogenesis of type I diabetes (Kitabchi et al., 1996; Physician's Guide to Insulin-Dependent (Type I) Diabetes, 1988). The association of certain kinds of HLA, abnormal immunological response, infection with pancreatrophic viruses (mumps, rubella, coxsackie virus, infectious mononucleosis, infectious hepatitis), toxins, and excessive stress may all be contributing factors that bring about destruction of the β-cell, which characterizes type I diabetes, the hallmark of which is insulin deficiency. In type I diabetes, an

Table 16-11. Biological Activities of Somatostatin

Body System	Inhibition of Secretion or Reduction
Endocrine	
Pituitary	Growth hormone, ACTH; thyrotropin
Pancreatic islets	Insulin; glucagon; pancreatic polypeptide
Gastrointestinal tract	Gastrin; pancreozymin; secretin; vasoactive intestinal peptide; gastric inhibitory polypeptide; motilin; gut glucagon-like immunoreactivity
Nonendocrine	
Gastrointestinal tract	Gastric acid secretion; pancreatic bicarbonate and enzyme release; gastric motility; gallbladder contraction
Liver	Splanchnic blood flow

Adapted from Montague, (1983).

ACTH, adrenocorticotropin

Sources and Fates of Glucose

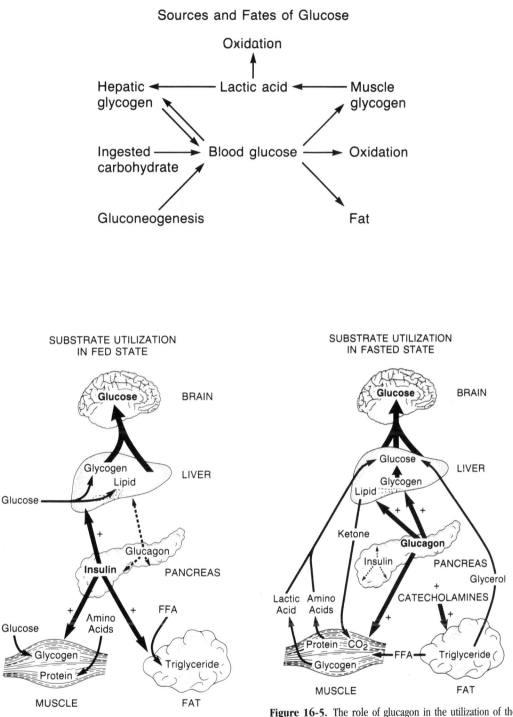

Figure 16-4. The role of insulin in the utilization of substrates in the fed state. An adequate amount of insulin ensures assimilation of glucose to lipid and glycogen in the liver, amino acid to protein in the muscle, and free fatty acid (FFA) into triglyceride in fat tissue. Reproduced with permission from Kitabchi et al., (1994).

Figure 16-5. The role of glucagon in the utilization of the substrate in the fasted state. Glucagon, catecholamines, and other counterregulatory hormone secretions predominate in starvation in conjunction with a decrease in insulin secretion. These events bring about glycogenolysis and gluconeogenesis in the liver, lipolysis in fat, and proteolysis in muscle. Reproduced with permission from Kitabchi et al., (1994).

increased incidence of antibodies to various organs, such as the thyroid, adrenal glands, and gastric cells, has been observed. Furthermore, antibodies to pancreatic islets have been detected by immunofluorescent techniques before the diagnosis of overt disease, and some investigators have reported the presence of insulin antibodies in newly diagnosed type I diabetics before therapy with insulin.

The term HLA is used to describe the major histocompatibility complex (MHC) in humans, which consists of two groups of closely linked genes on the short arm of the sixth chromosome. Certain HLA types (HLA-DR3 and HLA-DR4) are highly correlated with IDDM in Caucasians, although not all diabetics have these HLA markers. On the other hand, HLA-DR2 seems to afford protection against type I, and HLA-DR3 correlates with the presence of circulating antibodies against islet cell antigen in newly discovered IDDM. These HLA types vary with race; for example, diabetes in Japanese correlates with HLA-BW54 and with HLA-DR4.

Type II Diabetes

Type II diabetes is 8 to 10 times more common than type I diabetes and accounts for greater overall morbidity. Genetic and environmental factors, aging, and adiposity play important roles; but viral disease, HLA type, and other immune factors apparently are not correlated. Analysis of identical twins with type II diabetes indicates about 90% concordance in the other twin. One subclassification of type II is maturity-onset diabetes of the young (MODY), or non-insulin-dependent diabetes of the young (NIDY), which seems to be transmitted as an autosomal dominant. This rare condition may or may not progress to frank diabetes.

Rates of insulin secretion and insulin levels in type II diabetes vary with age, the duration of diabetes, dietary regimen, prior glycemic control, and adiposity. Thus, a newly discovered obese type II diabetic has a high basal insulin level and fewer insulin receptors in insulin-sensitive target tissues (downregulation of receptors). These patients usually present with a fasting blood glucose value <140 mg/dL and increased secretion of second-phase insulin (*hyperinsulinemia*). With the progression of the disease, insulin secretion is reduced and the fasting plasma glucose gradually increases; so when the latter value ranges between 160 and 200 mg/dL, basal insulin levels and the number of insulin receptors may both be in the normal range. When the blood glucose concentration exceeds 200 mg/dL, there is generally a significant reduction of insulin secretion (secondary to glucose toxicity in the pancreas) and increased insulin resistance brought about by defects at postreceptor sites.

Insulin resistance (Reaven, 1988), which is present in both type I and type II diabetes, may be multifactorial; some of these factors are summarized in Table 16-12.

Pathophysiology of DKA and HHNS

The basic underlying defect leading to DKA or HHNS is an absolute or relative deficiency of insulin result-

Table 16-12. Mechanism of Apparent Insulin Resistance

Type of Defect	Mechanism(s)
Prereceptor	Circulating antiinsulin factors: antibodies against insulin "counterregulatory" hormones Abnormal insulin synthesis Accelerated insulin degradation
Receptor number or affinity or both	Primary defects Circulating antireceptor antibodies (membrane receptors) Physiological regulatory mechanisms (i.e., downregulation or upregulation) Absent target issue
Postreceptor events	Detective receptor, a second-messenger activity Accelerated destruction of insulin intracellularly Distal steps in insulin action

ing in the inability of glucose to enter insulin-sensitive tissues (e.g., muscle, liver, adipose tissue) and a failure to suppress gluconeogenesis (Montague, 1983). The pathophysiology of these two metabolic derangements closely parallels that of alarm reactions, such as stress, starvation, injury, and burns, in which the body marshals all its defenses to protect the brain from hypoglycemia. Because the brain can metabolize only glucose during the early phase of injury or starvation, catecholamines play an important role in ensuring adequate availability of glucose. This is accomplished by numerous metabolic events that occur with excess catecholamines, namely:

1. *Hyperglycemia:* Increased glycogenolysis brought about by conversion of glucose 6-phosphate to glucose in the liver, secondary to stimulation of adenylate cyclase by catecholamines, causes hyperglycemia.

2. *Lactate production:* The pathway of glycogenolysis in the muscle is also facilitated by catecholamines, but because muscle lacks the enzyme glucose 6-phosphatase, glucose 6-phosphate cannot be converted to glucose but rather is shunted to pyruvate and then to lactate. Excess lactic acid leads to an increased anion gap $[(Na^+ + K^+)\text{-}(Cl^- + HCO_3^-)]$, decreased bicarbonate reserve, and acidemia.

3. *Increased lipolysis:* Triglyceride breakdown in adipose tissue is stimulated, resulting in increased serum FFA.

The events depicted in Figure 16-6 are triggered by the diminution of net effective circulating insulin with resultant hyperglycemia. Increasing hyperglycemia triggers a second series of events characterized by increased levels of counterregulatory, catabolic hormones, such as glucagon, adrenocorticotropin (ACTH), cortisol, and possibly growth hormone.

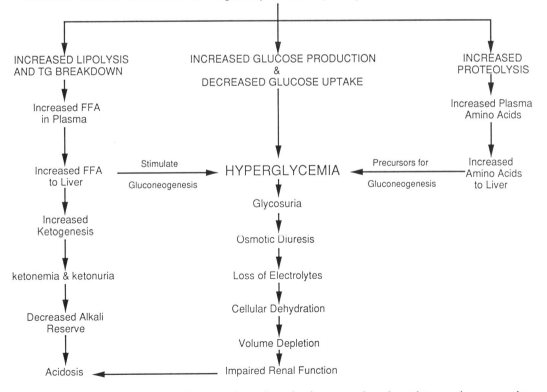

Figure 16-6. Metabolic consequences of diabetic ketoacidosis (DKA). Decreased insulin and increased counterregulatory hormones (glucagon, catecholemines, and cortisol). FFA, free fatty acids. Modified from Kitabchi and Fisher (1981).

Therefore, adequate glucose production is ensured through increased gluconeogenesis by the action of glucagon and cortisol, which is accomplished by activation of muscle proteases, leading to the release of amino acids (mainly alanine) that provide substrate for gluconeogenesis and conversion from a carbohydrate- to a fat-metabolizing system through activation of gluconeogenic enzymes.

Plasma glucose levels rise further and osmotic diuresis ensues, leading to dehydration caused by the hyperosmolar effect of the elevated blood glucose concentration. Switch to a fat-based metabolism occurs as insulin deficiency in the presence of catecholinemia leads to the release of FFA into the circulation. The FFA are metabolized to ketone bodies (β-hydroxybutyrate and acetoacetate) in the liver, which are then used as alternate energy substrates. As metabolic decompensation progresses, the rate of ketone body production eventually exceeds the rate at which they are used, and the resulting ions are neutralized by buffers, chiefly HCO_3^-. Acidosis develops as the buffering capacity of the blood is reduced.

Figure 16-7 provides a detailed summary of the biochemical alterations occurring with DKA. The combination of insulin deficiency with increased lev-

els of counterregulatory hormones leads to an increase in the cAMP-dependent protein kinase activity, in turn setting off a modification of metabolism in the three major insulin-sensitive tissues (fat, muscle, and liver) through a cascade phenomenon. Increased FFA production from lipolysis, combined with increased concentrations of glucagon and cAMP and insulin deficiency, leads directly to increased ketogenesis, independent of malonyl-coenzyme A (CoA). At the same time, accelerated conversion of fatty acyl-CoA to triacylglycerol and the decreased clearance of very low density lipoprotein and chylomicrons from the blood lead to hypertriglyceridemia. In the liver, the presence of increased FFA may directly reduce glycolysis by decreasing the activities of the rate-limiting enzymes of glycolysis: hexokinase, phosphofructokinase, and pyruvate kinase. Also, the increased glucagon/insulin ratio may lower the level of hepatic fructose-1,6-biphosphate activity through the action of cAMP-dependent protein kinase. Through activation of a series of rate-limiting enzymes (fructose-1,6-biphosphatase, phosphoenolpyruvate carboxykinase (PEPCK), glucose 6-phosphatase, and pyruvate carboxylase) increased gluconeogenesis in the liver occurs in DKA. PEPCK is

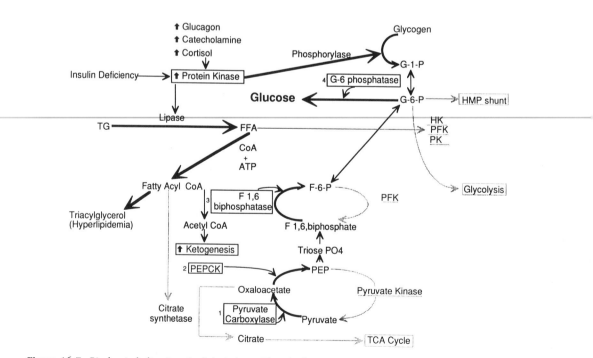

Figure 16-7. Biochemical alterations in diabetic ketoacidosis leading to increased gluconeogenesis, lipolysis and ketogenesis, and decreased glycolysis.

particularly sensitive to the inhibitory effects of insulin. Glucagon, by raising cAMP levels, activating phosphorylase and stimulating cAMP-dependent protein kinase, stimulates glycogenolysis and the breakdown of glycogen to glucose 1-phosphate in the liver. Glucagon also stimulates the conversion of glucose 6-phosphate to glucose by activation of liver glucose 6-phosphatase, which coincidentally reduces the flow of glucose 6-phosphate through the hexose monophosphate shunt. In this manner, both glycogenolysis and gluconeogenesis are increased in uncontrolled diabetes, accounting for a significant part of the hyperglycemia observed in DKA. Thus, insulin deficiency in DKA results in hyperglycemia, not only as a result of diminished glucose metabolism in insulin sensitive tissues but also because of inappropriate hepatic glucose output. All these events are reversed with insulin therapy.

It may be considered that HHNS is at one end of a spectrum of metabolic disturbances associated with insulin deficiency, with DKA being at the other end. The pathogenesis of the HHNS syndrome remains unclear, but fluid losses are more severe than in DKA, and, thus, a more pronounced state of hyperosmolarity develops. Because the increase in the levels of the counterregulatory hormones is less exaggerated than occurs in DKA, and there is a greater residual level of insulin in HHNS (enough to prevent lipolysis but not enough to facilitate glucose uptake and prevent gluconeogenesis), lipolysis and increased FFA release do not occur; hence, plasma glucose rises, but FFA and ketones do not.

Chronic Complications of Diabetes

Major chronic complications of diabetes in both type I and type II patients consist of microvascular disease, including nephropathy and retinopathy, macrovascular disease, such as atherosclerotic heart disease, and neuropathy, which appears to be caused by abnormal metabolic events. Although the detailed mechanisms responsible for the complications of diabetes are not clear, it has long been thought that these clinical complications, particularly the microvascular ones, are the results of metabolic disturbances caused either by relative or absolute insulin deficiency. Genetic and environmental factors may also play important roles. The recent Diabetes Control and Complications Trial (DCCT) clearly linked glycemic control to complications, especially those associated with microvascular disease (eye and kidney disease), but also neuropathy, which is probably secondary to metabolic derangements.

Many of the diabetic complications involve tissues such as the kidney cortex, nervous tissue, retina, and RBC, that are insensitive to insulin and therefore can take up glucose freely. In these tissues the intracellular glucose concentration is determined mainly by the ambient glucose concentration; therefore, a high intracellular glucose concentration may occur as a result of inadequate insulin and resultant high blood glucose levels. Figure 16-8 depicts pathways of the overuse of glucose in insulin-insensitive tissues (RBC, kidney, nervous tissue). The accumulation of excess glucose leads to formation of polyol (in nervous tissue) or glycosylated hemoglobin (in RBC). The latter reaction proceeds through formation of a Schiff base between the aldehyde form of the sugar and the free amino groups in protein (hemoglobin), followed by an Amadori rearrangement of the Schiff base to a ketoamine derivative that is stabilized by cyclization and formation of a hemiketal structure (Fig. 16-9). Irreversible glycosylation of hemoglobin A forms hemoglobin A_{1c}, which occurs slowly through the 120-day life span of the RBC at a rate proportionate to the blood glucose concentration. Therefore, measurement of hemoglobin A_{1c} provides an index of previous glycemic control (see the following section). Increased glycosylation of protein during periods of elevated serum glucose could also be responsible for excessive production of glycoprotein. It has been suggested that increased glycosylation of protein in peripheral nerve or kidney basement membrane may be related to the conditions that characterize neuropathy and nephropathy, respectively, in diabetics (Spiro, 1996).

In conclusion, it is becoming clear that hyperglycemia may increase the rate of glycosylation of many tissue proteins and may, in part, account for some of the chronic complications of diabetes. A direct relationship of increased glycosylation to tissue lesions has not been demonstrated, however.

The relationship of macrovascular complications to glycosylation events is not clear, but it may be the result of multiple factors, including environmental, metabolic, and genetic. Although the DCCT study was of type I diabetics, it is reasonable to presume that better glycemic control in type II diabetes will have a similar beneficial effect.

Pathways of Glucose Overutilization in Diabetes

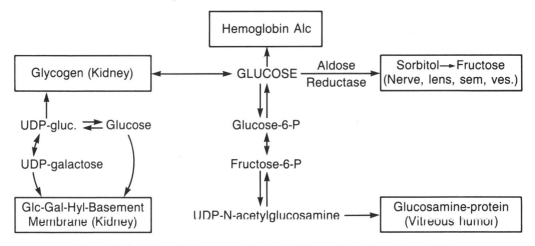

Figure 16-8. Pathway of glucose overutilization in diabetes. *Adapted from* Spiro, (1996).

Assessment of Glycemic Control

In past years, measurement of urine glucose was the only means a person with diabetes had to monitor glucose control. Unfortunately, this measurement correlated poorly with blood glucose values and was often misleading. Many inexpensive and accurate devices are now available for the diabetes patient to perform self-glucose monitoring with only a drop of blood from a finger stick. These tests take advantage of test strips impregnated with the enzyme glucose oxidase and small, easily portable battery-operated meters, some of which have a memory for more than 200 readings, recorded by day and time of the test. In addition, physicians can determine a hemoglobin A_{1c} which will provide a clue to recent glycemic levels (Bunn, 1981). Hemoglobin A_{1c} in normal subjects is usually 4 to 6%, whereas in diabetics it can increase to as much as 20%. Falsely low levels may be seen in patients with anemia, especially hemolytic anemias with shortened RBC half-life, and in patients with abnormal hemoglobins, such as sickle cell disease, as they will have less glycation. Falsely high levels of glycated hemoglobin may be seen in patients with high levels of fetal (F) hemoglobin.

Chemical Reaction

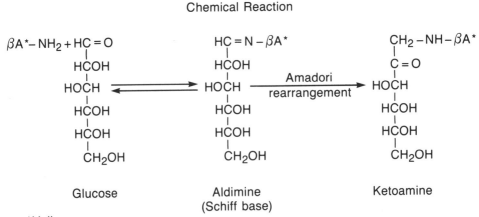

Figure 16-9. Glycosylated hemoglobin in humans. Valine. *Adapted from* Bunn, (1981).

THERAPY

The treatment of DKA consists of insulin and fluid and electrolyte therapy to replace prior and ongoing losses of body water, sodium, chloride, and potassium. Insulin not only promotes entry of glucose into muscle, liver, and adipose tissue, but it blocks gluconeogenesis and lipolysis and stimulates lipogenesis. Thus, insulin helps restore the body to an anabolic or fed state (Table 16-7, Fig. 16-4) by action at multiple sites. As hyperglycemia is treated, glycosuria and the accompanying obligatory loss of water and electrolytes are reversed. Metabolism of glucose to bicarbonate and inhibition of ketogenesis allow restoration of the major buffering system of the body and return to a normal pH. Bicarbonate therapy, therefore, is not required in DKA (although when the serum pH is <7.0, most physicians will give small amounts of HCO_3^- intravenously), and the rise in HCO_3^- serves as a guide to the response to treatment. The amount of insulin used to treat DKA is also controversial. Until recently, pharmacological amounts (50–100 U every 1 or 2 hours) were employed by many physicians in the belief that DKA was associated with marked resistance to insulin. Current treatment in most centers consists of physiological amounts of insulin (5–10 U/h) until plasma glucose levels are in the 150–250 mg/dL range, followed by the introduction of intravenous glucose along with insulin every 2 to 4 hours until complete recovery, which usually occurs within 24 hours.

The form of day-to-day treatment of DM depends on several factors. By definition, type I diabetes requires insulin therapy, and modern treatment plans strive to simulate normal physiology insofar as is possible. Most type I patients require, in addition to careful diet planning, insulin at least twice daily (e.g., a combination of short-acting "regular" insulin with an intermediate-acting insulin such as neutral protamine Hagedorn or Lente) to achieve adequate glycemic control. More intensive therapy using multiple daily insulin injections and use of a portable battery-operated pump for continuous subcutaneous insulin infusion (CSII) are increasingly popular. Implantation of mechanical devices that monitor glucose levels and provide insulin or glucagon appropriately or transplantation of intact pancreas or islets are promising experimental approaches to treatment.

Attempts to produce a lasting remission of type I

DM by use of the immunosuppressive agent cyclosporin early in the course of the disease have been disappointing. Currently, a large national study is under way to investigate the feasibility of preventing type I diabetes in subjects at risk by induction of immunolgical tolerance. Although the importance of altered immune mechanisms in the etiology of type I diabetes cannot be denied, much experimental work remains to be done before the value of such therapy can be assessed.

Type II diabetes occurring in the obese person may respond to diet and weight reduction alone That failing, a variety of oral hypoglycemic agents, the sulfonylureas, are available that act by stimulating endogenous insulin secretion acutely. After several months of therapy, however, insulin levels return to pretreatment values despite continued improvement of glucose control, implying that these agents have extrapancreatic as well as pancreatic effects on the metabolism of glucose. Although 60 to 70% of type II patients show an initial satisfactory response to sulfonylurea therapy, 3% per year will have secondary failure and require insulin for treatment. The recent introduction of a nonsulfonylurea drug, metformin, in the United States has added another useful therapy for some type II patients. Whereas it is theoretically possible to normalize glucose metabolism with insulin in all patients with type II diabetes, many patients, particularly those who are obese, are extremely insulin resistant and difficult to treat satisfactorily, even with very large amounts of insulin. Prevention of diabetes may be the most prudent in persons at high risk for NIDDM (i.e., by ethnicity, impaired glucose tolerance, previous history of gestational diabetes or morbid obstetric history, upper body adiposity, and family history of diabetes).

QUESTIONS

1. Contrast the utilization of substrates by brain, liver, muscle, and fat in the fed and fasted states and indicate the major hormone mediators in each case.
2. What are the principal actions of insulin in reversing the abnormalities of DKA?
3. Which type of diabetes is more prone to DKA? Why?
4. Contrast the effects of insulin with those of glucagon on carbohydrate and lipid metabolism.
5. What are the events leading to hyperglycemia in DKA?
6. Is there any evidence that the chronic complications of diabetes are related to hyperglycemia?

REFERENCES

Bunn HF. Evaluation of glycosylated hemoglobin in diabetic patients. *Diabetes* **30:**613–617, 1981.

DCCT Research Group: The effect of intensive treatment of diabetes on the development and progression of long term complications in insulin-dependent diabetes mellitus. *N Engl J Med* **329:**977–986, 1993.

Harris MI, Hadden WC, Knowler WC, Bennett PH: Prevalence of diabetes and impaired glucose tolerance and plasma glucose levels in U.S. Population aged 20–74 yr. *Diabetes* **36:**523–534, 1987.

Kitabchi AE, Fisher JN: Insulin therapy of diabetic keto-acidosis: Physiologic versus pharmacologic doses of insulin and their routes of administration, *in* Brownlee M (ed): *Handbook of Diabetes Mellitus,* vol 5. New York, Garland Press, 1981, pp 95–149.

Kitabchi AE, Fisher JN: Diabetes mellitus, *in* Conn R (ed): *Current Diagnosis.* Philadelphia, WB Saunders, 1991, pp 766–774.

Kitabchi AE, Wall BM: Diabetic ketoacidosis. *Med Clin North Am* **79:**9–37, 1995.

Kitabchi AE, Duckworth WC, Stentz FB: Insulin synthesis, pro-insulin and C-peptide, in Rifkin H, Porte D (eds): *Diabetes Mellitus,* 4th ed. New York, Elsevier Science Publishing Co., 1990, pp 71–88.

Kitabchi AE, Fisher JN, Murphy MB, Rumbak MJ: Diabetes ketoacidosis and hyperglycemic hyperosmolar nonketotic state, *in* Kahn CR, Weir G (eds): *Joslin's Diabetes Mellitus Textbook,* 13th ed. Philadelphia, Lea and Febiger, 1994, pp. 738–770.

Kitabchi AE, Murphy MB, Sherman AR, et al.: Diabetes mellitus, *in* Ling FW, et al. (eds): *Primary Care in Gynecology,* Baltimore, Williams & Wilkins, 1996, pp. 279–298.

Medical Management of Non-Insulin-Dependent (Type II) Diabetes, ed 3. American Diabetes Association, 1994. Alexandria, VA.

Montague W (ed): *Diabetes and Endocrine Pancreas: A Biochemical Approach.* New York, Oxford University Press, 1983.

National Diabetes Data Group: Classification and diagnosis of diabetes mellitus and other categories of glucose intolerance. *Diabetes* **28.**1039–1057, 1979.

National Diabetes Data Group: *Diabetes in America,* 2nd ed. NIH Publication No. 95-1468, 1995.

Physician's Guide to Insulin-Dependent (Type I) Diabetes., Alexandria, VA American Diabetes Association, 1988.

Reaven GM: Banting lecture 1988: role of insulin resistance in human disease. *Diabetes* **38:**1595–1607, 1988.

Spiro RG: Search for a biochemical basis of diabetic micro-angiopathy. *Diabetogia* **12:**1–14, 1996.

Part III

Metabolism of Complex Molecules

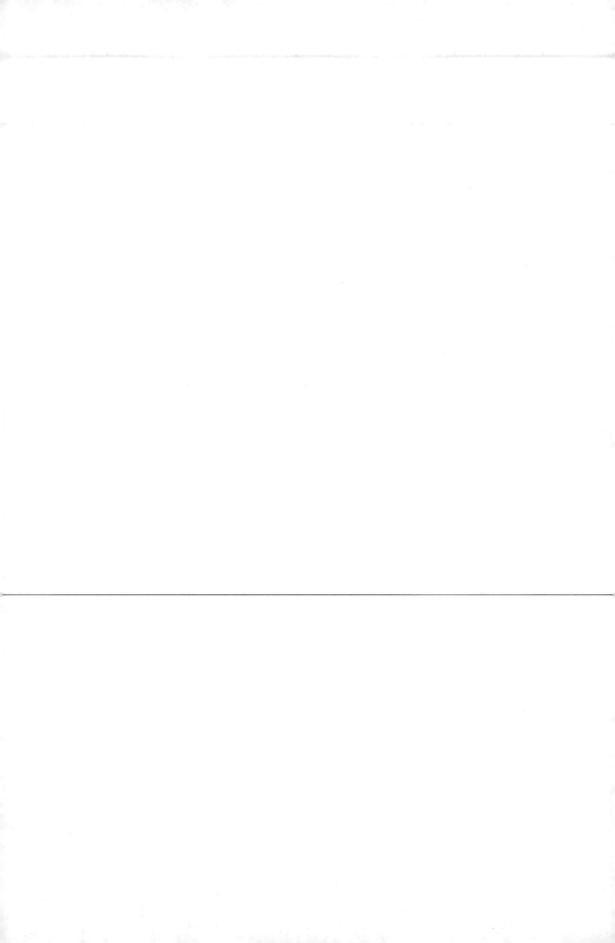

17

Rhabdomyolysis and Acute Renal Failure

KAZUHARU MURAKAMI

CASE REPORT

On the morning of August 8, 1988, a 78-year-old man fell while working in his garden. He was lying under the blazing sun for 3 hours before being discovered by his family. He could not walk by himself, and his urine was the color of red wine and had a pH of 6.0. After being admitted to the hospital because of disturbances of consciousness and muscular weakness, he was diagnosed as having *oliguric* (reduced urine secretion) renal failure according to the following criteria: elevations in serum creatinine and blood urea nitrogen (BUN) and a urinary volume of less than 200 mL per 24 hours (normal, 1000–1500 mL). Physical examination at the hospital showed that he was alert and oriented. He complained of pain in his thighs, but no muscle swelling was apparent. His body temperature was 37.2°C (normal, 36.0–37.0°C); blood pressure, 138/70 mm Hg (normal, <160/95 mm Hg); and pulse, 72/min (normal, 60–90/min). Edema was noted in his face and lower extremities, and abrasions were found on his extremities. Chest radiographs showed *pneumonic consolidation* (indicative of alveoli filled with fluid produced by inflamed tissue) on the right upper field of his lung. Proteinuria and *microhematuria* (the presence of blood in the urine) were present, and the urine sediment showed red blood cells (40–50/high power fields, HPF) and white blood cells (10/HPF). Serum electrolytes were as follows: sodium, 132 mEq/L (normal, 136–146 mEq/L), potassium, 5.0 mEq/L (normal, 3.6–5.0 mEq/L); chloride, 104 mEq/L (normal, 99–110 mEq/L); and calcium, 3.6 mEq/L (normal, 3.9–5.0 mEq/L). Other laboratory studies yielded the following values: BUN, 161 mg/dL (normal, 8–20 mg/dL); serum creatinine, 10.7 mg/dL (normal, 0.6–1.5 mg/dL); glutamic oxalacetic transaminase (GOT), 177 U/L (normal, 5–40 U/L); lactic dehydrogenase (LDH), 1117 U/L (normal, 180–460 U/L); creatine phosphokinase (CPK), 6200 IU/ml (normal <80 IU/ml). Myoglobin was detected in the serum, 1.5 mg/dL (normal, <0.003 mg/dL) and urine, 102 mg/dL (normal, <0.002 mg/dL). Blood gas analysis showed severe metabolic acidosis: pH, 7.35; Pa_{CO_2}, 23.3 mm Hg (normal, 35–45 mm Hg); Pa_{O_2} 73.6 mm Hg (normal, 83–108 mm Hg); HCO_3^-, 12.8 mEq/L (normal, 22–28 mEq/L). The patient's base excess (BE) was −10.2 mEq/L (normal, −2 to +2 mEq/L). The base excess represents the concentration of titratable base minus the concentration of titratable acid when titrating the blood with a strong acid or base to a pH of 7.40 at a p_{CO_2} of 40 mm Hg at 37°C. A positive BE value indicates a relative deficit of non-carbonic acid, whereas a negative BE value indicates a relative excess of non-carbonic acid. Hemodialysis was initiated to treat the acute renal failure induced by rhabdomyolysis. In addition, the respiratory infection was treated with antibiotics. It was suspected that the cause of the rhabdomyolysis was heat stress, dehydration, and infection (pneumonia). About 10 days later, *polyuria* (excessive secretion of urine) appeared, and the BUN and the serum creatinine levels fell gradually. Because the patient had regained virtually normal renal function, dialysis was discontinued.

DIAGNOSIS

Rhabdomyolysis, the destruction of skeletal muscle, is usually associated with weakness, stiffness, pain, and swelling. It almost always leads to marked elevations of muscle cell constituents in the serum or urine, in particular enzymes (e.g., CPK, GOT, LDH, aldolase), proteins (e.g., myoglobin), or electrolytes (potassium, phosphorus) or as pigmenturia (myoglobinuria). It is well known that rhabdomyolysis and myoglobinuria are associated with acute renal failure.

MOLECULAR PERSPECTIVES

Pathogenesis of Rhabdomyolysis

Rhabdomyolysis can be induced by numerous factors with crush syndrome, excessive use of skeletal muscle, and heat-induced disorders being the most common. Alcoholism, infections, metabolic disorders, myopathies, and certain drugs (for instance, heroin and amphetamines) also can induce rhabdomyolysis. Table 17-1 lists the causes of rhabdomyolysis.

Traumatic

The *crush syndrome* is exemplified by injuries incurred during combat. It comprises two separate entities: *hypovolemia* (a decrease in the volume of circulating blood) and acute renal failure (ARF) (Mitchel and Freeman, 1969). Hypotension may exacerbate the renal effects of myoglobin released from damaged muscle, thereby causing ARF.

Myoglobinuric ARF may occur after severe physical exertion (Jackson, 1970). This condition is common in military recruits subjected to vigorous exercise, such as squat-jumping, marching, or running. It is characterized by pain, swelling, and tenderness caused by skeletal muscle necrosis associated with the passage of dark pigmented urine and the onset of renal failure. These events may occur in any setting of unaccustomed exercise and is not limited to military training.

Arterial embolization (obstruction of an artery) followed by ischemic myopathy, myoglobinemia, myoglobinuria, and renal failure has also been reported. It typically occurs with emboli that occlude major blood vessels that serve the lower extremities, and it is characterized clinically by severe pain, tissue *ischemia* (localized tissue anemia), and rigidity

Table 17-1. Causes of Rhabdomyolysis

Excessive muscular activity	Drugs
Contact sports	Heroin
Noncontact sports	Amphetamines
Seizures	D-lysergic acid diethylamide (LSD)
Delirium tremens	Salicylate overdose
Status asthmaticus	Toxins
Direct muscle injury	Carbon monoxide
Trauma	Mercuric chloride
Burns	Snake bite
Ischemia	Infections
Compression	Bacterial, viral
Vascular occlusion	Genetic disorders
Sickle cell trait	Abnormal carbohydrate metabolism
Air embolism	Abnormal lipid metabolism
Immunological diseases	Muscular dystrophies
Dermatomyositis	McArdle's disease
Polymyositis	Tarui's disease
Metabolic disorders	Miscellaneous
Diabetes mellitus	Idiopathic
Hypokalemia	Extreme temperature
Hypernatremia	Electric shock
Myxedema	

of the affected limbs along with massive local edema. The ischemia results in coldness, *hypesthesia* (impaired tactile sensitivity), pallor, and cyanotic mottling of the extremities. Rigidity of the extremities may be explained by an ischemic myopathy involving several muscle groups. Massive *myoedema* (a lump in a muscle) occurs within 12 to 24 hours after the occlusion of a major vessel and has a nonpitting woody consistency. As in the crush syndrome, myoedema and the release of myoglobin into the systemic circulation follow the restoration of blood flow to an ischemic muscle. Myoglobinuria appears 10 to 12 hours after the occlusion occurs and is dependent on myoglobin release from ischemic muscle. Although most cases of ischemic myopathy with rhabdomyolysis are associated with arterial insufficiency, a number of other causes have been suggested, including metabolic (e.g., diabetes mellitus), inflammatory, and toxic etiologies for myonecrosis as well as elective ligation of the inferior vena cava. Venous pooling and hypotension secondary to diminished venous return, along with compression of the arterial vasculature resulting from increased interstitial pressure, contribute to the myoglobinuric ARF. Vigorous muscle contractions occurring during *status epilepticus* (convulsive state pertaining to or affected with epilepsy), *status asthmaticus* (dyspneic state pertaining to or affected with asthma), or prolonged labor during pregnancy have also resulted in ARF. Muscular contraction, trauma, and coma all contribute to the development of ARF after epileptic seizures. The vigorous contraction of respiratory muscles during status asthmaticus and the associated dehydration are thought to be a result of ARF.

Nontraumatic

Nontraumatic rhabdomyolysis with ARF describes that form of renal disease occurring secondary to myoglobinuria without evidence of surgical intervention or trauma (Grossman et al., 1974; Koffler et al., 1976). Most commonly encountered in patients with a history of heroin or alcohol overdose, this form of ARF may account for 5 to 7% of all cases of ARF. Table 17-2 presents a partial listing of causes of nontraumatic rhabdomyolysis. Other known causes include diabetic ketoacidosis, burns, malignant hypertension, and poisoning from ingestion of copper sulfate, mercuric chloride, or zinc phosphate.

Table 17-2. Myoglobin-induced Acute Renal Failure

Traumatic
   Crush syndrome, postexertional, ischemic
   Grand mal seizures

Nontraumatic
   Myopathy
      McArdle's disease, Tarui's disease
      Alcoholism
   Prolonged Coma
      Drug overdose (alcohol, narcotics, heroin)
      Hyperosmolar
   Hyperpyrexia and heat stroke
   Severe electrolyte abnormalities
      Hypokalemia, hypophosphatemia
      Idiopathic paroxysmal myoglobinuria

Myopathy

A variety of diseases affecting muscle have also been associated with rhabdomyolysis and myoglobinuric ARF. Muscle enzyme deficiencies such as in McArdle's disease (myophosphorylase deficiency) (McArdle, 1951), Tarui's disease (phosphofructokinase deficiency) (Tarui et al., 1965), and carnitine palmitoyltransferase deficiency are all associated with rhabdomyolysis and ARF. McArdle's disease is related to impaired glycogen breakdown, with a resultant increase in muscle glycogen stores. Serum lactate levels fail to rise with ischemic exercise, a finding also characteristic of patients with phosphofructokinase deficiency. The major symptoms in patients with McArdle's syndrome are usually evident from early life and consist of muscle pain and stiffness after exercise. It is inherited as an autosomal-recessive trait and has been associated with seizure activity, nausea, and vomiting, all of which may contribute to ARF. Myoglobinuria may occur in up to 50% of patients with McArdle's disease, but frank ARF is rare. In addition to the above enzymic defects, a family with a hereditary deficiency of LDH M-subunit and exercise-induced rhabdomyolysis was recently described. Other muscle diseases associated with rhabdomyolysis and ARF, but only rarely, include *dermatomyositis* and *polymyositis* (chronic, progressive inflammatory disease associated with erythmatous rash on the forehead, and neck and others that affect the striated muscle, skin, and other connective tissues of the body).

Muscle disease may occur in patients with alcoholism, and myoglobinuric ARF has been reported in some alcoholics. Alcoholic myopathy may present with a spectrum of muscle involvement, ranging from asymptomatic chronic myopathy with sustained elevations of serum CPK levels to acute rhabdomyolysis and ARF. The acute syndrome, characterized by pain and swelling of large muscle groups, usually occurs during a drinking party and correlates roughly with the quantity of ethanol consumed. Myoglobinuria is found in 50% of these patients, half of whom will progress to ARF. The mechanism responsible for alcoholic myopathy is probably related to an altered cell membrane permeability indicated by both morphologic and enzymatic changes. *Hypokalemia* (low potassium level in serum), *hypophosphatemia* (low phosphate level in serum), and *hypomagnesemia* (low magnesium concentration in serum) are common in alcoholics and appear to potentiate alcoholic myopathy.

Prolonged Coma

Prolonged coma and drugs have been shown to result in myoglobinuric ARF (Cadnapaphornchai et al., 1980). Many drugs have been implicated. Drug-associated rhabdomyolysis is generally attributed to the development of pressure-induced myonecrosis during periods of depressed consciousness. Drugs that lead to this condition include heroin, chlorpromazine, barbiturates, and alcohol. Factors that contribute to the induction of rhabdomyolysis in patients using these drugs that are usually associated with coma include hypotension, hypothermia, metabolic acidosis, depression of cellular metabolism, decreased muscle perfusion secondary to hypotension, and hypoxia due to respiratory depression.

Hyperpyrexia and Heat Stroke

Most often, ARF associated with hyperpyrexia is reported in association with heat stress and exercise (Vertel and Knochel, 1967). The ARF associated with heat stress has been shown to be due to rhabdomyolysis and occurs most often under circumstances likely to interfere with glycolysis, including fever and hypokalemia. The serum potassium concentration is usually depressed in the early stage of heat stroke. Potassium plays a role in creatine *phosphorylation* (high energy phosphate bond storage) necessary for energy-dependent protein synthesis and the maintenance of ion gradients and the muscle cell membrane potential. Experimental induction of

potassium depletion in dogs causes an acute degeneration of skeletal muscle, supporting a role for potassium in predisposing an individual to *myonecrosis* (necrosis of muscle).

Infections

Certain infections are among the less well-known factors precipitating myoglobinuria. Volume depletion resulting from microorganism-elicited vomiting or diarrhea is an important contributing factor that may determine whether ARF will supervene. Patients who are volume-depleted tend to excrete an acidic urine, which potentiates the nephrotoxicity of filtered myoglobin. In addition, patients with muscle injury produce large amounts of uric acid, which precipitates in acidic urine, and may participate in the pathogenesis of ARF.

Severe Electrolyte Abnormalities

The hypokalemia responsible for myonecrosis has been related to drug therapy (diuretics, amphotericin B), licorice ingestion, alcohol consumption, gastrointestinal potassium loss, renal tubular acidosis, and exercise in hot weather. Knochel and Schlein (1972) reviewed the effects of potassium deficiency on skeletal muscle. The combination of potassium depletion and exercise may be extremely detrimental to skeletal muscle metabolism.

Myoglobinemia and Myoglobinuria

Myoglobin, one of the main muscle constituents, is a heme protein that closely resembles hemoglobin. Its molecular weight of 17,800 is about 25% that of hemoglobin (molecular weight, 68,800). In healthy individuals, the myoglobin content of skeletal muscle is 4 mg/g wet weight (Kagen, 1973). In normal plasma the myoglobin concentration ranges from 0 to 0.003 mg/dL. Fifty percent of plasma myoglobin is bound to α_2-globulin at myoglobin concentrations below 23 mg/dL. A renal threshold of 0.5 to 1.5 mg/dL exists for myoglobin. The *renal threshold* refers to the concentration of a substance in plasma at which it begins to be excreted in the urine. Therefore, the plasma level of myoglobin must exceed 1.5 mg/dL before it is excreted into the urine. At plasma concentrations between 1.5 and 23 mg/dL, about 50% of the circulating myoglobin is filtered.

Before the urine becomes discolored by myoglobin, however, the urine level of myoglobin must exceed 100 mg/dL. The following variables thus determine whether myoglobinuria is visible: (1) the plasma level of myoglobin relative to the renal threshold; (2) the extent of the plasma protein binding of myoglobin; (3) the glomerular filtration rate; and (4) the urine flow rate.

Clinical Features in Rhabdomyolysis

In many patients with rhabdomyolysis, the serum creatinine concentration is disproportionately elevated with respect to that of BUN (Knochel, 1981). Such a disproportionate elevation of the creatinine level probably results from the escape of massive amounts of creatine phosphate from damaged muscle; the release of creatine phosphate, which is subsequently converted to creatinine, results in a daily rise in the serum creatinine concentration above the 0.5 to 1.0 mg/dL/day range usually seen in ARF. Patients with rhabdomyolysis may have a rate of increase in serum creatinine of 2 mg/dL/day or more. A BUN: creatinine ratio below 10 has been reported and should suggest the presence of rhabdomyolysis. One of the most characteristic electrolyte abnormalities induced by rhabdomyolysis is severe *hyperkalemia* (high concentration of potassium in serum). The release of potassium ions from damaged muscle cells may produce extreme hyperkalemia, especially in patients with acidemia or oliguria. Uncontrollable hyperkalemia is a frequent indication of the need for these patients to undergo dialysis. Hypocalcemia also appears early following rhabdomyolysis and usually becomes prominent after the first 24 hours (Knochel, 1981). The reduction in serum calcium probably results from deposition of calcium in damaged muscles. Phosphate leakage from damaged muscle cells causes hyperphosphatemia and, in turn, provokes the precipitation of calcium phosphate in soft tissues, blood vessels and the eyes (Knochel, 1981). Most patients with rhabdomyolysis show evidence of disseminated intravascular coagulation, which might contribute, in part, to a reduction in renal blood flow and glomerular filtration rate. Disseminated intravascular coagulation is a symptom characterized by a reduction in the elements involved in blood coagulation due to their use in widespread blood clotting within the vessels. It is not clear, however, whether it results

from a liberation of thromboplastin from damaged muscle (Blachar et al., 1981). Thromboplastin promotes the conversion of prothrombin to thrombin, thereby promoting blood clotting.

Nephrotoxicity of Myoglobin and Other Muscle Constituents

Controversy exists regarding the nephrotoxicity of myoglobin itself. Many studies have suggested that myoglobin is relatively nonnephrotoxic but that it becomes highly toxic when dehydration, acidemia, or both coexist. Aciduria is regarded as a prerequisite for myoglobin nephrotoxicity, and it is thought that dehydration and a concentrated urine potentiate the nephrotoxic effects of myoglobin in the presence of an acidic urine. At or below a urine pH of 5.6, myoglobin produces ferrihemate (hematin, a porphyrin chelate of iron [III]) (Bunn and Jandl, 1966), which seems toxic to the kidney as well as to the vascular and reticuloendothelial systems (Anderson et al., 1942; Braun et al., 1970).

Mechanisms of Renal Failure

One possible explanation for ARF resulting from myoglobinemia is the induction of intratubular obstruction by the local precipitation of heme pigments, which may also be promoted in acidic urine. Cellular debris and *pigmented casts* (solid reproductions of an enclosed space of renal tubules) are prominent histologic findings in myoglobinuric ARF. Controversy still exists regarding the detailed mechanisms responsible for the development of acute renal failure in myoglobinuria. Suggested mechanisms for producing and maintaining renal failure include: (1) a primary reduction of glomerular hemodynamic changes or reduced glomelular permeability; (2) tubular obstruction by casts; and (3) backleakage of filtrate across damaged tubular epithelia. Figure 17-1 shows a theoretical model for the development of acute renal failure.

An alternative mechanism for producing or maintaining renal failure involves altered hemodynamics, that is, a primary reduction of GFR caused by cortical and glomerular hemodynamic changes or reduced glomelular permeability. Mediators of the initial vasoconstrictive event have not been identified conclusively but suggestions include the following: (1) increased sympathetic nervous system activity;

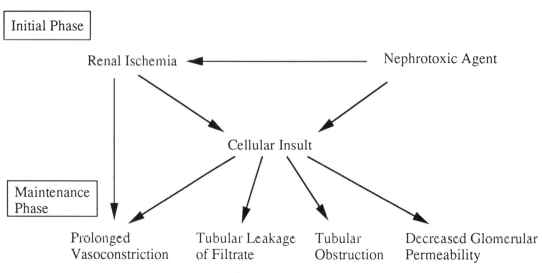

Figure 17-1. Summary of the pathogenesis of acute renal failure.

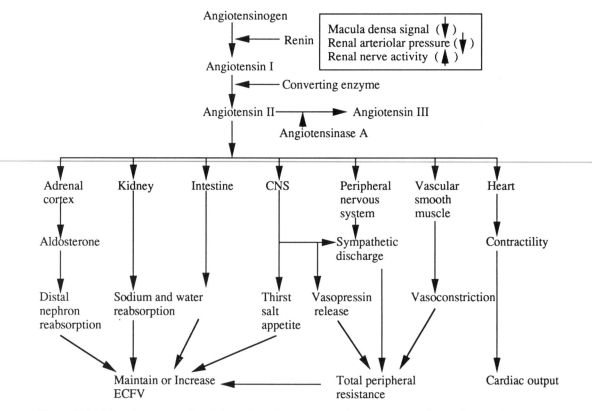

Figure 17-2. Schematic representation of the renin-angiotensin system showing major regulators of renin release. The biomedical cascade leading to A II, and the major effects of A II. CNS, central nervous system; ECFV, extracellular fluid volume.

(2) activation of the renin-angiotensin system (Fig. 17-2); (3) depressed renal prostaglandin synthesis; and (4) elevated plasma vasopressin concentration. Prior administration of phenoxybenzamine (a potent α-adrenergic blocking agent) in the glycerol model of ARF in the rat attenuates, but does not prevent, the development of renal failure, suggesting a partial contribution of increased sympathetic nerve activity to renal vasoconstriction. An increased activity of the renin-angiotensin system might directly affect the renal blood vessels (i.e., via angiotensin II receptors in glomeruli) or act indirectly through tubuloglomerular feedback to reduce GFR. Changes in renal or circulating prostaglandins were recently implicated in the pathogenesis of pigment-induced ARF. Inhibition of prostaglandin synthetase has been demonstrated to worsen glycerol-induced ARF, and infusions of prostaglandins have a beneficial effect in this same experimental model. These studies suggest that considerations of vasoconstrictor agents, such as the renin-angiotensin system, without attention to concomitant changes in a vasodilator system (prostaglandins), may lead to erroneous interpretation of results (Fig. 17-3). Endogenous vasopressin levels in the rat have been shown to increase 40-fold 2 hours after glycerol injection. This level exceeds that required to induce vasoconstriction. Administration of exogenous vasopressin in vasoconstrictive doses increases the severity of experimentally-induced ARF. Although a decrease in glomerular permeability has not been studied in myoglobinuric ARF, the identification of angiotensin II and vasopressin receptors on mesangial cells raises the possibility of a link between these agents and glomerular capillary filtration surface area. Early swelling of glomerular epithelial and mesangial cells 30 minutes after glycerol injection supports the speculation that reduced glomerular permeability plays a role in the initiation of myoglobinuric ARF.

THERAPY

In rhabdomyolysis associated with exertion, marked dehydration may be present, which can lead to shock. Aggressive fluid replacement with saline is essential. Because hyperkalemia is more common and more severe in myoglobinuric acute renal failure, early administration of Kayexalate (a potassium-exchange sulfonate resin, sodium polystyrene sulfonate) is prudent. After restoration of body fluids, mannitol, furosemide, or both can be administered intravenously in an attempt either to mitigate acute renal failure or to convert oliguric to nonoliguric renal failure. Urinary alkalinization with sodium bicarbonate or sodium lactate is reasonable but

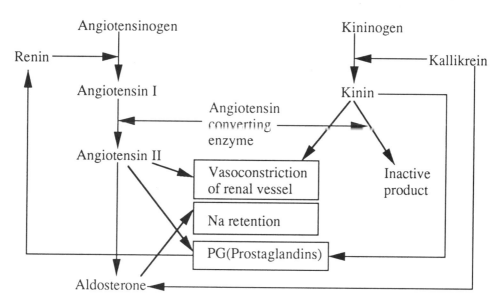

Figure 17-3. Interaction between renin-angiotensin system and prostaglandin, kinin, and kallikrein systems.

should be done carefully so as not to provide excessive amounts which can cause heart failure due to overhydration. In patients whose urine flow increases in response to mannitol or furosemide, urine pH is usually above 6, obviating the need for alkali administration. Both hemodialysis and peritoneal dialysis are effective in patients with acute renal failure.

QUESTIONS

1. What is the definition of rhabdomyolysis?
2. What are the molecular properties of myoglobin and which of those are likely to play a role in nephrotoxicity?
3. What are the most effective approaches to the therapy of rhabdomyolysis?
4. What are some of the markers of muscle damage that are found in serum?
5. What is the role of CPK in the diagnosis of myocardial infarction (heart attack)?
6. How would you distinguish myoglobinuria resulting from Tarui's disease versus heat stroke?

REFERENCES

Anderson WAD, Morrison DB, Williams EF Jr: Pathologic changes following injections of ferrihemate (hematin) in dogs. *Arch Pathol* **33**:589–602, 1942.

Blachar Y, Fong JSC, de Chaderevian JP, Drummond KN: Muscle extract infusion in rabbits: A new experimental model of the crush syndrome. *Circ Res* **49**:114–124, 1981.

Braun SR, Weiss FR, Keller Al, Ciccone JR, Preuss HG: Evaluation of the renal toxicity of heme proteins and their derivatives: A role in the genesis of tubule necrosis. *J Exp Med* **131**:443–460, 1970.

Bunn HF, Jandl JH: Exchange of heme among hemoglobin molecules. *Proc Natl Acad Sci USA* **56**:974–978, 1966.

Cadnapaphornchai P, Taher S, McDonald FD: Acute drug-associated rhabdomyolysis: An examination of its diverse renal manifestations and complications. *Am J Med Sci* **280**:66–72, 1980.

Grossman RA, Hamilton RW, Morse BM: Nontraumatic rhabdomyolysis and acute renal failure. *N Engl J Med* **291**:807–811, 1974.

Jackson RC: Exercise-induced renal failure and muscle damage. *Proc R Soc Med* **63**:4–8, 1970.

Kagen LJ: *Myoglobin: Biomedical, Physiological, and Clinical Aspects.* New York, Columbia University Press, 1973.

Knochel JP: Rhabdomyolysis and myoglobinuria, *in* Suki WN, Eknogen G (eds): *The Kidney in Systemic Disease*, 2nd ed. New York, John Wiley & Sons, 1981, 263–264.

Knochel JP, Schlein EM: On the mechanisms of rhabdomyolysis in potassium depletion. *J Clin Invest* **51**:1750–1758, 1972.

Koffler A, Frieder, RM, Massry SG: Acute renal failure due to non-traumatic rhabdomyolysis. *Ann Intern Med* **85**:23–28, 1976.

McArdle B: Myopathy due to a defect in muscle glycogen breakdown. *Clin Sci* **10**:13–33, 1951.

Mitchel RM, Freeman J: Crush syndrome: The management of hypovolemia and renal complications. *Aust NZ J Surg* **39**:155–159, 1969.

Tarui T, Okuno G, Ikura Y, Tanaka, T, Suda M, Nishikawa M: Phosphofructokinase deficiency in skeletal muscle. A new type of glycogenesis. *Biochem Biophys Res Commun* **19**:517–523, 1965.

Vertel RM, Knochel LP: Acute renal failure to heat injury. An analysis of ten cases associated with high incidence of myoglobinuria. *Am J Med* **43**:435–451, 1967.

18

Abetalipoproteinemia: A Disorder of Lipoprotein Assembly

ALAN T. REMALEY AND CATHERINE M. BULEY

CASE REPORT

A 22-year-old woman was referred to her physician after a routine cholesterol screening test revealed a markedly decreased plasma cholesterol concentration of 0.45 mmol/L (normal, 3.88–5.25 mmol/L). Fractionation of the patient's plasma cholesterol showed a significantly decreased level of low-density lipoprotein (LDL) cholesterol (0.03 mmol/L; normal, 1.3–3.4 mmol/L) and only a moderately decreased level of high-density lipoprotein (HDL) cholesterol (0.39 mmol/L; normal, 0.8–2.4 mmol/L). The patient did not complain of any symptoms except numbness in her feet and occasional difficulty in maintaining balance. Her past medical history was positive for two long-standing problems: malabsorption and decreased night vision. The patient's history of malabsorption dates back to her childhood, when she was first diagnosed with celiac disease. A gluten-free diet, however, did not alleviate her symptoms and was discontinued. Instead, by avoiding fatty foods the patient's symptoms of malabsorption significantly improved. The patient first noted difficulty with night vision over 6 years ago, when she was first learning to drive a car. Since that time her night vision has gradually deteriorated.

Physical examination showed that the patient had decreased deep-tendon reflexes and decreased vibratory and proprioceptive senses in her lower extremities. The patient was also observed to have *gait ataxia* (inability to coordinate muscles involved in

walking) and a positive *Rhomberg sign* (loss of balance when standing with eyes closed). On an opthamologic exam, the patient was found to have a bilateral *pigmented retinopathy* (noninflammatory disorder of the retina). Further laboratory testing showed a slightly prolonged prothrombin time and a decreased hematocrit. Numerous *acanthocytes*, "star shaped" red blood cells, were seen on a blood smear (Fig. 18-1). The reticulocyte count was also noted to be increased and the erythrocyte sedimentation rate decreased. Quantitation of plasma apolipoprotein levels showed an absence of apolipoprotein (apo) B, the principal protein of chylomicrons, very low density lipoprotein (VLDL), and LDL. The patient's parents, who were in good health, both had a normal level of apoB. Finally, a diagnosis of abetalipoproteinemia was made after small intestinal biopsy showed normally formed villi filled with a large number of intracellular droplets that stained positive for fat. The patient was treated with vitamin A, E, and K supplements.

DIAGNOSIS

As illustrated in this case, patients with abetalipoproteinemia are frequently misdiagnosed. Furthermore, there is usually a long delay until they are correctly diagnosed and treated. The rarity of the disease and the large number of seemingly unrelated symptoms and laboratory abnormalities make abetalipopro-

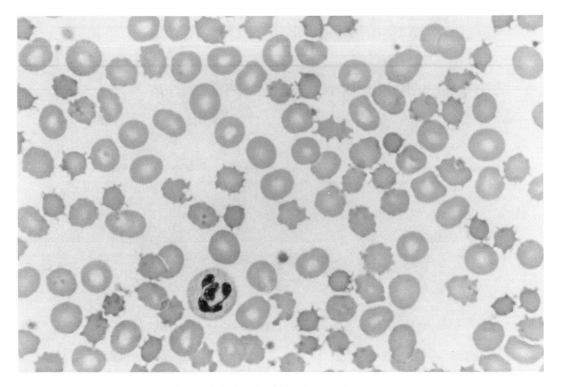

Figure 18-1. Peripheral blood smear of acanthocytes.

teinemia difficult for the physician to recognize. Fortunately, the increasing use of cholesterol screening programs should facilitate the early diagnosis of this disease, which is critical if the irreversible neurologic damage that occurs in untreated cases is to be prevented. Any patient with a low plasma cholesterol concentration associated with malabsorption and neurologic symptoms should be evaluated for abetalipoproteinemia.

The primary biochemical defect in abetalipoproteinemia is the absence of apoB, the principal protein of the large lipoprotein particles, namely chylomicrons, VLDL and LDL. Besides accounting for the low level of plasma cholesterol, the absence of apoB results in fat malabsorption, which eventually leads to fat-soluble vitamin deficiencies. It is the fat-soluble vitamin deficiencies, particularly vitamin E deficiency, that are responsible for most of the clinical and laboratory abnormalities seen in patients with abetalipoproteinemia.

The first symptom of abetalipoproteinemia, malabsorption, usually occurs in the first few years of life. The malabsorption problem is often misdiag-

nosed as celiac disease; however, it is due to an inability of the small intestine to absorb fats, and the symptoms can be greatly alleviated by avoiding fatty foods. Fats, such as cholesterol and fatty acids, are at first readily absorbed, but because of the absence of apoB production, any absorbed fat cannot be secreted into the lymphatic system. This results in lipid engorgement of the enterocytes of the small intestine, a phenomenon that is readily apparent when biopsy sections of the small intestine are stained for fat. The role of apoB in fat absorption is in packaging any absorbed fat into chylomicron particles for secretion. Because of the hydrophobic nature of fats, they cannot be directly secreted but are secreted as a complex with apoB-containing lipoproteins. ApoB is the major structural protein of chylomicrons and acts like a detergent in maintaining the solubility of lipids in plasma. It is therefore the absence of apoB that causes the fat malabsorption in abetalipoproteinemia.

After several years of fat malabsorption, patients with abetalipoproteinemia eventually develop fat-soluble vitamin deficiencies. Usually by early adulthood, patients develop a mild deficiency of vitamins A and K. The decreased night vision experienced by the patient in this case is due to vitamin A deficiency. Vitamin K deficiency is often detected by abnormal coagulation tests, such as a prolonged prothrombin time. Vitamin K is necessary for the synthesis of several coagulation factors, namely, factors II, VII, IX, and X. Patients with abetalipoproteinemia can develop problems with *hemostasis* (the stoppage of blood flow), but it is usually not severe. Patients with abetalipoproteinemia do, however, develop a severe deficiency of vitamin E, which causes most of the symptoms seen in abetalipoproteinemia. Although vitamin E is known to be an antioxidant that can prevent the oxidation of numerous biochemical substances, particularly lipids containing unsaturated carbon-carbon double bonds, the exact intracellular role of vitamin E and the mechanism for the cellular damage one sees in vitamin E deficiency are not known. The tissue most affected by vitamin E deficiency is neural tissue, thus accounting for the neurologic abnormalities in abetalipoproteinemia. Pathologically, vitamin E deficiency is manifested by a demyelination of the long axons of the spinal cord. Initially, this resulted in the mild neurologic abnormalities observed in the patient in this case report of decreased deep-tendon reflexes and loss of vibratory and proprioceptive senses. If left untreated, the vitamin E deficiency will eventually lead to irreversible damage to the axons of the spinocerebellar tracts, which results in ataxia, spasticity, and severe muscle contractions. Pigmented retinopathy is also an outcome of vitamin E deficiency, and left untreated will progress to blindness. Because of the association of pigmented retinopathy with ataxia, abetalipoproteinemia is frequently misdiagnosed as Friedreich's ataxia, an ophthalmologic and neurologic disease of unknown etiology.

Hemotologic abnormalities, particularly the presence of acanthocytes, are often clues to the presence of abetalipoproteinemia. *Acanthocytes* are abnormally formed red blood cells and have a "star-shaped" appearance (Fig. 18-1). Acanthocytes form in abetalipoproteinemia because the decreased level of plasma cholesterol leads to an abnormal cholesterol:phospholipid ratio in the plasma membrane, which in turn causes a change in the shape of the red blood cell. Acanthocytes are susceptible to hemolysis and can also cause anemia and a compensatory *reticulocytosis* (increased production of new

red blood cells). The decreased *sedimentation rate* (the rate of red cell sedimentation during centrifugation) is due to the abnormal shape of the red blood cells and their decreased ability to self-aggregate (*rouleaux*) into the more rapidly sedimenting cell clusters.

In summary, the diagnosis of abetalipoproteinemia does not require any specialized testing. It is based largely on a consistent clinical picture in association with a low plasma cholesterol concentration and apoB deficiency. A small intestinal biopsy is useful for confirming the diagnosis.

MOLECULAR PERSPECTIVES

Whereas the first clinical description of abetalipoproteinemia was made by Bassen and Kornzweig (1950) in 1950, the major biochemical abnormality, apoB deficiency, was not discovered until 1960. ApoB is a large protein of approximately 549,000 kd consisting of alternating hydrophilic and hydrophobic protein domains that wrap around the surface of a lipoprotein particle. It occurs in two forms: apoB-100 and apoB-48. ApoB-100 is the full-length version; in humans, it is synthesized by the liver and is found on VLDL and LDL particles. ApoB-48 is 48% of the size of apoB-100, hence its name. It is synthesized in the intestine and found on *chylomicrons*, the lipoprotein particles that deliver lipids from the intestine to the liver. Both apoB-100 and apoB-48 are produced from a single gene; however, apoB-48 is produced by the translation of only the 5'-end of the apoB mRNA, which encodes for only the amino-terminal portion of apoB-100 protein. In an unusual mechanism (Powell et al., 1987), the mRNA of apoB-100 is edited after transcription to produce a stop codon in the middle of the gene, which, when translated, results in the shorter apoB-48 protein (Fig. 18-2). This step is catalyzed by a cytidine deaminase, which creates a stop codon by specifically changing a single, specific deoxycytosine residue at position 6666 into a deoxyuracil base. As a result, a glutamine codon is changed into a stop codon (Teng et al., 1993).

Like the synthesis of other secretory proteins, the translation of apoB occurs on ribosomes attached to the endoplasmic reticulum (Boren et al., 1993; Kane and Havel, 1989). Because of the hydrophobic protein domains of apoB, the latter remains attached to

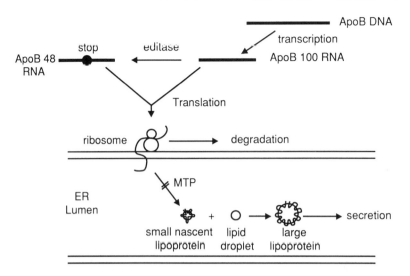

Figure 18-2. Apolipoprotein B (ApoB) biosynthesis and lipoprotein assembly. MTP, microsomal triglyceride transfer protein; ER, endoplasmic reticulum.

the endoplasmic reticulum membrane until it binds enough lipid to form a small nascent lipoprotein particle (Fig. 18-2). A protein called *microsomal triglyceride transfer protein* (MTP) facilitates the transfer of cholesteryl esters, phospholipids, and triglycerides from the endoplasmic reticulum to apoB, enabling apoB to detach from the membrane of the endoplasmic reticulum (Watterau et al., 1992). This step is one of the major sites of regulation of apoB synthesis and secretion. ApoB mRNA is nearly constitutively expressed, and apoB production is regulated instead by the ability of apoB to bind lipid and form a lipoprotein particle that is competent for secretion. In a mechanism that is not completely understood, if there is not sufficient lipid available and apoB cannot form a lipoprotein particle, then apoB undergoes intracellular degradation by proteases. In this way the availability of dietary or endogenously synthesized lipid controls the rate of apoB production. Once the nascent lipoprotein particle forms, it is enlarged by fusion with lipid droplets that are produced in the smooth endoplasmic reticulum, where most lipid biosynthesis occurs. The enlarged lipoprotein particle is then transported to the Golgi Complex where additional lipid is added. Apoprotein B is finally modified by glycosylation, and then the mature lipoprotein particle is secreted into the lymphatic system.

Originally, the defect in abetalipoproteinemia was thought to be caused by a mutation in the gene for apoB that caused a decreased rate of transcription (Linton et al., 1993; Gregg and Watterau, 1994). Several studies, however, have detected increased amounts of apoB mRNA in cells of patients with abetalipoproteinemia. Furthermore, restriction fragment length polymorphism (RFLP) studies of families with abetalipoproteinemia have shown that the defective gene is not linked with apoB. It has also been shown that apoB protein is synthesized in abetalipoproteinemia but not secreted from the cell, thereby suggesting a defect in lipoprotein assembly. It was recently shown that MTP activity is absent in patients with abetalipoproteinemia. MTP has been conclusively shown to be the primary defect resulting from a point mutation in the coding portion of the gene. In the absence of MTP activity, apoB cannot be packaged with lipid and therefore cannot be released from the endoplasmic reticulum membrane. The normal intracellular degradative pathway that controls apoB secretion post-translationally is thus likely to be responsible for degrading apoB. The result of this defect is that apoB, in both the intestine and liver, cannot be produced, thereby preventing chylomicrons, VLDL, and LDL from being secreted. The absence of these lipoproteins from blood accounts for the hypocholesterolemia in abetalipoproteinemia.

The inability of the intestine to form chylomicrons

and to secrete the absorbed fat results in the lipid accumulation in enterocytes and eventually in fat malabsorption and fat-soluble vitamin deficiencies. The malabsorption of fat, however, does not explain the preferential vitamin E deficiency, which is responsible for most of the symptoms that arise in persons with abetalipoproteinemia. In the presence of bile salts, vitamin E is absorbed by the small intestine (Fig. 18-3). Because vitamin E does not have a separate transport system and because it is hydrophobic, it is normally transported in the plasma by lipoproteins, particularly apoB-containing lipoproteins. Initially, vitamin E is packaged in the enterocyte, along with neutral lipids, into the core of the chylomicrons produced by the intestine. Chylomicrons are produced after a meal and act primarily as carriers of dietary fat. They exist in the circulation for only a relatively short time before they are removed by the liver. In this way, most of the absorbed vitamin E is delivered to the liver, and only a small proportion of it is delivered to peripheral tissues (Fig. 18-3). Vitamin E in the liver is then repackaged into the core of VLDL particles before secretion. The recapture and repackaging of vitamin E is facilitated by a tocopherol binding protein, which selectively repackages the alpha-tocopherol

form of vitamin E, which is the biologically active form of the vitamin. The secreted VLDL particle is converted to LDL in the plasma. The subsequent uptake of LDL by peripheral tissues then results in the delivery of most of the vitamin E to those extra-hepatic sites. Patients with abetalipoproteinemia develop severe vitamin E deficiency because they are defective in three steps in this pathway. First, along with the other fat-soluble vitamins, the fat malabsorption decreases the absorption of vitamin E (Fig. 3, step 2) (Rader et al., 1993; Kayden and Traber, 1993). In addition, the small amount of vitamin E that may be absorbed cannot be efficiently secreted by the intestine because of the defect in chylomicron secretion (step 3). Finally, any vitamin E that is delivered to the liver also cannot be secreted because of the defect in VLDL secretion (step 5). Vitamins A and K are also packaged into chylomicrons after absorption from the lumen of the intestine, but, unlike vitamin E, they have a separate transport system in the blood and are not dependent on VLDL for their transport. Because the absorption of vitamins A and K is affected only at steps 2 and 3, patients with abetalipoproteinemia do not develop severe deficiency of these vitamins. The other defects in the vitamin E transport pathway (Fig. 18-3) are due to *choles-*

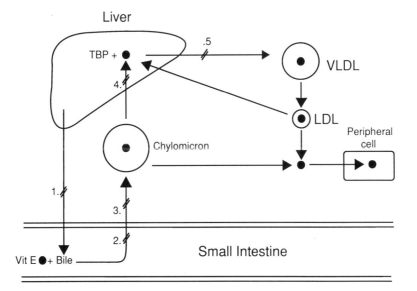

Figure 18-3. Intestinal uptake and plasma transport of vitamin E (●): 1, bile secretion into the lumen of the intestine; 2, vitamin E absorption by enterocytes; 3, incorporation of vitamin E into chylomicrons; 4, hepatic extraction of vitamin E from the blood by tocopherol binding protein (TBP); and 5, VLDL secretion. VLDL, very low density lipoprotein; LDL, low-density lipoprotein.

tasis (a failure of bile flow), the absence of bile (step 1), or familial vitamin E deficiency, which is due to a defect in the tocopherol binding protein molecule (step 4).

Several related diseases of apoB metabolism can have the clinical appearance of abetalipoproteinemia (Table 18-1). Patients with hypobetalipoproteinemia can have all of the same symptoms as abetalipoproteinemia, although they are usually less severe. The defect is due to various mutations in the apoB gene that result in truncated forms of the apoB protein. These truncated forms are usually secreted but are rapidly catabolized, resulting in a very low level of plasma apoB. In normotriglyceridemic abetalipoproteinemia, lipoprotein particles containing apoB-48, but not apoB-100, are secreted. For some of these patients, the defect is not linked to the apoB gene locus, whereas for others it is due to an apoB gene mutation that fortuitously results in a truncation protein that is approximately the same size as apoB-48. Finally, in chylomicron retention disease, apoB-100-containing lipoprotein particles are produced and secreted, but there is a defect in apoB-48 secretion that results in chylomicron retention by enterocytes.

THERAPY

The key to the successful treatment of abetalipoproteinemia is early diagnosis. Supplementation of the diet with fat-soluble vitamins will prevent the manifestations of the disease. Delayed treatment will prevent the progression of the disease but will not reverse any long-standing neurologic damage. The most critical vitamin to supplement is vitamin E: The severe neurologic and ophthalmologic abnormalities in our patient are due primarily to vitamin E deficiency. Massive oral doses are needed to overcome the multiple biochemical blocks in the pathway of vitamin E transport and metabolism in abetalipopro-

teinemia. Because plasma vitamin E levels will not accurately reflect the effectiveness of vitamin E supplementation, end-organ assays, such as determination of the level of vitamin E in adipose tissue, are the best way to monitor vitamin E therapy. Adjunct therapy with vitamin A and K is also recommended. Vitamin A is useful in restoring night vision and in alleviating the retinopathy. Vitamin K should be administered if there is evidence of a hemostasis problem. Vitamin D, another fat-soluble vitamin, is not deficient in abetalipoproteinemia and therefore does not need to be included in the therapy.

The symptoms of malabsorption can be readily treated by modifying the diet. Most abetalipoproteinemia patients learn on their own to limit their fat intake to prevent their symptoms of malabsorption from occurring. Surprisingly, despite the major changes in their plasma lipoprotein profile, patients with abetalipoproteinemia do not appear to suffer any consequences of abnormal plasma lipid delivery. Apparently, other apolipoproteins can perform some of the same functions in the plasma as apoB. Perhaps because of the low level of plasma cholesterol, patients with abetalipoproteinemia are not at an increased risk of cardiovascular disease.

QUESTIONS

1. In addition to lipoproteins, what is the other major proteinaceous carrier of hydrophobic substances in the blood, and what does it transport?
2. Discuss the possible reasons why apoB is prone to proteolysis when present in the endoplasmic reticulum membrane but not when it forms a lipoprotein particle.
3. Discuss two reasons why patients with abetalipoproteinemia do not develop vitamin D deficiency.
4. ApoB-100 consists of alternating protein domains of hydrophilic and hydrophobic amino acids. In contrast, most other apolipoproteins consist of amphipathic helices, which are alpha-helices that contain hydrophobic amino acids on one face and hydrophilic amino acids on the

Table 18-1. Disorders of Apolipoprotein B (ApoB) Biosynthesis and Secretion

Name	Genetics	apoB Defect	Etiology
Abetalipoproteinemia	Recessive	No apoB-48 or 100	Absence of MTP
Hypobetalipoproteinemia	Codominant	Variable	ApoB mutation
Normotriglyceridemic abetalipoproteinemia	Recessive	No apoB-100	ApoB mutation
Chylomicron retention disorder	Recessive	No apoB-48	Unknown

MTP, microsomal triglyceride transfer protein.

other. Speculate about the structure and orientation of these protein domains with respect to the lipid constituents of lipoproteins for both types of apolipoproteins.

5. Patients with hypobetalipoproteinemia secrete truncated forms of apoB that form smaller and denser lipoprotein particles than apoB-100. Explain the possible mechanism.

6. Explain why abetalipoproteinemia is a clinically recessive disorder, whereas hypobetalipoproteinemia is a codominant disorder.

7. Discuss other possible sites of defects in apoB biosynthesis for the diseases shown in Table 18-1.

8. Patients with defects in tocopherol binding protein can be readily treated by frequent administration of vitamin E, together with frequent meals throughout the day. Explain in terms of the kinetics of chylomicron metabolism why a single daily dose of large amounts of vitamin E is an ineffective treatment for these patients.

REFERENCES

Boren J, Wettesten M, Rustaeus S, Andersson M, Olofsson S-O: The assembly and secretion of apoB-100-containing lipoproteins. *Lipoprotein Metab Health Dis* **21**:487–493, 1993.

Bassen FA, Kornzweig AL: Malformation of the erythrocytes in a case of atypical retinitis pigmentosa. *Blood* **5**:381–387, 1950.

Gregg RE, Wetterau JR: The molecular basis of abetalipoproteinemia. *Curr Opin Lipidol* **5**:81–86, 1994.

Kane JP, Havel RJ: Disorders of the biogenesis and secretion of lipoproteins containing the B apolipoproteins, *in* Scriver CR, Beaudet AL, Sly WS, Valle D: (eds): *The Metabolic Basis of Inherited Diseases.* New York, McGraw-Hill, 1989, pp 1853–1885.

Kayden HJ, Traber MG: Absorption, lipoprotein transport, and regulation of plasma concentrations of vitamin E in humans. *J Lipid Res* **34**:343–358, 1993.

Linton MF, Farese RV, Young SG: Familial hypobetalipoproteinemia. *J Lipid Res* **34**:521–541, 1993.

Powell LM, Wallis SC, Pease RJ, et al.: A novel form of tissue-specific RNA processing produces apolipoprotein B-48 in intestine. *Cell* **50**:831–836, 1987.

Rader DJ, Brewer HB: Abetalipoproteinemia: New insights into lipoprotein assembly and vitamin E metabolism from a rare genetic disease. *JAMA* **270**:865–869, 1993.

Teng B, Burant CF, Davidson NO: Molecular cloning of an apolipoprotein B messenger RNA editing protein. *Science* **18**:1816–1819, 1993.

Wetterau JR, Aggerbeck LP, Bouma M-E, et al.: Absence of microsomal triglyceride transfer protein in individuals with abetalipoproteinemia. *Science* **258**:999–1001, 1992.

Low-density Lipoprotein Receptors and Familial Hypercholesterolemia

SIMEON MARGOLIS

CASE REPORT

A 30-year-old male chemist visited his physician because of intermittent chest discomfort. He had been entirely well until he experienced an episode of substernal tightness 3 months previously after enjoying a heavy meal in a restaurant. He subsequently noted similar substernal tightness on two occasions while shoveling snow. The chest discomfort lasted about 10 minutes and disappeared when he rested. After talking to his brother, who had been recently hospitalized with a *myocardial infarction* (heart attack), the patient decided to seek medical attention.

Three years before, the patient had been told that his plasma cholesterol level was >400 mg/dL and had been advised to restrict his intake of fat and cholesterol. He had not followed this recommendation, however. He has no history of hypertension, diabetes, or heart disease. He drinks one beer after dinner almost every day and has never smoked. His job is not highly stressful. The review of systems was completely normal. He was taking no medications. There is no family history of diabetes or hypertension. His father had an elevated serum cholesterol and died of a heart attack at age 41. His mother is alive and healthy. His only sibling had a myocardial infarction at age 34; his most recent cholesterol was 372 mg/dL. His 4-year-old son and 2-year-old daughter are well, but the daughter's cholesterol was 265 mg/dL when routine blood tests were obtained during an acute illness.

Physical examination revealed a white man, 175.6 cm (5 ft 9 in) tall and weighing 69 kg (152 lb). He appeared neither acutely nor chronically ill but showed some anxiety about his condition. Vital signs included blood pressure of 124/68 mm Hg (normal, <140/90), pulse 84 beats per minute (normal, 80–100) and regular respirations of 16 per minute (normal, 15–26). His skin was warm and dry. Examination of his head showed nothing abnormal, with no *arcus corneae* (a whitish ring-shaped deposit in the cornea) or *xanthelasmas* (a fatty irregular yellow nodule on the skin of the eyelid, neck, or back). The fundi showed no hypertensive retinopathy or lipid deposits. There was no jugular venous distention and the carotid pulses were strong and equal bilaterally with no *bruits* (abnormal sounds heard on auscultation). The thyroid was normal in size and texture, and the lungs were clear. The point of maximal impulse, indicating heart size, was in the fifth intercoastal space in the midclavicular line (normal). S-1 and S-2 were normal. A grade II/VI systolic ejection murmur was heard at the apex. The abdomen showed no organomegaly, masses, or tenderness. The rectal examination was negative for masses and *stool quaiac* (a test for blood in feces). The extremities revealed no *edema* (accumulation of fluids in tissues), clubbing of fingers, or joint abnormalities. All peripheral pulses were normal. Nontender nodular masses, noted over both Achilles tendons, had rough, irregular surfaces (Fig. 19-1). The neurological examination was normal.

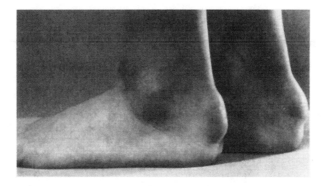

Figure 19-1. Achilles tendon xanthomas.

Complete blood count, electrolytes, blood urea nitrogen (BUN) creatinine, glucose, calcium, phosphorus, aspartate aminotransferase (AST), alanine aminotransferase (ALT), alkaline phosphatase, bilirubin, uric acid, serum protein, albumin, serum protein electrophoresis, and urinalysis results were all within normal limits. Thyroid function tests were also normal. Fasting cholesterol level was 446 mg/dL (normal, <200 mg/dL), triglycerides 128 mg/dL (normal, <200 mg/dL), and high-density lipoprotein (HDL) cholesterol 38 mg/dL (average in men, 45 mg/dL). A chest radiograph showed a normal heart size and no pulmonary lesions. Electrocardiogram revealed inverted T waves in leads 1, AVL, V4, V5, and V6 (abnormal).

After undergoing a positive exercise stress test, he underwent coronary *angiography* (roentgenographic visualization of blood vessels), which showed 50% narrowings of the left anterior descending and circumflex coronary arteries. His angina was treated medically with a beta blocker and sublingual nitroglycerin. He was seen by a dietician for a cholesterol-lowering diet and started on simvastatin, 20 mg a night.

DIAGNOSIS

This normotensive, nondiabetic patient who has never smoked suffered from classic angina pectoris with significant coronary artery disease at the age of 30 years. Hypercholesterolemia and a family history of premature coronary heart disease are his only coronary risk factors. The family history of premature coronary heart disease (father and brother) and hypercholesterolemia (father, brother, and daughter) makes it likely that some form of familial hyperlipidemia predisposes this family to premature coronary heart disease.

Before reaching a diagnosis of primary hyperlipidemia, secondary causes of hypercholesterolemia should be ruled out, including hypothyroidism; nephrotic syndrome; chronic renal failure; diabetes; use of glucocorticoids, accutane, or estrogen; Cushing's disease; primary biliary cirrhosis; or other types of obstructive liver disease, dysglobulinemias (systemic lupus, multiple myeloma, macroglobulinemia), and acute intermittent porphyria. His clinical features and laboratory tests clearly indicate that he does not have secondary hypercholesterolemia.

Familial hypercholesterolemia (FH), familial combined hyperlipidemia, familial dysbetalipoproteinemia (type III hyperlipidemia), and familial defective apoprotein B-100 are four forms of familial hyperlipidemia associated with premature coronary heart disease (Davignon et al., 1991). Caused by a mutation in the gene for the receptor for low-density lipoprotein (LDL), FH is inherited as an autosomal-dominant trait, and several of his family members have elevated levels of total and LDL cholesterol. Familial combined hyperlipidemia is characterized by overproduction of apoprotein (apo) B-100 and very low density lipoprotein (VLDL). Affected family members have about an equal likelihood of having elevations in cholesterol alone, triglycerides alone, or both cholesterol and triglycerides. Familial combined hyperlipidemia can be suspected when LDL apo B-100 levels are high compared with LDL cholesterol levels, but family studies are required to establish the diagnosis.

In patients with dysbetalipoproteinemia, an abnormal apoprotein E results in elevations of both cholesterol and triglycerides as a result of the delayed removal of intermediate density lipoprotein (referred to as IDL, VLDL remnants, or beta-VLDL) and chylomicron remnants. There are three isoforms of apoprotein E: E2, E3, and E4. E2 and E4 each differ from the most common isoform E3 by a single amino acid substitution. Patients who inherit two genes for E2 tend to develop dysbetalipoproteinemia because E2 binds poorly to its receptor. Patients with dysbetalipoproteinemia have another as yet unidentified abnormality because the E2/E2 pattern is present in about 1% of the population, but dysbetalipoproteinemia is far less common. This disorder is associated with accelerated peripheral vascular disease as well as premature coronary heart disease. The diagnosis is made by showing that the ratio of cholesterol on VLDL (isolated by ultracentrifugation) to total plasma triglycerides is ≥0.3. The recently identified syndrome of familial defective apo B is caused by a mutation in the gene for B-100 that prevents normal binding of LDL to its receptor (Innerarity et al., 1987). This dominantly transmitted disorder has clinical characteristics identical to FH.

Familial combined hyperlipidemia is the most common of these disorders; it occurs with a frequency of about 1% in the general population and is present in about 30% of patients with early coronary heart disease. The prevalence of FH is estimated at 0.2% in the white population but is much higher in some populations. About 3 to 6% of patients with early coronary heart disease have FH. Both dysbetalipoproteinemia and defective apo B are far less common.

One important physical finding in this patient is the presence of Achilles tendon xanthomas, which are usually diagnostic of FH. Tendon xanthomas may be absent, however, in patients with FH, especially at younger ages. Some patients with dysbetaliproteinemia may have tendon xanthomas, but they are absent in those with other types of familial hyperlipidemia. Tendon xanthomas are also seen in two other conditions, both rare. *Cerebrotendinous xanthomatosis,* a form of normolipidemic xanthomatosis associated with premature atherosclerosis and various neurological manifestations, is caused by a defect in bile acid synthesis that leads to increased levels of plasma and tissue cholestanol, a catabolic product of cholesterol metabolism. *Sitosterolemia,* another rare disorder resulting from excessive absorption and accumulation of plant sterols from the diet, may also cause tendon xanthomas and premature vascular disease.

Because FH is characterized by a defect in the LDL receptor, elevated levels of plasma LDL cholesterol are uniformly observed and form the standard means for diagnosis. Ultracentrifugation techniques, available only in specialized laboratories, can be used to measure LDL cholesterol, but it can also be estimated by the following formula:

LDL Cholesterol = total cholesterol

$$- \left(\text{HDL cholesterol} + \frac{\text{triglyceride}}{5} \right)$$

This empirical formula cannot be used in patients with dysbetalipoproteinemia or when the plasma triglycerides are >400 mg/dL.

In this patient,

LDL Cholesterol = 446 mg/dL

$$- \left(50 \text{ mg/dL} + \frac{128 \text{ mg/dL}}{5} \right) = 370 \text{ mg/dL}$$

Based on guidelines proposed by the National Cholesterol Education Program, cholesterol levels are considered normal when <200 mg/dL, high when >240 mg/dL, and borderline when between 200 and 239 mg/dL. (Comparable values in children are as follows: normal <170 mg/dL, borderline 171 to 200 mg/dL, and high >200 mg/dL). A normal LDL cholesterol is less than 130 mg/dL. The diagnosis of heterozygous FH in this patient is supported by his high total and LDL cholesterol levels, the presence of tendon xanthomas, the lack of evidence for any cause of secondary hyperlipidemia, the normal triglyceride levels (although patients with FH can have elevated triglycerides), and the strong family history of premature coronary heart disease and hypercholesterolemia. As in the present case, adults with heterozygous FH usually have cholesterol levels between 300 and 550 mg/dL. Cholesterol values this high can occur in some patients with dysbetalipoproteinemia, but the plasma cholesterol seldom exceeds 350 mg/dL in patients with familial combined hyperlipidemia.

MOLECULAR PERSPECTIVES

To appreciate the consequences of a defect in the LDL receptor in FH, it is necessary to understand the normal metabolism of LDL and other lipoproteins.

Lipoprotein Structure and Composition

The plasma lipids consist of triglycerides, cholesterol, phospholipids, and free fatty acids. Free fatty acids are released from adipose tissue and carried by albumin. Because of their insolubility in aqueous solutions, all the other lipids are transported in combination with proteins, which together constitute the plasma lipoproteins. The *lipoproteins* are spherical particles with a central core of the more water-insoluble lipids (triglycerides and cholesteryl esters) and a surface coat of proteins and the more polar lipids (cholesterol and phospholipids). The size and density of each lipoprotein is determined by the amount of lipid in the central core.

Ultracentrifugation of plasma from an overnight-fasted person separates the lipoproteins into three major classes according to their differences in density (Table 19-1): VLDL, density <1.006 g/mL; LDL, density 1.019–1.063 g/mL; and HDL, density 1.063–1.21 g/mL. Small amounts of IDL, density 1.006–1.019 g/mL) may also be present. A fourth major class of lipoproteins, chylomicrons, are normally present in the plasma for only 1 to 8 hours after a fat-containing meal. Because they float on top of plasma, chylomicrons can be detected by examination of plasma after overnight refrigeration. Triglycerides are the major components of chylomicrons (85–90%) and VLDL (55–65%). Consequently, hypertriglyceridemia is due to an elevation in chylomicrons, VLDL, or both. Cholesterol and cholesteryl esters account for about half of the mass of LDL. Hypercholesterolemia, in the absence of elevated triglycerides, is almost always due to increased concentrations of LDL. Proteins make up about 50% of the mass of HDL.

The protein components of lipoproteins are called *apoproteins* and have a variety of essential functions (Table 19-2). Apo AI, the major protein of HDL, activates lecithin:cholesterol acyltransferase (LCAT) and thus plays an important role in the conversion of free cholesterol to cholesteryl esters, which are transferred from HDL to other lipoproteins by cholesteryl ester transfer protein (CETP), an exchange protein for cholesteryl esters and triglycerides. Apo B-100 is required for the transport of triglycerides from the liver on VLDL and is vitally important for the binding of LDL and IDL to LDL receptors. Apo B-48, produced exclusively in the intestinal mucosa, which contains a premature stop codon in the mRNA for apo B-100, is essential for intestinal triglyceride transport and assists in chylomicron remnant uptake by its hepatic receptor. Apo CII activates lipoprotein lipase, which then hydrolyzes the triglycerides of VLDL and chylomicrons. Apo CIII may inhibit the binding of some lipoproteins to hepatic receptors. Apo E is an important determinant of the affinity of apo-E-containing lipoproteins, including IDL and chylomicrons remnants, for their apo E hepatic receptors. Lp(a) is an LDL-like lipoprotein (Lp) that contains a large protein called apo(a) covalently attached to apo B-100 through a disulfide linkage. High levels of Lp(a) are associated with an increased risk of coronary heart disease, probably because the structural similarity of apo(a) to portions of plasminogen interferes with the removal of blood clots by the fibrinolytic protein plasmin, which is formed from plasminogen.

Epidemiological evidence indicates that HDL protects against coronary artery disease, whereas LDL is an atherogenic lipoprotein. There is growing evidence that increased levels of LDL apo-B (referred to

Table 19-1. Characteristics of Plasma Lipoproteins

Lipoprotein Class	Density (g/mL)	Electrophoretic Mobility	Diameter (Å)	Major Component	Apoproteins
CM	<1.006	Origin	800–5000	Dietary triglycerides	Major: CI-III Minor: AI-II, B-48
VLDL	<1.006	Pre-β	300–800	Endogenous triglycerides	Major: B-100, CI-III Minor: E
IDL	1.006–1.019	β and pre-β	250–350	Cholesteryl esters, triglycerides	Major: B-100 Minor: CIII, E
LDL	1.019–1.063	β	180–280	Cholesteryl esters	Major: B-100
HDL	1.063	α	50–120	Protein	Major: AI-II Minor: CII, E

CM, chylomicrons; VLDL, very low density lipoprotein; IDL, intermediate density lipoprotein; LDL, low-density lipoprotein; HDL, high-density lipoprotein.

Table 19-2. Classification of Lipoprotein Proteins (Apoproteins)

Apoprotein	Size (no. of amino acids or MW)	Site of Synthesis	Special Function
AI	243	Liver, intestine	Activates LCAT
AII	154	Liver, intestine	
AIV	MW 26,000	Intestine	
B-100	MW 550,000	Liver	Hepatic triglyceride transport
B-48	MW 250,000	Intestine	Intestinal triglyceride transport; binding to apo B receptor
CI	57	Liver	
CII	78	Liver	Activates lipoprotein lipase
CIII	79	Liver	Inhibits binding to liver receptors
D	MW 22,000		Exchange protein for cholesterol esters and triglycerides
E	MW 33,000	Liver	Binds to apo B and apo E receptors

MW, molecular weight; LCAT, lecithin: cholesterol acyltransferase; apo, apoprotein.

as *hyperapobetalipoproteinemia*) predispose to coronary heart disease despite normal LDL cholesterol levels. It is unclear whether elevated levels of triglycerides are an independent risk factor for coronary heart disease, but hypertriglyceridemia is at least an indirect risk factor because it is almost always associated with low levels of HDL cholesterol.

Effects of LDL on the Arterial Wall

The deposition of LDL cholesterol into the arterial wall has long been recognized as the first step in the development of the arterial plaques characteristic of atherosclerosis. This process is initiated by oxidation of the unsaturated fatty acids of LDL by free radicals formed in tissues during normal metabolic processes. Oxidation of these fatty acids leads to chemical modifications of apo B-100, which then binds to scavenger receptors present on reticuloendothelial cells and macrophages within the intima of the arterial wall. The unregulated uptake of oxidized LDL by macrophages results in the formation of cholesteryl-ester-rich foam cells, the central feature of early fatty streaks that eventually progress to form atherosclerotic plaques. Other long-term effects of oxidized LDL include stimulation of monocyte entry into the arterial wall, inhibition of their egress, and alteration of the properties of the endothelial cells lining the arterial wall. More recent studies have identified acute effects of oxidized LDL on endothelial cells,

including enhanced adhesion of monocytes and platelets, promotion of thrombosis, inhibition of fibrinolysis, and decreased production of nitric oxide, which acts to causes vasodilation of coronary arteries in response to exercise. High levels of oxidized LDL may cause coronary arteries to constrict, rather than dilate, during exercise or stress and thus contribute to the symptoms of angina.

Lipoprotein Metabolism

As shown in Figure 19-2, there are endogenous and exogenous pathways for lipoprotein metabolism.

The Exogenous Pathway

Chylomicrons are formed in the intestine to transport dietary lipids into the bloodstream. Lipoprotein lipase, an enzyme bound to the endothelial surfaces of capillaries in many extrahepatic tissues, particularly adipose tissue and skeletal and cardiac muscle, splits most of the triglycerides in the core of chylomicron particles. As triglycerides are removed, significant amounts of the surface apoproteins (apo As and apo Cs) and lipids (cholesterol and phospholipids) are transferred to HDL. The resulting chylomicron remnants, containing primarily apoprotein B-48 and apoprotein E, are recognized by hepatic remnant receptors and are rapidly removed from the circulation by the liver.

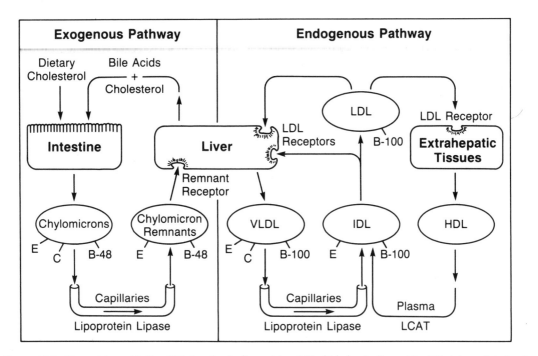

Figure 19.2. Lipoprotein metabolism LDL, low-density lipoproteins; HDL, high-density lipoprotein; IDL, intermediate-density lipoprotein; LCAT, lecithin:cholesterol acyltransferase.

The Endogenous Pathway

Triglycerides synthesized in hepatocytes are secreted from the liver as VLDL, which contain apoproteins B-100, C, and E. Just like triglycerides in chylomicrons, VLDL triglycerides are hydrolyzed by lipoprotein lipase in extrahepatic tissues. The hydrolysis of triglycerides converts VLDL to IDL, that dissociate from the endothelium and return to the circulation. The IDLs are converted to LDLs, by hepatic triglyceride lipase or removed directly by receptors in the liver and peripheral tissues. When IDLs are converted to LDLs, most of the triglycerides and all of the apoproteins except B-100 are lost. The B-100-containing LDLs bind to LDL receptors and are taken up by extrahepatic tissues and liver. Nascent, disc-shaped HDLs are mainly synthesized in the liver and intestine but can also be formed during the conversion of VLDL and chylomicrons to IDL and chylomicron remnants. HDL transports cholesterol from peripheral tissues to the liver, and HDL is required for the removal of excessive surface cholesterol and phospholipids from chylomicrons and VLDLs during their catabolism. LCAT, a plasma enzyme secreted by the liver, transfers a fatty acid from lecithin to cholesterol to form lysolecithin and cholesteryl esters. Lysolecithin is removed by albumin. The cholesteryl esters move into the central core of the nascent HDLs to form the mature spherical HDL particles. These cholesteryl esters are carried to the liver either directly on HDL or after transfer to VLDL, IDL, and LDL by CETP. After they are taken up by the liver, cholesteryl esters are hydrolyzed to free cholesterol, which is excreted in the bile or converted to bile acids. These actions of HDL prevent the accumulation of cholesterol in body tissues.

Normal LDL Metabolism

The LDL Receptor Pathway

Tissue uptake of LDL is mediated by a cell surface receptor (Brown and Goldstein, 1986; Goldstein and Brown, 1990). The ligand for this receptor on LDL is apoprotein B-100. The LDL receptors recognize both apo B-100 and apo E. The affinity of the LDL receptor for apo E is 20-fold greater than for apo B-100 (Innerarity et al., 1987). The IDL, containing both apo B-100 and apo E, binds to the LDL receptor with a higher affinity than LDL, which contains only apo B-100. In normal humans, however, only a fraction of IDL is taken up by LDL receptors; most IDL escapes uptake and is converted to LDL by hepatic triglyceride lipase.

The LDL receptor gene spans about 45 kb of DNA and is divided into 18 exons and 17 introns. It is located near the end of the short arm of chromosome 19. Although the genes for apo E, apo CI, and apo CII are also on chromosome 19, they are on the long arm of the chromosome, distant from the gene for the LDL receptor. The receptor is initially synthesized in the rough endoplasmic reticulum as a precursor containing immature carbohydrate side chains and having a molecular weight of 120 kd. Its molecular weight increases to 160 kd as the receptor undergoes elongation of its O-linked carbohydrate chains in the Golgi apparatus. The mature receptor then moves to and is inserted into the plasma membrane. Human fibroblasts are estimated to contain from 10,000 to 20,000 LDL receptors. The variable number of receptors in other cells depends in part on their cholesterol requirements.

The mature LDL receptor, a glycosylated protein of 839 amino acids, spans the plasma membrane of the cell and can be divided into five domains (Fig. 19-3). Beginning at the extracellular amino-terminal end of the protein, the first domain of 322 amino acids is enriched in disulfide-bonded cysteine (15%) and contains the LDL-binding site. The 350 amino acid residues in the second domain are homologous with the precursor of epidermal growth factor. The third domain of 48 amino acids reaches the plasma membrane; it is rich in serine and threonine and contains the O-linked glycosylated side chains. The following domain of 22 amino acids spans the plasma membrane. The fifth, the cytoplasmic and carboxy-terminal domain, includes the signal for movement of the receptor to coated pits and thus is required for the internalization of LDL by receptor-mediated endocytosis.

As shown in Figure 19-4, receptor-mediated endocytosis occurs after LDL binds to the LDL receptor. The receptors for LDL have been shown by electron microscopy to localize to *coated pits,* indented segments of cell membrane enriched with the protein clathrin, that occupy only 2% of the cell surface but contain 50 to 80% of the LDL receptors. These pits facilitate the endocytosis of receptor-bound LDL by

invaginating into the cell and forming an endocytic vesicle (*endosome*) surrounded by a cage-like lattice formed by clathrin molecules. Within the endosome, the LDL receptor dissociates from LDL and recycles back to the cell surface, where it can again serve to internalize LDL. The endosome then fuses with lysosomes, where an acidic cholesteryl ester hydrolase splits the cholesteryl esters to produce free cholesterol and proteolytic enzymes hydrolyze the apoprotein to amino acids. The LDL provides cholesterol for cell membranes in many cells and substrate for steroid hormone synthesis in the adrenal cortex, ovary, and testis. The cholesterol derived from LDL also regulates three metabolic functions (Fig. 19-5): First, cholesterol suppresses endogenous cholesterol synthesis by inhibition of 3-hydroxy-3-methylglutaryl-coenzyme A reductase (HMG-CoA reductase), the rate-limiting enzyme in cholesterol biosynthesis. Cholesterol synthesis begins with condensation of two acetyl-CoA units to form acetoacetyl-CoA. Condensation with an additional acetyl-CoA leads to the synthesis of HMG-CoA, which is converted to mevalonate by HMG-CoA reductase (Fig. 19-5). Second, cholesterol activates acyl-coenzyme A:cholesterol acyltransferase (ACAT), a microsomal enzyme that forms cholesteryl esters that are stored as cytoplasmic lipid droplets. Third, cholesterol turns off the synthesis of the LDL receptor in the endoplasmic reticulum. All these important steps of metabolic regulation serve to maintain cellular cholesterol homeostasis. As expected, cholesterol synthesis and uptake are enhanced and cholesteryl ester synthesis is reduced when cultured fibroblasts are exposed to a medium that does not contain LDL.

The liver contains at least two independent lipoprotein receptors: LDL receptor and chylomicron remnant receptors. The former is responsible for binding endogenous lipoproteins such as LDL and IDL and is under tight regulation, especially by cellular cholesterol content, in the liver as well as in other tissues. By contrast, the chylomicron remnant receptor is not downregulated by an increase in the cholesterol content of hepatocytes.

In humans the number of hepatic LDL receptors is increased by the administration of L-thyroxine, bile acid-binding resins, and HMG-CoA reductase inhibitors; in animals LDL receptors are also increased by estradiol and starving; feeding, especially saturated fats, decreases LDL receptors. Chylomicrons and VLDL that contain apo E bind poorly to LDL recep-

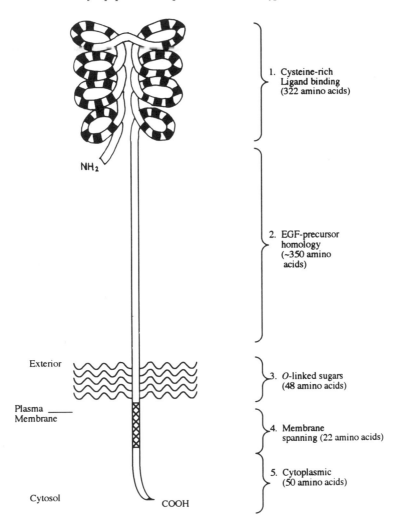

Figure 19-3. The five domains in the structure of the human low-density lipoprotein (LDL) receptor. The amino acid sequence of the protein was deduced from the sequence of the cloned cDNA. The receptor is a dimer of two identical 839-residue polypeptides. From the amino-terminus, these domains are: (1) a 322 amino acid segment that is extremely rich (15%) in disulfide-bonded cysteine and that contains the ligand binding site; (2) 350 residues which are (unexpectedly) homologous to the precursor of the growth hormone epidermal growth factor; (3) a region just outside the plasma membrane rich in serine and threonine residues, and the site of O-linked glycosylation; (4) a membrane-spanning segment; and (5) the 50 carboxyl-terminal residues that project into the cytoplasm. Adapted from Yamamoto et al: *Cell* **39**:27, 1984.

tors because they also contain apo CIII, which may mask the receptor-binding site on apo E and interfere with binding to the LDL receptor. Apoprotein B-48 on chylomicrons and their remnants is not a ligand for the LDL receptor.

Hepatic receptors for chylomicron remnants, which recognize particles containing apo B-48 and apo E, are not affected by genetic alterations in LDL receptors, as they are under separate genetic control. It appears that apo E is an important determinant of the affinity of lipoproteins for both receptors; through the interaction of apo E with its neighboring apo B-48, exogenous lipoproteins containing apo B-48 are directed to chylomicron remnant receptors, while endogenous apo B-100-containing IDLs are directed to LDL receptors. Needless to say, because LDL contains only apo B-100, it binds exclusively to LDL receptors.

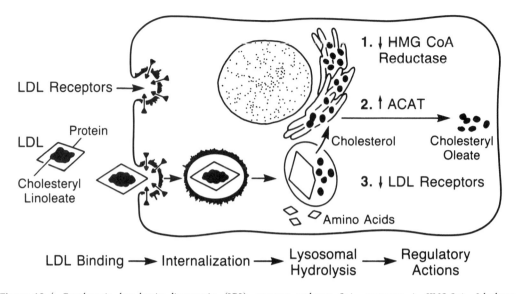

Figure 19-4. Extrahepatic low-density lipoprotein (LDL) receptor pathway. CoA, coenzyme A; HMG-CoA, 3-hydroxy-3-methylglutaryl-CoA; ACAT, acyl-coenzyme A:cholestrol acyltransferase.

One unique feature of hepatic cholesterol metabolism, compared with that of extrahepatic tissues, is the synthesis of bile acids and the biliary excretion of cholesterol and bile acids. Cholesterol hydroxylation by cholesterol 7α-hydroxylase (Fig. 19-5), the rate-limiting enzyme in bile acid synthesis, is followed by further hydroxylations of the cholesterol rings and shortening of its hydrocarbon side chain to form roughly equal amounts of the two major primary bile acids, cholic and chenodeoxycholic acids. Bile acids are excreted into bile along with free cholesterol and lecithin. This cholesterol-bile acid pathway provides the liver with another mechanism to regulate cholesterol metabolism. Factors activating cholesterol 7α-hydroxylase are expected to increase LDL receptors by depleting the free cholesterol pool in the liver. Application of this pathway to the therapy of FH will be discussed in the Therapy section. Another pathway for the removal of cholesterol from the liver is its secretion via VLDL.

Removal of LDL from the Circulation by LDL-Independent Mechanisms

In vivo turnover studies have used ^{125}I-labeled LDL and LDL chemically modified by cyclohexanone on arginine residues or by hydroxyacetaldehyde on lysine residues. The modified LDLs do not bind to the LDL receptor and are taken up by LDL-receptor-independent mechanisms. The turnover studies showed that normal persons catabolize 45% of their LDL pool per day. About 30% of the LDL pool is removed by the LDL receptor pathway described herein, but 15% of the LDL is removed by scavenger receptors and receptor-independent pathways (bulk endocytosis, low-affinity pathways) that principally take place in macrophages and histiocytes of the reticuloendothelial system. At least two distinct scavenger receptors have been characterized: One binds acetylated LDL, the other binds oxidized LDL. These receptors differ from the LDL receptor, they do not bind native LDL, and their synthesis is not downregulated by cholesterol accumulated within the cell.

Genetic Defect in the LDL Receptor in Patients with Familial Hypercholesterolemia

Mutations in the gene for the LDL receptor cause FH. (Davignon et al., 1991). Clinically, the defect is characterized by elevated plasma LDL levels and deposition of LDL-derived cholesteryl esters in tendons (*xanthomas*) and arteries (*atherosclerosis*). It is inherited as an autosomal-dominant trait with a gene dosage effect. Homozygotes are more severely affected than heterozygotes.

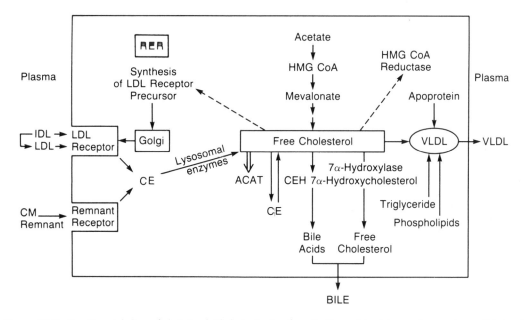

Figure 19-5. Hepatic metabolism of cholesterol. Cholesteryl esters from the lipoproteins taken up by receptor-mediated endocytosis are hydrolyzed by lysosomal enzymes to release free (unesterified) cholesterol, which in turn reduces the synthesis of the precursor of LDL receptors, decreases HMG-CoA reductase activity, and enhances ACAT activity. Cholesterol can also be synthesized from acetate through HMG-CoA reductase, the rate-limiting enzyme in cholesterol biosynthesis. Free cholesterol, either from lipoproteins or from endogenous synthesis, can be esterified by ACAT and stored as cholesteryl esters, which may be hydrolyzed by a neutral cholesterol ester hydrolase. Cholesterol and cholesteryl esters can be packaged into VLDL particles and secreted into the bloodstream. Free cholesterol can also be excreted directly into the bile or converted to bile acids through cholesterol 7α-hydroxylase, the rate-limiting enzyme in bile acid synthesis. RER, Rough endoplasmic reticulum; CE, cholesteryl esters; CM, chylomicrons; IDL, intermediate-density lipoprotein; VLDL, very low-density lipoprotein; LDL, low-density lipoprotein; HMG-CoA, 3-hydroxy-3-methylglutaryl-coenzyme A; ACAT, acyl-coenzyme A:cholesterol acyltransferase; CEH, cholesterol ester hydrolase; ---, inhibition; →, stimulation.

One in about 500 persons is heterozygous for FH. Heterozygotes can often be diagnosed at birth by measuring plasma LDL cholesterol from umbilical cord blood. Heterozygotes may have LDL cholesterol levels two to three times normal. These persons produce only half the normal number of functional LDL receptors. The symptoms of premature coronary atherosclerosis usually develop in the third or fourth decade of life, with a peak incidence in the fourth and fifth decades. Heterozygotes for FH account for about 5% of all cases of myocardial infarction; about 85% suffer a myocardial infarction by the age of 60. About half of the FH heterozygotes have significant peripheral vascular disease. Murmurs are frequently heard over the abdominal aorta and femoral, iliac, and carotid arteries. Tendon xanthomas typically involve the Achilles tendon and tendons on the dorsum of the hand, elbows, and knees. In one study of a large number of FH heterozygotes, 80% had Achilles

tendon xanthomas; xanthomas of the extensor tendons of the fingers were present in only about one third. About 20% of these patients complain of recurrent, short-lived episodes of pain in the area of the Achilles tendon. Cholesterol deposits in the eyelids (*xanthelasmas*), which were present in 30% of these patients, and in the cornea (*arcus lipoides corneae*), present in 50%, are not helpful in making the diagnosis.

About one person per million inherits two mutant alleles for the LDL receptor. At present, more than 150 different mutant alleles have been recognized in the LDL receptor gene, and mutations have been found in all domains of the gene. Persons who inherit two different mutant alleles at the LDL receptor gene locus are still defined as homozygotes to designate the severely affected offspring of two heterozygous parents. As mentioned earlier, immediately after synthesis, precursors of the receptor protein move from the rough endoplasmic reticulum to the Golgi apparatus for carbohydrate processing. The mature receptors then reach the plasma membrane and cluster in coated pits. Five functional genetic defects have been demonstrated in the LDL receptor, and the different effects of these mutations on LDL receptor function may explain the heterogeneity of the clinical expression in patients with FH. Most frequent are class I mutations, in which there is no synthesis of recognizable LDL receptor protein. Class II mutations involve impaired transport of precursors to the Golgi; as a result, the carbohydrate chains of the receptors fail to mature, and movement to the cell surface is delayed or stopped completely. "Receptor-negative" patients generally have class I or class II mutations. In class III mutations, receptors are processed normally and move to the cell surface, but they fail to bind LDL. In class IV mutations, the receptors do not cluster in coated pits because of a defect in the cytoplasmic domain of the receptor. These mutations are referred to as *internalization defects* because the receptor binds LDL but is unable to internalize it. Class V mutations result in an inability of the receptor to recycle back to the plasma membrane after LDL is removed in lysosomes.

As mentioned, some homozygotes may be heteroallelic genetic compounds; that is, they have two different mutant alleles at the LDL receptor locus. The final result is impaired binding or internalization of LDL. Receptor-negative FH homozygotes have no functional LDL receptors, whereas those who are receptor-defective have 2 to 25% of the normal amount of receptor activity. The former have higher LDL cholesterol levels and an earlier onset of coronary heart disease and coronary deaths. Frequently, homozygotes develop coronary atherosclerosis before the age of 10 years, and myocardial infarction has been reported as early as 18 months of age. They frequently succumb to complications of myocardial infarction before the age of 30 years. Planar cutaneous xanthomas are often present at birth and always develop within the first 6 years of life. Xanthomas in the interdigital webs of the hands, tendon xanthomas, xanthelasma, and arcus corneae are also present. Severe aortic stenosis, resulting from cholesterol deposition in the aortic valve, occurs in about half of FH heterozygotes and can lead to congestive heart failure and death. The mitral valve can also be affected, but far less often.

The elevated LDL levels in patients with FH are clearly related to decreased LDL catabolism in both hepatic and extrahepatic tissues as a result of the defect in the LDL receptor pathway. IDL particles, which bind to the same receptors, are also catabolized abnormally by the liver, and it has been suggested that the reduced hepatic uptake of IDL further raises LDL levels because of increased conversion of IDL to LDL. The reduced clearance of IDL may lead to hypertriglyceridemia in some patients with FH.

When ^{125}I-labeled VLDL is given intravenously to patients with homozygous FH, the removal of the labeled IDL from plasma is markedly delayed and the conversion to ^{125}I-labeled LDL is enhanced. This observation further supports the hypothesis that a deficiency of hepatic LDL receptors leads to both LDL overproduction (by increased shunting of IDL to LDL) and decreased LDL degradation (by defective hepatic and extrahepatic LDL receptor pathways). A therapy that increases the number of hepatic LDL receptors would therefore be a reasonable approach to the treatment of FH.

Despite the defect in the LDL receptor, FH patients have normal plasma levels of chylomicrons and their remnants because they have normal levels of lipoprotein lipase to catabolize chylomicron triglycerides and normal hepatic receptors for the uptake of chylomicron remnants. On the other hand, their HDL cholesterol levels tend to be low.

As indicated earlier, normal subjects catabolize 30% of their LDL pool per day by the LDL receptor and 15% of their LDL pool by LDL-receptor-independent pathways. In heterozygotes with FH, 10 to 15% of the LDL pool is catabolized by the LDL receptor and 15% by the scavenger pathway. The FH homozygotes with undetectable LDL receptors degrade 15% of their LDL pool daily through the scavenger pathway. Thus, the scavenger pathway clears 15% of the circulating LDL in both normal and FH patients. Because the total body pool of LDL is two to three times greater than normal in heterozygous FH and six times normal in homozygous FH, scavenger cells are thought to remove six times more LDL cholesterol from plasma daily in homozygotes and two to three times more in heterozygotes than in normal persons. This large amounts of LDL-derived cholesteryl esters accumulate in tendon macrophages (*xanthomas*), bone marrow histiocytes, hepatic Kupffer cells, splenic macrophages, and blood vessel walls.

Because a reduction in the intracellular cholesterol pool effectively increases the number of LDL receptors and LDL catabolism, further understanding of the regulation of the intracellular cholesterol pool in hepatic and extrahepatic cells would provide additional clues to the management of patients with FH.

THERAPY

Although the focus of this chapter is on the treatment of elevated total and LDL cholesterol levels, it is critical to identify and treat *all* risk factors for coronary heart disease, especially in those with FH or elevated cholesterol levels due to any cause (Havel and Rapaport, 1995). The danger of additional risk factors is more than additive among persons with more than one risk factor. Cessation of cigarette smoking eliminates its risk within a few years. Control of high blood pressure reduces the incidence of coronary heart disease only modestly, but it dramatically lowers the likelihood of a stroke.

Rationale for Treatment

Efforts to prevent or slow the development of coronary heart disease are defined as *primary prevention* when carried out in persons with no known coronary heart disease or as *secondary prevention* when carried out in patients with established coronary heart disease. Many intervention trials have examined the effects of lowering plasma cholesterol for both primary and secondary prevention.

The Lipid Research Clinic's Coronary Primary Prevention Trial provided the first clear-cut evidence for a benefit of lowering cholesterol levels in primary prevention. This study compared the ion-exchange resin cholestyramine-plus diet with the placebo-plus diet in about 4000 middle-aged men with no known coronary disease. Over an average period of 7 years, the drug-treated group had a 19% reduction in coronary events, such as sudden death and myocardial infarction. Coronary events were decreased by 2% for every 1% reduction in plasma cholesterol, but there was no decrease in overall mortality. The more recent West of Scotland Study (Shepherd et al., 1995) placed 6595 men with no history of coronary heart disease on either placebo or the cholesterol-lowering drug pravastatin. During an average follow-up period of 4.9 years, the pravastatin-treated group

had a 31% lower incidence of myocardial infarction or death from coronary heart disease and a significant 22% decrease in overall mortality.

A number of secondary-prevention trials have used coronary angiography to examine the anatomy of the coronary arteries before and after 2 to 4 years of various measures to lower LDL cholesterol. The cholesterol-lowering therapies have included extremely low-fat diets alone, moderate diets plus multiple or single drugs, and ileal bypass surgery. Overall, these studies showed significant slowing of plaque progression as well as regression of plaques in the treated group compared with controls. Although these studies included fewer women than men, similar results were obtained in both men and women. In a similar study in Scandinavia 4444 subjects (19% women) with a history of coronary heart disease were followed for a median period of 5.4 years on either placebo or the cholesterol-lowering drug simvastatin. Compared with the placebo group, those treated with simvastatin had a 34% reduction in the risk of a major coronary event, 37% lower requirement for angioplasty or bypass surgery, and a significant 30% reduction in all causes of mortality. Coronary events were reduced significantly in both men and women, but the overall mortality for women was the same in the simvastatin and placebo groups.

Together these intervention trials provide strong evidence for the benefits of lowering total and LDL cholesterol in both primary and secondary prevention.

Guidelines for Treating Hypercholesterolemia

The Adult Panel of the National Cholesterol Education Program (1993) recommended that decisions on the treatment of hypercholesterolemia be based on a combination of the LDL cholesterol level and the presence or absence of risk factors. People with known cardiovascular disease (coronary heart disease, cerebrovascular disease, or peripheral vascular disease) or diabetes are considered at very high risk. *High risk* is defined by the presence of two or more of the risk factors delineated in Table 19-3. In very high-risk patients, the target is to achieve an LDL cholesterol <100 mg/dL. In such patients a diet is started if the LDL cholesterol exceeds 100 mg/dL, and drug treatment is recommended if the diet does

Table 19-3. Risk Factors for Coronary Heart Disease[a]

Men aged >45 yr
Women aged >55 yr or following a premature menopause
Family history of premature coronary heart disease in a father, brother, or son before age 55 mother, sister, or daughter before age 65
Cigarette smoking
Hypertension or treatment for hypertension
HDL cholesterol <35 mg/dL

[a] If the HDL cholesterol >60 mg/dL, 1 risk factor can be subtracted from the above total. High risk is defined by a score of 2 or more risk factors.

not lower the LDL cholesterol to <100 mg/dL. In high-risk patients a diet is recommended when the LDL cholesterol is greater than 130 mg/dL, and drug treatment should be considered if the diet does not lower the LDL cholesterol <160 mg/dL. A cholesterol-lowering diet is recommended for low-risk patients if their LDL cholesterol exceeds 160 mg/dL. Drug treatment should be considered if the diet does not lower the LDL cholesterol: (1) below 220 mg/dL in men aged 35 years of age and in premenopausal women, or (2) below 190 mg/dL in men older than 35 and in postmenopausal women.

Dietary Measures

In general, patients with hypercholesterolemia should first be treated with a diet that limits the intake of saturated fats to <7% of calories and cholesterol to <200 mg per day (Levine et al., 1995). These restrictions are best accomplished by limiting the use of meats, dairy products, and eggs and replacing them with poultry, fish, margarine, and monounsaturated cooking oils. Oils rich in oleic acid, such as olive or canola oils, are recommended because they lower cholesterol but are less readily oxidized than the polyunsaturated oils derived from corn, soy beans, or safflower. Water-soluble fiber, for example, from oat bran and psyllium seeds (contained in products like Metamucil), can lower total LDL cholesterol levels by 5 to 10%; however, FH homozygotes do not respond to dietary manipulations, and heterozygotes respond less well than those with other types of hypercholesterolemia. Because diet alone seldom lowers LDL levels by more than 10% in FH heterozygotes, it is always necessary to add a pharmacological agent to obtain a satisfactory reduction of LDL cholesterol. The prolonged retention time of LDL in the circulation of patients with FH

may increase the likelihood of LDL oxidation. Although there is still no proof of any benefits from a high intake of antioxidants to prevent LDL oxidation, it is reasonable for FH patients to follow a diet rich in the antioxidants beta-carotene and vitamin C. Some physicians also recommend a daily 400 IU pill of vitamin E, an antioxidant difficult to obtain from foods in this amount.

Pharmacological Agents for FH Heterozygotes

HMG-CoA Reductase Inhibitors

The HMG-CoA reductase inhibitors (commonly referred to as *statins*) are the most effective drugs now available to lower total and LDL cholesterol (Treasure et al., 1995). They increase the number of LDL receptors and the removal of LDL from the circulation by inhibiting cholesterol biosynthesis and thereby lowering the intracellular concentration of cholesterol. The four statins approved in this country (lovastatin, pravastatin, simvastatin, and fluvastatin) can decrease LDL cholesterol by 50%, reduce triglycerides by about 10%, and raise HDL cholesterol by 6 to 8%. The statins are well tolerated; side effects (gastrointestinal symptoms, increased liver enzymes, and myositis) occur in about 2% of patients. In fact, in several trials the frequency of side effects in the placebo-treated subjects was the same as in those treated with simvastatin or pravastatin. Long-term risks are still possible because the statins have only been used for about 8 years. In the two studies cited above, however, there was no increased incidence of cancer or any other disorders during the 5- to 5.5-year duration of the trials.

Bile Acid Sequestrants (Ion-Exchange Resins)

Two nonabsorbable cationic resins, cholestyramine and colestipol, bind bile acids in the intestine and eliminate them in the stools. Because the fall in circulating levels of bile acids caused by the resins enhances cholesterol 7α-hydroxylase activity (see Fig. 19-4), hepatic bile acid synthesis and excretion may be increased by as much as 10-fold. The resultant fall in the pool of hepatic-free cholesterol leads to increased synthesis of hepatic LDL receptors and increased activity of HMG-CoA reductase. Despite the increase in cholesterol synthesis, the enhanced removal of LDL from the circulation, coupled with the greater conversion of cholesterol to bile acids, reduces the plasma LDL cholesterol concentration and the total body pool of cholesterol during treatment of FH homozygotes with bile acid sequestrants. The HDL cholesterol levels are unchanged or increased slightly. Patients with hypertriglyceridemia should not be treated with ion-exchange resins, which can raise triglyceride levels.

Because they are not absorbed from the intestine, the bile acid sequestrants are quite safe, and they are the only drugs that might be considered for use in children. The major side effect of constipation and the inconvenience of taking large amounts of resin powders have limited the compliance with these two drugs.

Nicotinic Acid (Niacin)

By reducing VLDL secretion from the liver, nicotinic acid decreases the formation of LDL. Nicotinic acid inhibits the hormone-sensitive lipase of adipose tissue and thereby reduces the flux of free fatty acids to the liver. This action partly explains its inhibition of VLDL triglyceride production. The drug does not alter the removal rate of LDL. Niacin not only lowers LDL cholesterol but reduces triglyceride levels and is the most effective drug available to raise HDL cholesterol levels, probably by decreasing HDL catabolism.

As the result of frequent side effects (flushing after each dose; nausea, upper abdominal pain and peptic ulcers; abnormal liver function tests; elevated uric acid levels and gout; and glucose intolerance), only about 40% of patients remain on niacin one year after the drug is started.

Probucol

Probucol is incorporated into the central core of LDL and enhances its removal from the circulation. This drug is not used commonly because its small reduction in LDL cholesterol levels (about 15%) is less than that observed with the drugs described above, and probucol lowers HDL cholesterol levels by a similar amount. A potentially positive effect of probucol is its strong antioxidant effect. In contrast to all the other cholesterol-lowering drugs, to date no clinical trial has shown that treatment with probucol protects against coronary heart disease.

Combined Drug Regimens

HMG-CoA Reductase Inhibitors and Bile Acid-Binding Resins

The addition of a bile-acid binding resin to a statin is the most effective drug combination to lower total and LDL cholesterol. By working together to lower intracellular cholesterol through different mechanisms, such a combination can effect significant further reductions in cholesterol levels with even a small dose of a resin combined with a full dose of one of the statins. Many patients with heterozygous FH can return their LDL to the normal range with this combination.

Bile Acid-Binding Resins and Nicotinic Acid

The resins speed LDL removal by increasing LDL receptors, whereas niacin decreases LDL production by reducing the formation of its VLDL precursor. The HDL levels are also increased by nicotinic acid. If tolerated by the patient, this combination can be an effective treatment for heterozygous FH.

Bile Acid Resins, HMG-CoA Reductase Inhibitors, and Niacin

This combination of three different drugs is effective in some patients who do not respond adequately to two drugs and who are able to tolerate the side effects of the regimen. The increased risk of severe myositis must be kept in mind when a statin and niacin are used together.

Ileal Bypass

Ileal-bypass surgery is effective in reducing LDL cholesterol levels in patients with heterozygous FH, but this form of treatment is not useful in homozygotes.

Treatment of FH Homozygotes

Many drugs that are efficacious in FH heterozygotes have limited value in homozygotes because of their severe LDL receptor defect. Some receptor-defective homozygotes, all of whom have at least a small number of functional receptors, may respond partially to the combination of an ion-exchange resin and a statin or nicotinic acid. Because of the relative ineffectiveness of drug treatment, a variety of nonpharmacologic methods have been used to treat FH homozygotes.

Plasma Exchange Therapy (Plasmapheresis)

Introduced in 1975, regular removal of the patient's plasma and replacement with donor plasma or albumin now constitute the most common therapeutic approach for FH homozygotes. Plasma LDL levels are temporarily lowered after each plasmapheresis, but they climb rapidly by the next treatment. Other problems include the inconvenience of frequent plasmapheresis and the removal of HDL along with LDL.

Apheresis

Apheresis involves the selective removal of LDL by passing patient plasma through a column that binds LDL to an immobilized antibody to LDL or precipitates it by the addition of heparin. These methods have proved effective in lowering LDL considerably, but they also suffer from the inconvenience of twice weekly to biweekly treatments. Moreover, none of the apheresis methods has been approved by the Food and Drug Administration for use in the United States.

Portacaval Shunt Surgery

End-to-side anastomosis of the portal vein to the vena cava has been used to treat more than 45 FH homozygotes. The procedure reduced total plasma cholesterol levels significantly in most patients and produced some regression in xanthoma size. The protective effect of this procedure on coronary heart disease has not been adequately studied.

Liver Transplantation

Liver transplants, accompanied by heart transplants in several young FH homozygotes with severe heart disease, have led to significant reductions in total and LDL cholesterol levels.

Gene Therapy

Studies are under way to incorporate normal LDL receptor genes into patients with FH. In the long run,

this approach offers the greatest hope for successful treatment of homozygous FH once the techniques of gene therapy are fully developed.

Prenatal Diagnosis

Prenatal diagnosis of FH can be done by amniocentesis. Measurement of binding, uptake, and degradation of ^{125}I-labeled LDL with cultured amniotic fluid cells can be diagnostic for the FH fetus and may establish an indication for therapeutic abortion. Three months after initiation of a diet and administration of 20 mg of simvastatin daily, our patient's cholesterol level fell to 335 mg/dL. The dosage of simvastatin was increased to 40 mg daily, and his cholesterol fell further to the range of 295 to 310 mg/dL. The addition of cholestyramine, three packets a day, lowered his cholesterol to 270 mg/dL. The patient was unable to tolerate the addition of niacin to this regimen. He has had minimal anginal symptoms while on medical treatment with a beta blocker and sublingual nitroglycerin when needed.

QUESTIONS

1. At what age should cholesterol-lowering treatment be started for the 2-year-old heterozygote daughter in our case report in an effort to prevent premature coronary heart disease?
2. Is the case-study patient at higher risk of stroke? If so, would the likelihood of stroke be reduced by maintaining LDL cholesterol levels consistently below 100 mg/dL?
3. What is the effect of estrogen on LDL and HDL cholesterol levels? Should women with heterozygous FH take birth control pills during child-bearing years and replacement estrogen after menopause?
4. What would you do if a FH heterozygote showed a good initial response to pravastatin but stopped taking the medication because she developed persistent insomnia?
5. Can you explain why people with diabetes might be considered at very high risk in this chapter even though the Adult Panel of the National Cholesterol Education Program only listed diabetes as one of the risk factors? Can you explain why obesity is not included as a risk factor?
6. HMG-CoA reductase inhibitors are used to block the production of cholesterol. Could the synthesis of any other biologically important products be inhibited by slowing the formation of mevalonate?

Acknowledgment: This chapter is a revision of a previous version of a chapter of the same title that was co-authored with Dr. James J.-S. Chen and which appeared in the first edition of this book.

REFERENCES

Brown MS, Goldstein JL: A receptor-mediated pathway for cholesterol homeostasis. *Science* **232**:34–47, 1986.

Davignon J, Roy M, Dufour R, et al.: Familial Hypercholesterolemia. Chapter 11 in *Primary Hyperlipoproteinemias* (Steiner G, Shafrir E, eds). McGraw-Hill, New York, 1991, pp. 201–234.

Goldstein JL and Brown MS: Regulation of the mevalonate pathway. *Nature* **343**:425–430, 1990.

Havel RJ, Rapaport E: Management of primary hyperlipidemia. *N Engl J Med* **332**:1491–1498, 1995.

Levine GN, Keaney JF Jr, Vita JA: Cholesterol reduction in cardiovascular disease. Clinical benefits and possible mechanisms. *N Eng J Med* **332**:512–521, 1995.

Innerarity TL, Weisgraber KH, Arold KS: Familial defective apolipoprotein B-100: low density lipoprotein with abnormal receptor binding. *Proc Natl Acad Sci USA* **84**:6919–6923, 1987.

Scandinavian Simvastatin Survival Study Group: Randomised trial of cholesterol lowering in 4444 patients with coronary heart disease: the Scandinavian Simvastatin Survival Study (4S). *Lancet* **344**:1383–1389, 1994.

Shepherd J, Cobbe SM, Ford I, et al. for the West of Scotland Coronary Prevention Study Group: Prevention of coronary hart disease with pravastatin in men with hypercholesterolemia. *N Engl J Med* **333**:1301–1307, 1995.

Summary of the second report of the National Cholesterol Education Program (NCEP) Expert Panel on Detection, Evaluation, and Treatment of High Blood Cholesterol in Adults (Adult Treatment Panel II). *JAMA* **269**:3015–3023, 1993.

Treasure, CB, Klein JL, Weintraub WB, et al. Beneficial effects of cholesterol-lowering therapy on the coronary endothelium in patients with coronary artery disease. *N Engl J Med* **332**:482–487, 1995.

Alport Syndrome (Hereditary Nephritis)

KARL TRYGGVASON AND YOSHIFUMI NINOMIYA

CASE REPORT

The patient, a 19-year-old boy with Alport syndrome, is the first of two children. His mother has had microscopic hematuria since childhood, but otherwise she has normal renal function. During the entire first pregnancy, the patient's then 27-year-old mother had *proteinuria* (excess protein in the urine) and microscopic *hematuria* (the presence of blood in the urine); her blood pressure was usually slightly above normal at about 130/90 mm Hg. There is no history of hematuria or kidney disease in her or her husband's family; however, the patient's younger sister has persistent microscopic hematuria without renal complications, as does her mother.

At age 1 year, the patient was having a checkup in connection with acute *otitis* (inflammation of the ear) and was found to have microscopic hematuria but no proteinuria. During follow-up checkups at ages 2 to 3, he was reported to have persistent hematuria, but his hearing was normal, and no ocular lesions were observed. When the boy was 4 years old, slight sensorineural hearing loss was first detected. At 2000 Hz there was a hearing loss at 30 decibels (dB), and in the 6000 to 8000 Hz range, a decreased hearing was recorded at 30 to 60 dB. The disease was then diagnosed tentatively as Alport syndrome. When he was 8 years old, the patient had a kidney biopsy taken. Light microscopy revealed diffuse proliferative changes in the glomeruli. Furthermore, electron microscopy revealed thinning and thickening as well as lamellation of the glomerular basement membrane (GBM), findings typical for Al-

port syndrome (Fig. 20-1). At this time the patient received his first hearing aid. When he was 12 years old, he was fitted with a bilateral hearing device for significant hearing loss.

With the exception of the hearing loss, the patient's general condition and development were normal until age 18 years. He performed well at school, and his kidney function was normal except for the persistent hematuria and proteinuria. At age 18 years, however, the patient's overall physical and clinical condition changed dramatically with clear development of kidney failure. His blood pressure rose to 190/94 mm Hg, and he was administered diuretic treatment. There was no *edema* (accumulation of fluid in connective tissue). His blood hemoglobin (Hb) had fallen to 118 g/L (reference value, 135–165), the hematocrit was 0.34 (normal, 0.40–0.54), and blood (B) erythrocytes were E12/L (normal, 4.5–6.5). Other values were serum (S)-Ca, 1.98 mmol/L (normal, 2.20–2.70); S-albumin, 21–30 g/L (normal 35–49); S-creatinine, 320 μmol/L (normal, 60–115); FS (fasting serum)-urea, 16.0 mmol/L (normal, 1.7–8.3); FS-phosphorus, 1.77 mmol/L (normal, 0.80–1.50); FS-cholesterol, 8.1 mmol/L (normal, 3.0–7.0); FS-triglycerides, 4.52 mmol/L (normal, 0.40–1.70); CB (capillary blood)-pH 7.27 (normal, 7.35–7.42); and CB-base excess (a unit used to characterize nonrespiratory acid-base imbalance. Base excess is positive when the imbalance goes in the alkaline direction and negative when it goes in the acid direction) −7.1 (normal, −2.5 to +2.5).

DNA analysis revealed a mutation in the gene for

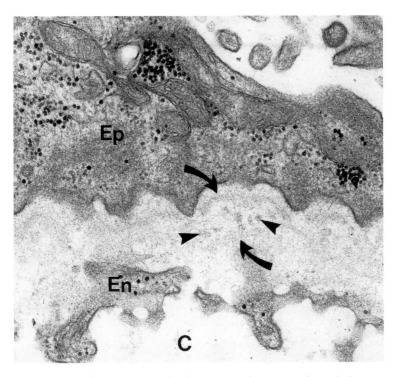

Figure 20-1. Electron micrograph of a glomerular capillary loop showing characteristic glomerular basement membrane (GBM) lesions in the Alport syndrome patient at age 8 years. The GBM has irregular thinning and thickening and electron-dense particles. C, capillary lumen; En, endothelial cell; Ep, epithelial cell; Arrow, thin split lamellated lamina densa of thickened GBM. Courtesy of Dr. Helena Auto-Harmainen, University Hospital of Oulu.

the $\alpha 5$(IV) collagen chain, which is an essential component of the type IV collagen structural framework of the GBM. The mutation is a C to T nucleotide change, which changes the CGA codon for arginine 373 to a premature TGA stop codon in the mRNA. The mutation results in a truncated, nonfunctional polypeptide chain, which apparently leads to a nonfunctional type IV collagen in the GBM. The mother and sister were shown to be heterozygous for the mutation.

Presently, at age 19 years, the general condition of the patient has worsened, although he recently finished high school with good grades. Recent laboratory values were Hb 90 g/L, hematocrit 0.27, B-erythrocytes 0.27 E12/L, S-Ca 2.19 mmol/L, S-albumin 28 g/L, S-creatinine 586 mmol/L, FS-urea 17.4, FS-phosphorus 1.63 mmol/L, FS-cholesterol 7.6 mmol/L, FS-triglycerides 3.08 mmol/L, CB-pH 7.25, and acid base excess −11.2. Additionally, there were significant hematuria and proteinuria. The present treatment is erythropoietin 3000 U ×3

(three times per day of medication) and diuretics. Hemodialysis treatment has not yet been initiated, and kidney transplantation has not yet been planned. It is apparent, however, that the disease is likely to progress to severe renal insufficiency so that those measures will soon have to be considered.

DIAGNOSIS

Recent progress in studies on the molecular genetics of Alport syndrome showing it to be caused by mutations in type IV collagen genes have demonstrated a clear need for new diagnostic criteria. This has become apparent as Alport syndrome has turned out to be phenotypically much more heterogeneous than previously anticipated.

According to Arthur Cecil Alport, who defined the syndrome in 1927, the hereditary hematuric nephritis now referred to as *Alport syndrome* is accompanied by hearing loss (Alport, 1927). Additional manifestations, such as ocular lesions, thrombocytopenia, and abnormal electron microscopic GBM findings, have also been reported. For decades, however, physicians have expected hearing loss to be an essential part of the syndrome. Flinter et al. (1988) proposed that the diagnosis of Alport syndrome should be made in hematuric patients who fulfill three of the following criteria: (1) familial history; (2) hearing loss; (3) ocular lesions; and (4) GBM abnormalities. There are, however, several examples of patients with progressive renal disease and mutations in type IV collagen genes who do not fulfill these criteria either. For example, inheritance cannot always be demonstrated because *de novo* mutations may account for up to 15% of the cases. Also, recent reports have clearly demonstrated that a large proportion of patients with renal failure and mutations in type IV collagen genes do not have hearing loss or eye manifestations. So, how should Alport syndrome be defined? We have recently proposed that the disease should be defined as progressive hematuria hereditary nephritis caused by mutations in type IV collagen genes (Heiskari et al., 1996). Present data indicate that these genes are the ones encoding the $\alpha3(IV)$, $\alpha4(IV)$, and $\alpha5(IV)$ chains of type IV collagen, that is, *COL4A3*, *COL4A4* and *COL4A5*, respectively. However, as pointed out by Gregory et al. (1996), physicians do not always have enough information to make a genetic diagnosis and require an operational definition as a basis for action. They have proposed a clinical definition requiring that four of 10 criteria be satisfied (Table 20-1). Based on the present knowledge, this definition should provide the diagnosis needed for clinical action. The ultimate diagnosis will always require DNA analysis.

MOLECULAR PERSPECTIVES

Basement Membranes

Basement membranes are flexible, thin (~100 nm thick) sheets of specialized extracellular matrix that underlie all epithelial cells and endothelial cells; they also surround individual muscle cells, fat cells, and Schwann cells. The basement membrane thus separates these cells from the underlying connective tissue matrix. In some tissues, such as the brain capillaries, the kidney glomeruli, and lung alveoli, a

Table 20-1. Criteria for the Clinical Diagnosis of Alport Syndrome[a,b]

1. Family history of nephritis of unexpected hematuria in a first-degree relative of the index case or in a male relative linked through any number of females.

2. Persistent hematuria without evidence of an another possibly inherited nephropathy such as thin GBM disease, polycystic kidney disease or IgA nephropathy.

3. Bilateral sensorineural hearing loss in the 2,000–8,000 Hz range. The hearing loss develops gradually, is not present in early infancy, and commonly presents before the age of 30 years.

4. A mutation in COL4An (where n = 3, 4, or 5).

5. Immunohistochemical evidence of complete or partial lack of the Alport epitope in glomerular, or epidermal basement membranes, or both.

6. Widespread GBM ultrastructural abnormalities, in particular, thickening, thinning, and splitting.

7. Ocular lesions including anterior lenticonus, posterior subcapsular cataract, posterior polymorphous dystrophy, and retinal flecks.

8. Gradual progression to ESRD in the index case or at least two family members.

9. Macrothrombocytopenia or granulocytic inclusions.

10. Diffuse leiomyomatosis of the esophagus, female genitalia, or both.

GBM, glomerular basement membrane; ESRD, end-stage renal disease.

[a]According to Gregory et al., 1996.

[b]Four of the 10 criteria should be fulfilled.

basement membrane lying between two cell layers functions as a highly selective filter. Basement membranes provide more than simple structural and filtering functions: They induce cell differentiation, determine cell polarity, influence cell metabolism, organize proteins in adjacent plasma membranes, and serve as specific highways for cell migration (Timpl and Brown, 1994).

The basement membrane is synthesized mainly by the cells that sit on it. As seen in the electron microscope, most basement membranes consist of two distinct layers: an electron-lucent layer (*lamina lucida or rara*) close to the basal plasma membrane of the cells, and an electron-dense layer (*lamina densa*). Some biologists use *basal lamina* to describe the thick basement membrane.

The molecular composition of the basement membrane varies from tissue to tissue and even from region to region in the same basement membrane; however, most mature basal laminae contain type IV collagen, the large heparan sulfate proteoglycan per-lecan, and the glycoproteins laminin and entactin (Timpl and Brown, 1994). Laminin is one of the first extracellular matrix proteins observed in a developing embryo. It is a large *cruciform* (cross-shaped) complex composed of three long polypeptide chains bound together by disulfide bridges. Like many other extracellular matrix molecules, it contains a number of functional domains: One binds to type IV collagen, one to heparan sulfate, one to entactin, and several others to laminin receptors on the surface of cells.

Glomerular Basement Membrane

The *glomerulus* is a vascular-epithelial organ that functions as an ultrafiltration unit for plasma (Fig. 20-2). Embryologically, it is formed by an invagination of a capillary-containing mesenchymal mass into an epithelial lining of a sac, namely, *Bowman's capsule*. The visceral epithelium contains a capillary network and becomes an internal part of the filtration membrane, whereas the parietal epithelium remains at the wall of the Bowman's capsule to collect

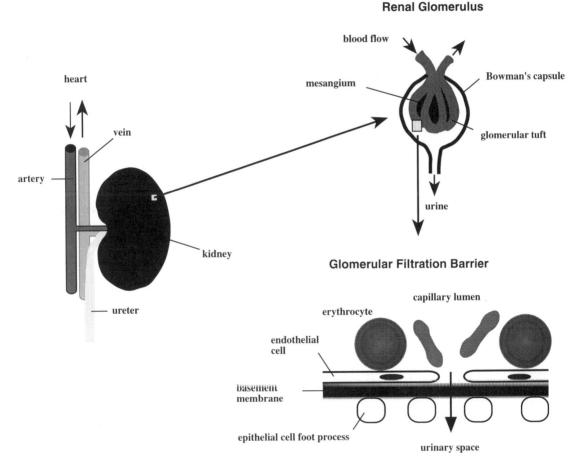

Figure 20-2. Schematic illustration of the kidney filtration units and the glomerular filtration barrier. Each kidney contains about one million ball-shaped glomeruli in which the filtration of blood filtration occurs. The glomerular capillaries divide and form a set of loops (glomerular tufts) located inside the Bowman's capsule. The filtration of blood occurs in the capillaries so that only small proteins and waste products, together with water, can pass into the urinary space. The actual filtration barrier consists of the fenestrated capillary endothelium, one glomerular basement membrane and the slit pores located in between the foot processes of the glomerular endothelial cells. The illustrations are not drawn to scale.

the plasma filtrate. The glomerular filtering membrane that filters plasma to make urine is called the *glomerular basement membrane* (GBM), which consists of: (1) a thin layer of fenestrated endothelial cells; (2) the basement membrane (~320 nm thick in the human adult); and (3) a thin layer of visceral epithelial cells (also called *podocytes*) (Fig. 20-1). Podocytes possess interdigitating processes and adher to the lamina rara externa of the basement membrane. The adjacent foot processes are separated by 20- to 30-nm-wide filtration slits, which make bridges by a thin diaphragm.

In terms of composition, the GBM is composed of the following: type IV collagen makes up about 50% of the dry weight of the GBM; laminin, which plays a role in the adhesion and attachment of cells to the matrix; a glomerular polyanion (mainly heparan sulfate proteoglycans) believed to be responsible for the charge-dependent filtration barrier; nidogen (entactin), a newly found glycoprotein; and several other glycoproteins. The major function of the glomerulus is filtration. The following two characteristics distinguish glomerular filtration from transcapillary exchange in other organs: (1) the glomerulus excludes almost completely from the filtrate those plasma proteins that are the size of albumin (molecular weight ~70,000, radius 3.6 nm) or larger; and (2) it exhibits an extraordinarily high permeability to water and low molecular weight solutes (e.g., glucose, amino acids, sodium ions). The filtration effect across the glomerulus depends on the size or radius of the molecules; filtration decreases as the effective molecular radius increases. In addition to size discrimination, the glomerulus discriminates between molecules according to their charge, allowing greater penetration of neutral and cationic molecules than of anionic molecules of the same size.

Type IV Collagen

The collagens are a family of highly characteristic fibrous proteins found in all multicellular organisms. A collagen molecule is composed of three α-chains that contain typical repeated structure of Gly-X-Y and forms a characteristic collagen triple helix. At present, 33 collagen α-chains encoded by separate genes are known, and 19 collagen types have been identified (Prockop and Kivirikko, 1995).

Type IV collagen was the fourth collagen type

found. It is more flexible than the fibrillar collagens. The triple helix of type IV collagen is interrupted in more than 20 regions, allowing multiple bends in an otherwise rigid molecule. This type of collagen is found only in basement membranes. The monomer of the type IV collagen network in basement membrane is a triple-helical molecule composed of three α-chains, two $\alpha1$ and one $\alpha2$ chains. Like the fibril-associated collagens, they are not processed after secretion from the cells but retain the terminal regions that prevent them from forming fibrils by side-to-side laterilization. Instead, they interact through their unprocessed terminal ends to assemble into a sheet-like multilayered meshwork (Fig. 20-3). Electron microscopic observations of type IV collagen assemblies suggested that these type IV collagen molecules associate by means of their carboxyl termini to form head-to-head dimers, which then form an extended lattice through amino-terminal interactions with another three type IV collagen molecules. The structure is further stabilized by numerous disulfide bridges and other covalent cross-links between the collagen molecules.

Recent studies of the molecular pathology of the basement membrane have led to the discovery of four new chains, $\alpha3$ to $\alpha6$, of type IV collagen, all of which were shown to be directly involved in the pathogenesis of diseases such as Goodpasture syndrome, Alport syndrome, and diffuse esophageal leiomyomatosis (Hudson et al., 1993).

Genes for Type IV Collagen

The mammalian type IV collagen genes have a unique arrangement (Fig. 20-4) in that they are located pairwise in a head-to-head fashion on three different chromosomes: chromosomes 13, 2, and X (Hudson et al., 1993). This implies that the six genes evolved through duplication and inversion of an ancestral gene. The paired genes subsequently underwent two further rounds of duplication, resulting in the three closely opposed pairs.

The type IV collagen genes are large (>100kb) and complex (>50 exons). Interestingly, the paired genes (e.g., the COL4A1 and COL4A2 genes that encode the $\alpha1(IV)$ and $\alpha2(IV)$ chains) share a common 130-base pair (bp) promoter region that contains *cis*-acting elements that have unidirectional and bidirectional transcription activities. The COL4A5 gene, coding for the $\alpha5(IV)$ chain, contains 52 ex-

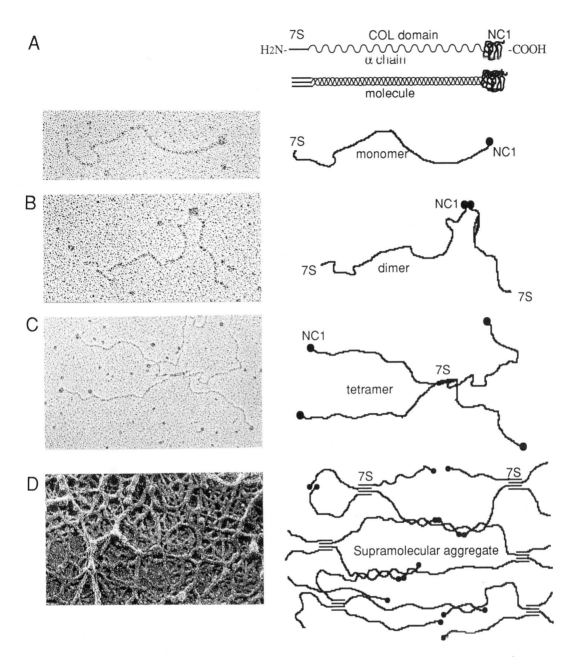

Figure 20-3. Electron micrographs of type IV collagen monomer, dimer, tetramer, and supramolecular aggregates after rotary shadowing and schematic illustrations of the structure and supramolecular assembly of type IV collagen. **A:** Each α chain has a 400-nm-long collagenous (COL) domain characterized by a frequently interrupted Gly-X-Y-repeat sequence, which is not shown. A glomerular noncollagenous domain (NC domain) is located at the carboxyl terminal end. The 7S domain is located at the amino terminal end. Three α chains (any of types α1, α2, α3, α4, α5, or α6) form a triple-helical molecule. The triple-helical molecule forms the building block (monomer) of the basement membrane meshwork. **B:** Individual monomers associate into dimers via disulfide bonds between NC domains or **C:** tetramers through disulfide bonds between the amino termini. **D:** The supramolecular network is formed by assembly of dimers and tetramers and is strengthened by lateral associations and partial winding of some molecules around each other. The other basement membrane components, such as laminin, proteoglycans, and entactin (nidogen), are bound to type IV collagen meshwork in an as yet unclarified manner. Courtesy of Dr. Eijiro Adachi, School of Medicine, Kitazato University.

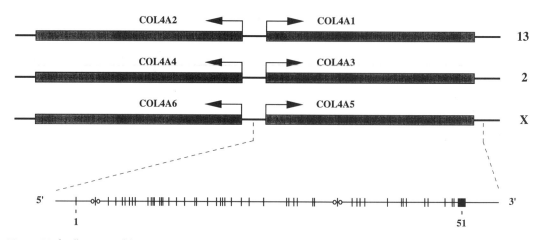

Figure 20-4. Illustration of the organization and chromosome location of the human type IV collagen genes. The genes coding for the six type IV collagen chains are located in pairs in a head-to-head manner on three different chromosomes. The genes are depicted as horizontal rectangles and the flanking regions by horizontal lines. For the *COL4A5* gene, the locations of exons are indicated by vertical bars and introns by horizontal line. The exons are numbered from the 5' end of the gene. Introns of unknown sizes are depicted by circles. *Reproduced from* Tryggvason and Heiskari (1995).

ons and spans 150 kb on chromosome X. The paired gene COL4A6 is located approximately 450 bp away from the COL4A5 gene and is also orientated head to head. The gene appears to be transcribed alternatively (Sugimoto et al., 1994).

Alport Mutations

Mutations have been described in the COL4A5 gene in more than 100 cases of X-linked Alport syndrome. Furthermore, a few mutations have been identified in the COL4A3 and COL4A4 genes in autosomal recessive forms of the disease. About 15% of the mutations are large gene rearrangements, such as deletions, insertions, inversions, or duplications, (for a review of Alport syndrome and the mutations that cause it, see Glassock et al., 1991; Tryggvanson and Heiskari, 1995). The remainder are small mutations, mainly single base changes, small deletions, insertions or duplications (Tryggvason and Heiskari, 1995). Almost all the mutations identified to date differ between families, which makes DNA-based diagnosis of Alport syndrome particularly difficult. The mutations can result in a complete absence of the protein (α chain) in question or in a malfunctional protein, which has been demonstrated by immunofluorescence staining of an Alport kidney using an α5(IV) chain-specific monoclonal antibody (Ninomiya et al., 1995). As a result, the structural

framework of the GBM, which requires type IV molecules containing these polypeptide chains, becomes structurally weak and disrupted.

THERAPY

General

Although the onset of hematuria occurs during early childhood, the disease usually progresses slowly. A large number of male patients enter terminal renal failure during adolescence (*juvenile form*), but the onset may occur beyond the age of 25 years (*adult type*). Usually, affected males and homozygous females develop end-stage renal disease before the fifth decade of life, whereas heterozygous females rarely develop renal failure. There is no satisfactory and curative conservative treatment available (Glassock et al., 1991). Patients developing end-stage renal disease are treated by hemodialysis, and also kidney transplantation whenever possible. About 5% of transplanted patients develop anti-GBM nephritis and reject the allografted kidneys.

Gene Therapy

As a result of the enormous advances in molecular genetics and biology research, gene therapy may be developing into a real possibility for the treatment of hereditary diseases in the future. Although gene therapy has not yet come of age as a viable therapeutic alternative, extensive research efforts are being made in that direction. Hereditary kidney diseases, such as Alport syndrome, primarily affecting the renal glomeruli, could potentially be treated by somatic gene therapy, which involves the introduction of normal cDNAs or complete genes for the $\alpha3(IV)$, $\alpha4(IV)$ or $\alpha5(IV)$ collagen chains into glomerular

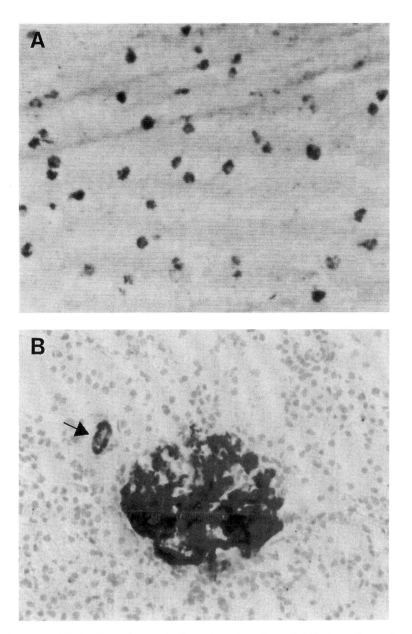

Figure 20-5. Expression of the Lac Z reporter gene in glomerular and capillary cells following perfusion of porcine kidney *in vivo*. About 85% of all glomeruli are positive for expression **(A)**, which appears to be in all cell types of the glomerulus **(B)**. Expression can also be seen in the endothelial cells of capillaries (arrow). In contrast, epithelial cells of the kidney tubuli are not positive, indicating that the reporter gene containing virus does not penetrate the glomerular basement membrane and reach the urinary and tubular spaces. *From* Parpala T, Heikkila P, Lukkarinen O, Tryggvason K (unpublished observation).

225

cells. Recent work has already shown it to be possible to transfer foreign genes into 85% of the glomeruli in vivo (Heikkilä et al., 1996). (Fig. 20-5). Thus, the stage has been set for actual gene therapy experiments in animal models of Alport syndrome. There are, however, many obstacles to be overcome before we can expect the disease to be cured in humans by gene therapy; but if gene therapy is going to become a viable alternative for the treatment of genetic diseases in general, it is likely to become an option for Alport syndrome.

QUESTIONS

1. Describe three major symptoms observed in Alport's syndrome patients.
2. How did scientists first find mutations in the COL4A5 gene from the Alport syndrome patients?
3. What is the function of the basement membrane?
4. What are RFLP, genetic markers, the human genome project, and positional cloning?
5. When you see a suspected Alport syndrome patient, what would you do to reach the final definitive diagnosis?
6. In genetic counseling you see a patient suffering from an inherited disorder; it is obvious that it is an inherited disease, since not only the patient but also his father and one of his brothers have a similar phenotype. However, nothing is yet described in textbooks about the gene responsible for the disorder. If you would like to investigate the responsible gene, what would you do? How would you approach the problem?

REFERENCES

Alport AC: Hereditary familial congenital haemorrhagic nephritis. *Br Med J* 1:504–506, 1927.

Flinter FA, Cameron JS, Chantler C, Houston I, Bobrow M: Genetics of classic Alport's syndrome. *Lancet* 2:1005–1007, 1988.

Glassock RJ, Cohen AH, Adler SG, Ward HJ: Secondary glomerular diseases, *in* Brenner BM, Rector FC, (eds): *The Kidney* Philadelphia, WB Saunders, 1991, pp 1331–1334.

Gregory MC, Terreros DA, Barker DF, Fain PR, Denison J, Atkin C: Alport syndrome—clinical phenotypes, incidence, and pathology, *in* Tryggvason K (ed): *Molecular Pathology and Genetics of Alport Syndrome.* S Karger AG, Basel, NY, 1996, pp. 1–28.

Heikkilä P, Parpala T, Lukkarinen O, Weber M, Tryggvason K: Adenovirus-mediated gene transfer into kidney glomeruli using an *ex vivo* and *in vivo* kidney perfusion system—First steps towards gene therapy of Alport syndrome. *Gene Therapy,* 3:21–27, 1996.

Heiskari N, Zhang X, Leinonen A, et al.: Identification of 17 mutations in ten exons in the COL4A5 collagen gene, but no mutations found in four exons in COL4A6. A study of 250 patients with Alport syndrome. *J Am Soc Nephrol,* 7:702–709, 1996.

Hudson BG, Reeders ST, Tryggvason K: Type IV collagen: Structure, gene organization, and role in human diseases. *J Biol Chem* 268:26033–26036, 1993.

Ninomiya Y, Kagawa M, Iyama K, Naito I, Kishiro Y, Seyer JM, Sugimoto M, Oohashi T, Sado Y. Differential expression of two basement membrane collagen genes, *COL4A6* and *COL4A5,* demonstrated by immunofluorescence staining using peptide-specific monoclonal antibodies. *J Cell Biol* 130:1219–1229, 1995.

Prockop DJ, Kivirikko KI: Collagens: Molecular biology, diseases and potentials for therapy. *Annu Rev Biochem* 64:403–434, 1995.

Sugimoto M, Oohashi T, Ninomiya, Y. The genes COL4A5 and COL4A6, coding for basement membrane collagen chains $\alpha5(IV)$ and $\alpha6(IV)$, are located head-to-head in close proximity on human chromosome Xq22 and COL4A6 is transcribed from two alternative promoters. *Proc Natl Acad Sci USA* 91:11679–11683, 1994.

Timpl R, Brown J: The laminins. *Matrix Biol* 14:275–281, 1994.

Tryggvason K, Heiskari N: Alport Syndrome. *in* Schlondorff D, Bonventere J (eds): *Molecular Nephrology: Kidney Function in Health and Disease.* New York, Marcel Dekker, 1995, pp 795–808.

21

Pancreatic Excocrine Insufficiency

PHILIP REYES AND WILLIAM R. GALEY, JR.

CASE REPORT

A.L., a 48-year-old housepainter, was admitted to the hospital complaining of severe "boring" epigastric pain radiating through to his midback, feeling tired, and passing foul-smelling and oily stools at an increased frequency. A.L. lost 20 lbs over the past 5 months as the diarrhea worsened. His appetite has been good, and he has been eating a well-balanced diet.

Mr. L has abused alcohol for about 22 years, mostly on weekends. He was admitted to the hospital four times in the last three years for severe epigastric pain. At the time of those admissions, his serum amylase and serum lipase levels were elevated but liver transaminase enzymes (aspartate transaminase [AST], 35 IU/L; alanine transaminase [ALT], 30 IU/L; normal range, 5–35 IU/L for both) were normal as was his total serum bilirubin concentration (1.2 mg/dL; normal range, 0.2–1.2 mg/dL). Serum gastrin levels were 50 pg/mL (normal range, 0–100 pg/mL). The esophageal, gastric, and duodenal mucosae appeared normal when upper gastrointestinal (GI) *endoscopy* (a method that permits examination of the esophageal, gastric, and duodenal tissues through a fiber-optic viewing device passed through the mouth) was done on the first and fourth admissions.

On the last admission, Mr. L appeared *cachectic* (thin and emaciated) and in obvious distress. He exhibited midepigastric tenderness but did not have an enlarged liver or spleen on examination. An abdominal roentgenogram (Fig. 21-1) was taken and showed *multifocal calcification* (many sites of cal-

cium salt deposits) of the pancreas. Serum amylase (25 IU/L; normal range, 30–110 IU/L) and lipase (20 IU/L; normal range, 23–300 IU/L) values were slightly below the lower limit of the normal range. Liver function tests, including AST and ALT, were normal except for serum gamma glutamyl transferase (GGT), which was moderately elevated at 140 IU/L (normal range, 5–85 IU/L). The serum bilirubin levels were normal, and no evidence of jaundice was seen. Analysis of the collected daily stool revealed 18 g of triglyceride (normal, <7 g), and microscopic examination showed undigested meat fibers. The patient's blood glucose was measured and found to be 230 mg/dL (normal range, 80–115 mg/dL). His *hematocrit* (the fraction of blood that is made up of red blood cells) was 36 (normal range, 42–57) with a mean cell volume of 106 fL (normal range, 81–99 fL). There was no evidence of blood in the stool as measured by a *stool guaiac* (a chemical test which reacts with the heme iron of hemoglobin) test. A glucose tolerance test showed a prolonged hyperglycemia, and insulin was found to be 4 μU/mL (normal range, 5–35 μU/mL). A D-xylose load test showed a 5-hour urinary excretion of 7 grams (normal, >5 g) with a 25-g oral dose. Serum vitamin B_{12} was measured at 100 pg/mL (normal range, 230–1140 pg/mL).

DIAGNOSIS

Midepigastric pain in a middle-aged person is commonly associated with gastric or duodenal ulcer, gallstones, pancreatitis, intestinal obstruction, or

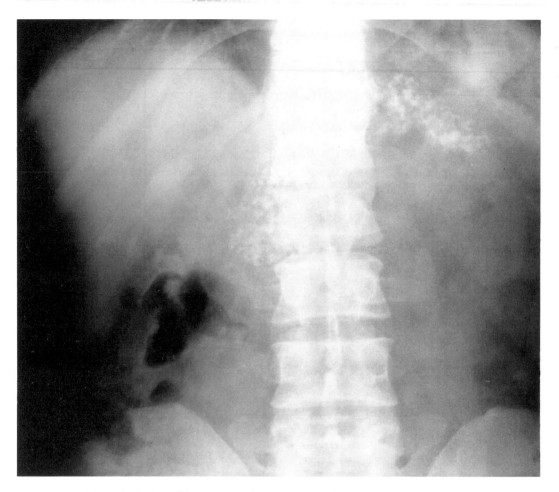

Figure 21-1. Abdominal radiograph of the patient. Visible are the vertebrae (running vertically in the center of photograph), top of the hips (bottom), and ribs (thin arched structures in upper half of figure). The dark spots in the lower left of the radiograph (lower right side of patient) are normal pockets of gas in the colon. The important clinical finding is the calcified pancreas seen as scattered white patches in the center and running up and to the right of the figure. The calcified pancreas with the patient's history is diagnostic of chronic pancreatitis.

colonic diverticulitis. The association of the pain with alcoholism and what appears to be a diarrhea associated with maldigestion (evidenced by the presence of triglycerides and meat fibers in the stool) strongly suggests pancreatic exocrine insufficiency. Furthermore, weight loss by an individual who is eating well is consistent with malabsorption of nutrients as a result of a maldigestion problem. Further evidence supporting an involvement of the pancreas is the *hyperlipasemia* (high blood level of lipase) and *hyperamylasemia* (high blood level of amylase) seen in previous episodes of what appears to be a continuing problem for this patient. Hyperamylasemia may arise from the inflammation of organs

other than the pancreas, such as the salivary glands, small intestine, or kidney, and can be produced by cancers of the lung, esophagus, and other organs. Although the analysis of serum amylase isozymes can be used to determine whether the amylase originated from the pancreas or other organs, this analysis is not commonly done. The recent improvement in the assay for serum lipase has made it a more appropriate enzyme to assess the potential pathology of the pancreas because the pancreas is the only important source of serum lipase activity.

Furthermore, whereas serum pancreatic amylase activity in a patient with pancreatitis can rise within a single day, levels commonly fall to near normal within three days even if the organ remains inflamed. Lipase activity often remains elevated for several days after the serum amylase level has normalized. The finding in the current hospitalization that serum amylase and lipase activities are somewhat *below* normal does not exclude the pancreas from consideration. On the contrary, these below-normal values most likely reflect the loss of the pancreas' ability to produce these and other digestive enzymes as a result of the chronic destructive nature of the disease process. This hypothesis is supported by the hyperglycemia and low circulating insulin levels, which suggest that the endocrine function of the pancreas has also been compromised in this patient as a result of the destruction of pancreatic tissue.

Steatorrhea (excess fat in the stool), evidenced by the "oily" stool and the 18 g of triglyceride in the daily stool collection, clearly indicates that dietary fat (primarily triglyceride) is not being completely digested. The presence of intact triglycerides and meat fibers in the fecal material suggests that the patient's problems are associated with maldigestion, not merely malabsorption, which is further supported by the D-xylose test showing that absorption is normal in Mr. L's small intestine. The D-xylose test is a measure of the area of the small intestine available for the absorption of nutrients and is accomplished by giving a standard oral dose of xylose and measuring the total amount of xylose (a nonmetabolized sugar) excreted in the urine over a standard amount of time.

Because the patient's liver function tests (AST, ALT, GGT) were near normal, his digestive problems would seem to be associated with the effect of alcohol abuse on the pancreas rather than a dysfunction of the exocrine liver secretion of bile salts. Steatorrhea may be caused by the liver's inability to produce bile salts, which are important in the digestion and absorption of fats. The moderate elevation of serum GGT, an enzyme induced by drugs such as alcohol, is most indicative of the continued abuse of alcohol by the patient.

The finding that the serum levels of bilirubin and enzymes found in the liver were not significantly elevated suggests that although Mr. L is an alcoholic, he has had little liver damage. Furthermore, it is unlikely that the pancreatitis he has experienced is due to a gallstone or cancer blocking the flow of pancreatic juice through the sphincter of Oddi into the bowel. If this were the case, the stasis of bile in the biliary duct would lead to increased serum levels of bilirubin and liver enzymes (AST, ALT, GGT).

The excessive secretion of HCl by the stomach is associated with the production of peptic ulcers and associated pain. Overproduction of HCl can lead to an abnormally low pH in the lumen of the small intestine, impeding digestion by pancreatic enzymes (which have near-neutral pH optima) and causing diarrhea. This may occur in Zollinger-Ellison syndrome, in which a gastrin-producing tumor causes excessive acid production. That this is not the case in our patient is evident from the observation that by endoscopy the gastric and duodenal mucosae appear normal and the serum gastrin levels are normal.

His fatigue may be because of his malnourished state but is more likely because of the *anemia* (lack of sufficient red blood cells) he is experiencing. The anemia appears to be the result of vitamin B_{12} deficiency rather than the loss of blood in that the red cells are larger than normal and the vitamin B_{12} levels in his blood are low (see Chapter 11, "Pernicious Anemia").

MOLECULAR PERSPECTIVES

Digestion and Absorption of Food

Overview

Food, for the most part, is composed of large or complex molecules (carbohydrates, proteins, fats) that cannot be absorbed by the intestinal tract. Accordingly, the function of digestion is to transform these chemical constituents into small and simple molecules that can be absorbed by the mucosal cells lining the intestines. Digestion is accomplished by a combination of: (1) mechanical disintegration of solid food (e.g., chewing and the churning action of stomach); and (2) degradation of food molecules by an array of hydrolytic enzymes. Mechanical action in the stomach converts food into a suspension of small particles known as *chyme*. Carbohydrates, proteins, and fats in these particles become readily accessible to the various pancreatic and intestinal hydrolases, commonly called *digestive enzymes*.

Although some degradation of carbohydrates and proteins occurs in the mouth and stomach, respectively, the vast majority of food molecules are degraded in the lumen of the small intestine. Moreover, the small intestine, sequentially comprising the duodenum, jejunum, and ileum, is also the site where virtually all of the digested food is absorbed. Most dietary nutrients, once absorbed, enter the hepatic portal vein and travel to the liver. They are then distributed by the bloodstream to the various tissues and organs of the body. On the other hand, most of the absorbed fat does not enter the hepatic portal system. Instead, fat is taken up by the lymphatic circulation for eventual delivery to the bloodstream.

Action of Digestive Enzymes

As already noted, food molecules are degraded by a variety of digestive enzymes. These enzymes are found in saliva, stomach secretions, and pancreatic secretions that enter the lumen of the duodenum.

Starch, the main digestible carbohydrate in the diet, is a polymer of glucose in which most of the monosaccharide units are linked by $\alpha(1\rightarrow4)$ glucosidic bonds. Some glucose units are joined by $\alpha(1\rightarrow6)$ bonds, forming branch points in the polymer. Starch is degraded by the enzyme α-amylase, an endosaccharidase, into a variety of products, including some glucose, disaccharides (maltose, isomaltose), maltotriose (a trisaccharide), and an oligosaccharide known as α-*limit dextrin*. The latter, on average, comprises eight glucose units and contains one or more $\alpha(1\rightarrow6)$ branch-point linkages. Isomaltose is another product of starch degradation that contains an $\alpha(1\rightarrow6)$ glucosidic bond.

Proteins are hydrolyzed by several proteases into a mixture of oligopeptides, dipeptides, and amino acids. The degradation of fats (mainly triglycerides), a process catalyzed by the enzyme lipase, produces free fatty acids and 2-monoglycerides.

Dietary disaccharides, primarily table sugar (sucrose) and milk sugar (lactose), the various disaccharide and oligosaccharide products of starch digestion, as well as oligopeptides and some dipeptides cannot be absorbed as such. Consequently, these molecules must undergo further digestion, primarily by hydrolases bound to the surface of the mucosal cells lining the small intestine. These so-called *brush-border enzymes* include various peptidases, sucrase, lactase, maltase, isomaltase, and α-limit dextrinase. The latter enzyme is responsible for cleaving the $\alpha(1\rightarrow6)$ bonds present in α-limit dextrin.

The principal final products of digestion are monosaccharides (mostly glucose, fructose, and galactose), amino acids, dipeptides, free fatty acids,

and 2-monoglycerides. These are the molecules actually absorbed by the intestinal mucosa.

Digestion and Absorption of Fat

The digestion and absorption of ingested fat deserve special mention, being more complex than the digestion and absorption of carbohydrates and proteins (see Fig. 21-2). As pointed out, dietary fat is composed mainly of triglycerides. Furthermore, fat digestion, like that of other nutrients, takes place primarily in the lumen of the small intestine and begins in the duodenum. Because of its water-insoluble nature, however, fat is present in chyme as a fat droplet-water emulsion, which is not the case for carbohydrates and proteins.

The most important enzyme involved in the digestion of triglycerides is *pancreatic lipase*. This enzyme is anchored to the surface of fat droplets by a pancreatic protein called *colipase*. Once anchored, pancreatic lipase cleaves two fatty acids from each triglyceride, leaving behind a 2-monoglyceride as the second major product of lipolysis.

To be absorbed by the intestinal mucosal cells, the fatty acids and 2-monoglycerides produced by lipolysis must first interact with *bile salts*, which are major constituents of bile. Cholesterol, released from dietary cholesterol esters by pancreatic cholesterol ester hydrolases, also interacts with bile salts, as do dietary lysophospholipids and fat-soluble vitamins. The association of these lipids with bile salts results in the formation of mixed micelles. The function of mixed micelles is to solubilize fatty acids and 2-monoglycerides (as well as cholesterol and other dietary lipids) and to transport these lipids through the unstirred water layer that overlies the surface of the intestinal epithelium. At the surface the micelles disaggregate and the lipids then enter the enterocytes by passive diffusion.

Fat absorption is usually an efficient process: 95% or more of ingested fat is absorbed when fat intake is moderate. Most fat absorption takes place in the upper portions of the small intestine (i.e., duodenum and jejunum). On the other hand, most of the bile salts are reabsorbed in the ileum, meaning that most bile salts remain in the lumen of the small intestine and can participate in several cycles of mixed micelle formation before they are reabsorbed.

Absorbed lipids normally undergo some metabolism within mucosal cells. For example, triglycerides are resynthesized from absorbed fatty acids (but

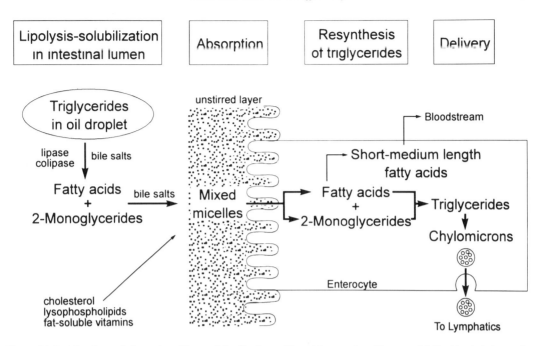

Figure 21-2. Digestion and absorption of ingested fat. The fatty acids and 2-monoglycerides are solubilized by their interaction with bile salts. The resulting mixed micelles transport these and other dietary lipids through the unstirred layer to the surface of the enterocyte. Following absorption, 2-monoglycerides (as well as lysophospholipids and cholesterol) are reesterified with long-chain fatty acids. The newly synthesized triglycerides, phospholipids, and cholesterol esters, together with fat-soluble vitamins, are packaged into chylomicron particles for delivery to the bloodstream via the lymphatic system. Ordinarily, fatty acids shorter than 10 or 12 carbon atoms are not metabolized by enterocytes. Instead, these fatty acids are released directly into the hepatic portal blood, travel to the liver, and eventually enter the general circulation bound to albumin.

usually only those longer than 10 or 12 carbon atoms) and 2-monoglycerides. Also, a portion of the absorbed cholesterol is re-esterified with fatty acids, as are lysophospholipids. The triglycerides, phospholipids, and cholesterol esters (as well as fat-soluble vitamins) are then incorporated into lipoprotein particles, known as *chylomicrons*, for delivery to the lymphatic system and then to the bloodstream. By contrast, absorbed fatty acids shorter than 10 or 12 carbon atoms are normally released directly into the hepatic portal vein. These latter fatty acids eventually enter the general circulation bound to albumin.

Role of the Pancreas in Digestion

Exocrine Function of the Pancreas

The pancreas is composed of two histologically distinct tissue types, allowing it to carry out two different and very important tasks (Habal, 1992). The *endocrine pancreas,* made up of islets of Langerhans, releases insulin, glucagon, and other hormones into the bloodstream. In this chapter we focus on the second important task of the pancreas, its exocrine function.

The *exocrine pancreas* plays an essential role in digestion by virtue of its capacity to secrete a fluid that is not only alkaline (about pH 8) but also rich in the hydrolytic enzymes needed to break down food molecules. As much as 1500 mL of this fluid, commonly known as *pancreatic juice,* is secreted into the lumen of the duodenum per day. The alkalinity of this fluid is due primarily to its relatively high concentration of HCO_3^-.

Because of its alkaline nature, pancreatic juice is able to neutralize gastric acid in duodenal chyme. Neutralization of gastric acid is absolutely necessary for proper digestion because pancreatic and brush-border hydrolases are virtually inactive in a strongly acidic environment. These digestive enzymes are maximally active under neutral or slightly alkaline conditions. Normally, chyme exhibits a near-neutral pH by the time it reaches the middle portion of the small intestine (i.e., jejunum).

Table 21-1 summarizes the properties and chemical composition of pancreatic juice. It is noteworthy that enzymes account for 90 to 95% of the total protein.

Pancreatic Zymogens and Proenzymes

Table 21-2 illustrates that the pancreas produces and secretes a wide selection of hydrolases, including α-amylase, proteases, lipolytic enzymes, and nucleases. Pancreatic juice contains additional proteins: prolipase and trypsin inhibitor. Colipase, once activated, is an important participant in the overall process of fat digestion.

Clearly, the pancreas must protect itself from the destructive effects of the hydrolases, especially proteases, that it produces and secretes. The occurrence of enzyme-inflicted damage to the pancreas, or *autodigestion,* is effectively prevented in two ways. First, all proteases are synthesized as inactive precursors, called *zymogens,* and are confined to intracellular vesicles. Second, protease action within the pancreas is prevented by a powerful inhibitor known as *trypsin inhibitor.* Not surprisingly, phospholipase A$_2$, which can disrupt cellular membranes by hydrolyzing membrane phospholipids to lysophospholipids, is also formed as an inactive proenzyme and confined to vesicles. The intracellular vesicles containing zymogens, proenzymes, and other precursor proteins are referred to as *zymogen granules.* Exocytosis of these granules is required for the release of these proteins by the pancreatic secretory cells.

Pancreatic zymogens and proenzymes (and other precursor proteins) are transformed into active forms only after being discharged into the lumen of

Table 21-1. Properties and Chemical Composition of Pancreatic Juice

Alkaline (pH ~8)
Isotonic
Complex Chemical Composition
Cations: Na$^+$, K$^+$, Mg^{2+}, Ca^{2+}
Anions: Cl$^-$, SO$_4^{2-}$, HPO$_4^{2-}$
HCO$_3^-$ (about 115 meq/L)
Digestive enzymes[a]
Other proteins

[a]See Figure 21-3.

Table 21-2. Principal Digestive Enzymes in Pancreatic Juice[a]

Carbohydrate digestion
α-amylase
Protein digestion
Trypsin (trypsinogen)
Chymotrypsin (chymotrypsinogen)
Elastase (proelastase)
Carboxypeptidases A and B (procarboxypeptidases A and B)
Trypsin inhibitor
Lipid digestion
Lipase
Colipase (procolipase)
Phospholipase A$_2$ (prophospholipase A$_2$)
Cholesterol ester hydrolase
Nucleic acid digestion
Ribonuclease
Deoxyribonuclease

[a]Zymogens, proenzymes, or precursor proteins are listed in parentheses

the duodenum. Activation involves the cleavage of one or more specific peptide bonds within each precursor protein molecule. The activation of all inactive proteins is accomplished by a cascade of reactions, initiated by the enzyme *enteropeptidase* (Fig. 21-3), previously called enterokinase, which is secreted by cells in the wall of the small intestine. Trypsin is formed from trypsinogen in the initial reaction. Once formed, trypsin catalyzes the proteolytic activation of the remaining protease zymogens and other precursor proteins, such as prophospholipase A$_2$ and procolipase. Trypsin, once present, can also catalyze its own formation from trypsinogen. The need for a trypsin inhibitor in pancreatic juice becomes evident when one considers the central role played by trypsin in the process of zymogen activation. In the intestinal lumen, however, this inhibitor is diluted by the chyme, thereby diminishing its effective concentration. The end result is that trypsin, no longer severely inhibited, is now able to carry out its important activation function.

Regulation of Pancreatic Secretion

The exocrine pancreas is made up of blind-ended, gland-like structures lined by acinar cells that drain into a system of ductules. The ductules merge into longer ducts, eventually converging into the main pancreatic duct. After joining the bile duct, the pancreatic duct empties into the duodenum through the sphincter of Oddi (Fig. 21-4). Acinar cells secrete a

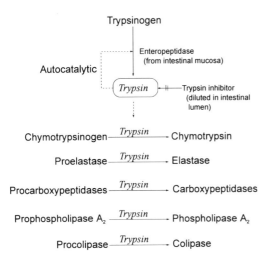

Figure 21-3. Activation of zymogens and other digestive precursor proteins secreted by the pancreas. Trypsin serves as the common activator of these precursor proteins. Activation normally occurs within the intestinal lumen and requires the cleavage of one or more specific peptide bonds. Trypsin, in turn, is generated when trypsinogen is activated by enteropeptidase, a protease secreted by the intestinal mucosa. Note that trypsin, once formed, activates more trypsinogen (i.e., acts autocatalytically). This scheme also points out that trypsin becomes active in the lumen of the intestine because trypsin inhibitor is diluted by chyme. This reversal of inhibition leaves trypsin free to carry out its crucial activation function.

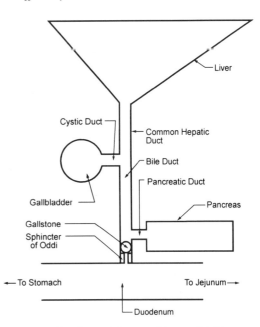

Figure 21-4. Schematic diagram of liver, gallbladder, pancreas, duodenum, and associated ducts. The diagram also illustrates how a gallstone might block the flow of bile and pancreatic juice into the duodenum.

fluid rich in digestive enzymes, whereas epithelial cells lining the ductules secrete a HCO_3^--rich fluid. Pancreatic juice arises by the combination of these two different fluids.

Secretion by the exocrine pancreas is stimulated by the intake of food and is mediated primarily by two hormones (secretin and cholecystokinin). Neural control is also involved. *Secretin,* produced by endocrine cells in the duodenal wall, stimulates the secretion of HCO_3^- by ductule epithelial cells. Cholecystokinin (CCK), also released by endocrine cells of the duodenum, acts primarily on acinar cells to stimulate the secretion of digestive enzymes and also causes the gallbladder to contract and to deliver its store of bile into the bile duct and consequently into the duodenal lumen through the sphincter of Oddi (see Fig. 21-4). Recall that bile is rich in bile salts and that the latter facilitate the digestion and absorption of dietary fat.

Inflammatory Disease of the Pancreas

Acute Pancreatitis

Pancreatic inflammatory disease (*pancreatitis*) may be acute or chronic in nature (Greenberger et al., 1991; Grendall and Cello, 1993). Acute pancreatitis is thought to cause little, if any, permanent damage to the pancreas. With proper treatment, patients normally recover within 1 to 2 weeks. Acute pancreatitis is associated with numerous risk factors or causes, alcohol abuse and gallstones being the most common in the United States. The pathogenic mechanism by which etiologic factors produce inflammation and disease is poorly understood. Nevertheless, it is widely held that autodigestion, caused by the inappropriate activation of zymogens and proenzymes within the pancreas, is a likely mechanism.

By causing cellular injury and death, tissue necrosis, and vascular leakage, autodigestion can account for the sudden onset of epigastric pain, and the markedly elevated levels of serum amylase and lipase seen in most of these patients. Incidentally, the rise in serum levels of these enzymes helps to remind us of an important biomedical concept; that is, cellular injury and death almost always lead to the release of intracellular enzymes into the bloodstream. Equally important is the finding that many enzymes are not evenly distributed among the various tissues and organs of the body. Thus, elevated serum enzyme levels have diagnostic value because they can often help identify the tissue site of disease in a patient.

Exactly why zymogens undergo activation within the pancreas is not known. It has been proposed that activation is somehow triggered by intermittent obstruction of pancreatic ducts or the sphincter of Oddi by proteinaceous plugs or gallstones, respectively. Alcohol is known to cause the formation of such plugs.

Chronic Pancreatitis and Pancreatic Exocrine Insufficiency

Chronic pancreatitis is a slowly progressive inflammatory disease involving permanent and cumulative damage to the pancreas. Pain may be severe, mild, or absent. Episodes of acute inflammation are not uncommon and are usually associated with epigastric pain and elevated serum levels of pancreatic enzymes. Because of the continued destruction of this organ, chronic pancreatitis invariably leads to significant losses of exocrine function. A condition formally known as *pancreatic exocrine insufficiency* arises when patients have suffered massive losses of exocrine function (Dimagnno, 1993). Not surprisingly, these patients often show normal or below normal levels of pancreatic enzymes in the serum.

Although the cause of chronic pancreatitis cannot always be established, chronic alcoholism and cystic fibrosis (in children) are the most common conditions associated with this disease in the United States (Marino and Gorelick, 1992). There seems to be little, if any, association with gallstones. As in the case of acute pancreatitis, alcohol is thought to favor the formation of protein plugs within pancreatic ducts. The pressure associated with chronic obstruction of these ducts can cause their dilation, eventually leading to tissue damage and fibrosis. The end result is often extensive calcification of pancreatic tissue. The mechanism by which this calcification arises is not well understood. Once again, the inappropriate activation of pancreatic zymogens is considered the primary event that triggers tissue destruction.

Consequences of Pancreatic Exocrine Insufficiency

We have already pointed out that chronic pancreatitis involves a progressive loss of pancreatic exocrine function. It is not surprising that the diminished capacity to secrete HCO_3^- and zymogens manifests itself as maldigestion and therefore malabsorption of fat and protein. This accounts for two diagnostic clinical findings: steatorrhea and the presence of undigested meat fibers in the stool. Malabsorption, however, does not usually occur until most of the exocrine function of the pancreas has been destroyed. We can say, therefore, that maldigestion-induced malabsorption of fat and protein is a classic symptom in patients with chronic pancreatitis of long duration.

Fat malabsorption may also reflect a reduced flow of bile into the duodenum (*cholestasis*) resulting from chronic inflammation, fibrosis, or cancer of the bile duct or spinchter of Oddi. This condition not only raises the serum level of alkaline phosphatase and other liver enzymes, such as alanine transaminase and aspartate transaminase, but also produces obstructive jaundice (seen as increased levels of circulating bilirubin.) In this case bilirubin is present primarily as the diglucuronide derivative (i.e., its conjugated or "direct reacting" form).

To make a correct diagnosis of pancreatic exocrine insufficiency, evidence must show that malabsorption is not the result of an abnormality or disease of the intestinal mucosa. This is usually done by showing that the absorptive capacity of the patient's small intestine is not impaired. To do so, one administers an oral dose of a test substance that does not require digestion and whose absorption, therefore, is not affected by the loss of pancreatic exocrine function. Furthermore, the test substance should be poorly metabolized, once absorbed, so that it can be quantitated in collected urine. D-xylose meets these requirements. Thus, a normal xylose absorption-excretion test is helpful in confirming a diagnosis of pancreatic exocrine insufficiency.

It may seem puzzling that the usual symptoms of exocrine insufficiency include fat and protein malabsorption but not carbohydrate malabsorption; however, this disparity can be largely explained by the known differences in the stability of pancreatic enzymes. Lipase is a very labile enzyme and is easily inactivated. For example, it is quickly denatured if the pH drops below 4. A pH this low within the lumen of the duodenum is not unusual in this disease because of the impaired secretion of HCO_3^-. Lipase is also very susceptible to digestion by pancreatic proteases, especially chymotrypsin (Thiruvengadam and Dimagnno, 1988).

Pancreatic proteases, although somewhat more stable than lipase, are also inactivated by low pH or proteolytic digestion. By contrast, α-amylase is relatively resistant to inactivation. Indeed, about 80 to 90% of these enzyme molecules are still active on reaching the ileum. Not surprisingly, considerably more lipase and protease activity is lost during the journey to the ileum.

Other factors should also be kept in mind when considering why fat malabsorption is much more common than carbohydrate malabsorption. First, α-amylase is also present in saliva; consequently, considerable starch digestion can take place in the mouth and stomach. Thus, it seems quite possible that action by salivary α-amylase is able to compensate for the markedly reduced levels of pancreatic α-amylase in the lumen of the small intestine. Second, studies have shown that the low intraduodenal pH associated with the loss of exocrine function can itself promote fat malabsorption. The explanation is that low pH is capable of precipitating bile salts, thereby reducing their effective concentration. Bile salts, of course, play a critical role in the formation of the micelles required for efficient fat absorption.

A low intraluminal pH will also reduce the activity of any lipase molecules that escape inactivation. Remember that the pH optima of digestive enzymes are in the neutral or slightly alkaline range.

A deficiency of pancreatic proteases, besides accounting for the incomplete digestion of meat fibers, also explains why many patients (about 40%) also suffer from vitamin B_{12} malabsorption. This vitamin cannot be absorbed until it is cleaved by proteases from its complex with R proteins present in saliva and gastric juice (see Chapter 11). Once released in the intestinal lumen, vitamin B_{12} forms a complex with intrinsic factor (produced and secreted by the stomach). The vitamin B_{12}:intrinsic factor complex then binds to its receptor on the mucosal surface of the ileum, where vitamin B_{12} is absorbed. Interestingly, the malabsorption of lipid-soluble vitamins is rarely seen in pancreatic exocrine insufficiency.

Loss of Endocrine Function in Chronic Pancreatitis

We have seen that the exocrine portion of the pancreas is the primary site of tissue destruction in chronic pancreatitis. Eventually, however, the islets of Langerhans begin to suffer damage as well. Once a sufficient fraction of the islets has been destroyed, the pancreas is no longer able to secrete adequate amounts of insulin in response to an oral load of glucose. Thus, hyperglycemia is a common finding in chronic pancreatitis patients who have sustained marked losses of pancreatic endocrine function.

The oral glucose tolerance test is widely used as a means of assessing the status of the endocrine pancreas. This test involves the ingestion of a standard dose of glucose, followed by the monitoring of blood glucose levels for about 2 hours. A normal test provides evidence that intestinal absorption as well as the endocrine pancreas are functioning properly. In patients with severe loss of pancreatic endocrine function, however, blood glucose rises to abnormally high values and returns to baseline levels more slowly than normal.

THERAPY

The treatment of pancreatitis focuses primarily on relieving pain, digestive enzyme supplementation, and stopping further harm to the pancreas by the cessation of alcohol use. Pain control may be accomplished using narcotic or non-narcotic drugs, injection of blocking agents into nerves enervating the pancreas, surgery, or simply oral supplementation of pancreatic digestive enzymes. This supplementation of enzymes appears to decrease pain by decreasing the stimulus for pancreatic secretion. This appears to result from the exogenous enzymes acting at the duodenal mucosa.

To correct the maldigestion and consequent malabsorption of nutrients, the mainstay of therapy is oral pancreatic enzyme supplementation (Lankish, 1993). Because the pancreatic enzymes, especially lipase, are susceptible to inhibition by the low pH of the stomach or digestion by the gastric pepsins (*en-*

dopeptidases), enteric-coated tablets of the pancreatic enzymes are often used. Additionally, drugs, such as cimetidine, that block acid production by the stomach are often used to prevent the acid inhibition and peptic digestion of the pancreatic enzymes. This approach is especially useful in the face of a pancreas that is compromised in its ability to produce the bicarbonate-rich and acid-neutralizing component of pancreatic juice as well as the pancreatic enzymes themselves.

In patients such as Mr. L, whose pancreas is no longer capable of carrying out its endocrine function of producing sufficient insulin to regulate glucose metabolism, it is necessary to provide insulin therapy. Occasionally, surgery is performed to remove blockages of the pancreatic ducts, which improves both the symptoms of pain and pancreatic enzyme insufficiency. Usually this surgery involves the removal of pancreatic stones if they are blocking the ductal system or excision of fluid-filled cysts that may be created in exacerbations of pancreatitis.

QUESTIONS

1. How might you explain the observation that maldigestion of fat and protein does not usually begin until at least 90% of the exocrine function of the pancreas has been destroyed?
2. Provide a likely molecular basis for the close association between cystic fibrosis in children and chronic pancreatitis.
3. What factors might limit the effectiveness of pancreatic enzyme replacement therapy? Explain your answers.
4. An elevated serum lipase level is said to be a more specific indicator of pancreatic disease than an elevated serum amylase level. If so, how might you explain this?
5. Why does triglyceride in the stool suggest that steatorrhea experienced by a patient is related to pancreatic insufficiency rather than the absorptive capacity of the small intestine?

REFERENCES

Dimagnno EP: A short, eclectic history of exocrine pancreatic insufficiency and chronic pancreatitis. *Gastroenterology* **104**:1255–1262, 1993.

Greenberger NJ, Toskes PP, Isselbacher KJ: Acute and chronic pancreatitis, *in* Wilson JD, Braunwald E, Isselbacher KJ, et al. (eds): *Harrison's Principles of Internal Medicine*, 12th ed. New York, McGraw-Hill, 1991, pp 1372–1383.

Grendall JH, Cello JP: Chronic pancreatitis, *in* Sleisenger MH, Fordran JS (eds): *Gastrointestinal Disease*, 5th ed. Philadelphia WB Saunders, 1993, pp 1654–1681.

Habal F: The pancreas, *in* Thomson ABR, Shaffer EA (eds): *First Principles of Gastroenterology*. Mississauga, Ontario, Canada, Astra Pharma Inc., 1992, pp 338–371.

Lankish PG: Enzyme treatment of exocrine pancreatic insufficiency in chronic pancreatitis. *Digestion* **5** (Suppl 2):21–29, 1993.

Marino CR, Gorelick FS: Scientific advances in cystic fibrosis. *Gastroenterology* **103**:681–693, 1992.

Thiruvengadam R, Dimagnno EP: Inactivation of human lipase by proteases. *Am J Physiol* **255**:G476–G481, 1988.

22

Lead Poisoning

GINJI ENDO AND SHIGERU TAKETANI

CASE REPORT

The patient, a 66-year-old man, had been employed in a secondary lead smelter for 44 years. The geometric mean of air lead concentrations at 10 points at his work sites was 0.26 mg/m³.

He complained of headache but denied vomiting, abdominal pain, constipation, loss of appetite, irritability, fatigue, or loss of muscular coordination. Also, he did not show the objective symptoms of pallor, clouding of consciousness, or *tetraparesis* (paralysis of extensor muscles with atrophy).

Results of laboratory studies disclosed the following values: blood lead levels, 66.4 μg/dL (normal, <20 μg/dL); urinary lead, 114 μg/24 hours (normal, <80 μg/24 hours); urinary δ-aminolevulinic acid (ALA), 18.3 mg/24 hours (normal, 1–7 mg/24 hours); and protoporphyrin in blood, 583 μg/dL (normal, 15–100 μg/dL) of erythrocytes. Hemoglobin was 12.6 g/dL (normal, 13.5–17.6 g/dL). Small erythrocytes or basophilic stippling erythrocytes in the peripheral blood were not observed.

Kidney functions were as follows: urinary protein, trace (normal, <30 mg/dL); blood urea nitrogen, 25 mg/dL (normal, 8–20); serum uric acid, 5.9 mg/dL (normal, 3.6–7.6); serum creatinine, 1.1 mg/dL (normal, 0.7–1.3); urinary *N*-acetyl-β-ᴅ-glucosaminidase (NAG) activity 7.0 U/L (normal, <5.0); urinary β₂-microglobulin, 92 μg/L (normal, 20–600); urinary α₁-microglobulin 9.5 mg/L (normal, 0.5–6.0). Liver function tests and analysis of plasma lipids did not show abnormal values.

The worker showed subclinical stages of lead poi-soning. The effects on the central and peripheral nervous systems were not clear; however, the effects of lead poisoning on heme biosynthesis were clearly manifested. Hemoglobin levels were decreased below the lower limit of normal by exposure to lead. The renal proximal tubular damage caused by lead was evident in the increase of urinary NAG activity and the increase in α₁-microglobulin excretion.

The worker had been engaged in lead-smelting work for long periods under higher air lead concentrations than the 0.15 mg/m³ level, which is the threshold limit value (TLV) of lead exposure recommended by the American Conference of Governmental Industrial Hygienists (ACGIH) (1993). The most important treatment for such a worker is to decrease his lead exposure by improving the occupational environment and industrial process. Although the worker wore a protective mask for dust, the effect was not sufficient to protect him against lead inhalation. A personnel protection plan should also be implemented to reduce his lead exposure.

DIAGNOSIS

In cases in which children ingest chips of lead-based paint in large quantities, an acute encephalopathy can develop, often accompanied by renal failure and severe gastrointestinal symptoms within a short time. Subclinical lead intoxication is dangerous to children because its effects emerge without associated symptoms. In most occupational exposure cases, however, lead is absorbed more slowly, over weeks or months, and the clinical course is subacute or chronic. Absorbed lead is toxic or deleterious to the central nervous system, peripheral nervous system, heme biosynthetic pathway (Kappas et al., 1989), kidneys, reproductive system, and gastrointestinal system.

The measurement of air concentrations of lead in the workplace is useful in evaluating the lead exposure of workers. The ACGIH recommends 0.15 mg/m^3 for the TLV of lead. The TLVs represent conditions under which it is believed that nearly all workers may be repeatedly exposed day after day without incurring adverse health effects. Investigation of the environment for lead sources is also useful in the prevention of lead poisoning in children (Center for Disease Control, 1991). Blood lead levels found in many physical examinations and symptoms of lead poisoning are the most reliable standardized indices of current lead exposure (Keogh, 1992).

Lead Mobilization Test

Calcium disodium ethylenediaminetetraacetic acid (CaNa$_2$EDTA) forms chelate complexes with heavy metals. The outcome of the provocative chelation test is determined by the amount of lead excreted following administration of CaNa$_2$EDTA. A lead mobilization test is used for children with initial confirmatory blood lead levels of 25 to 44 μg/dL and for adults in whom nonspecific symptoms appear long after cessation of lead exposure. The patient empties the bladder, and CaNa$_2$EDTA is infused over one hour at a dosage of 500 mg/m^2 of body surface in 5% dextrose. An 8-hour CaNa$_2$EDTA mobilization test is considered positive if the lead excretion ratio (lead excretion for 8 hours (μg): CaNa$_2$EDTA (mg)) is >0.6.

Central Nervous System

The manifestations of lead neurotoxicity are highly age and dose dependent. Acute encephalopathy, characterized by diffuse pathogenic changes and cerebral edema, including lethargy, seizures, intermittent *stupor* (cloudiness of consciousness) with lucid intervals, and *ataxia* (a loss of the power of muscular coordination), is usually associated with abdomen and peripheral nervous system symptoms when blood lead levels exceed 150 μg/dL. The subencepalopathy is manifested by cognitive dysfunction,

memory loss, mood changes, and neural behavioral abnormalities, including headaches, sleep disturbance, irritability, anorexia, lassitude, weakness, and loss of libido. These symptoms are usually associated with prolonged elevation of lead levels above 80 to 100 μg/dL. Because of the nonspecific symptoms, patients are often not correctly diagnosed.

Children's nervous systems are more sensitive than those of adults. In the guidelines for management of childhood lead poisoning, the Center for Disease Control (CDC) have concluded that blood lead levels in excess of 10 μg/dL (0.481 μmol/L) are associated with increased risks of neurotoxicity. The signs of the neurotoxicity early in development, including prenatal development, are in memory and attention, including lower intelligence quotient (IQ) scores.

Peripheral Nervous System

Polyneuropathy from lead is more severe in motorial nerves than in sensory nerves. Lead targets motor axons and produces axonal degeneration and segmental demyelination. Demyelination of long nerves produces a prolonged nerve conduction time and subsequent paralysis of extensor muscles with atrophy (wrist drop or foot drop). Subclinical neuropathy, evidenced by a decrease in ulnar nerve motor conduction velocity, is occasionally seen at blood lead levels above 30 to 40 μg/dL.

Heme Synthesis and Hematological Effects

Anemia secondary to impaired heme synthesis is usually observed when blood lead levels exceed 80 μg/dL, and reduced hemoglobin production results when blood lead levels exceed 50 μg/dL (Moore et al., 1980). The presence of basophilic stippled erythrocytes is associated with severe anemia in cases with greater intoxication and iron deficiency. Pyrimidine 5'-nucleotidase (Py-5-N) inhibition by lead may be responsible for the basophilic stippling of erythrocytes. Increased urinary ALA and elevated coproporphyrins are observed in blood when lead levels exceed 40 μg/dL. Zinc protoporphyrin (ZPP) elevation is observed at blood lead levels greater than 20 μg/dL, and ZPP levels of 100 μg/dL of blood or 250 μg/dL of erythrocytes correspond to blood lead levels of 50 μg/dL. Decreases in ALA dehydratase and

Py-5-N activities are associated with blood lead levels above 10 to 15 μg/dL.

Renal Effects

The effects of lead on the renal proximal tubule have been observed with manifestations of the Fanconi syndrome, a constellation of transport defects in the proximal tubule, that results in excessive urinary excretion of amino acids, glucose, phosphate, uric acids, and proteins (Chia, 1994). Intranuclear inclusion bodies that contain high concentrations of lead are observed in the biopsy of renal tubular cells from exposed workers. NAG is a lysosomal enzyme that is rich in proximal tubular epithelial cells. α_1-Microglobulin is a low molecular weight glycoprotein which passes freely through the glomerulus, whereupon it is reabsorbed by proximal tubular cells. Increases of NAG activity and α_1-microglobulin in urine reflect proximal tubular damage or dysfunction and are occasionally seen when blood levels of lead exceed the 20 to 40 μg/dL range. Prolonged exposure to lead causes the irreversible pathological findings of diffuse interstitial or peritubular fibrosis in the proximal tubules. Chronic forms of end-stage renal disease and renal failure with gout or hypertension follow many years of excessive lead exposure.

Reproductive System

Lead is associated with increases in spontaneous abortion, stillbirth, and infant mortality. Because lead readily passes the placenta and accumulates in the fetus, a mother's lead burden can cause serious damage to the cognitive development of her child. Women aged less than 45 years should not engage in work that would entail lead exposure and should strive to keep their blood lead levels below 10 μg/dL. In males, a decrease in the sperm count and an increase of abnormal sperm occur with lead intoxication, but the blood lead levels at which reproductive damage occurs in males is not known.

Gastrointestinal Systems

Lead *colic* (severe abdominal pain) and sporadic vomiting are observed in acute intoxication with blood lead levels >100 μg/dL. Vomiting, diarrhea, constipation, loss of appetite, and *dysphoria* (a state of feeling unwell) of the epigastrium are also observed at lower levels of intoxication. Lead-blue lines in the gingival margin are deposits of lead sulfide that are made from lead dust by bacterial metabolism. Black stools are also due to lead sulfide and are observed in cases of heavy exposure to lead.

Other Organs

A defect in vitamin D synthesis is seen in children with blood lead levels as low as 12 μg/dL. Vitamin D synthesis in renal tubular cells is affected by lead because it interferes with a heme-containing hydroxylase enzyme that converts 25-hydroxyvitamin D_3 to 1,25-dihydroxyvitamin D_3.

Lead lines are also observed in roentgenograms as increased density by lead absorbance at the metaphyseal plate of growing long bones. These are generally seen in chronic cases in children associated with excess 50 μg/dl for a prolonged period.

MOLECULAR PERSPECTIVENESS

Lead exerts a variety of deleterious effects on intracellular biochemical pathways. Protein and nucleic acid synthesis are adversely affected and alterations of cellular ion transport and metabolism occur, resulting in a general reduction in cell division. These changes are nonspecific and of little value in monitoring human lead exposure. The effect of lead on the biosynthesis of heme is of particular interest, however, as physiologically significant and easily measurable changes occur at comparatively low lead levels (Moore et al., 1980). One of the most sensitive indicators of lead toxicity is the decreased activity of ALA dehydratase, the enzyme that catalyzes the second step of the heme biosynthetic pathway present in the cytosol of erythrocytes (Fig. 22-1). ALA dehydratase is a octamer that consists of eight identical subunits each one having a molecular mass of 36 kd. It is induced during erythroid differentiation. ALA dehydratase in mammalian erythrocytes and liver is maximally active *in vitro* in the presence of Zn and sulfhydryl compounds, such as 2-mercaptoethanol, cysteine, reduced glutathione, and dithithreitol. Catalytic activity is quickly lost when oxidation of its sulfhydryl groups takes place on exposure of the enzyme to oxygen or sulfhydryl inhibitors or by removal of Zn by chelation with EDTA. Lead displaces

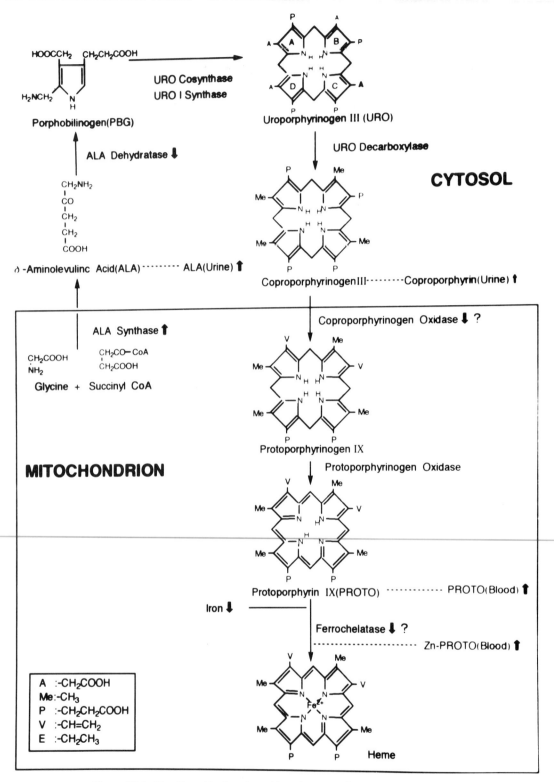

Figure 22-1. The effect of lead on heme biosynthesis. Details are covered in the text.

Zn from the enzyme, thereby inactivating it. Lead-inhibited ALA dehydratase can be reactivated *in vitro* by the addition of Zn or dithiothreitol, both of which decrease the binding of lead to the enzyme. Thus, the reversal of the lead inhibition of ALA dehydratase by zinc is a sensitive index of excess lead exposure.

Recently, cDNAs encoding human, rat, and mouse ALA dehydratases have been cloned, and cysteine and histidine residues at the Zn-binding site in the catalytic center of the protein were revealed. The genes for human and mouse ALA dehydratase have also been identified. The structural analysis of the gene for mouse ALA dehydratase revealed that the gene in AKR and DAB/2 mice was amplified, a finding consistent with the observations that the activity of ALA dehydratase in inbred mouse strains AKR and DAB/2, which are resistant to lead poisoning, is high compared with those in any other mice strains. These findings indicate that the gene dosages among mouse strains are correlated with ALA dehydratase activity and imply that the amount of the transcript of ALA dehydratase in mouse can be a critical factor in lead toxicity.

Inhibition of ALA dehydratase by lead results in excess urinary excretion of ALA with little or no increase in porphobilinogen, a product of the ALA dehydratase reaction (Fig. 22-1). The increase in urinary ALA is preceded by an increase in ALA in the blood. In addition to ALA dehydratase inhibition by lead, an increase in the activity of ALA synthase, the first enzyme in the heme biosynthetic pathway, also results in the excess excretion of ALA. An elevation of the activity of ALA synthase, the rate-limiting enzyme in the pathway of heme biosynthesis, in lead intoxication is considered one of the signs of the depression of heme synthesis because ALA synthase is subject to negative feedback regulation by the pathway's end-product, heme. Two distinct isoforms of human ALA synthase were recently identified, one a nonerythroid-type enzyme with a molecular mass of 66 kd, and the other erythroid tissue-specific with a mass of 58 kd. Both enzymes share highly conserved amino acid sequences, implying that they have the same catalytic site and follow the same mechanism. The expression of nonerythroid-type ALA synthase is inhibited by heme at both the transcriptional and posttranscriptional level; however, heme does not regulate the expression of erythroid-specific enzyme. Therefore, the activity of ALA synthase in erythropoietic cells does not change in lead poisoning; nor does

its activity appear to be correlated with the extent of increase in urinary ALA.

Lead exposure is a well-known cause of elevated levels of urinary coproporphyrin and red cell Zn-protoporphyrin, and these metabolites are often used to monitor occupational lead exposure. The urine porphyrin present when there is lead exposure was identified as coproporphyrin III. Until routine atomic absorption methods became available for the analysis of blood and urine lead, urine porphyrin analysis was widely used for many years to monitor industrial lead exposure. Excess coproporphyrin excretion is a less sensitive indicator of lead poisoning than are the other effects of lead on the heme pathway. Increased urine coproporphyrin III excretion is thought to be the result of direct inhibition of coproporphyrinogen oxidase by lead (Fig. 22-1). In considering the mechanism responsible for the elevated urine coproporphyrin level, the preferential accumulation of lead in the kidneys may be important. In experimental animals exposed to lead for long periods, kidney mitochondrial enzymes such as malate dehydrogenase and glutamate dehydrogenase were inhibited, whereas the same enzymes in liver mitochondria were not affected. Therefore, the increased urine coproporphyrin level in lead exposure may result from a localized decrease of coproporphyrinogen oxidase in the kidneys. Furthermore, lead may affect the intracellular transport of porphyrins. Coproporphyrinogen oxidase is located in the intermembrane space of the mitochondria, whereas its substrate, coproporphyrinogen, is produced in the cytosol by uroporphyrinogen decarboxylase. The mechanism by which coproporphyrinogen is moved from the cytosol and then through the outer membrane of mitochondria is unknown. The mitochondrial outer membrane is freely permeable to compounds with molecular weights as high as 2000 to 3000. When coproporphyrinogen reaches the inside of the outer membrane of a mitochondrion, coproporphyrinogen oxidase may transport it to the inner membrane, where the penultimate enzyme of the heme biosynthetic pathway, protoporphyrinogen oxidase, is located. If lead did interfere with the transport of coproporphyrinogen from the cytosol to either the outer membrane or to the inner membrane, the excess substrate could be the source of the increased urine coproporphyrinogen. The mechanism responsible for the elevation of urinary coproporphyrin is unclear.

Increased erythrocyte protoporphyrin resulting from industrial lead exposure was first described in 1946, when blood levels of lead 12 times the upper limit of the reference range were observed in lead-smelter workers. It was hypothesized at that time that lead might interfere with the utilization of iron in the synthesis of hemoglobin. Once the discovery was made that ferrochelatase is an iron-chelating enzyme that catalyzes the insertion of ferrous ion into proto-porphyrin, inhibition of the enzyme's activity by lead *in vitro* was shown soon thereafter. Subsequent investigations have confirmed that the elevation of red cell protoporphyrin by lead poisoning is the direct result of the inhibition of ferrochelatase (Taketani, 1994). As methods to measure porphyrins were developed, it was discovered that it is Zn-protoporphyrin, rather than free protoporphyrin, that accumulates in the red cells of lead-intoxicated individuals. Specifically, Zn-protoporphyrin is converted into free protoporphyrin by the acid treatment used in the clinical laboratory to extract porphyrins from tissues.

Recent studies demonstrated that ferrochelatase exhibits both zinc- and iron-chelating activities. The affinity of ferrochelatase for zinc ions is somewhat higher than for ferrous ions, and zinc ions are used when ferrous ions are not available. Thus, the critical factor in Zn-protoporphyrin accumulation is the lack of available ferrous ions rather than the direct inhibition of ferrochelatase by lead. The effects of lead on iron transport may be more important than the inhibition of ferrochelatase by lead. Lead actually inhibits the uptake of iron from plasma transferrin by reticulocytes. Furthermore, because ferrochelatase utilizes ferrous ions but not ferric ions as substrate, the reduction of ferric ions is an essential step of heme biosynthesis. The reduction of ferric ion must occur near the active site of ferrochelatase because ferrous ions thus formed are quite unstable and reoxidize rapidly to the ferric state. The mitochondrial NADH oxidation system, which corresponds to Complex I of the respiratory chain, is involved in the reduction of ferric ions and is sensitive to inhibition by lead. Several mitochondrial enzymes, including those that are elements of the respiratory chain and oxidative phosphorylation apparatus, are also inhibited by lead. Accordingly, such inhibitions could result in an insufficient supply of ferrous ions to ferrochelatase. In addition, lead directly impairs a number of membrane-associated

biochemical functions by upsetting the structural integrity of organelles such as mitochondria. The location of ferrochelatase in the inner membrane may render this enzyme especially vulnerable to mitochondrial membrane damage. Alternatively, if membrane permeability is changed and the concentration of zinc ions in mitochondria is increased by lead, zinc may readily reach the active site of ferrochelatase, whereupon Zn-protoporphyrin formation occurs. Although these hypotheses can explain the effects of lead on heme biosynthesis, the biochemical basis for many other manifestations of lead poisoning remains obscure.

Lead causes metabolic abnormalities unrelated to the heme biosynthetic pathway. *Plumbism* (chronic lead poisoning) is associated with an acquired deficiency of pyrimidine-specific 5'-nucleotidase in red blood cells. A hereditary form of this enzyme deficiency, like lead intoxication, leads to hemolysis and basophilic stippling of erythrocytes. In both instances, the enzyme deficiency impairs dephosphorylation of pyrimidine 5'-nucleoside monophosphates to soluble products that can diffuse from red cells. Pyrimidine nucleotides then accumulate and block RNA degradation, thereby giving rise to the appearance of basophilic stippling (the appearance of spots) in erythrocytes.

The ultimate effect of lead on a red blood cell is to disrupt the plasma membrane of the cell. The normal life span of erythrocytes is about 120 days. In cases of hemolytic anemia, the the mean life span of the cells is reduced. This shortening of the red cell life span is thought to result from the direct toxic effects of lead on the plasma membrane of the cell. Lead inhibits (Na^+, K^+)ATPase activity in erythrocytes. Incubation of erythrocytes *in vitro* with high concentrations of lead (80–150 µg/dL) causes leakage of large quantities of potassium ions. This loss of K^+ is irreversible and is the result of lead's interference with this energy-requiring ion pump. At the same time, because there is little change in the influx of sodium ions into the cells, the concentration of sodium ions in lead-poisoned erythrocytes is increased. Ultimately, this results in cell shrinkage. The loss of potassium ions increases the mechanical fragility of the red blood cells and causes them to lyse.

As explained, the kidneys are especially vulnerable to lead poisoning because they readily accumulate lead. The earliest pathological evidence of lead exposure in kidneys is the appearance of intracellular inclusion bodies and alterations in mitochondrial morphology. The appearance of the inclusion bodies is most common in the lining cells of the proximal tubules. The eosinophilic electron-dense bodies are composed mostly of a sulfhydryl-rich lead: protein complex. These complexes appear after a brief exposure to lead and before any overt alteration of kidney function. The inclusion bodies are thought to serve a temporary protective storage function in that the lead is complexed in a nondiffusible form, thereby reducing the amount of free lead available to disrupt essential cell functions. Two lead-binding proteins with molecular masses of 11.5 kd and 63 kd are present in the cytosol of rat kidneys. The induction of a novel 32-kd protein in lead-exposed renal epithelial cells was recently demonstrated. These proteins may be involved in the formation of the inclusion bodies one sees in kidneys in lead intoxication. Lead can also induce the production of renal metallothionein, a zinc- and cadmium-binding protein. The induction of metallothionine by metals probably serves to detoxify the latter. Nonetheless, the extent of metallothionein induction by lead in kidney is less than that achieved with other metals such as zinc and cadmium.

Lead poisoning can result in permanent brain damage, and high-level lead exposure during childhood can cause various neurological problems and sometimes even irreversible mental retardation. Exposure to subclinical levels of lead produces intelligence deficits, poor academic achievement, hyperactivity, and deficient fine motor control as well as short stature and decreased weight. The symptoms of acute encephalopathy, a syndrome of severe neurological symptoms that may culminate in coma and death, usually appear over several days and are seen when the blood level of lead exceeds 60 μg/dL. These neurological abnormalities produced by lead are related to the ability of the metal to either inhibit or mimic the action of calcium.

Low lead levels enhance the spontaneous or basal release of neurotransmitters from presynaptic nerve endings. Lead-induced release of neurotransmitters also occurs in the central nervous system (Silbergeld, 1992). *In vitro* incubation of synaptosomes prepared from rat brain with micromolar concentrations of lead increases the spontaneous release of dopamine, acetylcholine, and γ-aminobutyric acid, concomitant with an increase in the efflux of cal-

cium. The enhanced calcium efflux is explained by stimulation of a plasma membrane efflux pump or the mobilization of intracellular calcium. Lead also inhibits evoked releases of neurotransmitters in the central nervous system. The evoked release of neurotransmitters, including dopamine and acetylcholine, requires the presence of extracellular calcium, and lead competitively blocks the voltage-sensitive calcium channel. Thus, if lead increases basal release of neurotransmitters and decreases the response of activated circuits, the precision of the relationship between stimuli and neural activity will be disrupted. Lead also impairs calcium action in nonexcitable tissues. Lead-induced accumulation of calcium has been observed in various cultured cells, such as rat brain microvessels, arterial smooth muscles, rat hepatocytes, and mouse bone cells.

Protein kinases, in respose to specific stimuli, phosphorylate proteins and thus alter the properties of these proteins to produce the physiological responses characteristic of the stimulating agents (Hemning et al., 1989). One family of protein kinases is activated by the calcium:calmodulin complex. Calmodulin is a calcium-binding protein. A member of this protein kinase family, namely, calmodulin-dependent protein kinase II, is highly enriched in neural tissues and may play a key role in the release of neurotransmitters (Fig. 22-2). Calmodulin has a higher affinity for lead than for calcium. Lead can substitute for calcium in at least the calmodulin-dependent process, thus activating a calmodulin-dependent phosphodiesterase, which promotes potassium ion loss from the cells. The ability of lead to interact with calmodulin and other calcium-binding proteins may be related to the similarity of the hydrated radii of these two divalent cations.

Protein kinase C, a calcium- and phospholipid-dependent enzyme associated with signal transduction, phsophorylates critical regulatory proteins that modulate of a number of cellular events, for example, cellular proliferation and differentiation (Hemning et al., 1989). In the nervous system, protein kinase C is involved in long-term potentiation in that activators of the enzyme enhance this process and inhibitors of the kinase block it. Because long-term potentiation is linked to memory storage, a disturbance may be reflected in learning and behavioral deficits in lead-poisoned children. Lead does activate protein kinase C, causing the translocation of this

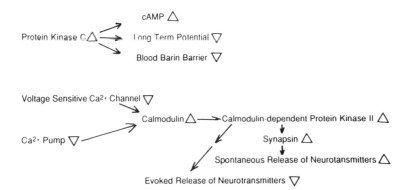

Figure 22-2. Two major linkages of lead neurotoxicity. △:Stimulation; ▽:Blockage.

enzyme from the cytosol to the membrane in intact microvascular cells (Markovac and Goldstein, 1988). The activation potency of lead is much greater than that of calcium. Thus, lead mimics calcium in the activation of protein kinase C. Lead also affects another second messenger, cyclic AMP, by altering postsynaptic catechoamine action and inhibiting *adenylate cyclase,* the enzyme that catalyzes the formation of cyclic AMP. Because protein kinase C phosphorylates the catalytic subunit of adenylate cyclase, lead, by activating protein kinase C, can influence other second-messenger systems.

Brain capillary endothelial cells are responsible for formation of the blood brain-barrier and are major sites of lead accumulation (Goldstein, 1988). Pathologic studies in children poisoned with lead have revealed a breakdown in the normally tight blood–brain barrier. The formation of the blood–brain barrier is the result of the special structure of brain microvessels made up of endothelial cells lacking fenestrae and transcellular channels. Certain ions, organic acids, and neuroactive amino acids are pumped from the brain across the endothelium into the blood. This permeability barrier differs from those in the other microvascular beds where ions and small organic molecules readily diffuse into tissue spaces and albumin traffics across the endothelium to be removed by lymphatic circulation. Exposure to lead (>4 μM) disrupts the blood–brain barrier as a result of a functional change in the state of the endothelium rather than as a result of cell necrosis.

The signals that initiate and maintain the function and integrity of the blood–brain barrier by endothelial cells appear to originate in astrocytes. Astrocytes are particularly vulnerable to the toxic effects of lead. Furthermore, immature astrocytes are more susceptible to lead than are the mature cells. The lead-induced abnormality in astrocytes plays a role in the loss of the special barrier properties normally possessed by brain endothelial cells. The development of resistance to lead encephalopathy in adult rats is associated with the removal of lead by mature astrocytes and its diversion of lead away from mitochondria to less vulnerable sites. Mitochondria, the sites of heme biosynthesis, oxidative phosphorylation, and intracellular calcium transport, are therefore a critical subcellular target in lead neurotoxicity, so the ability to protect these sites is important for maintaining the functional integrity of mature astroyctes.

It is thought that lead directly affects intracellular second-messenger activity in endothelial cells. Protein kinase C may function in the differentiation of brain endothelial cells and its marked sensitivity to inhibition by lead points to this enzyme as a potential target of lead toxicity. Based on the finding that exposure of microvessels prepared from the brains of immature rats to lead results in translocation of protein kinase C from the cytosol to the membrane, the activation of protein kinase C may be mediated by lead's ability to mimic or mobilize calcium. The sequence of proliferation and differentiation of brain endothelial cells may be disrupted; these events could explain, in part, the defects in barrier function that occurs in acute lead encephalopathy.

THERAPY

The CDC (1991) provides guidelines for the prevention of lead poisoning in children. If a large number of children in a community have blood lead levels ≥10 μg/dL, community-wide interventions should be considered by the appropriate agencies. To be successful, community-level intervention must involve at least five types of activities: (1) screening and surveillance; (2) risk assessment and integrated prevention planning; (3) outreach and education; (4) infrastructure development; and (5) hazard reduction.

Management of lead hazards in the environment of an individual child should begin at a blood lead level of 15 μg/dL. Environmental case management includes: (1) educating parents about the sources, effects, and prevention of lead poisoning; (2) investigating the environment to identify lead sources and effectively communicating the results of this investigation; (3) taking immediate measures to reduce lead exposure; (4) enacting long-term intervention to reduce lead exposure; and (5) evaluating the efficacy of the intervention.

Children with blood lead levels ≥20 μg/dL need to undergo a complete medical evaluation, whether or not symptoms are present. Special attention should be given to a detailed history that includes clinical symptoms, the child's activity level, the existence of *pica* (the ingestion of nonfood substances), and the child's nutritional status. A child should be given a neurological examination, a psychosocial and language development examination, a lead mobilization test, evaluation of iron status, and other special diagnostic tests; however, there is no consensus regarding the medical management of children with blood lead levels <45 μg/dL.

Asymptomatic children with blood lead levels ≥45 μg/dL should receive chelation therapy with CaNa$_2$EDTA, which must be diluted to a concentration of <0.5% either in dextrose and water or in 0.9% saline solution. A dosage of 1,000 mg/m^2/day can be given intravenously by continuous infusion or in two divided doses a day over 30 to 60 minutes. Individual courses should be limited to 5 days, and repeated courses should be given at a minimum of 2- to 5-day intervals. During treatment, evaluations of renal and hepatic function and determination of serum electrolyte levels should be done regularly.

Symptomatic children with blood lead levels ≥45 μg/dL or asymptomatic children with blood lead levels ≥70 μg/dL represent an acute medical emergency. The children are given both 2,3-dimercapto-1-propanol (British antilewisite BAL, a chelator) and CaNa$_2$EDTA. The treatment is begun with a dose of 75 mg/m^2 of BAL given by deep intramuscular injection; BAL should be administered only at a daily dosage of 450 mg/m^2 in divided doses of 75 mg/m^2 every hour.

In the case of workers, environmental assessment should be done for all work sites to measure the lead content of dust and fumes. Action levels may be one tenth of the 0.15 mg/m^3 of the TLV recommended by the ACGIH and should call for environmental interventions and a medical evaluation of workers. The most important action is immediate improvement of the work environment and the industrial process. A local exhaust apparatus is important to decrease lead dust or fumes. Air pollution should be prevented by filtration of dust collectors. Rest rooms should be equipped with mats to remove mud from shoes, a brush to remove mud from work clothes, and washbowls or showers and gargling equipment. Smoking, drinking and eating should be prohibited in the work place. Dust-guard masks should be worn in lead-polluted working places.

Adults with mild to moderate symptoms and with blood lead levels of >50 μg/dL should be given a daily dosage of CaNa$_2$-EDTA 1000 mg/m^2/day for 5 days, each dose being divided into two or three injections by the intramuscular or intravascular route. A second course is based on blood lead response. A drug-free interval of 2 to 3 weeks should precede a repeat course.

When there is severe lead encephalopathy, or when blood lead levels exceed 100 μg/dL, adults should be administered both BAL and CaNa$_2$EDTA. BAL, 300 mg/m^2, is given daily in a dose every 4 hours by the route of intramuscular administration. CaNa$_2$-EDTA, 1500 mg/m^2, is administered daily every 4 hours by the intravascular administration. Both drugs are given for 5 days. If blood lead and clinical conditions respond to therapy, BAL can be eliminated in 2 or 3 days. The dosage of CaNa$_2$-EDTA for adults should not exceed 2000 mg/daily.

Women aged under 45 years should be banned from lead-handling work. A blood lead level of 10 μg/dL is also of concern in pregnant women because of exposure of the fetus to lead.

QUESTIONS

1. Lead poisoning of children is more severe than that of adults. What are the reasons why a child would be more sensitive to the neurotoxic effects of lead?

2. What enzyme in the heme biosynthetic pathway is the most sensitive indicator of lead poisoning? What is the mechanism of lead toxicity in the erythrocyte?

3. Where is coproporphyrinogen oxidase located? How is the enzyme related to the increase of urinary coproporphrin in lead poisoning?

4. Zn-protoporphyrin in erythrocytes is a useful marker of lead poisoning. What mechanisms are involved in the accumulation of Zn-protoporphyrin by lead?

5. Which has a higher affinity for ferrocheratase, zinc ion or ferrous ion, and what is the pathophysiologic significance of this difference of affinities?

REFERENCES

American Conference of Governmental Industrial Hygienists. *Documentation of the threshold limit values and biological exposure indices,* 6th ed. Cincinnati, Ohio, ACGIH, 1993, pp 847–851, BEI-99-104.

Center for Disease Control: *Preventing Lead Poisoning in Young Children.* Atlanta, Georgia, U.S. Department of Health and Human Services/Public Health Service, Center for Disease Control, 1991.

Chia KS: Subclinical nephrotoxicity of inorganic lead: a review. *J Occup Med Singapore* **64:**41–49, 1994.

Goldstein GW: Endothelial cell-astrocyte interactions, a cellular model for the blood–brain barrier, *Ann NY Acad Sci* **529:**31 39, 1988.

Hemning HC, Narin AC, McGinness TL, Huganir RL, Greengard P: Role of protein phosphorylation in neural signal transduction. *FASEB J* **3:**1583–1592, 1989.

Kappas A, Sassa S, Galbraith RA, Nordmann Y: The porphyrias, *in* Scriver CR, Beaudet AL, Sly WS, Valle D (eds): *The Metabolic Basis of Inherited Disease.* New York, McGraw-Hill, 1989, pp 1305–1365.

Keogh JP: Lead, *in* Sullivan JB, Krieger GR (eds.) *Hazardous Materials Toxicology, Clinical Principles of Environmental Health,* Baltimore, Williams & Wilkins, 1992, pp 834–844.

Markovac J, Goldstein GW: Picomolar concentrations of lead stimulate brain protein kinase C. *Nature* **334:**71–73, 1988.

Moore MR, Meredith PA, Goldberg A. Lead and heme biosynthesis, *in* Singhal RL, Thomas JA (eds): *Lead Toxicity.* Baltimore, Urban & Schwarzenberg Inc., 1980, pp 79–118.

Silbergeld EK: Mechanisms of lead neurotoxicity, or looking beyond the lamppost. *FASEB J* **6:** 3201–3206, 1992.

Taketani S: Molecular and genetic characterization of ferrochelatase. *in* Fujita H (ed): *Regulation of Hemeprotein Synthesis,* Dayton, AlphaMed Press, 1994, pp 41–54.

23

Peroxisomal Disorders: Zellweger Syndrome and Adrenoleukodystrophy

YASUYUKI SUZUKI AND TADAO ORII

CASE REPORT

Patient 1

A female child with Zellweger syndrome was born to nonconsanguineous parents at 38 weeks' gestation. She weighed 2652 g and her Apgar score was 7 at 1 min after birth. There was no family history of early infant death or of spontaneous abortion. Soon after delivery, she was admitted to the hospital for severe *hypotonia* (reduced tension of muscles), feeding difficulty, and convulsions.

Physical examinations revealed characteristic facial *dysmorphism* (anatomical malformation), including a large fontanelle (5 × 5 cm), frontal *bossing* (swelling), shallow supraorbital ridges, *hypertelorism* (excessive width between the eyes), a low nasal bridge, and a high arched palate. *Hepatomegaly* (enlarged liver) (4 cm below the ribs), jaundice, and palmar simian crease were also identified. Neurologically, she was virtually immobile, with arms and legs abducted (Fig. 23-1A). Absence of Moro, sucking and deep tendon reflexes, horizontal *nystagmus* (rapid oscillation of the eyeballs), and convulsions refractory to treatment with anticonvulsants were observed.

The following were the results of routine laboratory tests at age 5 months (normal range): white blood cell count, 9800/mm³ (6000–12,000); hemoglobin, 9.4 g/dL (9.0–14.0); platelet count, 228,000/mm³ (131,000–362,000); total protein, 5.7 g/dL (6.0–8.0); total bilirubin, 1.9 mg/dL (0.3–1.0); direct bilirubin, 1.2 mg/dL (0.0–0.3); serum glutamate:oxaloacetate transaminase (sGOT), 904 IU/L (7–35); serum glutamate:pyruvate transaminase (sGPT), 233 IU/L (7–30); lactate dehydrogenase (LDH) 625, IU/L (160–420); thrombotest (measurement of coagulation factors II, VII, and X), 21% (>70%); creatine kinase, 32 IU/L (40–200); myelin basic protein, 1.3 ng/mL (<4); neuron-specific enolase, 13 ng/mL (<10). Roentgenography of the patella revealed the presence of calcific stippling (Fig. 23-1B). T_2-weighted cranial magnetic resonance imaging (MRI) revealed enlargement of posterior horns of lateral ventricles. The electroencephalogram showed a 5 to 6 Hz slow-wave burst and multifocal spikes. Auditory brainstem-evoked potentials showed no response.

The very long chain fatty acid (VLCFA) composition of serum sphingomyelin of the patient revealed a marked increase of tetracosanoic acid (C24:0), pentacosanoic acid (C25:0), and hexacosanoic acid (C26:0) (Fig. 23-2, Table 23-1). The rate of C24:0 oxidation and the level of dihydroxyacetone phosphate (DHAP) acyltransferase activity in cultured skin fibroblasts from the patient were severely decreased (Table 23-1). Electron microscopic examination of the liver biopsy (Fig. 23-3) and immunofluorescence staining of fibroblasts (Fig. 23-4) revealed the absence of peroxisomes. These findings led to the diagnosis of Zellweger syndrome.

Psychomotor development was severely retarded.

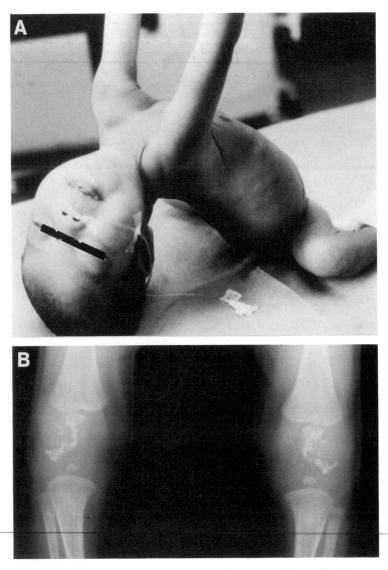

Figure 23-1. Severe hypotonia, typical facial appearance **(A)**, and calcific stippling of the patella **(B)** in patient 1 with Zellweger syndrome.

The patient acquired neither social smile nor head control. Hepatic dysfunction and respiratory insufficiency progressed, and the patient died at the age of 5 months. The major autopsy findings were *polymicrogyria* (abnormal smallness of the brain's convolutions) of the brain, neuronal *heterotopia* (abnormal location), poor myelination in the white matter, hepatic fibrosis, and renal cortical microcysts.

Patient 2

The patient with X-linked adrenoleukodystrophy (ALD), a 10-year-old boy, was the first-born child of unrelated healthy parents. He had an uncle with adrenomyeloneuropathy manifesting spastic *paraparesis* (partial paralysis of the lower limbs). The patient developed normally until age 7 years 5 months, when he became inattentive and did not

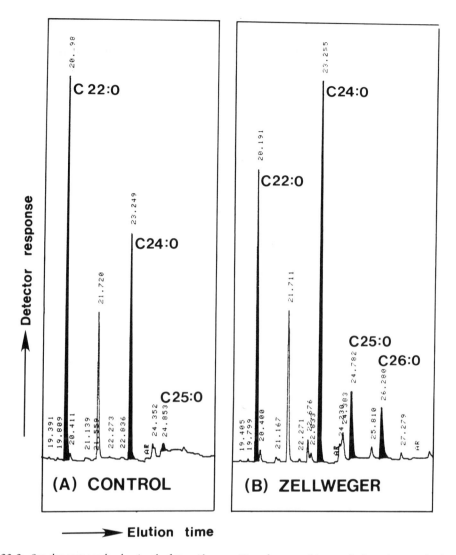

Figure 23-2. Gas chromatography showing the fatty acid composition of serum sphingomyelin from the control subject **(A)** and from the Zellweger patient 1 **(B)**. Note the prominent peaks of C24:0, C25:0, and C26:0 in B. Numbers on the peaks indicate elution time in minutes.

Table 23-1. Results of Biochemical Studies

	VLCFA in sphingomyelin			C24:0	
Subject	C24/C22	C25/C22	C26/C22	Oxidation[a]	DHAP-AT[b]
Patient 1	2.700	0.244	0.276	24	0.11
Patient 2	1.341	0.053	0.038	116	1.19
Control	<0.844	<0.024	<0.012	432 ± 112	1.64 ± 0.56
	(n = 155)			(n = 24)	(n = 10)

VLCFA, very long-chain fatty acids; DHAP-AT, dihydroxyacetone phosphate acyltransferase activity.

[a] pmol/h/mg protein.

[b] nmol/h/mg protein.

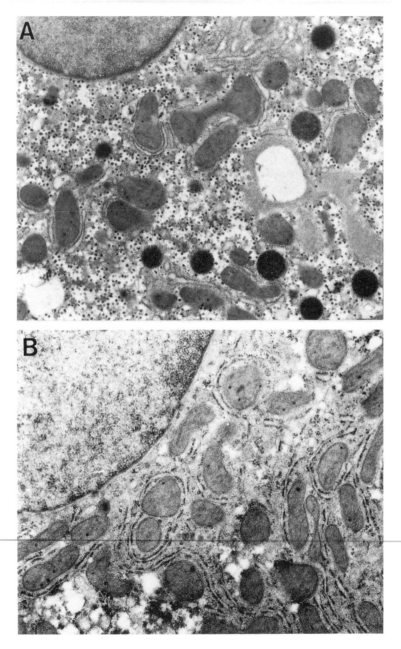

Figure 23-3. Electron micrograph of liver biopsy from the control subject (**A**) and patient 1 (**B**). Peroxisomes are darkly stained with 3,3′-diaminobenzidine tetrachloride. Peroxisomes are absent in patient 1.

respond to his mother's voice. He began to stumble easily 2 months later.

At the age of 7 years 8 months, when he came to the hospital, his gait was *ataxic* (uncoordinated movements). Deep-tendon reflexes and muscle tonus were increased. Babinsky reflex was negative but toe *clonus* (convulsive spasms) was positive. He was

dull of apprehension. Visual acuity was normal, but visual field could not be tested. Other physical findings, including cranial and autonomic nerve function, sensation of skin, muscle power, and fundoscopic examination, were normal.

The following were the results of laboratory tests (normal range): white blood cell count, 4600/mm³

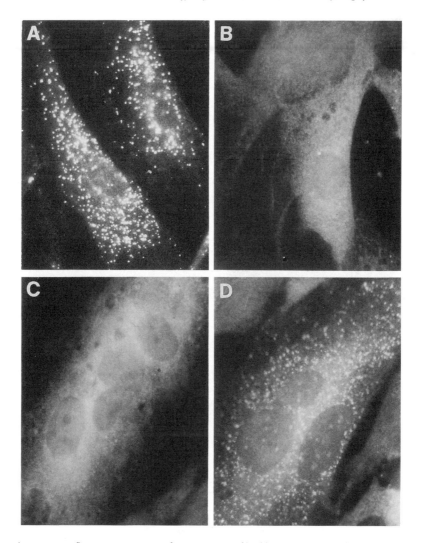

Figure 23-4. Indirect immunofluorescence staining of peroxisomes in fibroblasts using anti-catalase immunoglobulin G. Numerous granules (peroxisomes) are visible in the control (**A**). The cytosol is diffusely stained and peroxisomes are absent in patient 1 (**B**). Uncomplemented fused cells have no peroxisomes (**C**), whereas complemented fused cells have peroxisomes in abundance.

(3900–9800); hemoglobin, 12.7 g/dL (13.5–17.6); platelet count, 227,000/mm³ (131,000–362,000); total protein, 6.9 g/dL (6.0–8.0); sGOT, 37 IU/L (7–35); sGPT, 62 IU/L (7–30); LDH, 482 IU/L (160–420); creatine kinase, 176 IU/L (40–200); lactic acid, 12.0 mg/dL (4–16); pyruvic acid, 1.1 mg/dL (0.3–0.9); immunoglobulin G (IgG), 1057 mg/dL (680–1620); IgA, 101 mg/dL (84–438); IgM, 95 mg/dL (57–288); myelin basic protein, 1.8 ng/mL (<4); neuron-specific enolase, 10 ng/mL (<10). Cerebrospinal fluid examination and adrenocortical function were normal.

T_2-weighted cranial MRI revealed high intensity areas in the bilateral parieto-occipital white matter (Fig. 23-5). Electroencephalography showed slow waves in both occipital areas. Sensory-evoked potentials, auditory brainstem-evoked potentials, and motor nerve conduction velocities were normal.

The VLCFA content of the serum sphingomyelin of the patient, the mother and the uncle were high (Table 23-1). The rate of C24:0 oxidation by cultured skin fibroblasts from the patient was decreased. Mutation analysis of the ALD protein gene revealed the presence of an exonic nonsense muta-

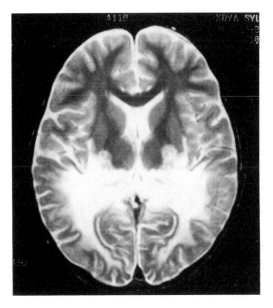

Figure 23-5. T_2-weighted cranial magnetic resonance imaging image of patient 2. Note the marked high intensity areas in the bilateral parieto-occipital white matter.

tion in the patient and the uncle. The mother, sister, and grandmother were carriers of this mutation. These findings supported the clinical diagnosis of X-linked ALD.

Following the diagnosis of X-linked ALD, treatment started with intravenous administration of immunoglobulin, restriction of dietary VLCFA, and oral administration of Lorenzo's oil consisting of 4 vol of glyceryl trioleate (C18:1) and 1 vol of glyceryl trierucate (C22:1). For the first several months, his motor ability was stable, and he could walk with support. Blood VLCFA levels decreased to the normal range; however, neurologic deterioration progressed thereafter. He became bedridden and blind at 8 years 6 months, difficulty in swallowing appeared, and response to the mother disappeared. He entered a decerebrated state at 10 years. During the administration of Lorenzo's oil, the platelet count decreased transiently (47,000/mm^3).

DIAGNOSIS

Zellweger Syndrome

Zellweger syndrome (Bowen et al., 1964) is the most severe phenotype of peroxisome-deficient disorders, and the diagnosis is made on the basis of characteristic clinical findings, multiple metabolic

dysfunctions, and an absence of peroxisomes. Differences between Zellweger syndrome and other milder forms of peroxisome-deficient disorders, such as neonatal adrenoleukodystrophy and infantile Refsum disease, are not clear-cut. Clinical classification does not correlate with genetic grouping, as described in the Molecular Perspectives section.

Severe hypotonia soon after birth (*floppy infant*) is the most prominent manifestation of Zellweger syndrome. Spontaneous movements are lacking and feeding difficulty occurs. Typical craniofacial dysmorphism, including a large anterior fontanel, high forehead, hypertelorism, *epicanthus* (a fold of skin extending from the root of the nose to the inner termination of the eyebrow), shallow supraorbital ridges, broad nasal bridge, low-set ears, high arched palate, and *micrognathia* (abnormally small jaws), is present. Neurologically, an absence of deep-tendon reflex, convulsions resistant to anticonvulsants, horizontal nystagmus, and severe psychomotor retardation are observed. Hepatomegaly and hepatic dysfunction gradually become obvious. Manifestations of renal involvement are not prominent, although renal cortical microcysts are characteristic pathological findings. Other clinical findings include calcific stippling in the patella (Fig. 23-1B), congenital heart disease, *pes equinovarus* (inversion and extension of the foot), undescended testis, and simian crease. The mode of inheritance is autosomal recessive. Most Zellweger patients die during early infancy.

Biochemical screening of Zellweger syndrome is usually made by gas chromatographic analysis of VLCFA. Accumulation of C24:0, C25:0, and C26:0 is prominent in tissues and body fluids such as brain, fibroblasts, and plasma (Fig. 23-2, Table 23-1). Other metabolic disturbances, including deficiency of plasmalogen and accumulation of intermediates of bile acid synthesis, phytanic acid, and pipecolic acid, are detected.

A defect of peroxisomes is identified in various tissues by means of electron microscopic examination (Fig. 23-3) and immunofluorescence staining of cultured fibroblasts with the use of anti-catalase IgG (Fig. 23-4). Biochemical assay of calatase latency in fibroblasts by means of digitonin titration is also useful.

Adrenoleukodystrophy

The diagnosis of X-linked ALD is based on the characteristic clinical course, the neuroradiological findings of leukodystrophy, and the accumulation of saturated VLCFA in various tissues and body fluids (e.g., serum) (Igarashi et al., 1976). The patients are male, and the defective gene is inherited by female carriers.

The phenotypes of X-linked ALD show diversity (Moser et al., 1995). The most common phenotype is childhood ALD, manifested usually at 4 to 8 years, whereupon the patient enters a vegetative state within a few years. Early symptoms of childhood ALD are often mistaken for minimal brain dysfunction, emotional disturbances, or subacute sclerosing panencephalitis. Patient 2 showed a typical clinical course of childhood ALD. In adolescent ALD, onset is between age 11 and 21 years, and the symptoms and progression are similar to those of childhood ALD. *Adrenomyeloneuropathy* in an adult-onset subtype characterized by spastic paraparesis, sphincter disturbances, and slow progressive decline over decades. Other subtypes, including adult cerebral form, cerebellar and brainstem dominant form, and Addison disease are known. Adrenocortical function studies are necessary for the detection of subclinical adrenocortical insufficiency. Patients with different phenotypes may be present within a kindred. The female carriers usually have no clinical symptoms.

Neuroradiological examinations are useful tools for the detection of leukodystrophy. The T_2-weighted MRI image shows a strikingly high-intensity signal in the parieto-occipital white matter, even in a relatively early stage of illness (Fig. 23-5). The computed tomography (CT) scan shows bilateral hypodensity in this region. Contrast-enhanced CT will reveal an enhancing peripheral zone of the hypodensity area that reflects the pathological changes. The brainstem auditory evoked responses, somatosensory responses, electroencephalogram, and conduction velocities in peripheral nerves are also informative.

Biochemical diagnosis of X-linked ALD is routinely made by gas chromatographic analysis of saturated VLCFA. Recently, the ALD gene was identified, as described in the section entitled Molecular Perspectives.

MOLECULAR PERSPECTIVES

Zellweger Syndrome

In the 1970s, biochemical abnormalities, such as elevated serum iron and pipecolic acid levels and defects in bile acid synthesis, were reported in patients with Zellweger syndrome. At that time, these metabolic disturbances were not considered to be caused by the peroxisomal defects. The absence of peroxisomes was identified in 1973.

The peroxisome, first identified in 1954 and named by DeDuve and Baudhuin, is a round or oval-shaped organelle bound by a single membrane. Peroxisomes are present in almost all eukaryotic cells. In humans, hepatocytes and renal tubular cells contain an abundance of large peroxisomes (0.5–1.5 μm). In other tissues, peroxisomes are smaller and are called *microperoxisomes*. Peroxisomes are absent or greatly reduced in number in tissues from patients with Zellweger syndrome (Goldfischer et al., 1973). *Catalase,* a marker enzyme of the peroxisomal matrix, is present in the cytosol. Electron microscopic examination and immunocytochemical detection using anti-catalase IgG are useful methods for detecting peroxisomes (Figs. 23-3 and 23-4). Recent studies using antibodies directed against peroxisomal membrane proteins revealed the presence of a ghost-like peroxisomal structure in Zellweger fibroblasts.

Accumulation of VLCFA, the most important biochemical abnormality in Zellweger syndrome as well as in X-linked ALD, was reported in 1982. Accumulation of VLCFA in Zellweger syndrome is much higher than in X-linked ALD, and it is linked to a defect in the proxisomal β-oxidation pathway (Fig. 23-6). The rate of C24:0 oxidation by Zellweger fibroblasts is severely reduced, and three β-oxidation enzymes (acyl-CoA oxidase, enoyl-CoA hydratase-3-hydroxyacyl-CoA dehydrogenase bifunctional enzyme, and 3-ketoacyl-CoA thiolase) are hardly detectable on immunoblot analysis. Precursors of these enzymes are normally synthesized on free polysomes, but their degradation occurs rapidly. Conversion of trihydroxycoprostanic acid into cholic acid and of dihydroxycoprostanic acid into deoxycholic acid takes place in the peroxisomal β-oxidation system. 2,4-Dienoyl-CoA reductase appears to have an important role in the degradation of unsaturated VLCFA, and its defect probably contributes to the accumulation of unsaturated VLCFA.

A deficiency of plasmalogen is also an important finding in patients with Zellweger syndrome. Dihydroxyacetone phosphate (DHAP) acyltransferase and alkyl-DHAP synthase, the enzymes that catalyze the first two steps of plasmalogen synthesis (Fig. 23-7), are deficient in Zellweger syndrome. Plasmalogen is a major component of the central nervous system

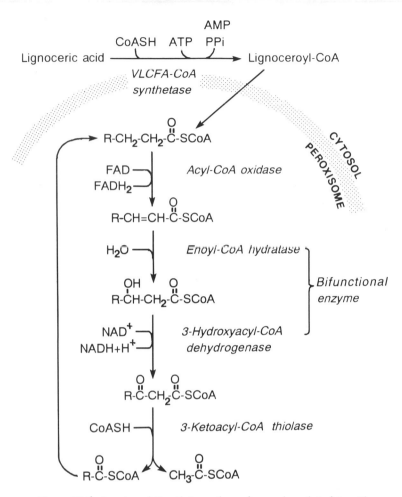

Figure 23-6. Peroxisomal β-oxidation pathways for very long-chain fatty acids.

and of various membranes. Although the function of plasmalogen is obscure, it may relate to myelination of neurons and protection of cells against photosensitized killing.

Phytanic acid oxidation activity is severely defective in Zellweger syndrome and in the case of classical Refsum disease with retinitis pigmentosa and neural deafness. Phytanic acid, exclusively derived from dietary foods, accumulates with advancing age. Phytanic acid is first α-oxidized to pristanic acid and then β-oxidized in peroxisomes (Fig. 23-8). Pipecolic acid oxidation is also defective in Zellweger syndrome. Docosahexaenoic acid (C22:6), which appears to be important for brain and retinal function, is also deficient.

These metabolic disturbances are considered to be caused by the absence of peroxisomes (Lazarow

and Moser, 1995). Peroxisomal enzymes cannot be transported into peroxisomes, probably as a result of defects in membrane integrity or in the protein-transport machinery of peroxisomes. Many kinds of enzymes, including β-oxidation enzymes, are degraded rapidly, and only a few kinds of enzymes (such as catalase) are stable in the cytosol.

To clarify the genetic relationship of peroxisome-deficient Zellweger syndrome and other milder variants, a complementation study by means of the somatic cell fusion method is required (Brul et al., 1988). Fused cells consisting of a specific pair of cell lines restore peroxisomal biogenesis (Fig. 23-4) and correct the biochemical abnormalities. Pathogenic genes for these cell lines are assumed to be different. To date, 10 complementation groups have been identified (Table 23-2), indicating that a con-

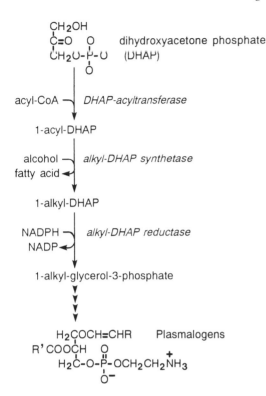

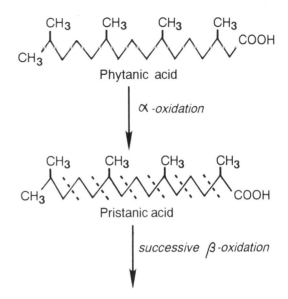

Figure 23-8. Pathways for phytanic acid degradation.

Figure 23-7. Pathways for plasmalogen biosynthesis. CoA, coenzyme A.

siderable genetic heterogeneity is present in Zellweger syndrome and that at least 10 genes are involved in the formation of normal peroxisomes. Furthermore, clinical classification does not correlate with genetic grouping.

In 1992 a gene responsible for Zellweger syndrome was cloned by means of the functional cloning method (Shimozawa et al., 1992). Mutant Chinese hamster ovary (CHO) cells with deficient peroxisomes were first isolated using ethylmethanesulfonate, a mutagenic agent. Next a rat liver cDNA library, constructed in a mammalian expression vector pcD2, was transfected into these cells. Revertant cells were selected by the photosensitized killing method in which plasmalogen-deficient cells were killed by the application of 12-(1'-pyrene)-dodecanoic acid and ultraviolet light. The plasmid in the selected cells was recovered and sequenced. The cloned cDNA had a 915-base-pair (bp) open reading frame that encodes 305 amino acids. The gene product, named *peroxisome assembly factor-1* (PAF-1), is a peroxisomal membrane protein

with a molecular weight of 35 kd and should play an important role in the biogenesis of peroxisomes and transport of various peroxisomal enzymes (Fig. 23-6). A complementation study revealed that the group F Zellweger syndrome patients belong to the same complementation group as that of the mutant CHO cells. When the human *PAF-1* cDNA is transfected into the group F Zellweger cells, peroxisomes appear and the biochemical defects are corrected. The human *PAF-1* gene is mapped to chromosome

Table 23-2. Complementation Groups of Peroxisome-deficient Disorders

Phenotype(s)	Complementation Group		
	Japan	U.S.A.	Netherlands
ZS, NALD, IRD	A	8	
ZS, NALD	B	7	
ZS, NALD	C	4	3
ZS	D	9	
ZS, NALD, IRD	E	1	2
ZS	F	10	5
ZS, NALD		2	4
ZS		3	
ZS		5	
ZS, NALD		6	

ZS, Zellweger syndrome; NALD, neonatal adrenoleukodystrophy; IRD, infantile Refsum disease.

Alphabet (A–F) and numbers (1–10) indicate the names of groups in each country.

8q21.1. A C → T transition at nucleotide position 355, which results in premature formation of the termination codon at [119]Arg, was identified homozygously in a group F Zellweger patient (patient 1). The mutant PAF-1 protein is truncated and assumed to be nonfunctional. The parents were heterozygotes for this mutation. Thus, one of the genes responsible for Zellweger syndrome is *PAF-1*.

A number of genes essential to the formation of functional peroxisomes remain to be determined. Vigorous efforts have been made to identify these genes by investigating the other peroxisomal membrane proteins, including the 70-kd peroxisomal integral membrane protein (70PMP) and several minor ones and genes involved in peroxisome biogenesis in yeast.

Adrenoleukodystrophy

Accumulation of saturated VLCFA, reported in 1976, is an isolated biochemical abnormality so far in X-linked ALD. This finding has been seen in tissues and body fluids of patients with different clinical phenotypes, including presymptomatic boys and asymptomatic female carriers. There is no difference in the degree of VLCFA accumulation between phenotypes. X-linked ALD and Zellweger syndrome are considered representative of the peroxisomal disorders. The former is a disease with single metabolic dysfunction and morphologically intact peroxisomes, and the latter is a disease with multiple metabolic dysfunctions and defective peroxisomes.

Fibroblasts from patients with ALD cannot degrade VLCFA, as in the case of Zellweger syndrome, although the severity of the β-oxidation defect and extent of VLCFA accumulation are less marked. Fatty acid accumulation is confined to saturated VLCFA. Interestingly, degradation of lignoceroyl-CoA (C24:0-CoA) is not impaired, but lignoceric acid degradation is deficient in ALD fibroblasts. These findings suggest that the metabolic defect in X-linked ALD is located in the step of CoA esterification of VLCFA. VLCFA-CoA synthetase (lignoceroyl-CoA ligase) activity is defective in ALD patients (Hashmi et al., 1986). Enzymes of the β-oxidation pathway are intact. Thus, lignoceroyl-CoA ligase had been considered a candidate enzyme for the primary cause of ALD.

Meanwhile, the gene for ALD is linked to those for red-green vision, glucose 6-phosphate dehydrogenase, and the DXS52 DNA probe, which recognizes polymorphic loci in the terminal region of the long arm of the X chromosome (Xq28). ALD patients manifest red-green color vision defects more frequently than controls, and abnormalities of the pigment genes are sometimes recognized. These findings indicate that the ALD gene resides in the neighborhood of the color-vision genes.

The ALD gene was cloned in 1993 by using the positional cloning method. Gene analysis of an ALD patient with blue-monochromatic color vision, and who had a complex gene rearrangement located upstream of the red color pigment gene, contributed greatly to the identification of the ALD gene. Genomic probes in this rearranged region revealed several gene deletions in ALD patients and also clarified a 4.2-kb mRNA in Northern blot analysis. These findings pointed to the presence of part of the ALD gene within this probe. The polymerase chain reaction (PCR) results, using primers from the putative exons in this probe, produced two cDNA fragments. The 2751-bp cDNA was isolated from the cDNA library using these fragments. The cloned cDNA coded the entire 745 amino acid sequence, named the *ALD protein*. Interestingly, the sequence of the ALD protein has a 38.5% amino acid identity with 70PMP, and both the ALD protein and 70PMP have an amino-terminal hydrophobic region and an ATP binding motif, indicating that the ALD protein is a peroxisomal membrane protein that belongs to the ATP-binding cassette superfamily of transporters (Mosser et al., 1993). The nucleotide sequence of the ALD protein is different from that of palmitoyl-CoA ligase, suggesting that the ALD protein is different from lignoceroyl-CoA ligase. The ALD protein seems to be related to the translocation of lignoceroyl-CoA ligase into peroxisomes (Fig. 23-9).

Since the identification of the ALD gene, various mutations, including large gene deletions, several missense mutations in the conserved region of ATP-binding site, nonsense mutations, and frameshift mutations leading to premature termination signal, have been identified. As expected from clinical observations, the same mutation was identified in patients with different clinical phenotypes within a kindred, suggesting that mutation of the ALD protein does not prescribe clinical phenotypes.

Many questions remain regarding the mechanisms responsible for the clinical symptoms and pathological findings of ALD. The most intriguing problem is that it is difficult to explain the onset of

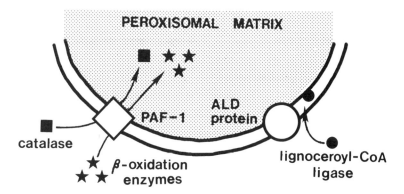

Figure 23-9. Hypothetical model of peroxisomal membrane proteins. Peroxisome assembly factor-1 (PAF-1) is required for translocation of many peroxisomal matrix enzymes including catalase and the β-oxidation enzymes. The adrenoleukodystrophy (ALD) protein is considered necessary for localization of lignoceroyl-coenzyme A (CoA) ligase.

leukodystrophy solely on the basis of the accumulation of VLCFA. Female carriers with high VLCFA levels and some biochemically diagnosed male patients do not manifest clinical symptoms. Perivascular infiltration of lymphocytes in the cerebral white matter suggests the involvement of immunological mechanisms. The reason why patients with different clinical phenotypes exist within a kindred is another important question. There appears to be no difference in the severity of a particular biochemical defect between patients with a severe phenotype and those with a milder one. Genetic segregation analysis suggests the presence of an autosomal modifier gene that may influence the severity of the phenotype.

THERAPY

Zellweger Syndrome

Treatment

Although there is no established treatment for Zellweger syndrome, symptomatic therapy for the neurologic disturbances and general management of the patient are important. Anticonvulsant medications for seizures, nasogastric tube feeding for nutritional management, assisted ventilation for respiratory failure, and vitamin K supplementation for the coagulation defect are necessary. Clinical trials including the restriction of dietary VLCFA, supplementation of plasmalogen, and administration of clofibrate, a peroxisome-proliferator, have not had positive results. Administration of docosahexaenoic acid (C22:6)

may have a favorable effect on neurologic disturbances.

Prevention

Genetic counseling is important for understanding and preventing Zellweger syndrome. A number of methods, including VLCFA analysis, measurement of C24:0 oxidation activity or DHAP-acyltransferase activity, immunoblot detection of peroxisomal enzymes, and immunocytochemical detection of peroxisomes, are available for the prenatal diagnosis of the disease using cultured amniocytes or chorionic villous cells. DNA analysis is feasible for the group F Zellweger syndrome.

Adrenoleukodystrophy

Treatment

Treatment of adrenoleukodystrophy consists of symptomatic therapy for the neurologic disturbances, steroid replacement therapy for the adrenal insufficiency, and specific treatment to prevent neurological deterioration. Symptomatic therapy includes counseling with a psychotherapist for the early symptoms of emotional and behavioral changes, medications for seizures and muscle spasms, and nasogastric tube feeding for pharyngeal dysfunction. Parent-support groups, for example, the United Leukodystrophy Foundation, exist in the United States. Glucocorticoid replacement therapy is required for patients with adrenal insufficiency.

Efforts have been made to develop specific treatments for ALD, and attempts to decrease VLCFA levels have been made. Restriction of foods containing VLCFA, such as dairy products like fat, nuts, seeds, and skin of vegetables, have failed to decrease serum VLCFA levels and have not altered the clinical course. Monounsaturated long-chain fatty acids (e.g., oleic acid and erucic acid) inhibit de *novo* biosynthesis of VLCFA in microsomes in cultured fibroblasts. Oral administration of erucic acid is effective in decreasing serum VLCFA (Rizzo et al., 1989). A clinical trial of Lorenzo's oil, consisting of one part of erucic acid and four parts of oleic acid, in combination with a VLCFA restriction diet, is under investigation in the United States (Moser et al., 1994). Prophylactic use of Lorenzo's oil in presymptomatic boys appears to decrease the rate of onset of the disease; however, improvement of neurologically affected patients is difficult to ascertain.

Bone marrow transplantation is expected to be an alternative treatment for ALD. It appears to be effective in mildly affected patients but may result in the further loss of neurological function. Long-term follow-up studies are necessary.

Prevention

As in the case of Zellweger syndrome, genetic counseling is important. Because the mode of inheritance of ALD is X-linked recessive and most of the patients' mothers are carriers, explanation of the disease to parents needs to be done carefully. The patient's mother sometimes blames herself or is blamed by the husband. Serum VLCFA analysis of family members is useful for the screening of female carriers and presymptomatic boys. The therapeutic trial of Lorenzo's oil for presymptomatic boys may be worthwhile, as described in the Therapy section. Prenatal diagnosis is performed by means of VLCFA analysis, measurement of VLCFA oxidation, linkage study, and mutation analysis of ALD protein gene using cultured amniocytes or chorionic villi.

QUESTIONS

1. Describe the metabolic function of peroxisomes and summarize the metabolic disturbances in Zellweger syndrome and ALD.
2. Compare the differences between peroxisomal and mitochondrial β-oxidation systems in the following aspects:

reaction sequences, enzymes, substrate specificity, cofactors, and biological significance.
3. What are the advantages and disadvantages of functional cloning and positional cloning compared with those of the conventional cloning strategy?
4. Both PAF-1 and the ALD protein are peroxisomal membrane proteins and the metabolic disturbances in both Zellweger syndrome and ALD are considered secondary phenomenon. Speculate on the functions of PAF-1 and ALD protein.
5. If an infant manifests severe hypotonia soon after birth and accumulation of VLCFA is documented, what should be the next step with regard to diagnosis and genetic counseling?
6. If a family with one child with ALD and a maternal grandfather with adult-onset adrenomyeloneuropathy inform you that they plan to have another child, how would you explain their genetic situation, risk of recurrence, interpretation of prenatal diagnosis, and medical care options for the next child?

REFERENCES

ZELLWEGER SYNDROME

Bowen P, Lee CSN, Zellweger H, Lindenberg R: A familial syndrome of multiple congenital defects. *Bull Johns Hopkins Hosp* **114**:402–414, 1964.

Brul S, Westerveld A, Strijland A, et al.: Genetic heterogeneity in the cerebrohepatorenal (Zellweger) syndrome and other inherited disorders with a generalized impairment of peroxisomal functions—A study using complementation analysis. *J Clin Invest* **81**:1710–1715, 1988.

Goldfischer S, Moore CL, Johnson AB, et al.: Peroxisomal and mitochondrial defects in the cerebro-hepato-renal syndrome. *Science* **182**:62–64, 1973.

Lazarow PB, Moser HW: Disorders of peroxisome biogenesis, *in* Scriver CR, Beaudet AL, Sly WS, Valle D (eds): *The Metabolic and Molecular Bases of Inherited Disease*. New York, McGraw-Hill Inc. 1995, pp 2287–2324.

Shimozawa N, Tsukamoto T, Suzuki Y, et al.: A human gene responsible for Zellweger syndrome that affects peroxisome assembly. *Science* **255**:1132–1134, 1992.

ADRENOLEUKODYSTROPHY

Hashmi M, Stanley W, Singh I: Lignoceroyl-CoA ligase: enzyme defect in fatty acid beta-oxidation system in X-linked childhood adrenoleukodystrophy. *FEBS Lett* **196**:247–250, 1986.

Igarashi M, Schaumburg HH, Powers JM, Kishimoto Y, Kolodney E, Suzuki K: Fatty acid abnormality in adrenoleukodystrophy. *J Neurochem* **26**:851–860, 1976.

Moser HW, Smith KD, Moser AB: X-linked adrenoleukodystrophy, *in* Scriver CR, Beaudet AL, Sly WS, Valle D (eds): *The*

Metabolic and Molecular Bases of Inherited Disease. New York, McGraw-Hill Inc. 1995, pp 2325–2349.

Moser HW, Kok F, Neumann S, et al.: Adrenoleukodystrophy update: Genetics and effect of Lorenzo's oil therapy in asymptomatic patients. *International Pediatrics* **9:**196–204, 1994.

Mosser J, Douar A-M, Sarde C-O, et al.: Putative X-linked adrenoleukodystrophy gene shares unexpected homology with ABC transporters. *Nature* **361:**726–730, 1993.

Rizzo WB, Leshner RT, Odone A, et al.: Dietary erucic acid therapy for X-linked adrenoleukodystrophy. *Neurology* **39:**1415–1422, 1989.

24

Inborn Errors of Urea Synthesis

SAUL W. BRUSILOW

CASE REPORTS

To emphasize the variability of clinical expression imposed by a biochemical abnormality that is a result of a mutation at one urea cycle locus (ornithine transcarbamylase), five cases are presented. Whereas the clinical backgrounds of these cases are dissimilar (a newborn infant, a 9-month-old boy, a 4-year-old girl, a postpartum woman, and an adult man), their clinical and biochemical courses are strikingly similar. They all demonstrate alterations in the level of consciousness, altered behavior, hyperammonemia, hyperglutaminemia, and a high pH and a low partial pressure of carbon dioxide, all of which are a consequence of high plasma concentrations of ammonium.

Case 1

A male infant was born after a full-term pregnancy and spontaneous vaginal delivery. He was well during the first 36 hours following birth but then was lethargic and irritable and had hyperactive deep-tendon reflexes. He was afebrile. A blood culture was drawn to rule out suspected sepsis and antibiotics were administered. Serum electrolytes were within normal limits except for a slightly decreased HCO_3^- concentration. The arterial blood pH was 7.50 (normal, 7.35–7.45) and the P_{CO_2} was 25 torr (normal, 35–45 torr); the blood urea nitrogen (BUN) level was 2 mg/dL (normal, 5–20 mg/dL). Chest radiograph performed because the baby was hyperventilating, was normal. Over the ensuing 24 hours, the lethargy progressed to stupor and then coma, requiring mechanical ventilation. Three days later the infant was transferred to a newborn intensive care unit, where the sepsis workup (including a lumbar puncture) was repeated. The head circumference was 2 cm greater than at birth. On day 5 the plasma ammonium level was measured and found to be 1800 μmol/L (normal, <35 μmol/L). Magnetic resonance imaging of the head revealed cerebral edema. While awaiting the results of plasma amino acid analyses and urinary orotic acid (orotate) analysis, hemodialysis was started; after 4 hours the plasma ammonium had decreased to 150 μmol/L. Despite control of his hyperammonemia, he remained in a deep coma with no evidence of spontaneous respiration or neurological function; life-support systems were discontinued after consultation with the family, and the infant died at 7 days of age. Plasma amino acid values revealed a glutamine level of 1500 μmol/L (normal, 550–650 μmol/L), no detectable citrulline (normal, 10–30 μmol/L), and an arginine level of 20 μmol/L (normal, 40–80 μmol/L). Urinary orotate was 100-fold greater than normal. Postmortem analyses of hepatic ornithine transcarbamylase (OTC) activity revealed it to be <2% of normal. A review of the family history, unfortunately in retrospect, showed that two of the mother's brothers had died in coma within the first week of life; *encephalitis* (inflammation of the brain) had been given as the cause of death.

Although this neonatal onset case is frequently,

but erroneously, cited as the characteristic of OTC deficiency it has become apparent over the past several years that OTC deficiency, the most common of the urea cycle disorders, occurs most often in older patients. The next four dramatic cases exemplify the late-onset expression of OTC deficiency.

Case 2

Before age 9 months, this boy's medical history was unrevealing and his development normal; however, at 9 months of age, following antibiotic treatment of otitis media, he was admitted to the hospital with a chief complaint of irritability, vomiting, and lethargy. Over a period of 24 hours, he rapidly progressed to coma and was unresponsive except to painful stimuli. He was afebrile. Notwithstanding normal liver transaminase values, a diagnosis of Reye syndrome was made and he was transferred to The Johns Hopkins Hospital. Laboratory studies on admission revealed a plasma ammonium level of 607 μmol/L; a plasma glutamine level, 1188 μmol/L; plasma citrulline level, 6 μmol/L; and urinary orotate excretion, 2669 μmol/mmol creatinine (normal, <2 μmol/L). Emergency treatment included intravenously administered sodium benzoate, phenylacetate, and arginine hydrochloride, after which his plasma ammonium values decreased to 153 μmol/L and 50 μmol/L 1 and 12 hours later and remained normal thereafter. A computerized tomography (CT) scan of the head revealed severe cerebral edema; coma persisted for 4 days. A liver biopsy revealed 5.7% of normal OTC activity and normal carbamyl phosphate synthetase activity.

Case 3

The patient was a 5-year-old girl whose neonatal course was uncomplicated as were her first 3 years of life. At 3 years of age she had a rather abrupt onset of episodes of "grogginess" approximately every 4 to 6 months, and they were often associated with combative behavior and biting but not associated with any discrete observable illness. During one of these episodes, she was admitted to a regional medical center, where the plasma ammonium level was noted to be increased but this finding was disregarded because ammonium levels were said to be "problematical." She was hospitalized for 5 days

during that episode and recovered after a course of intravenous fluids. Three weeks before admission to The Johns Hopkins Hospital, the patient had been "in and out of grogginess." She was sent home from school because of excessive sleepiness. During this episode, she had the previously observed aggressive outbursts that included awakening her parents by biting. She was admitted to a local hospital and was found to be lethargic, agitated, and ataxic. She was afebrile. Her plasma ammonium level was 193 μmol/L; her arterial blood gases were, pH 7.45, P_{CO_2}, 30 torr. Within 48 hours she became unresponsive to all but painful stimuli and required mechanical ventilation. A nearby regional hospital was unable to accept her for admission, and she was flown to Baltimore by air ambulance. During her transfer she developed decorticate posturing and a fixed and dilated pupil. On arrival she was deeply comatose, unresponsive, and on a ventilator. Her plasma ammonia and glutamine levels were 314 μmol/L and 1321 μmol/L, respectively. Her urine orotate was five-fold greater than normal. A brain computed tomographic (CT) scan revealed cerebral edema. She was promptly treated with intravenous benzoate/phenylacetate and arginine; 24 hours after admission her plasma ammonia concentration was 34 mmol/L. Based on these laboratory measurements, a diagnosis of OTC deficiency was made. Over the ensuing week she gradually improved, became ambulatory and communicative, but it became apparent that she was cortically blind. Three weeks after admission, her vision improved and she was discharged. Her most recent school evaluation suggests that she has changed from a bright interactive 5-year-old girl to a withdrawn, confused, inattentive child.

Case 4

A 21-year-old white woman gave birth to a 2.76 kg male infant at 38 weeks of gestation; pregnancy and delivery were uneventful. At 8 days postpartum, she developed headache and confusion and became uncommunicative. She was admitted to the psychiatric service where a diagnosis of postpartum depression was made. Twenty-four hours later she became comatose and had generalized tonic-clonic seizures, decorticate posturing, and papilledema. She was afebrile. She was transferred to the medical service, where the initial diagnosis was subarachnoid bleeding. Serum electrolytes, liver transaminase, and bilirubin levels were normal, as were the studies of cerebrospinal fluid and coagulation. Arterial pH was 7.44; p_{CO_2}, 31 torr; plasma ammonium level, 226 μmol/L. A CT scan of the head was normal. An electroencephalogram (EEG) revealed slow waves and the absence of *epileptiform* (resembling that of epilepsy) activity. Despite treatment with *lactulose,* (a cathartic disaccharide used to treat central nervous system dysfunction accompanying liver disease) the plasma ammonium level increased to 411 μmol/L and she became progressively more comatose with evidence of cerebral edema and increased intracranial pressure. Despite supportive therapy, hemodialysis, and treatment with benzoate and phenylacetate (all of which led to a rapid reduction of the plasma ammonium level to 40 μmol/L), she died with massive cerebral edema. Postmortem OTC activity in the liver was 5.5% of normal. Carbamyl phosphate synthetase I activity was normal. Postmortem examination of the brain revealed severe cerebral edema, manifested by flattening of the *gyri* (convoluted ridges of the brain) and herniation of the cerebellar tonsils; the brain was otherwise grossly normal. A review of the patient's medical history revealed a 3-day episode of coma at the age of 5 years.

Case 5

This 30-year-old white man was admitted to a local hospital for lethargy, confusion, and forgetfulness. Over the ensuing 5 days, he continued to be disoriented with vomiting, loss of memory, ataxia, and slurred speech; a diagnosis of encephalopathy of unknown etiology was made. Physical examination at the time of admission was normal with the exception of the neurologic exam. He was afebrile. The patient was unable to perform simple arithmetic tasks and had poor short- and long-term memory. Asterixis was noted. Initial laboratory tests, including liver function tests, were within normal limits. The plasma ammonia level measured on day 5 of admission was 104 μmol/L, rising to 194 μmol/L the following day. The patient gradually improved and was discharged several days later with a diagnosis of Reye syndrome. He subsequently had a positive allopurinol test that in this clinical setting, was diagnos-

tic for OTC deficiency. Within this pedigree there are six other late-onset OTC-deficient males.

DIAGNOSIS

The first case exhibits the clinical course common to all neonatal-onset urea cycle disorders. The following are the important points: (1) the infant is almost always full-term; (2) clinical symptoms usually starting after the 24 hours of age because it takes time for ammonium to accumulate (during pregnancy the placenta clears ammonium from the blood of the fetus and the maternal liver detoxifies it); (3) respiratory *alkalosis* (evidence of overbreathing caused by hyperammonemia occurs); (4) high plasma ammonium concentration is present; (5) *glutamine,* a "storage site" for ammonium, accumulates; (6) there is an absence (or nearly so) of plasma citrulline (the product of the OTC reaction); (7) coma can occur, and (8) orotic aciduria (a pyrimidine) occurs as a consequence of accumulation of *carbamyl phosphate* (the substrate for ornithine transcarbamylase), which promotes pyrimidine biosynthesis. The history of male deaths in the maternal line strongly supports the diagnosis of OTC deficiency, an X-linked disorder.

Four cases of late-onset OTC deficiency (the most commonly occurring urea cycle disease) are included to emphasize the great phenotypic and genetic variability of this inborn error of metabolism. Thus, it may be assumed that because OTC deficiency is an X-linked disease, the variability in males is a function of a mutation at the OTC locus that permits the synthesis of some OTC activity. Variability in females is best explained by the phenomenon of random X-chromosome inactivation; when a large proportion of a female's active X-chromosome has a mutation at its OTC locus, the female then has a limited ability to synthesize OTC. Hence she will have a restricted ability to synthesize urea and will be vulnerable to hyperammonemic encephalopathy.

Patients with defects in carbamyl phosphate synthetase (CPS), argininosuccinic acid synthetase (AS), or argininosuccinase (AL), all of which are autosomal recessive disorders, show clinical pictures similar to those of the above cases, the severity being a function of the amount of residual enzyme activity; careful evaluation of plasma amino acid analyses with attention to the substrates and products of each urea cycle enzyme (Fig. 24-1) will reveal differences that readily distinguish these defects from one another. Of particular importance is evaluation of the plasma citrulline concentration. In AS deficiency it is extremely high (>2000 μmol/L) compared with ALD, in which the plasma citrulline level is approximately 300 to 500 μmol/L and is associated with extraordinarily high concentrations of argininosuccinic acid (>1000 μmol/L). Inspection of the metabolic pathways (Fig. 24-1) will reveal that these changes are simply a function of the accumulation of the substrates of the particular enzymes. The laboratory features of carbamyl phosphate synthetase deficiency are identical to those of OTC deficiency, except for a normal level of orotate excretion.

Deficiency of arginase (ARG) manifests itself differently. Severe hyperammonemia in the newborn period is uncommon. The major manifestations of mental retardation and spastic paralysis of the lower extremities gradually appear in the first year of life and ultimately become obvious. The diagnosis is made after finding increased plasma arginine levels and decreased concentrations of arginase in erythrocytes. In addition, orotic aciduria may be found, presumably because inactivity of ART limits intramitochondrial ornithine synthesis, which in turn becomes a rate-limiting factor in OTC activity; the result

is carbamyl phosphate accumulation and activation of pyrimidine biosynthesis.

Although hyperammonemia and hyperglutaminemia clearly result from an abnormality of a specific urea cycle enzyme, many other genetic diseases may be responsible for hyperammonemic coma in the newborn period and later that closely resemble the urea cycle defects but can easily be distinguished from them. These diseases result in the accumulation of propionic acid (caused by propionyl-CoA carboxylase deficiency) and methylmalonic acid (caused either by methylmalonyl-CoA racemase or methylmalonyl-CoA mutase deficiencies). The degradation of the amino acids valine, threonine, isoleucine, and methionine gives rise to these intermediates. Both propionic acid (as propionyl-CoA) and methylmalonic acid (as methylmalonyl-CoA) competitively inhibit the utilization of acetyl-CoA in the synthesis of *N*-acetylglutamate (NAG), which is an absolute allosteric effector of CPS. When any of these inhibitors accumulate, carbamyl phosphate synthesis is impaired and hyperammonemia results. These diseases are usually easily recognizable because the accumulation of organic acids is sufficiently great to titrate plasma bicarbonate levels with an accompanying decrease in blood pH, findings quite different from urea cycle enzyme defects where the blood pH

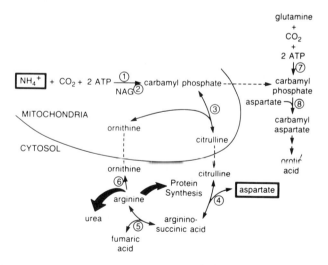

Figure 24-1. Urea synthesis in the liver. Dashed lines represent transport of metabolite across membrane. Enzymes involved are represented by circled numbers. (1) Carbamyl phosphate synthetase I (CPS I). (2) *N*-Acetylglutamate (NAG), an obligatory effector of CPS I. NAG is synthesized in the mitochondria by NAG synthetase from acetate and glutamate. Organic acids are competitive inhibitors of this reaction. (3) Ornithine transcarbamylase (OTC); (4) argininosuccinate synthetase (AS); (5) argininosuccinate lyase (AL); (6) arginase (ARG); (7) carbamyl phosphate synthetase II (CPS II); (8) aspartate transcarbamylase; ATP, adenosine triphosphate.

is increased. Analysis of the patients urine by gas-liquid chromatography and mass spectroscopy will usually reveal the metabolic defect.

MOLECULAR PERSPECTIVES

The survey of the urea cycle is divided into three sections. The first examines normal urea synthesis; the second, regulation of urea synthesis; and the last, abnormalities of urea synthesis. To begin, the routes of nitrogen entry into the urea cycle and the five enzymes that constitute this cycle are examined (Brusilow and Horwich, 1995).

Biochemistry of the Urea Cycle

Unlike the carbon, hydrogen, or oxygen atoms of dietary fats and carbohydrates, which can be stored in large amounts as body fat, there is no storage form of nitrogen; nitrogen contained in amino acids not used for net biosynthetic purposes must be excreted to avoid the accumulation of toxic nitrogenous products. Vertebrates have evolved a number of products for excretion of waste nitrogen. Aquatic animals, for example, excrete nitrogen as ammonium and thus are labeled ammoniatelic. Birds are *uricotelic;* that is, they excrete their waste nitrogen as uric acid. Mammals, including humans, are *ureotelic;* that is, they excrete waste nitrogen as urea.

The urea molecule contains two nitrogen atoms, both of which are derived from the free amino acid pool. One nitrogen atom is derived from aspartate (Fig. 24-1), a product of the transamination of oxaloacetate by glutamate. Although it is clear that ammonium is the source of the other nitrogen atom (Fig. 24-1), it is not certain from what amino acid it is derived. Although it is assumed that ammonium is derived from the oxidative deamination of glutamate via hepatic glutamate dehydrogenase, this has not been proved. Other possible sources of ammonium include hepatic deamination of glycine, serine, threonine, histidine or purine nucleotides, or deamination of glutamine, which is known to be synthesized in muscle and may be transported to the liver via the bloodstream.

Five enzymes are involved in the synthesis of urea: Two are located in the mitochondrial matrix of the liver cell; the remaining three occur in the cytosol.

Why these reactions are separated is unclear, but compartmentation, in general, is known to confer dimensions of both specificity and metabolic regulation upon the cell.

The first step of the urea cycle is catalyzed by the intramitochondrial enzyme carbamyl phosphate synthetase I (CPS I) (Fig. 24-1). A complex enzyme of subunit molecular weights of 165 kd. CPS I has been isolated in both monomer and dimer forms. Curiously, it constitutes nearly 20% of all mitochondrial matrix protein. The small intestine also has CPS I activity.

The synthesis of carbamyl phosphate requires two high-energy phosphate bonds per molecule of carbamyl phosphate formed. It also requires magnesium in two forms: bound as MgATP for substrate and free magnesium ions that stimulate enzyme activity. Additionally, N-acetylglutamate (NAG) is an obligatory allosteric effector of CPS (Fig. 24-1).

CPS I has been mapped to the short arm of chromosome 2. The cDNA is quite large and contains a 5' untranslated end of 139 bases, an open reading frame of 4500 nucleotides, and a 3'-untranslated sequence of 905 nucleotides followed by a polyA tract. The protein subunit contains a cleavable 38 amino acid leader peptide, which directs the subunit for mitochondrial import.

Carbamyl phosphate condenses with ornithine within the mitochondria to form citrulline via a reaction catalyzed by the enzyme OTC (Fig. 24-1). OTC is a trimer, with each subunit being 35 kd. The concentration of OTC in the mitochondrial matrix is ~10% that of CPS; however, its specific activity is 25 times greater. Although the reaction is reversible, the equilibrium favors citrulline formation at 37°C. OTC is also found in the small intestine. OTC is located on the short arm of the X-chromosome. The gene itself is 85 kilobases (kb) long and has 10 exons. The cDNA is 1600 nucleotides in length of which 1062 encode the protein subunit. Similar to the case of CPS 1, the subunit contains a leader peptide of 32 amino acids that directs the subunit for mitochondrial import.

Carbamyl phosphate is also the substrate for a cytosolic enzyme, aspartate transcarbamylase (Fig. 24-1). Formed via CPS II in the cytosol with glutamine as nitrogen donor, carbamyl phosphate is used by aspartate transcarbamylase to form pyrimidine precursors, particularly orotic acid. When intramitochondrial carbamyl phosphate accumulates (see Case Reports) it diffuses into the cytosol, where it serves as a substrate for pyrimidine synthesis, thereby accounting for the orotic aciduria seen in OTC deficiencies (Fig. 24-1).

The third step of the urea cycle takes place in the cytosol (Fig. 24-1). Citrulline, the product of the second step, first diffuses out of the mitochondria into the cytosol, where it condenses with a molecule of aspartate in a reaction catalyzed by argininosuccinate synthetase (AS).

This reaction consumes two high-energy phosphate bonds, as does the first step of urea synthesis, although in this case the two-high energy phosphate bonds come from a single molecule of ATP, which is split, yielding AMP and pyrophosphate. The subsequent splitting of pyrophosphate by pyrophosphatase pulls this reversible reaction to the right. Argininosuccinate synthetase is a tetramer composed of 48 kd subunits. Argininosuccinic acid synthetase is located on the long arm of chromosome 9 and is 63 kb in size. Its 16 exons encode a cDNA of 1600 bases. The AS gene is characterized by having many pseudogenes dispersed to 14 different loci.

Argininosuccinase lyase (AL) catalyzes the fourth step in ureagenesis; it cleaves argininosuccinate to arginine and fumaric acid. It has been mapped to the long arm of chromosome 7. The protein subunit is encoded by a cDNA of 1389 bases. Curiously, AL contains many similarities to the structural proteins (delta crystallins) found in the lens of the eye.

The final step of the urea cycle, the hydrolysis of arginine to form urea and regenerate ornithine, is catalyzed by arginase (ARG). ARG is probably a 120 kd trimer, each of whose subunits is approximately 35 kd in size. Because the hepatic activity of arginase is very high, hepatic levels of arginine are quite low. Arginase is also found in kidney and erythrocytes. The gene (11.5 kb) is found on the long arm of chromosome 6 and contains 8 exons coding for 322 amino acids.

Regulation of the Urea Cycle

The urea cycle serves two purposes. First, it contains many of the biochemical reactions required for the synthesis of arginine. In this regard it should be noted that, unlike normal persons in whom arginine is a nonessential amino acid, arginine is an essential amino acid in patients with urea cycle defects (other than arginase deficiency).

Second, the urea cycle incorporates into the waste product urea nitrogen atoms (normally derived from dietary protein nitrogen) that are not retained for net biosynthetic purposes. The amount of urea synthesized by an individual is closely related to dietary nitrogen intake and net protein synthesis. For example, in adult men and women in whom nitrogen balance is neutral, all dietary nitrogen must be excreted; there is no "storage" form of nitrogen. Rapidly growing infants, however, retain much of their dietary nitrogen for growth and therefore excrete much less of their dietary nitrogen as urea than do adults; they are said to be in positive nitrogen balance.

Enzyme induction plays an important role in the synthesis of urea and may explain how larger and larger amounts of dietary nitrogen are converted to urea. When rats were fed progressively larger amounts of protein, the activity of all their urea cycle enzymes increased in coordinate fashion (Shimke, 1962).

Although such enzyme induction plays a role in long-term regulation of urea synthesis, there are a number of candidate molecules that are thought to be responsible for short-term regulation; these include the ammonium ion itself, *N*-acetylglutamate (an allosteric activator of carbamyl phosphate synthetase), arginine, and ornithine. The relative importance of these molecules in inducing the urea cycle enzymes is controversial.

Although all the enzymes required for urea synthesis are found in the liver, the overall conversion of nitrogen to urea involves extrahepatic and intrahepatic compartmentation. For example, the presence of carbamyl phosphate synthetase and ornithine transcarbamylase activity in the intestine leads to the synthesis of citrulline, which is transported to the kidney, where it is converted to arginine. Within the liver itself, the urea cycle enzymes are confined to the periportal hepatocytes, whereas other liver enzymes may be found elsewhere; for example, ornithine aminotransferase is found in the perivenous hepatocytes.

THERAPY

Because the biochemical defect in patients with urea cycle disorders is at the level of the synthesis of *waste nitrogen* (defined as dietary nitrogen not used for biosynthetic purposes), the goal of therapy is two-fold. First, the requirement for waste nitrogen synthesis (urea synthesis) should be reduced by decreasing dietary nitrogen intake. Second, new pathways for the synthesis and excretion of waste nitrogen should be exploited. There are several strategies available to fulfill this latter approach.

It has long been known that the administration of *benzoate* (the salt of benzoic acid) and *phenylacetate* (the salt of phenylacetic acid) to humans activates the biosynthesis of two nitrogen-containing compounds, hippurate (a glycine-benzoate conjugate) and phenylacetylglutamine (a phenylacetate-glutamine conjugate), respectively. The net effect of these reactions is to divert nitrogen destined for urea synthesis to hippurate and phenylacetylglutamine (Fig. 24-2). A very important and practical feature of these compounds is their nitrogen content; on a molar basis, phenylacetate supports the production of phenylacetylglutamine which has two nitrogen atoms as compared to hippurate (the benzoate conjugate) which contains only one nitrogen atom. For this reason, benzoate therapy has been abandoned

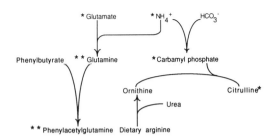

Figure 24-3. The pathways of waste nitrogen synthesis in patients with argininosuccinic acid synthetase deficiency when treated as described in the text. Supplementary dietary arginine supports the continued synthesis of citrulline; hence its excretion as a waste nitrogen product. Phenylbutyrate functions as described in Figure 24-2. The asterisks denote nitrogen atoms destined for waste nitrogen excretion in citrulline* and phenylacetylglutamine**.

except for the intravenous dosage form; however, because phenylacetate has a long-deserved reputation for its repugnant odor (it is employed as a defensive weapon by the stinkpot turtle) phenylacetate is now supplied as a pro-drug, phenylbutyrate (the salt of phenylbutyric acid), which is beta-oxidized *in vivo* to phenylacetate.

Phenylbutyrate therapy is now the mainstay of management of deficiencies of CPS and OTC as well as argininosuccinic acid synthetase (Fig. 24-3). In argininosuccinic acid synthetase deficiency, dietary

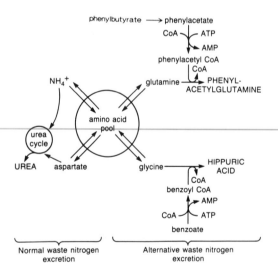

Figure 24-2. Incorporation of nitrogen from the amino acid pool into urea compared with phenylacetylglutamine and hippuric acid. Note that the synthesis of phenylacetylglutamine or hippurate incorporates nitrogen from the free amino acid pool, thereby diverting nitrogen from the defective urea synthetic pathway. Because phenylacetate has a repugnant odor, phenylbutyrate, which is beta-oxidized to phenylacetate, is now prescribed as a pro-drug. AMP, adenosine monophosphate; ATP, adenosine triphosphate; CoA, coenzyme A.

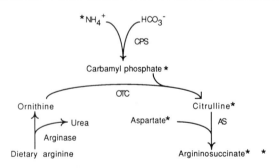

Figure 24-4. The pathway of waste nitrogen synthesis in patients with argininosuccinase deficiency when treated as described in the text. Supplementary dietary arginine supports the continued synthesis of argininosuccinate and hence its excretion as a waste nitrogen product. Asterisks denote the number of waste nitrogen atoms contained in various substrates and products.

supplements are supplied to promote the biosynthesis and excretion of citrulline; citrulline then serves as a vehicle for waste nitrogen excretion. It should be noted that citrulline only contains one waste nitrogen atom and it is derived from carbamyl phosphate.

Figure 24-4 shows the strategy exploited in the treatment of argininosuccinase deficiency. In this disease it should be noted that the accumulated product (the substrate for the enzyme), argininosuccinic acid, carries the two nitrogen atoms that are destined for urea. By providing a continuous source of dietary arginine, argininosuccinic acid may continuously be synthesized and excreted, thereby serving as a substitute vehicle for urea as a waste nitrogen product.

QUESTIONS

1. How many ATP molecules are required for the synthesis of urea from ammonium ions and bicarbonate?
2. Explain the rationale behind the use of phenylacetate therapy for the treatment of urea cycle defects.
3. Why is ammonium ion toxic to the central nervous system?

REFERENCES

Brusilow SW, Horwich AL: Urea cycle enzymes, *in* Scriver C, Beaudet A, Sly W, Valle D (eds): *The Metabolic and Molecular Basis of Inherited Disease,* 7th ed., New York, McGraw-Hill, 1995, 1187–1232.

Shimke RT: Adaptive characteristics of urea cycle enzymes in the rat. *J Biol Chem* **237**:459–468, 1962.

α_1-Antitrypsin Deficiency

SARAH JANE SCHWARZENBERG AND HARVEY L. SHARP

CASE REPORT

The patient, now a 28-year-old white man with α_1-antitrypsin deficiency, received a combined liver-kidney transplant for cirrhosis complicated by portal hypertension, renal insufficiency secondary to *membranoproliferative glomerulonephritis,* (a progressive inflammation of the glomeruli of the kidney with proliferation of mesangial cells and thickening of glomerular capillary walls and narrowing of the capillary lumina) and combined restrictive and obstructive pulmonary disease at age 18 years.

Jaundice and *pruritus* (localized itching) were observed when the patient was age six weeks old and resolved spontaneously after about 2 months. He was hospitalized for pneumonia at age 20 months, and an enlarged liver was noted. A percutaneous needle biopsy specimen from the liver was interpreted to show postnecrotic cirrhosis, although reevaluation of the biopsy specimen showed the presence of periodic acid-Schiff (PAS)-positive, diastase-resistant globules (Fig. 25–1). He was then referred to our institution at age 2.5 years for liver transplantation.

At our initial evaluation, the physical examination revealed a well-developed young boy in no acute distress. He was not jaundiced; however, it was notable that he had a protuberant abdomen with a liver edge palpable 3 cm below the right costal margin in the midclavicular line. The liver was nontender and hard. The spleen was palpable 6 cm below the left costal margin. No other abnormalities were noted.

The child's laboratory tests revealed a normal hematological picture except for a platelet count of 122,000/mm³ (below normal). He had normal liver enzymes except for a serum glutamic: oxaloacetic transaminase (SGOT) of 197 u/mL (slightly increased). Both his blood urea nitrogen (BUN) and creatinine levels were normal. The patient's serum protein electrophoresis was abnormal, with a low serum albumin of 2.9 g/dL and an α_1-globulin band that was barely visible. Because of this latter finding, protease inhibitor (Pi) phenotyping was done on the child and his family. The child was found to be PiZZ, whereas both parents had the heterozygote or PiMZ phenotype.

The child's subsequent course was one of gradual hepatic deterioration. At age 3 years, he was first noticed to have *ascites* (intra-abdominal fluid accumulation). His deterioration progressed slowly until the age 6 years, when severe ascites and peripheral edema necessitated the initiation of *spironolactone* (a potassium-sparing diuretic) therapy. Several admissions to the hospital were required over the next 6 years as serum albumin values <2.0 g/dL resulted in profound exacerbations of ascites and scrotal edema. Albumin infusions were occasionally necessary to control these episodes. During this time the patient also had two episodes of primary *peritonitis* (intraperitoneal infection) and one episode of α-streptococcal sepsis.

By age 11 he began to manifest a decrease in renal function, as measured by a creatinine clearance of 71 mL/min (normal, 105 mL/min). He also developed a protein-losing nephropathy with a 24-hour urinary protein excretion of 600 mg that increased to 14 g after albumin infusions (normal

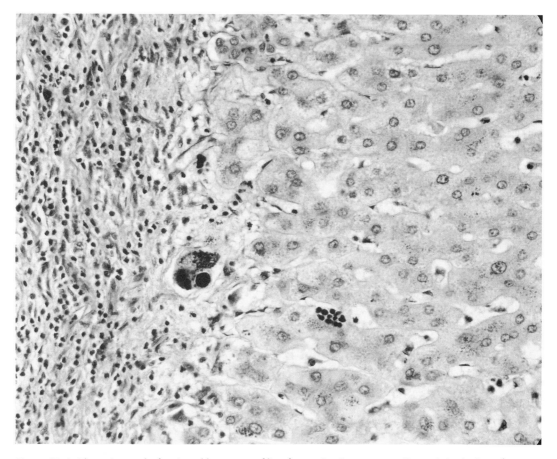

Figure 25-1. Photomicrograph of periportal hepatocytes of liver from patient in case report. Note variation in size and presence of cytoplasmic globules. The stain used is periodic acid-Schiff's after diastase.

urinary protein excretion is 100 mg/24 h). Because of abnormal coagulation study results, renal biopsy was deferred; however, the clinical picture was consistent with the membranoproliferative glomerulonephritis seen in α_1-antitrypsin deficiency.

At age 12, the patient was admitted with acute chest pain from a left spontaneous *pneumothorax* (air within the pleural cavity), which required hospitalization and chest tube insertion, but he recovered without sequelae. After resolution of this problem, pulmonary function testing revealed findings consistent with both severe airway obstruction and destruction of alveolar lung tissue, consistent with emphysema. No further pulmonary problems occurred until the patient was age 16, when he developed extrinsic asthma with occasional episodes of bronchospasm. Pulmonary function studies at that time, although improved from those immediately following his

pneumothorax, still revealed combined obstructive and destructive lung disease.

Also about age 12, the patient began to experience episodes of acute hepatic encephalopathy. The first of these episodes was the most severe. The patient entered the hospital in a confused and disoriented state with an elevated ammonia level. The immediate problem was easily controlled with neomycin (a nonabsorbable antibiotic that kills intestinal, ammonia-forming bacteria) enemas. During this admission, gastrointestinal bleeding developed, exacerbating the hyperammonemia (serum ammonia, 450 mg/dL). The patient gradually slipped into grade IV hepatic coma with fundoscopic changes consistent with increased intracranial pressure. *Coagulopathy* (an increased bleeding tendency) prevented the placement of an intracranial pressure monitor. He was treated empirically for presumed cerebral edema associated with acute hepatic encephalopathy with hyperventilation, a mannitol drip, and barbiturate coma. The patient recovered without neurological sequelae. Despite protein restriction (1.0 g protein per kilogram of body weight per day), the patient had two other milder episodes of hyperammonemia over that year, resulting in a trial of α-keto analogues of amino acids to treat his malnutrition. Although his condition improved, the role of this experimental therapy in his clinical course is unclear. The protocol under which the α-keto analogues were obtained expired without recurrence of the patient's hyperammonemia. He continued on limited protein intake, neomycin, and lactulose, with periodic monitoring for subclinical hepatic encephalopathy by electroencephalography.

Despite these disorders associated with his α_1-antitrypsin deficiency, he maintained an active life, attending school and camping with his parents. By the age of 16 his renal condition had deteriorated considerably, with a creatinine clearance of only 23 mL/min. He was therefore accepted as a candidate for a combined liver-kidney transplant. After a 2-year wait for an immunologically compatible donor, the transplant was successfully performed at age 18 years at the University of Minnesota Hospitals. He completed high school and is now employed full-time and in good health.

DIAGNOSIS

α_1-Antitrypsin is a circulating antiprotease controlled by codominant alleles. Homozygosity for an abnormal α_1-antitrypsin variant (the Z allele) predisposes individuals to lung, liver, and, less commonly, kidney disease. The preceding case report is typical of the most severe manifestations of this deficiency.

Whereas liver disease may become manifest at any age, from infancy to extreme old age, emphysema is unusual in childhood, presenting more commonly in the adult α_1-antitrypsin-deficient individual (Perlmutter and Pierce, 1983). Indeed, it represents the most common manifestation of the deficiency. The emphysema associated with α_1-antitrypsin deficiency (representing about 1% of all cases of emphysema) develops at a relatively early age with an equal distribution between men and women. Emphysema usually presents with shortness of breath (*dyspnea*) and

chronic cough. Pneumothorax may result from the bursting of an emphysematous bleb. The emphysema associated with α_1-antitrypsin deficiency is indistinguishable from nonfamilial forms, although chronic bronchitis and the associated cough occur less frequently than in other forms of emphysema. There is a wide range of disability associated with the pulmonary complications of α_1-antitrypsin deficiency, from completely asymptomatic individuals to chronic pulmonary cripples. Unfortunately, once emphysema becomes symptomatic in the α_1-antitrypsin-deficient individual, it usually pursues a relentless course.

Although the liver disease associated with α_1-antitrypsin deficiency may develop at any age, children usually have liver disease as their first manifestation of the disease. About 10 to 20% of PiZZ infants are first seen for neonatal *cholestatic* (failure of bile flow) liver disease. A child with α_1-antitrypsin deficiency may grow and develop normally for a while (this time varies with the individual patient) before manifesting the complications of cirrhosis. About 25% of children who initially develop cholestasis will recover and never experience further complications associated with chronic liver disease.

Clinically, cirrhosis associated with α_1-antitrypsin deficiency is similar to that seen in other forms of childhood liver disease. Malnutrition, coagulopathy, and complications of portal hypertension, including splenomegaly, variceal hemorrhage, and ascites, develop to a varying degree. In the absence of infection or an episode of dehydration, both of which may precipitate hepatic deterioration, a patient may survive for years with cirrhosis and adequate hepatic function. In α_1-antitrypsin deficiency, jaundice after 6 months of age is usually an ominous finding that suggests a significant deterioration in clinical status within a year. A decrease in hepatic synthetic capacity accompanies this deterioration, manifested by a decrease in coagulation factors synthesized by the liver.

Renal disease represents a rare clinical complication of this deficiency, resulting in massive protein loss, hypoalbuminemia, and renal failure. The kidney disease is an immunological disorder occurring only in patients with liver disease and resulting in a membranoproliferative glomerulonephritis with α_1-antitrypsin antigen present as well as complement and immunoglobulins. It should not be confused with the nonspecific spotty asymptomatic glomerulonephritis or hepatorenal syndrome commonly seen in cirrhosis.

In summary, three clinical situations should alert the clinician to the possibility of α_1-antitrypsin deficiency:

1. Cholestasis in infancy (see Fig. 25-2).
2. Cirrhosis of unproven etiology at any age.
3. Emphysema early in life, especially if predominantly basilar.

The diagnosis may first be suspected during direct observation of the cellulose acetate serum protein electrophoresis, in which the α_1-globulin band is small or undetectable in the α_1-antitrypsin-deficient person. Because α_1-antitrypsin represents 90%, of the total α_1-globulin peak, depression of this peak usually represents a deficiency of that protein. The trypsin-inhibitory capacity, a functional measure of the amount of trypsin inhibited by 1.0 mL of serum, and the α_1-antitrypsin level, measured by radial immunodiffusion assay, are both similarly depressed, usually to levels <40% of normal. Screening tests are not completely reliable, nor do they permit accurate genetic counseling; therefore, abnormal levels of α_1-antitrypsin on screening examination should lead to more specific diagnostic tests. The diagnostic test of choice is Pi typing, in which isoelectric focusing is used to separate the various α_1-antitrypsin species in the individual's serum by charge differences. Comparison with sera of known Pi type per-

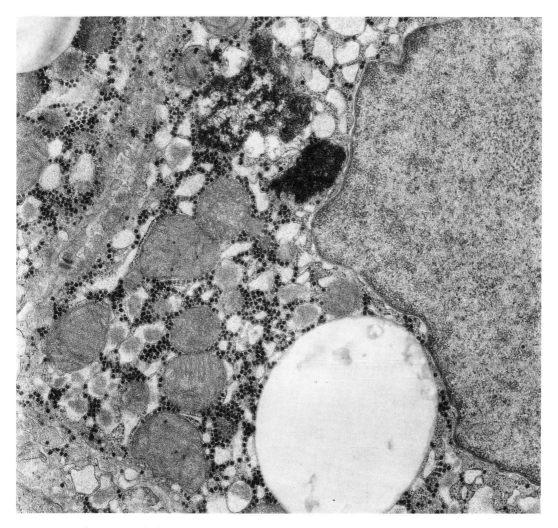

Figure 25-2. Photomicrograph of a portion of a hepatocyte from a cholestalic infant with PiZ phenotype. Amorphous α_1-antitrypsin (AT) in the transitional zone between rough and smooth endoplasmic reticulum. B, bile, T, triglyceride droplet.

mits identification of the phenotype of the individual.

Liver biopsy is important in the evaluation of α_1-antitrypsin-associated liver disease because it facilitates a more accurate prognosis. The patient with α_1-antitrypsin deficiency may have one of several histological pictures. In the neonate with α_1-antitrypsin deficiency, the liver may have evidence of fibrosis or cirrhosis, and some specimens will demonstrate a paucity of the intrahepatic bile ducts; however, the usual histological finding in the neonate is proliferation of the intrahepatic bile ducts simulating the histological picture of extrahepatic biliary *atresia* (absence of bile ducts). There are usually few giant cells (*multinucleated hepatocytes*) seen. α_1-Antitrypsin deficiency is therefore an important diagnosis to exclude in the evaluation of the child suspected of extrahepatic biliary atresia, as it may mimic this disease clinically and histologically. Patency of the extrahepatic biliary tree may be demonstrated by radionuclide scanning, detection of bile in duodenal contents, or cholangiography.

On light microscopy, PAS-positive, diastase-resistant globules representing the retained α_1-antitrypsin protein are found in periportal hepatocytes. These globules represent the abnormal α_1-antitrypsin not transported from the endoplasmic reticulum. These inclusions are fairly pathognomonic of the deficiency state and can be verified with α_1-antitrypsin antibody stains; they are also seen in heterozygote individuals (PiMZ).

Although the average child with α_1-antitrypsin deficiency needs no more pulmonary evaluation than careful periodic examinations, PiZZ individuals with symptomatic pulmonary disease require more specific evaluation. The first step in evaluating patients suspected of having emphysema is the chest roentgenogram, which may show hyperinflation, flattened diaphragms, the presence of bullae, and narrowing of the pulmonary arteries. As basal emphysema is more common in α_1-antitrypsin deficiency, the lower zones of the lungs are more commonly involved. Even with normal radiographic findings, pulmonary function tests may reveal early emphysematous changes. The α_1-antitrypsin-deficient patient may have a decrease in forced expiratory volume with an increase in total lung capacity and functional residual capacity. These findings are probably the results of a combination of obstructive lung disease with a decrease in the elasticity of the lung.

The patient in our case report illustrates the clinical presentation and course of α_1-antitrypsin deficiency. The spectrum of disease in α_1-antitrypsin deficiency is broad (Perlmutter, 1994); the patient presented has several of the manifestations of a disease with an insidious but progressive course. The differential diagnosis of this patient, at the age of diagnosis (about 3 years of age), would include chronic active hepatitis, congenital hepatic fibrosis, choledochal cyst, primary sclerosing cholangitis, and cystic fibrosis. One must always determine the α_1-antitrypsin level when confronted with chronic liver disease, with Pi typing, confirms, to confirm the diagnosis of α_1-antitrypsin deficiency.

MOLECULAR PERSPECTIVES

α_1-Antitrypsin is a 51,000-Da protein produced primarily by the hepatocyte, but it is also produced by macrophages and perhaps intestinal and kidney cells. The α_1-antitrypsin gene is 12.2 kb long and located on the long arm of chromosome 14. Sequence similarities to other serine protease inhibitors has established the existence of a large evolutionarily related gene family, including α_1-antichymotrypsin, antithrombin III, thyroid and corticosteroid binding proteins, and the protease nexins. The gene consists of seven exons and six introns. The protein is encoded by exons II–V, with the three small exons Ia, Ib, and Ic being transcribed but not translated. The transcriptional start site varies depending on the cell type in which transcription occurs.

The translation product of the α_1-antitrypsin gene contains a 24-amino acid peptide at the amino-terminus, which forms a leader sequence. The polypeptide is cotranslationally translocated to the endoplasmic reticulum where the signal peptide is cleaved and high mannose glycosylation residues are added. As the glycoprotein completes its transit through the endoplasmic reticulum to the Golgi apparatus, the terminal mannose residues of the oligosaccharide moities are cleaved and secondary glycosylation residues, including sialic acid, are added. The mature glycoprotein is packaged in the Golgi and secreted into the serum. The secreted protein contains variability in the secondary carbohydrate side chains, which produces a microheterogeneity, causing the glycoprotein to resolve into multiple bands when subjected to acid protein electrophoresis.

The function of this serine protease is to protect tissues from proteolytic enzymes released during the normal inflammatory response. Although α_1-antitrypsin has some activity against most serum proteases, inhibition of elastase by irreversible binding appears to be its primary role. This inhibition appears to result from an irreversible reaction between α_1-antitrypsin and elastase at the reactive center of the molecule, a methionine residue at position 358. Consistent with its function as an antiprotease, an increase in serum levels of α_1-antitrypsin occurs in inflammatory states, including malignancy, bacterial infections, and severe burns. It also rises during certain changes in hormonal conditions, as in pregnancy and during treatment with estrogen-containing birth control pills. The relative protein content of the various bands changes with inflammation, perhaps reflecting variability in the percentage of glycosylation. This may represent an adaptation permitting more rapid synthesis and secretion of α_1-antitrypsin in inflammation.

The Pi locus is highly pleomorphic, with more than 60 different alleles identified. The nomenclature of the Pi locus is based on the electrophoretic mobility of the various Pi types at pH 4.9. PiMM represents the homozygous normal allele; letters alphabetically before M designate anodal variants, and those after M designate cathodal variants. Null alleles also exist that produce no detectable serum α_1-antitrypsin. Most of these variant alleles produce no change in α_1-antitrypsin serum levels or function. As both alleles are expressed in codominantly controlled conditions, heterozygosity for the Pi locus may be identified electrophoretically. This is important for family studies of α_1-antitrypsin deficient patients. Identity of allelic variants may be confirmed by DNA sequencing.

Although many variant forms of the antiprotease exist, the most common alleles associated with deficiency are the S and Z variants, both producing proteins migrating cathodal to the normal protein. Homozygosity for these variants (PiZZ and PiSS genotypes), as well as compound heterozygosity (PiSZ), are all associated with deficient serum levels of α_1-antitrypsin. PiZZ individuals have about 10 to 20% of the normal level of α_1-antitrypsin, whereas PiSZ individuals have about 35% of the normal level.

The rare person with homozygosity or compound heterozygosity of the null gene with one of these alleles has severe deficiency.

These abnormal Pi alleles are most commonly found in individuals of European descent. Approximately 3% of Europeans are heterozygotes for the Z allele, whereas about 7% carry the S gene. The Z allele tends to be found more commonly in northern Europeans, whereas southern Europeans tend to have the S allele at a slightly higher frequency. The incidence of serious α_1-antitrypsin disease is about one in 2000 among persons of northern European extraction.

The Z variant, which has been studied most extensively, has a single base pair mutation, leading to the production of a protein in which lysine is substituted for glutamic acid at position 342. Primary glycosylation residues are added to the Z-variant polypeptide in the endoplasmic reticulum, but subsequent transport out of the endoplasmic reticulum is impaired. This trapping of the relatively insoluble Z-α_1 antitrypsin may be the result of the capacity of Z-α_1 antitrypsin to undergo spontaneous polymerization under nondenaturing conditions. Additionally, at least one α_1-antitrypsin variant, null$_{Hong Kong}$ (a truncated form which is retained similarly to Z-α_1 antitrypsin), is associated with the molecular chaperone, calnexin, which normally functions in protein folding. This latter observation may also explain the retention and degradation of Z-α_1 antitrypsin in the liver. The PiZZ individual has large amounts of intrahepatic α_1-antitrypsin protein that is not released into the circulation, thereby accounting for the markedly reduced serum levels of α_1 antitrypsin (Lomas et al., 1992). The Z protein that is released into the serum has the ability to inhibit elastase and has a half-life similar to that of the M protein. Carriers for this allele (PiMZ) have serum α_1-antitrypsin levels about 60% of normal, with small α_1-antitrypsin-containing globules visible in their hepatocytes. Other rare phenotypes associated with both low serum levels of α_1-antitrypsin and hepatic globules include PiM$_{Malton}$ and PiM$_{Duarte}$.

The S variant has a mutation at amino acid position 264, where valine is substituted for glutamic acid. The S-α_1-antitrypsin appears to have normal protease-inhibitory activity but is degraded intracellularly prior to secretion. The null alleles (PiQ) produce no immunologically or functionally active protein; there are several such allelic variants described, generally involving deletion of large portions of the α_1-antitrypsin gene.

Deficiency of α_1-antitrypsin produces an imbalance in the ratio of protease to protease inhibitor, resulting in emphysema (Perlmutter and Pierce, 1983). Both alveolar macrophages and polymorphonuclear leukocytes contain proteases, including collagenase and elastase. During the normal inflammatory response in the lung, as might occur with infection or cigarette smoking, these phagocytic cells migrate to the lung alveoli, releasing their proteases. Antiproteases in the lung of a normal person, including α_1-antitrypsin, would keep the activity of these agents localized to the site of the inflammation, allowing them to scavenge proteases and thereby protect alveolar tissue. In the lungs of PiZZ individuals, an imbalance exists in the ratio of protease to protease inhibitor. This deficiency is exacerbated by the inactivation of any α_1-antitrypsin present by oxidants released by neutrophils or cigarette smoke and by modification of α_1-antitrypsin function by neutrophilic proteases, which allows the proteases, particularly elastase, to attack the alveolar tissue, producing the emphysematous lesion.

Cigarette smoking markedly increases the risk of emphysema in PiZZ homozygotes. Cigarette smoke causes the release of neutrophil chemotactic factor, increasing the number of protease-containing neutrophils in the lung. Release of elastase from these cells is increased in the presence of cigarette smoke. Finally, as stated previously, cigarette smoke oxidizes the reactive-site methionine in α_1-antitrypsin, reducing its inhibitory capacity. In a study of 22 nonsmokers homozygous for α_1-antitrypsin deficiency living in areas free of urban air pollution, it was found that the onset of emphysema was later than in smokers (51.4 years for smokers compared with 71 years for nonsmokers). More nonsmokers were completely free of symptoms or had only mild symptoms in their sixth or seventh decades. Thus, emphysema associated with α_1-antitrypsin deficiency is not due simply to a genetic defect, but it requires an environmental stimulus as well.

The pathophysiology of liver disease associated with α_1-antitrypsin deficiency is not as well understood (Ibarquen et al., 1990). Studies in transgenic animals and clinical analysis of human disease suggest that the globules of Z-α_1-antitrypsin trapped in the endoplasmic reticulum of the liver are either directly damaging to the hepatocyte or facilitate damage by infection or toxins. The increased incidence of viral hepatitis documented in patients with heterozygous Z-α_1-antitrypsin deficiency and liver disease, however, suggests that the deficiency in protease inhibition may also contribute to the development of liver disease.

Many questions remain regarding α_1-antitrypsin-associated disease. The mechanism by which Z-α_1 antitrypsin globules injure or permit injury of the liver is unknown. The importance of α_1-antitrypsin in the regulation of other proteases deserves study; for example, the observation that α_1-antitrypsin participates in regulation of protein C raises questions about deficient persons. Clinical studies to explore the role of α_1-antitrypsin deficiency in lung disease in young patients and to compare liver disease in neonates and adults are important. Finally, clinical studies to explore the natural history of heterozygosity for α_1-antitrypsin and its effect on a person's health remain necessary.

THERAPY

Once emphysema develops, little specific therapy is available. Standard treatment of the patient with emphysema consists of supportive care, including early antibiotic treatment of all pulmonary infections. If, on pulmonary function testing, any reversibility of the airway obstruction can be effected with bronchodilators, these may be used. As the pathogenesis of α_1-antitrypsin deficiency-associated emphysema is related to cigarette smoking, it is important to counsel the patient to stop smoking. This is the only measure known to increase life expectancy for these patients.

Many attempts have been made to provide replacement therapy for α_1-antitrypsin-deficient individuals. Past studies using synthetic substitutes for α_1-antitrypsin have proved unsuccessful because of side effects associated with these compounds. Protocols for transfusion therapy have required large plasma volumes for treatment of each patient. Fractionation techniques have made it possible to recover active α_1-antitrypsin from blood. Use of this product for intravenous replacement therapy in deficient persons has shown that it is possible to increase levels in the serum to those of PiMZ heterozygotes; theoretically, such levels should protect against the development of emphysema. Pulmonary lavage of these patients showed that functional α_1-antitrypsin reaches the alveolar structures. Recombinant α_1-antitrypsin, now available, would reduce the risk of transfusion-related viral hepatitis. Studies have shown that the recombinant product can be administered as an aerosol. It diffuses across the respiratory epithelium, enters the lung lymph, and eventually reaches the systemic circulation. Unfortunately, it is not known whether these therapies have any influence on the development or progression of emphysema. Further carefully controlled, multicenter trials are necessary to answer this question before this therapy can be recommended for these patients.

Liver disease is managed conventionally, maintaining appropriate nutritional support and managing the complications of portal hypertension and hepatic failure as they occur. We counsel heterozygote parents of a PiZZ child to stop smoking cigarettes because of the danger passive cigarette smoke represents to the lungs of their PiZZ child. Definitive therapy of liver disease is limited to successful liver transplantation. There is no evidence of recurrence of liver disease after successful liver transplant. Theoretically, one would assume that liver transplantation, by changing the patient's Pi type, would prevent the development of lung disease; however, studies necessary to prove this hypothesis have not been done. The effect of α_1-antitrypsin replacement therapy on liver disease has not been studied.

Gene therapy offers the hope that the disease might eventually be completely controlled. The human α_1-antitrypsin gene has been successfully introduced into rat hepatocytes, which, when transplanted into a rat liver, expressed the protein in small quantities. This strategy would most likely be successful in preventing the development of emphysema; however, it is unclear whether it would cure the liver disease. If liver disease is dependent on the presence of unsecreted Z-α_1-antitrypsin, adding the normal α_1-antitrypsin gene would not stop its development or progression. Investigators in this field are working to develop techniques of targeted homologous recombination to replace completely the α_1-antitrypsin exon containing the PiZ mutation. Patients thus treated would express only the M-α_1-antitrypsin.

We recommended that all relatives of a patient

with α_1-antitrypsin deficiency be Pi-typed because relatives of the proband may have the PiZZ genotype. These patients may be free of disease at the time of discovery but may have clinically unsuspected PiZZ liver or lung disease. For future counseling of the family, it is important to identify the Pi type of the patient accurately and to identify heterozygotes. Although measurement of α_1-antitrypsin immunogenically or functionally is accurate, there may be some difficulty identifying PiMZ heterozygotes with these methods because they have α_1-antitrypsin levels that may rise to normal levels during inflammation. One must therefore rely on Pi typing, which should be done by an institution familiar with the many α_1-antitrypsin alleles.

Until recently, the only method of *in utero* diagnosis available to families in which both parents were heterozygotes was fetoscopy with fetal blood sampling. Although reliable, this method was dangerous to the fetus. Prenatal diagnosis can now be done on fibroblasts collected by amniocentesis or by chorionic villus biopsy by polymerase chain reaction amplification and analysis of the mutated region of the gene. Thus, it is now possible to offer parents low-risk early diagnosis of α_1-antitrypsin deficiency *in utero*.

Counseling of the families of a PiZZ person requires a careful explanation of the principles of codominant inheritance. Parents who are both PiMZ heterozygotes have a one in four risk of having a PiZZ child in any subsequent pregnancy. Unfortunately, it is not possible to predict whether a PiZZ child will be among the 10 to 15% of PiZZ individuals with early liver disease. Thus, the family's decision to undergo *in utero* diagnosis of α_1-antitrypsin deficiency is a complex one.

QUESTIONS

1. Describe a possible clinical course for the patient described in the case report in the perinatal period.
2. The mother of the child in the case report was PiMZ. Discuss the likely results of a serum trypsin-inhibitory assay and a liver biopsy in the mother. If her trypsin inhibitory capacity was found to be 75% of normal, how would you explain it?
3. If the parents of the proband sought genetic counseling from you in a subsequent pregnancy, what information would you give them?

4. If a drug existed that specifically stimulated the transcription of mRNA for α_1-antitrypsin in the liver, would this be a reasonable therapy for PiZZ individuals? Why or why not? Would your recommendation be different for the PiSS patient?
5. As the patient described reaches maturity, what would your recommendation be for his future career? Why?

REFERENCES

Ibarguen E, Gross CR, Savik SK, Sharp HL: Liver disease in alpha-1-antitrypsin deficiency: Prognostic indicators. *J Pediatr* **117**:864–870, 1990.

Lomas DA, Evans DL, Finch JT, Carrell RW: The mechanism of Z α_1-antitrypsin accumulation in the liver. *Nature* **357**: 605–607, 1992.

Perlmutter DH: The SEC receptor: A possible link between neonatal hepatitis in α_1-antitrypsin deficiency and Alzheimer's disease. *Pediatr Res* **36**:271–277, 1994.

Perlmutter DH, Pierce JA: The α_1-antitrypsin gene and emphysema. *Am J Physiol* **257**:L147–L162, 1983.

26

Gaucher Disease: A Sphingolipidosis

JOHN K. SCARIANO AND ROBERT H. GLEW

CASE REPORT

The patient is a 34-year-old woman of Ashkenazic Jewish ancestry. On admission to the hospital at age 4 years (September 1967), a bone marrow biopsy revealed the presence of Gaucher cells (Fig. 26-1), and she was diagnosed as having Gaucher disease. White blood cell (WBC) β-glucosidase assays were performed on the patient and her immediate family members in December 1973. Her parents and only sibling had heterozygote levels of WBC β-glucosidase; the patient's β-glucosidase value was only 19% of the control mean level, confirming the diagnosis of Gaucher disease on a biochemical-enzymatic basis. In addition, she was found to have an elevated level of serum acid phosphatase (ACP) activity, which is also a characteristic of Gaucher disease patients.

At age 15 years, splenomegaly had greatly extended into the pelvis and right lower quadrant of the abdomen; she underwent splenectomy in June 1978 for persistent *thrombocytopenia* (low platelet count). Her spleen weighted 2070 g (normal range, 100–170 g). Biopsies of lymph nodes and liver revealed the presence of Gaucher cells. Following splenectomy, her platelet count rose from 80×10^9 to 291×10^9/L (normal range, 140×10^9–440×10^9/L), and her hemoglobin had increased from 12.5 to 15.0 g/dL (normal range, 13.5–16.0 g/dL).

Following splenectomy, she did extremely well until August 1978, when she noticed pain in her left hip. She subsequently developed a limp on the left side and resorted to the use of crutches to minimize the pressure placed on the left hip. Even with the use of crutches, however, she continued to have pain when walking. Prolonged sitting also caused her discomfort, particularly when rising. Radiological examination (Fig. 26-2) revealed the classic picture of Gaucher disease osteonecrosis of the left hip, with significant collapse of the head of the femur. In May 1983 she elected to undergo hip replacement surgery. The patient underwent resection of the left femoral head and insertion of a total hip replacement device and acetabular implant. Radiographic examination in 1990 demonstrated evidence of a bone marrow-expanding disease that included diffuse marrow replacement in the right knee. Surgery to replace the acetabulum of the left hip was performed in March 1990.

Starting in June 1990, the patient was administered Ceredase (the commercial name of a glucocerebrosidase preparation) at a dosage of 15 U/kg every 2 weeks. In September, when it was determined that the patient's insurance company was willing to provide coverage for enzyme replacement therapy, the dosage was increased to 30 U/kg every 2 weeks. Four months later, although the patient's hematological parameters (hemoglobin, hematocrit, and platelet count) had improved somewhat, they had not normalized. Nevertheless, she reported increased stamina and a sense of well-being following Ceredase administration. The regimen was changed to 15 U/kg every week in an attempt to reduce fluctuations in the patient's energy level. One year later, in February 1992, the dosing schedule was altered to 7.5 U/kg twice per week in an effort to

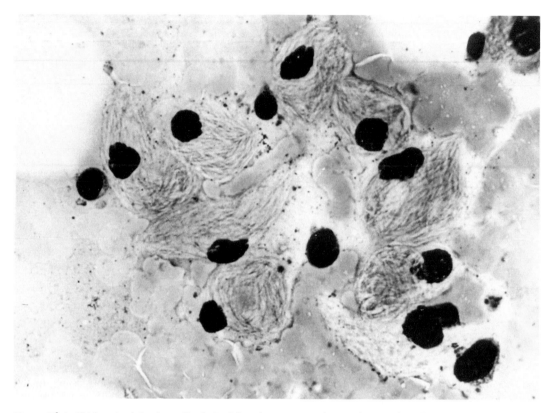

Figure 26-1. Wright-stained Gaucher cells obtained from bone marrow showing the typical wrinkled appearance of the cytoplasm. ($\times$ 175).

maintain more consistently the patient's stamina level. In June the dosage was decreased by half, which resulted 3 months later in the patient reporting increased fatigue. At that time, an indwelling catheter was placed in the patient as a port for providing venous access, and her dosage was increased to 5.5 U/kg twice a week.

The patient experienced several bone crises during the first year of treatment, but the duration and intensity were less severe than before enzyme replacement. Following the first year of treatment, a progressive reduction in bone pain was noted. With subsequent attempts to titrate down the Ceredase dosage, the patient reported a gradual return of bone pain. She also felt less energetic. These symptoms decreased after her dosage was returned to 11 U/kg every week. As shown in Table 26-1, over the

Table 26-1. Therapeutic Response to Enzyme Replacement Therapy

Therapeutic Response	December 1988	October 1992
Liver volume (cc)	3151	2271
RBC count (10^6/mm³)	3.87	4.67
Hemoglobin (g/dL)	12.4	13.9
Hematocrit (%)	36.8	42.6
MCV (fL)	95	91
Platelet count (10^3/mm³)	133	326
MPV (fL)	10.3	93.0

RBC, red blood cells; MCV, mean cell volume; MPV, mean platelet volume.

course of 4 years of treatment there was an improvement in the patient's hematological indices, including significant increases in platelet count and size. Furthermore, there was a notable reduction of liver volume.

Figure 26-2. Radiograph of the patient's normal-appearing hip taken in 1979 (**a**) and a collapsed and necrotic left femoral head in 1983 (**b**).

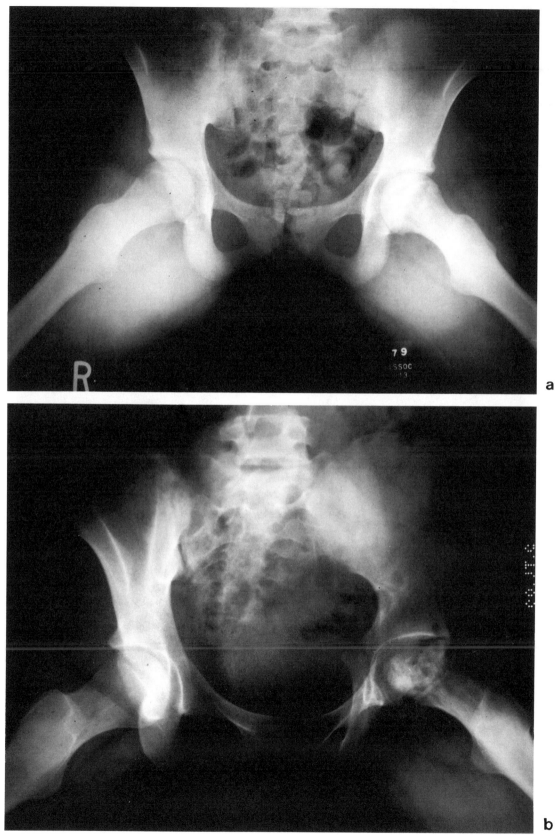

a

b

DIAGNOSIS

The diagnosis of Gaucher disease is most often confirmed by a pathologist who identifies the highly characteristic "Gaucher cells" in a stained aspirate of bone marrow. Gaucher cells, which are pathognomonic for Gaucher disease, are mononuclear cells of the macrophage-reticuloendothelial system (Figs. 26-1 and 26-3). They occur in abundance in sites of the reticuloendothelial system, namely, the spleen, liver, and bone marrow, and elsewhere in small numbers, usually in the lymph nodes and lungs. In the neurological forms of Gaucher disease, these unique storage cells are found in the brain as well as in the visceral organs and are located primarily in perivascular areas of the brain. When stained with the Wright stain, Gaucher cells appear as large cells with an abundant cytoplasm that has the appearance of wrinkled tissue paper. The nucleus is usually oval and positioned eccentrically. The wrinkled, striated appearance of the cytoplasm is due to the accumulation of the glucocerebrosidase-rich storage material

referred to as *Gaucher deposits* (Fig. 26-1) (Brady and Barranger, 1983). The diagnosis of Gaucher disease, as well as the identification of asymptomatic heterozygous carriers, can be confirmed biochemically on the basis of enzyme assays (Glew et al., 1982; Glew et al., 1985).

Two enzyme abnormalities of diagnostic value are seen in patients with Gaucher disease: a marked deficiency in tissue glucocerebrosidase and an elevation in serum ACP. The elevation in ACP activity occurs in most but not all cases of Gaucher disease; therefore, the diagnosis of Gaucher disease cannot be ruled out based only on the serum ACP value being in the normal range. Nevertheless, the finding of an elevated serum ACP value should heighten suspicion of Gaucher disease (actually, 95% of Gaucher disease patients exhibit an elevated serum ACP value).

In addition to the fact that the serum ACP value is not always increased in Gaucher disease, another reason not to use this procedure to make a definitive diagnosis is that the test is not specific for Gaucher

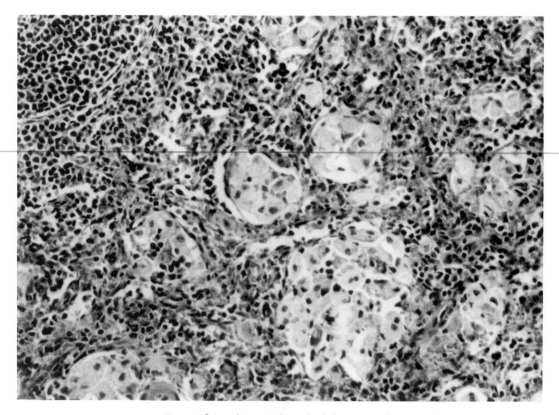

Figure 26-3. Splenic Gaucher cells, light micrograph.

disease; sera from persons with other lysosomal storage diseases (e.g., Niemann-Pick disease) also contain elevated serum levels of ACP activity.

On occasion, the bone marrow aspiration procedure provides no sample (a "dry" tap) or the aspirate contains limited numbers of Gaucher cells, which can obscure the diagnosis. Additionally, bone marrow aspiration provides no information regarding the carrier state of the individual. Consequently, the definitive biochemical test for Gaucher disease is the glucocerebrosidase determination. Two different β-glucoside substrates are used for this purpose: the natural substrate, glucocerebroside; and the artificial, nonphysiological substrate, 4-methylumbelliferyl-β-D-glucopyranoside (MUGlc). Although the assay can be performed on any tissue, the tissues of choice are peripheral blood leukocytes, which can be isolated conveniently in less than 2 hours by a dextran-settling procedure, and cultured fibroblasts grown from a punch biopsy of the skin. The antenatal diagnosis of Gaucher disease can also be performed, in which case one cultures amnion cells obtained by amniocentesis.

In the case of the glucocerebroside-dependent assay, it is convenient to use [³H]-glucocerebroside labeled in the glucose moiety. In the reaction below, the substrate, [³H]-glucocerebroside, is soluble in chloroform and insoluble in water, while the radiolabeled product of the reaction, [³H]-glucose, is water-soluble:

$$[^3H]\text{-Glucocerebroside} + H_2O \rightarrow [^3H]\text{-glucose} + \text{ceramide}$$

After incubating the substrate and tissue extract at 37°C in the appropriate buffer (0.2 *M* sodium acetate, pH 5.5) and in the presence of some activator lipid (e.g., sodium taurocholate, 2% wt/vol), the reaction is terminated by extraction of the incubation medium with CHCl₃-methanol (2:1 vol/vol); the top layer (the water phase) containing [³H]-glucose is counted in a liquid scintillation spectrometer to give a measure of the extent of reaction. Extracts from tissues from persons with Gaucher disease will usually generate <10% as much [³H]-glucose as controls.

Because most clinical laboratories find it inconvenient to use the radiolabeled authentic substrate assay, investigators have established β-glucosidase assay conditions that allow estimation of the relative

glucocerebrosidase content of human tissues when nonphysiological β-glucosides serve as the glucocerebrosidase substrate. The artificial substrate of choice, and the one in widest use today, is MUGlc, which is cleaved by lysosomal glucocerebrosidase, the deficient enzyme in Gaucher disease (Daniels and Glew, 1982). This substrate is nonfluorescent, but one of the products of the reaction, 4-methylumbelliferone, is intensely fluorescent at alkaline pH (Fig. 26-4). Thus, the extent of reaction can be estimated by determining the quantity of fluorescence generated by a particular tissue extract using a fluorimeter and a standard solution of 4-methylumbelliferone for calibration purposes.

Unfortunately, however, a second β-glucosidase is present in most human tissues, particularly leukocytes. The problem is that this second β-glucosidase does not cleave glucocerebroside and is not deficient in most cases of Gaucher disease, but it does cleave the artificial substrate MUGlc. Fortunately, the inclusion of bile salts like sodium taurodeoxycholate in the assay medium inhibits the activity of the second β-glucosidase, while stimulating the activity of lysosomal glucocerebrosidase. Thus, the nonphysiologic β-glucoside can be used to estimate the relative glucocerebrosidase content of leukocytes and fibroblasts.

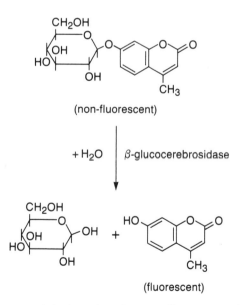

CH₂OH

(non-fluorescent)

+ H₂O | β-glucocerebrosidase

CH₂OH

(fluorescent)

Figure 26-4. The β-glucoside reaction illustrating using the artificial substrate MUGlc. 4-methyl-β-D-glucopyranoside (MUGlc).

It should be emphasized that although the glucocerebroside-dependent glucocerebrosidase and MUGlc-β-glucosidase assays have proved 100% effective in diagnosing Gaucher disease, neither assay has been completely reliable in identifying Gaucher disease heterozygotes; experience has shown that about one of every 10 obligate heterozygotes will be incorrectly assigned to the "control" category.

Molecular diagnosis of Gaucher disease relies on the identification of mutations within the glucocerebrosidase gene. An extract of DNA from leukocytes of afflicted patients is often amplified by means of the polymerase chain reaction, and alterations may be identified on sequencing the complete cDNA. Analysis of restriction length fragment polymorphism is particularly useful in detecting the ⁴⁴⁴Leu→Pro mutant, as this substitution creates an additional cleavage site for two restriction endonucleases. A newer and clever method uses an amplification refractory system based on allele-specific or sequence-specific oligonucleotide primers. In this methodology, the polymerase chain reaction will not occur unless a sequence of defined specificity is present on the gene. It is possible to design appropriate primers that are specific for any characterized mutation.

MOLECULAR PERSPECTIVES

Gaucher disease is the most common of the sphingolipidoses, a group of related genetic diseases that result from the impaired lysosomal enzyme function. Figure 26-5 shows the relationships among the lysosomal enzymes that constitute the pathway of sphingolipid catabolism. The substrates and products that constitute the pathway are linked by a series of irreversible reactions that remove a sugar moiety, a sulfate residue, or a fatty acid; all these reactions are hydrolytic, and the product of one reaction becomes the substrate for the next enzyme in the sequence. In the case of sugar residues, the oligosaccharide domains are disassembled by removing the monosaccharides one at a time from the nonreducing end of the sugar chain. All reaction sequences converge on ceramide, which is degraded in turn by an amidase called *ceramidase*.

The lysosomal hydrolases occur in two places in the organelle; some, like glucocerebrosidase, are firmly associated with the lysosomal membrane, whereas others, like hexoseaminidase A, exist largely in soluble form in the lysosomal matrix. All the enzymes that constitute the sphingolipid-catabolic pathway are glycoproteins.

Another common property of the lysosomal hydrolases is that they exhibit maximum activity at a relatively acid pH (i.e., pH 4.0–5.5), hence the term *acid hydrolase*. The presence of an adenosine triphosphate (ATP) driven proton pump maintains the internal milieu of the lysosomes of most cells at or near pH 5.2.

With these general comments, let us return to Gaucher disease specifically. All tissues of the patient under discussion, like every patient with Gaucher disease, are markedly deficient in lysosomal glucocerebrosidase activity. Glucocerebrosidase normally catalyzes the reaction shown in Figure 26-6. As a result of insufficient glucocerebrosidase activity, the substrate for the deficient enzyme accumulates in cells where glucocerebroside precursors are being catabolized. The patient in the case report had only about one-fifth the normal amount of glucocerebrosidase. Most of the glucocerebrosidase stored in the liver, spleen, and bone marrow is derived from the catabolism of membranes of WBC and red blood cells (RBC). Most WBC have a short life span and are degraded in macrophages of the reticuloendothelial (macrophage) system. Membrane sphingolipids of senescent RBC also contribute glucocerebroside precursors to the sphingolipid-catabolic pathway. In Gaucher disease, as the oligosaccharide chains of the sphingolipids are catabolized, metabolism is aborted at the level of glucocerebroside and the lipid molecules self-associate to form bilayers, which in turn stack up as membranous sheets. Because of the insolubility of glucocerebroside in water and body fluids, the lipid cannot be readily excreted in the urine, and only a relatively low rate of excretion occurs by way of the hepatic-biliary route. Thus, glucocerebroside molecules aggregate in the lysosomes of cells where they are generated, (Fig. 26-7) and, in the case of spleen and liver, give rise to splenomegaly and hepatomegaly. The enlarged spleen and liver destroy RBC, WBC, and platelets prematurely, thereby contributing to the anemia, leukopenia, and thrombocytopenia, respectively, that are common in patients with Gaucher disease.

The storage cells in the bone marrow have a myelophthisic effect; that is, they crowd out the normal hematopoietic tissues. As a result of Gaucher

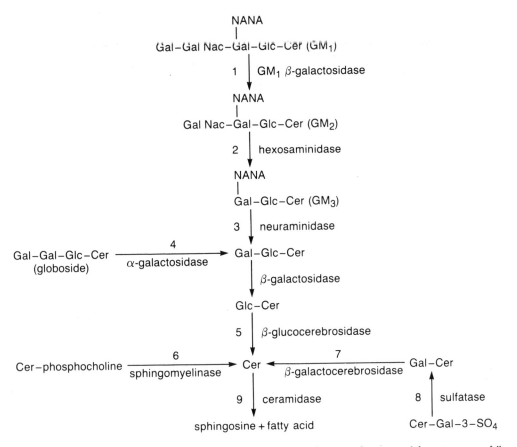

Figure 26-5. The pathway of sphingolipid catabolism. Diseases that result from specific enzyme deficiencies are as follows: (1) GM, gangliosidosis; (2) GM$_2$ gangliosidosis (Tay-Sachs disease); (3) sialidosis; (4) Fabrys disease; (5) Gauchers disease; (6) Niemann-Picks disease; (7) Krabbes disease; (8) metachromatic leukodystrophy; (9) Farbers disease. Cer, Ceramide; Glc, glucose; Gal, galactose; GalNAc, N-acetylgalactosamine; NANA, N-acetylneuraminic acid.

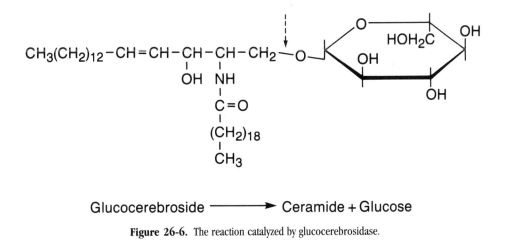

Figure 26-6. The reaction catalyzed by glucocerebrosidase.

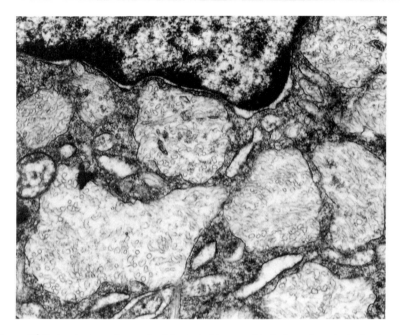

Figure 26-7. An electron micrograph of the typical lysosomal inclusions of a splenic Gaucher cell.

cell accumulation in the bone marrow, Gaucher patients often suffer from skeletal involvement; this includes frequent fractures and bone and joint pain, particularly in the femur, and is accompanied by swelling and tenderness of the surrounding tissue. Osteonecrosis and collapse of the femoral head occur in many patients, often severe enough to require hip replacement surgery, as exemplified by the subject of the case report. Frequently seen in younger patients undergoing rapid bone growth is the "Erlenmeyer flask" deformity, which arises from expansion of the cortex of the distal femur (Hill et al., 1993).

Patients suffering from Gaucher disease are usually placed in one of three clinical subtypes (Table 26-2). Type 1, the form of the disease originally described by Gaucher, is also termed *adult form* or *chronic nonneuropathic* Gaucher disease. The adult form of the disease usually follows a chronic, progressive course characterized by hepatosplenomegaly, anemia, thrombocytopenia, and erosion of the long bones. The range of clinical severity is great; some patients suffer intensely before their third decade of life, whereas others remain undiagnosed into their sixth or seventh decade of life. Chronic nonneuropathic Gaucher disease, which is distinguished from the types 2 and 3 forms of the disease by the lack of neurological involvement in these patients, is detected most frequently in members of the Ash-

Table 26-2. Clinical Features of the Gaucher Phenotypes

Clinical Features	Type 1	Type 2	Type 3
Onset	Child/adult	Infancy	Juvenile
Hepatosplenomegaly	+	+	+
Hypersplenism	+	+	+
Bone crises/fractures	+	−	+
Neurodegenerative course	−	+++	++
Death	Childhood	<2 yrs.	3rd to 4th decade
Ethnic predilection	Ashkenazic	Panethnic	Swedish (Norrbottnian)

kenazic Jewish population, occurring at a rate of 1 in 2500.

The patient described in the present report has the type 1 form of Gaucher disease and is spared central nervous system (CNS) involvement. In infants with the type 2 form of the disease, often referred to as *malignant, infantile,* or *acute neuropathic* Gaucher disease, the brain contains Gaucher cells and CNS involvement is extensive. These infants usually die before the age of 2 years. Type 2 Gaucher disease is characterized by neurological involvement, failure to thrive, *strabismus* (lack of parallelism of the visual axes of the eyes), muscle hypertonicity (*spasticity*), and retroflexion of the head. Type 3 Gaucher disease is referred to as the *juvenile,* or *subacute neuropathic* form. Although type 3 patients usually live longer than type 2 patients, they, too, suffer from neurological involvement. Gaucher cells are present in neuronal and nonneuronal tissues from type 3 patients, whose condition, while similar to that of type 2 patients, is usually less severe.

The accumulation of storage lipid in lysosome-rich cells of the reticuloendothelial system produces secondary effects, one of which is the elevated ACP activity usually seen in the blood of patients with Gaucher disease. As the lysosomes become progressively engorged with glucocerebroside, they eventually rupture and spill their contents into the blood.

Because glucocerebrosidase is firmly embedded in the lysosomal membrane, solubilization requires extraction with detergents such as Triton X-100 or bile salts (e.g., sodium cholate). Subsequent separation of enzyme protein and detergents using a butanol-extraction step renders glucocerebrosidase soluble in aqueous media and also removes endogenous, natural lipid activators, such that demonstration of activity *in vitro* now requires inclusion of some phospholipid or bile salt in the assay medium (Basu and Glew, 1984; Basu et al., 1984).

Glucocerebrosidase has a subunit molecular weight (MW) of ~67,000, and these inactive subunits have a tendency to aggregate into catalytically active dimers, tetramers, and even larger forms. Its pH optimum is in the range of 5.0 to 5.8, and the specific activity of the enzyme depends on the nature of the lipid activator used in the assay. Glucocerebrosidase has a rather strict specificity for β-D-glucosides; it will cleave the glucose moiety from glucocerebroside as

well as from nonphysiological substrates like MUGlc and *p*-nitrophenyl-β-D-glucopyranoside, but it has little or no activity toward β-D-galactosides or β-D-xylosides. When nonphysiological β-D-glucoside substrates are used, the activity measured is referred to as *β-glucosidase activity.*

With regard to activators of catalytic activity, glucocerebrosidase is particularly responsive to acidic lipids and an 11,000 MW heat-stable glycoprotein referred to historically as *heat-stable factor* (HSF) and more recently as *sphingolipid activator protein* (SAP). The membrane lipids that are most effective in reconstituting glucocerebrosidase are acidic phospholipids, like phosphatidylserine and phosphatidylinositol, and gangliosides, like GM_1. These acidic lipids activate glucocerebrosidase by increasing the maximum velocity (V_{max}) and decreasing the Michaelis constant (K_m), and, at least in dilute aqueous buffers, activation is associated with conversion of the enzyme from a low to a high molecular weight form.

In terms of molecular genetics, the human glucocerebrosidase gene is located within band q21 of the long arm of chromosome 1. It consists of 7604 base pairs (bp) that reside in 11 exons that are separated by 10 introns (Fig. 26-8). A consensus sequence representing an inducible promoter occurs immediately upstream of two independent start codons. The 5.6 kilobase (kb) primary transcript is processed and translated into a polypeptide containing 497 amino acids, with an approximate molecular mass of 67,000 Da. Five consensus sequences for *N*-linked oligosaccharide chain glycosylation sites (Asn-X-Ser or Asn-X-Thr) are present in the primary structure of the enzyme, four of which are occupied by complex-type oligosaccharide chains containing mannose, fucose, galactose, *N*-acetylglucosamine, and sialic acid (Fig. 26-9). The active site of glucocerebrosidase is localized to the carboxyl terminal region of the enzyme and is coded for by exons IX and X. Aspartate[443] participates in the catalysis of glucocerebroside hydrolysis; this corresponds to base 1448 in the cDNA sequence.

A glucocerebrosidase pseudogene is located 16 kb downstream from the functional gene. Although it has many sizable intronic and exonic deletions and contains several nonsense and missense point mutations, it is actively transcribed from a weak promoter but not expressed. Genomic DNA from Gaucher patients, which codes for dysfunctional glucocerebro-

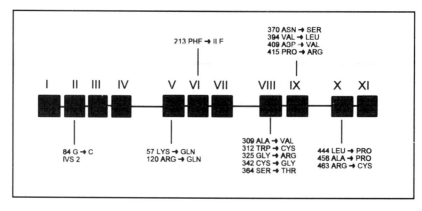

Figure 26-8. Sites of mutations in six of the 11 exons (Roman numerals) of the human glucocerebrosidase gene.

sidases, frequently includes mutations constitutively present in the pseudogene, suggesting recombination as a cause of some forms of the disease.

To date, 36 different alleles have been associated with Gaucher disease, including both *private* (unique) and *public* (common) mutations. *Homoallelic* disease is the result of inheriting precisely the same mutation from both parents. *Heteroallelic,* or complex, defects arise when an alteration in one allele coexists with a different mutation (or mutations) in the corresponding allele. Interestingly, the heteroallelic, or complex, genotypes are frequently correlated to severe forms of the disease, especially the neuronopathic phenotypes; For example; alterations of amino acids in positions 409, 444, and 456 in one allele, coexisting with a mutation of amino acid 444 in the other allele, is common in type 2

disease (Brady et al., 1993). Nonsense mutations that shift the reading frame of the gene or destroy recognition sites for mRNA processing ribonucleoproteins also produce more often the serious expressions of the disease; these kinds of mutations are exclusively heteroallelic. Homoallelic nonsense mutations would give rise to a null phenotype, a complete absence of functional glucocerebrosidase, and most likely would result in death *in utero*.

One or more of three aberrations account for 80% of the mutations in Gaucher patients. The most commonly encountered alteration is a missense point mutation in which guanine is substituted for adenine at position 1226 in exon IX of the cDNA sequence (Fig. 26-8); this results in replacement of an asparagine by a serine residue at amino acid position 370. Type 1 patients who are homoallelic for this mutation have relatively mild disease, and, with the exception of slight splenomegaly, many are relatively asymptomatic. If a type 1 patient manifests the mutation in a complex or heteroallelic form, the disease is more severe and progressive, but neurological complications do not occur. Of particular interest is the observation that the presence of a single [370]Asn→Ser substitution in one allele precludes the development of primary CNS involvement, no matter what mutation is present in the complementary allele. It seems that the level of residual catalytic activity of this mutant glucocerebrosidase is sufficient to metabolize glucocerebroside and prevent its accumulation in the brain but is insufficiently high to metabolize the larger quantities of glucocerebroside generated from leukocyte and erythrocyte turnover in the spleen.

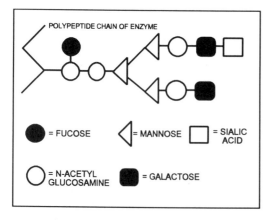

Figure 26-9. Schematic representation of the complex *N*-linked oligosaccharides contained in glucocerebrosidase.

Another common mutation involves the substitution of cytosine for thymine at nucleotide 1448 in the cDNA, causing proline to be substituted for leucine at amino acid position 444 precisely within the active site region of the enzyme. It is thought that such a substitution affects substrate binding in the catalytic center. This mutation is homoallelic in the rare Norrbottnian variant of the disease (type 3) and also in Japanese patients with type 1 Gaucher disease.

A frameshift mutation (84GC) involving the insertion of an extra guanine residue at cDNA nucleotide position 84 truncates the protein on translation (Fig. 26-8). Alternatively, a missense mutation localized in the boundary region between intron II and exon II, (IVSG$^+$ A$^+$) causes the loss of a splicing donor recognition site for mRNA processing. This alteration is common among the Ashkenazic Gaucher population. The 84GC, and IVSG$^+$ A$^+$ mutations are exclusively heteroallelic (Beutler, 1993).

THERAPY

Before the successful implementation of enzyme replacement therapy was initiated in 1990, which has dramatically improved the quality of life for many suffering from Gaucher disease, the therapy, like that of the other sphingolipidoses, remained largely supportive, aimed at lessening the impact of the various manifestations of the disease process. Because the splenomegaly associated with Gaucher disease often results in anemia and thrombocytopenia, the latter placing the individual at risk for bleeding diathesis, splenectomy was eventually performed on almost all patients. Although some physicians contend that postponing splenectomy as long as possible reduces the age of onset and rate of development of bone and liver involvement, there is little evidence to support this position. Surgical intervention, for example, the implantation of a hip prosthesis in the woman discussed in this chapter, often results in decreased bone pain and increased mobility. Six years after her left hip was reconstructed, the patient's artificial hip is functioning well and she is free of pain at the site.

In 1966, just a year or two after the enzymatic basis of Gaucher disease was identified, Brady and co-workers proposed a novel protocol for treating the disease, namely, the intravenous infusion of exogenous glucocerebrosidase. Eight years later, the earliest attempts at enzyme supplementation were undertaken using native glucocerebrosidase purified from human placenta. Despite the modest reductions in plasma and hepatic glucocerebroside levels that were achieved with a single infusion of glucocerebrosidase, the outcome of the initial treatment was disappointing because the infused enzyme did not effectively penetrate into the affected cells (i.e., macrophages) where the offending glycolipid is stored. The principal obstacle was the rapid clearance of the infused enzyme from the circulation via selective uptake by hepatocytes. Because glucocerebroside accumulates in the reticuloendothelial system of patients with Gaucher disease, a strategy was needed to target the placental enzyme specifically to macrophages (Brady and Furbish, 1982). At about the same time, lectin-like receptors on the plasma membrane of macrophages were identified that selectively bind glycoproteins whose oligosaccharide chains terminate in α-linked mannose residues. It was subsequently shown that macrophages use a receptor-mediated endocytotic mechanism to internalize glycoproteins that contain exposed mannose residues at the nonreducing ends of their oligosaccharide chains. Hepatocytes, in contrast, express surface receptors that bind galactose-terminated glycoproteins (Furbish et al., 1981).

Native placental glucocerebrosidase contains four oligosaccharide chains, all of which terminate with sialic acid (Fig. 26-9). To optimize glucocerebrosidase uptake by macrophages, the enzyme must be treated sequentially with neuraminidase, β-galactosidase and β-N-acetylglucosaminidase, a process that results in the exposure of mannose residues (Barton and Brady, 1991).

In the early 1990s, macrophage-targeted glucocerebrosidase supplementation proved to be a highly effective and safe therapy for most cases of Gaucher disease. Several accounts describe a gradual resolution of the clinical features of the disease, an overall decrease in lipid accumulation in organs and the circulation, and a dramatic improvement in the quality of life of the patients (Parker et al., 1991). No adverse effects following treatment were reported. As seen in Table 26-1, the patient in the present report showed improvement in hematological parameters and a significant reduction in liver volume after enzyme replacement therapy.

A typical therapeutic regimen involves biweekly infusion of 60 IU of macrophage-targeted glucocerebrosidase per kilogram of body weight administered intravenously over 9 to 12 months to types 1 and 3 Gaucher patients who still have their spleens intact. To treat the more severe forms of the disease, a weekly infusion regimen is advised. In most cases, therapy results in a significant decrease in splenic volume and in the level of circulating glucocerebroside. Generalized improvement in hematologic variables follows clearance of Gaucher cell infiltrates from the bone marrow. In a few subjects there is slow and partial recovery from skeletal complications. Patients gain weight, grow taller, and experience increased vigor, decreased bone pain, satiety, and chronic fatigue. Normalization of hematological parameters occurs after 3 to 4 months of enzyme supplementation, including elevations in hemoglobin concentration and platelet count, an increase in the survival time of autologous labeled red blood cells, and decreased percentage of reticulocytes. Clearance of Gaucher infiltrates from the bone marrow, and as much as a 60% reduction of splenic volume is thought to underlie the basis of such changes. Analysis of bone marrow aspirates of patients receiving enzyme supplementation therapy reveals qualitative changes in Gaucher cells, specifically a reduction in size and a decrease in lipid content. Amelioration of hematological variables is dose-dependent; discontinuing therapy causes the hematological indices to revert to pretreatment values.

The cost of treating a single patient with glucocerebrosidase is several hundred thousand dollars per year, raising several concerns regarding compensation because insurance plans may refuse to authorize coverage. Such a prohibitive cost often places a severe financial burden on patients in this country and makes enzyme replacement therapy in less developed nations an impossibility.

Human cDNA containing the glucocerebrosidase gene was recently overexpressed in Chinese hamster ovary (CHO) cells, providing a source of enzyme that is free of potentially pathogenic contaminants (it takes tons of placental tissue per year to purify therapeutic quantities of enzyme). Because CHO cells are eukaryotic, they synthesize fully glycosylated forms of glycoproteins. A double-blind, random parallel trial of the placental-derived and CHO-expressed recombinant glucocerebrosidase demonstrated no significant differences in clinical efficacy or cost between the two sources; however, there was a 20% higher occurrence of anti-glucocerebrosidase immunoglob-

ulin G antibodies in the sera of patients receiving the placental enzyme. This increase may be a result of increased denaturing of the protein, which occurs in the many organic solvent extraction steps required to purify the placental enzyme (Grabowski et al., 1995).

A formidable challenge remains in targeting glucocerebrosidase to the involved cells in the CNS of patients with type 2 disease. Intraventricular infusion and temporary alteration of the blood–brain barrier have been suggested, but at this time no effective delivery strategy has yet been formulated for the neuronopathic Gaucher phenotype.

QUESTIONS

1. What are some of the ethical questions that would arise if: (a) one attempted to implement a screening program to detect carriers of Gaucher disease that employed a biochemical test with a diagnostic specificity of 0.95? (b) A woman was encouraged to undergo amniocentesis to determine if the fetus was affected?
2. How would you go about determining the nature of the phospholipid in the lysosomal membrane that is the true *in vivo* activator of glucocerebrosidase?
3. What is the cause of elevation in serum acid phosphatase activity in Gaucher disease?
4. What is the major source of the accumulated glucocerebroside in Gaucher disease? In what form is the accumulated lipid stored in the lysosome?
5. How would you assess whether glucocerebrosidase replacement therapy was effective in a teenager with Gaucher disease?
6. What consequences of immunoglobulin production against glucocerebrosidase might occur in a patient receiving placental enzyme replacement therapy?
7. What is the cause of the pancytopenia associated with Gaucher disease?
8. Assume you have discovered a new mutation at base position 276 in the glucocerebrosidase gene. How would you use this information to design a polymerase chain reaction based assay for the presence of this mutation in the parents and siblings and siblings of the index case?

REFERENCES

Barton NW, Brady RO, et al.: Replacement therapy for inherited enzyme deficiency—macrophage-targeted glucocerebrosidase for Gaucher's disease. *N Eng J Med* **324**:1464–1470, 1991.

Basu A, Glew RH: Characterization of the phospholipid requirement of a rat liver β-glucosidase. *Biochem J* **224**:515–524, 1984.

Basu A, Glew RH, Daniels LB, et al: Activators of spleen glucocerebroside from controls and patients with various forms of Gaucher's disease. *J Biol Chem* **259**:1714–1719, 1984.

Beutler E. Gaucher disease as a paradigm of current issues regarding single gene mutations of humans. *Proc Natl Acad Sci USA* **90**:5384–5390, 1993.

Brady RO, Furbish FS. Enzyme replacement therapy: Specific targeting of exogenous enzymes to storage cells, *in* Martonosi AN (ed): *Membranes and Transport,* vol. 2. New York, Plenum Press 587–592, 1982.

Brady RO, Barranger JA. Glucosylceramide lipidosis: Gaucher's disease, *in* Stanbury JB, Wyngaarden JB, Frederickson DS, et al. (eds): *The Metabolic Basis of Inherited Disease.* New York, McGraw-Hill, 842–856, 1983.

Brady RO, Barton NW, Grabowski GA. The role of neurogenetics in Gaucher disease. *Arch Neurol* **50**:1212–1224, 1993.

Daniels LB, Glew RH. β-glucosidase assays in the diagnosis of Gaucher's disease. *Clin Chem* **28**:569–577, 1982.

Furbish FS, Steer CJ, et al.: Uptake and distribution of placental glucocerebrosidase in rat hepatic cells and effects of sequential deglycosylation. *Biochim Biophys Acta* **673**:425–434, 1981.

Glew RH, Basu A, Prence EM, et al.: Biology of disease—lysosomal storage diseases. *Lab Invest* **52**:250–269, 1985.

Glew RH, Daniels LB, Clark LS, et al.: Enzymic differentiation of neurologic and nonneurologic forms of Gaucher's disease. *J Neuropathol Exp Neurol* **41**:630–641, 1982.

Grabowski GA, Barton NW, et al.: Enzyme therapy in type 1 Gaucher disease: comparative efficacy of mannose-terminated glucocerebrosidase from natural and recombinant sources. *Ann Intern Med* **122**:33–39, 1995.

Hill SC, Parker CC, et al.: MRI of multiple platyspondyly in Gaucher disease. *Arch Neurol* **50**:1212–1224, 1993.

Parker RI, Barton NW, et al.: Hematologic improvement in a patient with Gaucher disease on long term-enzyme replacement therapy: Evidence for decreased splenic sequestration and improved red blood cell survival. *Am J Hematol* **38**:130–137, 1991.

27

I-Cell Disease

JAMES P. CHAMBERS AND JULIAN C. WILLIAMS

CASE HISTORY

The patient (Fig. 27-1) was a 38-week gestation product of a 22-year-old $G_1P_1Ab_0$ (gravida 1, first pregnancy; para-delivery, first delivery; abortion, 0) woman and her 31-year-old first-cousin partner. Pregnancy was complicated by *oligohydramnios* (deficiency in the amount of amniotic fluid); an amniocentesis revealed a normal male karyotype. The infant was delivered by cesarean section because of maternal *preeclampsia* (development of hypertension due to pregnancy). Apgar scores were 8/9, weight 2200 g (5%), and length 18.5 in (5%). On newborn examination, *microcephaly* (a broad nasal bridge with anteverted nostrils), *micrognathia* (smallness of the jaws, especially the underjaw), *hypospadias* (a defect in the wall of the urethra), and undescended testes were seen. A tentative diagnosis of Smith-Lemli-Opitz syndrome was postulated. By 9 months of age, marked developmental delay was noted. Repeat evaluation revealed bilateral inguinal hernias, dysmorphic features with *synophrys* (growing together of the eyebrows), and thick upper lip with gum hypertrophy; limitation of motion at the knees, hips, elbows and wrists; *camptodactyly* (bending of fingers), rib flaring, hepatosplenomegaly, corneal clouding, and hypotonia, in addition to those findings reported at birth. A lysosomal enzyme screen indicated elevated plasma and urine enzymes and sialyloligosaccharides in the urine. These findings and the physical examination are consistent with a diagnosis of I-cell disease.

DIAGNOSIS

In 1967 DeMars, while studying a group of suspected Hurler patient biopsies, made the seminal observation in one patient of the presence of an abundance of cytoplasmic "inclusions" (DeMars and Leroy, 1967). These cells were so distinctive compared with cells cultured from other patients with similar clinical symptoms that DeMars coined the appellation *I-cell*. Subsequently, I-cell disease was classified as a mucolipidosis (designated *ML-II*) by Spranger and Wiedemann, a group of recessively inherited lysosomal storage diseases characterized by intracellular accumulation of acid mucopolysaccharides, sphingolipids, or glycolipids in visceral and mesenchymal cells (Spranger and Wiedemann, 1970). I-cell disease is suspected clinically by the phenotype and is confirmed biochemically. The I-cell disease infant is usually small for gestational age and is clinically differentiated from Hurler's syndrome by earlier onset of signs and symptoms, the absence of excessive mucopolysacchariduria, short stature, and the rapidly progressive course leading to death usually by age 4. The disease progresses with the child developing coarse facial features with puffy eyelids, prominent epicanthal folds, flat nasal bridge, anteverted nostrils, *macroglossia* (enlargement of the tongue), and severe skeletal abnormalities. Craniofacial abnormalities, restricted joint movement with generalized hypotonia, congenital hip dislocation, hernias, and bilateral *talipes equinovarus* (clubfoot) may be observed in the neonatal period. Gin-

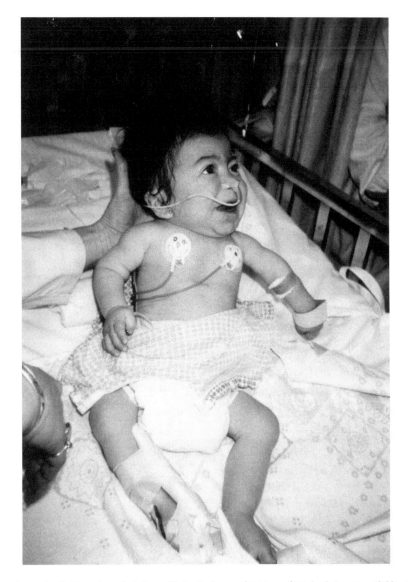

Figure 27-1. A 9-month-old Hispanic male infant with I-cell disease (Division of Medical Genetics, Children's Hospital, Los Angeles).

gival hypertrophy is more striking than in the Hurler syndrome. Hard, firm subcutaneous nodules may represent accumulation of storage material. By 6 months of age, psychomotor retardation is usually obvious. Joint immobility progresses with development of claw-hand deformities and kyphoscoliosis. Hepatomegaly is prominent, but splenomegaly is minimal. Corneal haziness may be present but is subtle, and corneal opacities due to the accumula-

tion of storage material are not as striking as in the Hurler syndrome.

Radiographically, I-cell disease is manifested in two successive stages of infancy, one observed in the neonatal period and the other at about 1 year of age. When detected at birth, peculiar radiographic changes of the bones reflect a more severe disturbance in bone development and growth and strongly resemble rickets or *osteomalacia* (softening and bending of the bones) as evidenced by the presence of rachitic-like (related to rickets) lesions and changes similar to those observed in hyperparathyroidism. The radiographic abnormalities found in older children appear to be more nonspecific and are typical of Hurler-like signs of *dysostosis multiplex* (roentgenographic abnormalities indicating bone changes at multiple sites).

The primary biochemical defect in I-cell disease, as well as in pseudo-Hurler polydystrophy, is in the enzyme uridine diphospho-*N*-acetylglucosamine: lysosomal enzyme *N*-acetylglucosamine-1-phosphotransferase (EC 2.7.8.17) and will be subsequently referred to as *phosphotransferase*. This metabolic error creates a secondary deficiency of most lysosomal enzymes, as described below. The reaction catalyzed by the phosphotransferase enzyme (reaction 1, Fig. 27-2) results in formation of the phosphodiester *N*-acetylglucosamine-1-phosphate-6-mannose, the intermediate in the synthesis of the mannose 6-phosphate recognition marker. Fibroblast phosphotransferase activity of parents of I-cell disease patients is 50% deficient compared with control fibroblasts, which is consistent with an autosomal recessive mode of inheritance of the I-cell mutation.

It has been proposed that I-cell disease and pseudo-Hurler polydystrophy are variants of the same disorder because fibroblasts from both these disorders are deficient in phosphotransferase activity. The difference is that in I-cell disease the deficiency is essentially total, whereas in pseudo-Hurler polydystrophy there appears to be a significant residual activity (approximately 10% of control values). Although two clinical presentations of I-cell disease have been described (i.e., the neonate and 6- to 12-month-old patient), correlation of the degree of deficiency of phosphotransferase activity with clinical severity in the two I-cell disease presentations remains controversial.

I-cell disease and pseudo-Hurler polydystrophy are characterized by excessive secretion of newly synthesized lysosomal enzymes into body fluids and concomitant loss of respective intracellular activities in fibroblasts. Shown in Table 27-1 are representative lysosomal enzyme activity levels in serum from I-cell disease and pseudo-Hurler polydystrophy patients, indicating significantly increased levels of lysosomal enzyme activity. Germane to the biochemical diagnosis is the characteristic pattern of lysosomal enzyme deficiency in cultured fibroblasts, that is, an increase in the ratio of extracellular to intracellular enzyme activity. Examination of I-cell fibroblasts (Table 27-2) reveals the characteristic increased ratio of extracellular to intracellular lysosomal enzyme activity consistent with the "excessive" secretion theme. It is interesting to note that not all lysosomal (i.e., intracellular) enzyme activities are decreased in I-cell fibroblasts; acid phosphatase and β-glucosidase are the exceptions (Table 27.2, see intracellular activity). In contrast, extracellular or se-

Table 27-1. Lysosomal Enzyme Activities in Serum from Patients with I-Cell Disease and Pseudo-Hurler Polydystrophy[a]

Enzyme	Controls	I-Cell	Pseudo-Hurler
β-Galactosidase	16.3	30.6	
α-Galactosidase	4.6	14.5	
α-Mannosidase	31.4	1116	3976
β-Glucuronidase	14.2	163	740
α-Fucosidase	235	5184	4389
Arylsulphatase A	14.2	1664	
α-Glucosaminidase	15.8	1531	76
β-Glucosaminidase	621	5040	4194

[a]Data were taken from a study by Poenaru et al. (1988). Galactosidase, mannosidase, glucuronidase, fucosidase, and glucosaminidase were assayed using the corresponding derivative of 4-methylumbelliferone. Arylsulphatase A was assayed using paranitrocatechol sulfate as substrate. Specific activity is expressed as nmol/h/ml of serum. Data shown are mean values.

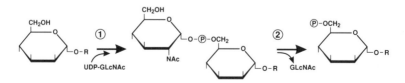

Figure 27-2. Synthesis of the mannose 6-phosphate recognition marker. R represents the 'high mannose' oligosaccharide of newly synthesized lysosomal enzymes. Reaction 1 is catalyzed by UDP-*N*-acetylglucosamine:lysosomal enzyme *N*-acetylglucosaminyl-1-phosphotransferase. Reaction 2 is catalyzed by *N*-acetylglucosamine-1-phosphodiester-*N*-acetylglucosaminidase.

Table 27-2. Intra and Extracellular Levels of Various Lysosomal Enzymes of Cultivated I-Cell Disease Fibroblasts[a]

Enzyme	Control	I-Cell Disease
Intracellular Activity		
α-Fucosidase	72	2.2
β-Galactosidase	584	6.7
α-Mannosidase	98	9.3
Neuraminidase	39	0.5
Acid Phosphatase	2,954	2,620
β-Glucosidase	162	148
Extracellular Activity		
α-Fucosidase	0.8	2.7
β-Glucuronidase	41	345
Hexosaminidase A	97	878
α-Mannosidase	2.3	24
β-Glucosidase	0.2	0.2

[a]Data were taken from a study by Ben-Yoseph et al. (1986). Whole-cell preparations were disrupted by sonication in water. Extracellular secretions from cultured fibroblasts were collected into serum-free medium for 24 hours. Hexosaminidase A activity was determined using the sulfated fluorogenic substrate (4-methylumbelliferyl derivative of β-GlcNAc-6-SO$_4$). Other lysosomal enzyme activities were determined using the respective commercially available fluorogenic substrates. Specific activities of enzymes (intracellular) are expressed as nanomoles substrate cleaved per milligram cell protein per hour. Activities in the medium (extracellular) were those secreted by 1 mg cell protein in 24 hours. Data shown are mean values.

Table 27-3. Prenatal Diagnosis: Levels of GlcNac-PO$_4$ Transferase and Various Lysosomal Enzymes in Amniotic Fluid and Cultivated Amniotic Fluid Cells[a]

Enzyme	Control	I-Cell Disease
Amniotic Fluid Cells[a]		
GlcNac-PO$_4$ Transferase	0.68	0.05
Intracellular Activity		
α-Fucosidase	478	22.3
β-Galactosidase	745	27.3
β-Glucosidase	136	278
β-Glucuronidase	244	17.4
Hexosaminidase A	1345	119
α-Mannosidase	190	14.7
β-Mannosidase	462	31.1
Extracellular Activity		
α-Fucosidase	53.4	285
β-Galactosidase	14.6	69.0
Hexosaminidase A	242	1843
α-Mannosidase	5.6	44.4
Amniotic Fluid[b]		
Hexosaminidase	155	1620
β-Glucuronidase	15.6	135
α-Fucosidase	18.0	140
α-Mannosidase	7.2	76
α-Galactosidase	0.78	2.4

[a]Data were taken from a studies conducted by Parvathy et al. (1989) and Besley et al. (1990). GlcNac-PO$_4$ transferase was assayed using UDP-[1-^{14}C]-N-acetylglucosamine, and α-methylmannoside as substrates (specific activity is expressed as nanomoles N-acetylglucosamine-1-phosphate transferred per milligram cell protein per hour). Extracellular secretions from cultured cells were collected into serum-free medium during a 24-hour period. Enzyme activity toward fluorogenic substrates was determined in cell sonicates and in serum-free media of cell cultures. Hexosaminidase A specific substrate (4-methyl-umbelliferyl-2-deoxy-2-acetamido-6-sulfo-β-D-glucopyranoside) was chemically synthesized. Intracellular activities are expressed as nanomole substrate cleaved per milligram cell protein per hour. Extracellular activities in cell cultures are expressed as the activity secreted into the medium per milligram of cell protein in 24 hours. Activities in amniotic fluid are expressed as nmol per h per mg protein. Data shown are mean values.

creted lysosomal enzyme activity of cultivated I-cell disease fibroblasts is significantly increased when compared to normal fibroblasts (Table 27.2, see extracellular activity).

Many tissues from I-cell patients exhibit normal levels of "intracellular" lysosomal enzymatic activities (e.g., brain, liver, kidney, and spleen). In the liver, lysosomal enzyme levels are normal except for diminished β-galactosidase and elevated β-hexosaminidase, β-xylosidase, and α-galactosidase. This fairly specific decrease in liver activity of β-galactosidase contrasts with the diminution of almost all lysosomal enzymes in cultured fibroblasts.

Prenatal diagnosis of I-cell disease has been based on greatly reduced phosphotransferase activity and abnormal intracellular-extracellular distribution of lysosomal enzymes in cultured amniotic fetal cells (Table 27-3). As indicated in Table 27-3, amniotic fluid cells secrete into the extracellular medium large amounts of lysosomal enzymes. Decreased levels of lysosomal enzymes in chorionic villus obtained by biopsy have also been observed in I-cell disease; however, the characteristic secondary effect, that is, the increased levels of lysosomal enzymes in the extracellular compartment, is only partially ex-

pressed or not expressed at all in chorionic villi, suggesting an alternative mechanism for the transport of lysosomal proteins. Although the diagnosis is made more reliably using cells obtained by amniocentesis, direct examination of the phosphotransferase activity of chorionic villi has been effectively used to diagnose I-cell disease prenatally. This approach affords a more rapid diagnosis than the 2 to 4 weeks required for diagnosis by amniocentesis.

Analysis of glycosphingolipids reveals elevations in trihexosylceramide (GL-3) and the ganglioside GM$_3$ (Fig. 27-3) but not in the massive accumulation associated with the glycosphingolipidoses. In the spleen, the only apparent lipid abnormality is an increase in the level of GM$_3$. The brain has normal levels of gangliosides, apart from a small increase in

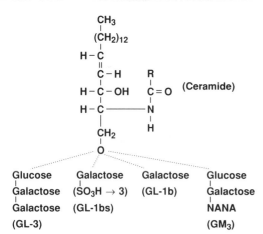

Glucose   Galactose   Galactose   Glucose
|
Galactose   (SO₃H → 3)   (GL-1b)   Galactose
|
Galactose   (GL-1bs)   NANA

(GL-3)   (GM₃)

Figure 27-3. Important glycolipids affected in I-cell disease. The dotted lines represent the respective β-linked glycosides; ceramide, 2-N-acylsphingosine; NANA, N-acetylneuraminic acid. GL-1bs is shown sulfated in the 3 position of galactose (SO₃H→3).

GM_3 and lower than normal concentrations of sulfatides GL-1bS and cerebrosides GL-1b (Fig. 27-3).

The histopathologic hallmark of I-cell disease is the presence of characteristic phase-dense, cytoplasmic, spherical (approximately 0.5–1.0 μm in diameter) vesicles (i.e., inclusions) (Fig. 27-4) surrounding the nucleus and juxtanuclear Golgi apparatus within the mesenchyme-derived tissues throughout the body. Ultrastructurally, the inclusions are bound by a single membrane and contain fibrogranular and membranous lamellar material. Are these inclusion bodies lysosomes or an unrelated organelle? Morphological and biochemical evidence indicates that the inclusion bodies are secondary lysosomes containing undigested material that has accumulated as a result of the deficiency of lysosomal enzymes.

Because of the extensive mesenchymal tissue involvement in I-cell disease, the observation of large amounts of unsulfated chondroitin in the cartilage matrix and compensatory decrease of chondroitin 4-sulfate has been viewed as suggesting possible abnormalities in the posttranslational assembly and subsequent modification of glycosaminoglycans; however, I-cell fibroblasts have been shown to: (1) internalize cell-surface proteoglycans; (2) remove glycosaminoglycan chains from the proteoglycan core protein; and (3) partially degrade heparan sulfate glycosaminoglycan chains in identical fashion as that

observed for normal fibroblasts (Brauker and Wang, 1987). Also suspect is the degradation of collagen (type I) in I-cell disease fibroblasts as a result of the greatly reduced levels of cathepsin B, which possesses potent collagenolytic activity; however, the rate of intracellular degradation of proline analogs by I-cell disease fibroblasts is comparable to rates of degradation observed for normal fibroblasts.

MOLECULAR PERSPECTIVES

The importance of lysosomal degradation is underscored by the fact that more than 35 lysosomal storage diseases have been described in humans, most of which arise from a deficiency of one of the lysosomal enzymes, leading to subsequent accumulation of the missing enzyme's substrate. Traditionally, these disorders have been viewed as arising from a mutation in a structural gene that codes for an individual lysosomal enzyme; however, the molecular theme of I-cell disease is that of "faulty" lysosomal targeting, the inability to transport (i.e., sort) lysosomal enzymes from their site of synthesis to the lysosome.

The important observation made by Hickman and Neufeld (1972) that I-cell fibroblasts are capable of *endocytosing* (the process by which cells take up macromolecules) lysosomal enzymes secreted by normal cells, but that normal cells are incapable of internalizing the enzymes secreted by I-cell fibroblasts, suggested that some kind of recognition marker for internalization of lysosomal enzymes is absent in I-cell fibroblasts. This recognition marker has been identified as mannose 6-phosphate (subsequently referred to as *man-6-P*).

The sorting (i.e., targeting of lysosomal enzymes to the lysosome) is part of a more general but very important question: How do cells transport proteins synthesized in the rough endoplasmic reticulum to diverse cellular destinations? The I-cell patient has proved invaluable in elucidating the complex nature of intracellular packaging and sorting of lysosomal enzymes. The physiological importance of this signal-mediated pathway is evident in that fibroblasts from patients with I-cell disease and pseudo-Hurler polydystrophy secrete rather than target most of their lysosomal enzymes.

To understand the molecular basis of I-cell disease, it is necessary first to examine the required processing of the carbohydrate moities, that is, oli-

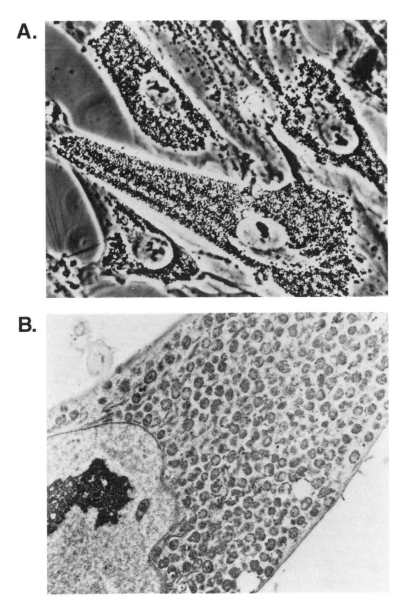

Figure 27-4. Microscopic examination of cultured I-cell skin fibroblasts. **A:** Phase contrast microscopy. **B:** Electron microscopy showing the inclusions (Photographs courtesy of Dr. Robert DeMars).

gosaccharide side chains, of lysosomal enzymes. For an excellent review that describes in detail the various structural and biosynthetic aspects of the oligosaccharides of glycoproteins, the reader should consult Kornfeld and Kornfeld (1985).

The biosynthetic pathways responsible for both membrane and secretory glycoproteins have been localized to specific lumenal regions of the Golgi and endoplasmic reticulum. As shown in Figure 27-5, the "core" oligosaccharide (three glucose, nine mannose, and two *N*-acetylglucosamine residues) is pre-assembled in an "activated" form and is transferred *en bloc* from a lipid-linked (dolichyl-pyrophosphate) carrier to distinct asparagine residues of the nascent polypeptide while the protein is being synthesized on membrane-bound polysomes. This transfer usually takes place before the folding of the polypeptide chain. Once glycosylation of the protein has occurred, processing of the oligosaccharide is initiated by trimming reactions that remove three glucose residues and one mannose unit. The proteins then move by vesicular transport to the Golgi, where they undergo a variety of additional post-translational modifications and are sorted for targeting to the proper destination, that is, to lysosome, secretory granule, or plasma membrane. It is during passage through the Golgi that the oligosaccharides on secretory and membrane glycoproteins are processed from "high mannose" to "complex" type side chains containing sialic-acid.

Specific lysosomal targeting is achieved via what is now referred to as the *man-6-P-dependent* sorting system and requires the concerted action of two key enzymes (Fig. 27-2). First, the previously mentioned enzyme, phosphotransferase, transfers *N*-acetylglucosamine 1-phosphate from the sugar nucleotide UDP-GlcNAc to the C-6 oxygen of selected mannose residues on asparagine-linked, high-mannose oligosaccharides of only lysosomal enzymes to give rise to a phosphodiester intermediate. A second enzyme, *N*-acetylglucosamine-1-phosphodiester α-N-acetylglucosaminidase (EC 3.1.4.45), cleaves the terminal α-N-acetylglucosamine residue to uncover a man-6-P group that serves as the required "recognition marker" component that leads to high-affinity binding to mannose 6-phosphate receptors (MPRs) in the Golgi. The MPRs and their bound ligands (i.e., lysosomal enzymes) are packaged into clathrin-coated vesicles that bud from the *trans* Golgi network and subsequently fuse with an acidic endosomal compartment, where the low pH promotes dissociation of receptor and ligand. Thus, these receptors mediate delivery of the "targeted" enzymes to endosomal compartments, where they are discharged and subsequently packaged into lysosomes (for reviews see Kornfeld, 1986; von Figura and Hasilik, 1986; Kornfeld, 1992). In I-cell disease, lysosomal enzymes are not modified by addition of man-6-P. Thus, they are not segregated by the MPRs into the appropriate transport vesicles in the *trans* Golgi network and instead are carried to the cell surface and secreted.

As previously shown in Figure 27-2, the phosphotransferase transfers *N*-acetylglucosamine-1-phosphate residues *en bloc* to the C-6 oxygen of particular mannose residues in "high mannose" oligosaccharide units of lysosomal enzymes. This reaction occurs in two stages: transfer of *N*-acetylglucosamine-1-phosphate to a mannose residue on the α-1,6 branch of a high-mannose oligo-

saccharide and addition of a second *N*-acetylglucosamine-1-phosphate to the α-1,3 branch thought to occur in a pre-Golgi compartment and the *cis* Golgi, respectively. A number of assay procedures have been described for the phosphotransferase using ^{32}P, ^{3}H, and ^{14}C-labeled UDP-GlcNAc (radioactivity is located in the GlcNAc moiety) as the *N*-acetylglucosamine-1-phosphate donor and a variety of acceptor substrates (e.g., β-hexosaminidase, glycopeptides, and α-methylmannoside). Using these substrates, a deficiency of phosphotransferase activity has been documented in fibroblasts, leukocytes, and organs from patients with I-cell disease and pseudo-Hurler polydystrophy.

Generally, phosphotransferase is assayed using α-methylmannoside as acceptor. After incubation, the reaction is terminated and the phosphodiester product of the transfer reaction (i.e., [^{14}C or ^{3}H]GlcNac-α-1-phospho-6-mannose-α-1-methyl) is chromatographically separated from the reaction components and the radioactivity determined. A general reaction scheme is presented below:

$$\text{UDP-}[^{3}\text{H}/^{14}\text{C}]\text{GlcNAc} + \text{Man}\alpha 1 \rightarrow \text{CH}_3 \rightleftarrows \text{UMP} +$$
$$[^{3}\text{H}/^{14}\text{C}]\text{GlcNAc}\alpha 1 \rightarrow \text{P-6Man}\alpha 1 \rightarrow \text{CH}_3$$

In vivo, the CH$_3$ group in the above reaction scheme is representative of the rest of the high-mannose oligosaccharide intermediate.

Of legion importance to the efficient targeting of enzymes to lysosomes is the ability of the phosphotransferase to recognize and bind with high affinity to a protein determinant that is common to lysosomal enzymes but absent from nonlysosomal glycoproteins. Because lysosomal enzymes do not share linear amino acid sequences, the phosphotransferase must specifically interact and recognize a conformation-dependent protein determinant that is expressed in 40 to 50 different lysosomal hydrolases while displaying low affinity for hundreds of other glycoproteins that contain identical high-mannose type oligosaccharides.

Elucidation of the requirements for phosphotransferase binding specificity has been given considerable attention. Much insight into this problem has been obtained from studies of cathepsin D, a bilobed lysosomal aspartylprotease that contains one asparagine-linked oligosaccharide per lobe. Using chimeric proteins containing either amino or carboxyl lobe sequences of cathepsin D substituted into a glycosylated form of the homologous secretory protein pepsinogen, the elements of a recognition domain have been identified that are thought to be shared among lysosomal enzymes and recognized by the phosphotransferase (a single lysine at position 203 and residues 265–292, which form a β-loop). A phosphotransferase recognition domain located on either lobe of the cathepsin/glycopepsinogen chimeric molecule is sufficient to allow phosphorylation of oligosaccharides on both lobes. It is interesting to note that the carboxyl lobe oligosaccharides of cathepsin D acquire two phosphates, whereas the amino lobe oligosaccharides only acquire one phosphate. Molecular modeling of the cathepsin D sequences inclusive of the lysosomal enzyme recognition domain indicates that these residues come together in three-dimensional space to form a surface patch on the carboxyl lobe of the molecule. The current thinking is that the phosphotransferase recognizes a number of topological features on the surface of the polypeptides destined for lysosomes, some combination of which is sufficient to produce an identifying signal.

Although much of the focus of I-cell disease centers around lysosomal enzyme carbohydrate processing, it is important to remember that lysosomal enzymes are synthesized as pre-proenzymes with amino terminal extensions that require further proteolytic processing. In addition to removal of the signal peptide in the endoplasmic reticulum, the newly synthesized protein may be subject to additional limited proteolysis during transport (Fig. 27-5). This proteolytic processing appears to be initiated in the prelysosomal compartments and is completed after the enzymes arrive in the lysosomes. In some cases there are further internal cleavages of the peptide as well as carboxyl-terminal processing. The biological significance of this processing is not well-understood but may play an early role in the sorting process (e.g., maintenance of the correct folding and conformation of the nascent protein that subsequently becomes a substrate for the phosphotransferase).

The high-affinity interaction between the phosphotransferase and lysosomal enzymes appears to be mediated primarily through protein-protein interactions. This is based on the fact that isolated high-mannose type oligosaccharide and glycopeptides are extremely poor phosphotransferase acceptor substrates. Furthermore, the phosphorylation of intact lysosomal enzymes is markedly inhibited by the inclusion of deglycosylated lysosomal enzymes in reaction mixtures, supporting the hypothesis that the phosphotransferase recognizes a protein domain that is common to all lysosomal enzymes but absent in nonlysosomal glycoproteins.

Newly synthesized lysosomal enzymes containing man-6-P residues are recognized by two distinct MPRs with molecular masses of 46 to 275 kd (for reviews see Kornfeld, 1992; Kornfeld and Mellman, 1989). The smaller 46-kd receptor requires divalent cations for its binding activity and is referred to as *cation dependent* (i.e., CD-MPR). In contrast, the larger 275-kd MPR does not require the presence of divalent cations for ligand binding and is referred to as *cation independent* (i.e., CI-MPR). In humans and in many other species, the larger receptor is identical to the receptor for the insulin-like growth factor II (IGF-II) and thus is referred to as the *man-6-P/insulin growth factor II receptor* (man-6-P/IGF-II).

The MPRs are distributed over several cellular compartments. A single pool of MPRs cycle constitutively between the Golgi, endosomes, and the plasma membrane. The major site for lysosomal enzyme sorting is the last Golgi compartment, referred to as the *trans Golgi network* (the *trans* Golgi reticulum, the *trans* tubular network, and Golgi endoplasmic reticulum-lysosome). In the *trans*-Golgi network, MPRs bind lysosomal enzymes and mediate their segregation from secretory proteins. At the plasma membrane, the man-6-P/IGF-II receptor binds and mediates endocytosis of extracellular ligands, whereas the CD-MPR appears not to function in endocytosis under physiological conditions despite being rapidly internalized from the cell surface (for review see Kornfeld, 1992). The distribution of MPRs in fibroblasts from some I-cell patients is abnormal, with the receptors found almost exclusively in Golgi cisternae and in coated vesicles located near the cisternae. Thus, defective receptors, as well as functional receptors wrongly distributed, represent possibly yet additional mechanisms that can result in the I-cell phenotype.

Whereas both types of MPRs bind man-6-P with the same affinity ($7\text{-}8 \times 10^{-6}$M), the man-6-P/IGF-II receptor binds diphosphorylated oligosaccharides with a significantly higher affinity than does the CD-MPR (2×10^{-9}M versus 2×10^{-7}M, respectively). Because oligosaccharides with two phosphomonoesters bind to the MPRs with an affinity similar

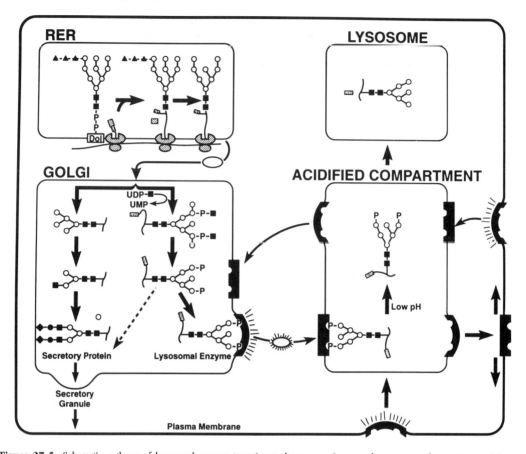

Figure 27-5. Schematic pathway of lysosomal enzyme targeting to lysosomes. Lysosomal enzymes and secretory proteins are synthesized in the rough endoplasmic reticulum (RER) and glycosylated by the transfer of a preformed oligosaccharide from dolichol-P-P-oligosaccharide (Dol). In the RER, the signal peptides (▨▨▨▨▨) are excised. The proteins are translocated to the Golgi, where the oligosaccharides of secretory proteins are processed to complex-type units and the oligosaccharides of lysosomal enzymes are phosphorylated. Most of the lysosomal enzymes bind to mannose 6-phosphate receptors (MPRs) (▬▬▬) and are translocated to an acidified prelysosomal compartment where the ligand dissociates. The receptors recycle back to the Golgi or to the cell surface, and the enzymes are packaged into lysosomes, where cleavage of their propieces is completed (▧▧▧▧). The P$_i$ may also be cleaved from the mannose residues. A small number of the lysosomal enzymes fail to bind to the receptors and are secreted along with secretory proteins. These enzymes may bind to surface MPRs in coated pits (⌣⌣⌣) and be internalized into the prelysosomal compartment. (■) N-Acetylglucosamine. (○) Mannose. (▲) Glucose. (●) Galactose. (♦) Sialic acid. *From* Kornfeld (1987). Used by permission of *FASEB J.*

to that observed for lysosomal enzymes, the high-affinity binding of lysosomal enzymes can be explained by a two-site model in which two phosphomannosyl residues on the lysosomal enzyme interact with the receptor. This interaction could be mediated either by two phosphomannosyl residues on the same oligosaccharide of the lysosomal enzyme or by single phosphomannosyl residues located on different adjacent oligosaccharides. It is generally agreed

that individual phosphomannosyl residues located on different oligosaccharides interact with the receptor with higher affinity than do two phosphomannosyl residues present on the same oligosaccharide.

Studies of the function of the CI-MPR in lysosomal enzyme transport have been facilitated by the identification of cell lines that lack this protein. Data derived from such studies demonstrate that this receptor is predominantly involved in the intracellular retention of lysosomal enzymes. Thus, cells that are CI-MPR negative or defective secrete large amounts of their newly synthesized lysosomal enzymes and are unable to endocytose extracellular ligands.

The function of the CD-MPR in lysosomal enzyme sorting had been for the most part considered primarily responsible only for residual sorting, that is, a minor role in lysosomal enzyme targeting to lysosomes. It now appears, however, that along with the CI-MPR, the CD-MPR plays a major role in intracellular targeting of lysosomal enzymes. Target disruption (where one allele of a gene is disrupted by homologous recombination and offspring of animals transmitting the disrupted gene are generated) studies of the CD-MPR have resulted in partial missorting of multiple lysosomal enzymes. Although both receptors function in combination to transport several lysosomal enzymes, it is possible that they are also responsible for targeting nonoverlapping subsets of a few enzymes. If the two MPRs bind the same phosphorylated oligosaccharides, then it is possible (or even likely) that their interactions with lysosomal enzymes are complex in nature, involving different, multiple phosphorylated oligosaccharides of varying accessibility.

Are signals on the MPRs needed for their rapid endocytosis from the cell surface and efficient sorting of the MPR-lysosomal enzyme complex in the Golgi? Such signals have been localized to the cytoplasmic tails of these proteins, and the internalization signal for the man-6-P/IGF-II receptor has been identified as Tyr-Lys-Tyr-Ser-Lys-Val, representing amino acid residues 24–29 from the amino terminus. The use of mutants has demonstrated that the conserved sequence near the COOH terminus of the cytoplasmic domain is important for CI-MPR function in sorting of lysosomal enzymes. It is conceivable, therefore, that mutations in this region could affect one or more molecular events underlying receptor trafficking. Furthermore, additional sorting signals may be present on different regions of the cytoplasmic domain of the CI-MPR. The CD-MPR contains at least two separate signals for rapid internalization in its 67-amino acid cytoplasmic domain. One signal includes Phe13 and Phe18; the other includes Tyr45. The Phe-containing signal consists of six amino acids (Phe-Pro-His-Leu-Ala-Phe); the Tyr-containing signal consists of four amino acids (Tyr-Arg-Gly-Val). The essential elements consist of an aromatic residue in the amino-terminal position separated from a bulky hydrophobic aromatic residue in the carboxyl-terminal position by two amino acids.

Does defective lysosomal catabolism in I-cell disease somehow feed back to affect the expression of lysosomal proteins and their receptors? Compared with control fibroblasts, two-fold increases in man-6-P/IGF-II receptors have been observed for fibroblasts from I-cell disease patients. This increase in receptor concentration stems from an increased rate of synthesis, not from differences of receptor stability. Interestingly, when they are exposed to insulin, growth factors I and II or tumor-promoting phorbol esters, I-cell fibroblasts respond differently than control fibroblasts. These observations indicate multiple regulatory sites in the man-6-P/IGF-II receptor pathway.

The discovery that CI-MPR and the IGF-II receptor are one and the same protein raised the fascinating possibility that this receptor may function in two diverse biologic processes: protein trafficking and transmembrane signalling. The results of several studies have shown that IGF-II mediates transmembrane signalling through an independent receptor. These responses include stimulation of glycogen synthesis, amino acid uptake, cell proliferation, Na^+/H^+ exchange, inositol triphosphate production, and Ca^{2+} influx.

In light of the increased number of man-6-P/IGF-II receptors in I-cell fibroblasts, the above interactions of IGF could have far-reaching effects. For example, I-cell disease has not been typically associated with abnormalities in phosphorous/calcium metabolism. The extensive skeletal deformities could involve impairment of mechanisms of orderly calcium deposition. Rather than resulting from a primary disorder of calcium metabolism, it is possible that the bone lesions in I-cell disease are secondary to altered lysosomal processing events in the kidney or liver.

Although both I-cell disease and pseudo-Hurler polydystrophy patients are deficient in phosphotransferase activity, they exhibit different patterns of intracellular and extracellular lysosomal enzyme activities in cultured skin fibroblasts, electrophoretic mobility, lectin binding properties, and responsiveness to sucrose loading. Complementation studies of fibroblasts from I-cell disease and pseudo-Hurler polydystrophy have yielded valuable insight into the biochemical basis of the observed heterogeneity. In these studies, fibroblasts from individual patients are fused with cells from other patients. Variants have been categorized on the basis of phosphotransferase activity toward α-methylmannoside as acceptor in the phosphotransferase assay as well as decreased secretion of lysosomal enzymes into the extracellular compartment.

Complementation studies of I-cell disease and pseudo-Hurler polydystrophy fibroblasts indicate three genetic groups (A, B, and C) exhibiting altered phosphotransferase activity and, presumably, involvement of three genes although intra-allelic complementation. Complementation group A is the largest and includes all I-cell disease and many pseudo-Hurler polydystrophy patients. The defects in patients from group A are thought to be alleles at the same locus and are characterized by a change in the catalytic portion of the phosphotransferase that renders it unable to use the artificial acceptor substrate (α-methylmannoside) used in the enzyme assay. In patients of complementation Group A, the phosphotransferase enzyme has been described as being smaller than normal, suggesting the absence of a catalytically important enzyme component. Groups B and C consist entirely of the less common pseudo-Hurler polydystrophy variants. Group B comprises patients with defective phosphotransferase catalytic function. The enzyme from patients with complementation group B phosphotransferase deficiency appears to be larger than normal, suggesting abnormal aggregation of the enzyme. Group C includes patients exhibiting a phosphotransferase with normal catalytic function toward α-methylmannoside but one that fails to recognize endogenous lysosomal enzymes as acceptor substrate. Thus, the enzyme recognizes the artificial acceptor substrate (α-methylmannoside), producing normal levels of enzyme activity. The mutation in group C is thought to affect a gene coding a noncatalytic phosphotransferase site or a component that is involved in the recognition of, or specific binding to, lysosomal enzyme precursors.

THERAPY

Currently, there is no cure for I-cell disease. Because it is an extremely rare disorder, there is probably no reason to consider genetic screening. If there is a positive family history, prenatal diagnosis should be carried out. Bone marrow transplantation has been proposed for the treatment of lysosomal storage diseases, and one case of I-cell disease has exhibited biochemical and clinical improvement following bone marrow transplantation (Yamaguchi et al., 1989). The precise mechanism underlying the improvement remains obscure because lysosomal storage diseases are not specific to blood cells. One plausible explanation is that cells derived from hematopoietic progenitors of the donor (that is, circulating leukocytes and tissue macrophages) can donate lysosomal enzymes to the deficient cells in all tissues of the host, either through secretion or direct cell-cell interactions.

Although the benefits of bone marrow transplantation at present are modest and considering that the risks and costs involved are high, its limited success has encouraged the prospect of gene replacement through transfection of hematopoietic progenitor cells with retroviruses. Retroviral vectors carrying cDNA encoding β-glucuronidase have been used to correct fibroblasts deficient in that enzyme (Wolfe et al., 1990). This is a promising general approach to the treatment of inborn errors of metabolism.

Acknowledgment: We thank Dr. Robert DeMars for providing the original photographs first describing the "I-cell." Additionally, we thank Dr. Robert H. Glew for his helpful comments and suggestions.

QUESTIONS

1. In certain cell types from I-cell disease patients (such as fibroblasts), lysosomal enzymes are secreted into the extracellular milieu rather than targeted to lysosomes. In contrast, other cells (such as hepatocytes, Kupffer cells, and leukocytes) contain nearly normal levels of lysosomal enzymes, even though these cells are also deficient in phosphotransferase activity. What do these observations suggest about the targeting of lysosomal enzymes in these different kinds of cells?
2. You are interested in devising a method for prenatal diagnosis of I-cell disease. Using the enzymes listed in Table 27-3, which of these enzyme activities would be most useful in this endeavor and why?
3. Acid sphingomyelinase is a lysosomal enzyme that catalyzes the breakdown of sphingomyelin to ceramide and phosphorylcholine. A deficiency of this enzyme leads to lysosomal accumulation of sphingomyelin in patients with Niemann-Pick disease. Recent data indicate that correct intracellular targeting of acid sphingomyelinase to lyso-

somes is dependent on the man-6-P-mediated pathway. Does this imply that the I-cell patient will present with Niemann-Pick symptoms? Can I-cell disease be viewed as a constellation of many lysosomal storage diseases?

4. In this chapter, we indicate that the metabolic error, that is, deficiency of phosphotransferase activity, in I-cell disease gives rise to a secondary phenotype of generalized diminished lysosomal enzyme activity. What other metabolic defect(s) in the man-6-P-mediated uptake system could result in such a phenotype, and how would you confirm the defect?

REFERENCES

Ben-Yoseph Y, Pack BA, Mitchell DA, et al. Characterization of the mutant *N*-acetylglucosaminyl-phosphotransferase in I-cell disease and Pseudo-Hurler polydystrophy: Complementation analysis and kinetic studies. *Enzyme* **35**:106–116, 1986.

Besley GTN, Broadhead DM, Nevin NC, Nevin J, Dornan JC: Prenatal diagnosis of mucolipidosis II by early amniocentesis. *Lancet* **335**:1164–1165, 1990.

Brauker JH, Wang JL: Nonlysosomal processing of cell-surface heparan sulfate proteoglycans. *J Biol Chem* **262**:13093–13101, 1987.

DeMars R, Leroy JG: The remarkable cells cultured from a human with Hurler's Syndrome: An approach to visual selection for *in vitro* genetic studies. *In Vitro* **2**:107–118, 1967.

Hickman S, Neufeld EF: A hypothesis for I-cell disease: defective hydrolases that do not enter lysosomes. *Biochem Biophys Res Commun.* **49**:992–999, 1972.

Kornfeld S: Trafficking of lysosomal enzymes in normal and disease states. *J Clin Invest* **77**:1–6, 1986.

Kornfeld S: Trafficking of lysosomal enzymes. *FASEB J* **1**:462–468, 1987.

Kornfeld S: Structure and function of the mannose 6-phosphate/insulin-like growth factor II receptor. *Annu Rev Biochem* **61**:307–330, 1992.

Kornfeld R, Kornfeld S: Assembly of asparagine-linked oligosaccharides. *Annu Rev Biochem* **54**:631–664, 1985.

Kornfeld S, Mellman I: The biogenesis of lysosomes. *Annu Rev Cell Biol* **5**:483–525, 1989.

Parvathy MR, Mitchell DA, Ben-Yoseph Y: Prenatal diagnosis of I-cell disease in the first and second trimesters. *Am J Med Sci* **297**:361–364, 1989.

Poenaru L, Castelnau L, Tome F, Boue J, Maroteaux P: A variant of mucolipidosis II. Clinical, biochemical and pathological investigations. *Eur J Pediatr* **147**:321–327, 1988.

Spranger JW, Wiedemann HR: The genetic mucolipidoses. Diagnosis and differential diagnosis. *Humangenetik* **9**:113–139, 1970.

von Figura K, Hasilik A: Lysosomal enzymes and their receptors. *Annu Rev Biochem* **55**:167–193, 1986.

Wolfe JW, Schuchman EH, Stramm LE, et al. Restoration of normal lysosomal function in mucopolysaccharidosis type VII by retroviral vector-mediated gene transfer. *Proc Natl Acad Sci USA* **87**:2877–2881, 1990.

Yamaguchi K, Hayasaka S, Hara S, Kurobane I, Tada K: Improvement of tear lysosomal enzyme levels after treatment with bone marrow transplantation in a patient with I-cell disease. *Ophthalmic Res* **21**:226–229, 1989.

28

Phenylketonuria: Biochemical Basis of a Clinically Heterogeneous Disorder

ALAN T. REMALEY

CASE REPORT

As part of a routine newborn screen, a 3.5-kg male infant was determined by a Guthrie test (see Diagnosis section) to have an increased plasma phenylalanine concentration. The infant was the first child of a marriage between first cousins and was born at 39 weeks after a normal pregnancy and delivery. The elevated plasma phenylalanine level was confirmed by a quantitative test to be at 484 μmol/L (normal, 70–200 μmol/L). By 12 days postpartum, the plasma phenylalanine concentration had increased to 1634 μmol/L; the plasma tyrosine level was 190 μmol/L (normal, 90–225 μmol/L). The patient was tentatively diagnosed as having phenylketonuria (PKU), a disorder of phenylalanine catabolism that results from a deficiency of phenylalanine hydroxylase. The patient was immediately placed on a diet low in phenylalanine; careful compliance with the diet and frequent monitoring of the plasma phenylalanine level resulted in the patient's plasma phenylalanine level being maintained below the lower limit of the normal range. The patient appeared to be developing normally until 4 months of age, when he developed truncal hypotonia and spasticity of the limbs. Despite being on a low phenylalanine diet, at 5 months of age the patient had several *grand mal* (epileptic) seizures.

Because of the patient's atypical course for PKU, further biochemical testing was performed. An oral phenylalanine loading test resulted in a plasma phenylalanine level of 1513 μmol/L (normal, <1200 μmol/L) at 6 hours and 242 μmol/L (normal, <200) at 24 hours. Biopterin, a cofactor for phenylalanine hydroxylase, was measured in the urine by the *Crithidia* bioassay and was found to be markedly elevated. By chromatographic analysis of the urine, the biopterin was found to be mostly in the inactive oxidized form of the cofactor, quinonoid dihydrobiopterin (qBH_2), and not in the active, reduced form of the cofactor, tetrahydrobiopterin (BH_4). Administration of BH_4, however, did not significantly lower the concentration of phenylalanine in the patient's plasma. A liver biopsy was performed, and enzyme assays for phenylalanine hydroxylase, GTP-cyclohydrolase, and pyruvoyltetrahydrobiopterin synthase revealed normal activity levels. In contrast, dihydropteridine reductase activity was not detected; this enzyme maintains the biopterin cofactor in the active, reduced state.

Because of the requirement for biopterin in neurotransmitter biosynthesis, urine levels of homovanillic acid, vanillylmandelic acid, and 5-hydroxyindoleacetic acid were measured and found to be abnormally low. In an attempt to correct a possible deficiency of neurotransmitters and the presumed cause of the persistent neurologic symptoms, the patient was treated with L-dopa (3,4-dihydroxyphenylalanine), 5-hydroxytryptophan, carbidopa, and folate. With this additional therapy, the patient's neurologic symptoms gradually resolved.

DIAGNOSIS

Phenylketonuria screening is the prototype of neonatal screening for the early diagnosis and treatment of genetic diseases (O'Flynn, 1992). The association of an elevated plasma phenylalanine level with mental retardation, the principal symptom of PKU, was first observed more than 50 years ago by Folling. The biochemical defect for the most common form of PKU was determined in 1953 to be a deficiency of phenylalanine hydroxylase. It was not until the early 1960s, however, when a screening test became available and, more importantly, an effective therapy could be offered, that PKU screening was routinely performed. Since the initial success of neonatal PKU testing, many other biochemical disorders are now routinely screened for in newborns.

Fortunately, because of the success of PKU screening and treatment, the clinical sequelae of PKU are rarely observed, and most cases are now diagnosed by testing in the clinical laboratory. The cardinal clinical feature of PKU is the mental retardation that gradually develops during the first year of life. If left untreated, patients with PKU can lose up to 1 IQ point per week and more than 50 IQ points in the first year. Because of the progressive and irreversible nature of the neurologic disease in PKU, it is important that PKU be diagnosed early and that therapy be initiated immediately.

Without the PKU screening test it is difficult to diagnose PKU clinically. The other clinical features of PKU are either not characteristic or are often too subtle to be recognized. There are several skin manifestations of the disease, such as eczema, pigment loss, musty odor, and scleroderma-like changes. Impaired physical growth and other features of neurologic disease, such as behavioral problems, delayed psychomotor development, and seizures, can all occur in untreated PKU.

One of the oldest and still most widely used screening tests for PKU is the Guthrie test. The Guthrie test is a semiquantitative bioassay that uses *Bacillus subtilis* bacteria, which, in the presence of a phenylalanine biosynthesis inhibitor, require exogenous phenylalanine for growth (Clark, 1992). The bacteria are mixed with an aliquot of a patient's blood specimen, and the growth of the bacteria is directly proportional to the amount of phenylalanine in the specimen. The false-negative rate of the Guthrie test has recently become a problem because of the practice of discharging newborns from the hospital within the first few days of birth. Ideally, the screening test should be performed at least 48 hours after birth, when the infant has had several feedings and has been exposed to dietary phenylalanine.

Subsequent confirmation of a positive screening test by a quantitative assay is necessary for several reasons. An elevated plasma phenylalanine level in newborns can be transitory and does not need to be treated. Transitory hyperphenylalaninemia is often associated with prematurity and is due to a maturational delay in the enzymes involved in the catabolism of phenylalanine. At the same time that the quantitative determination of phenylalanine is done, tyrosine is also measured to distinguish PKU from disorders of tyrosine catabolism. Patients with disorders of tyrosine catabolism also have an elevated plasma phenylalanine level, but unlike PKU patients, their plasma tyrosine level is also increased. Quantitative measurement of phenylalanine is also used to categorize PKU patients into one of two clinical phenotypes. Patients whose plasma phenylalanine concentration exceeds 1200 μmol/L are considered to have classic PKU and will develop all of the characteristic signs and symptoms of PKU. Patients whose plasma phenylalanine concentration is below 600 μmol/L are classified as having benign hyperphenylalaninemia, because their phenylalanine level is below the threshold at which symptoms appear. These patients usually do not need to be treated, but because of the irreversible nature of the neurologic damage in classic PKU, they are often initially treated until confirmatory tests, such as the phenylalanine loading test. In this test, patients ingest a fixed amount of phenylalanine and the subsequent rise and clearance of plasma phenylalanine over time can be used to classify patients with hyperphenylalaninemia.

Determination of the level of plasma phenylalanine is sufficient to make a correct diagnosis and decide on the need for therapy in most cases of hyperphenylalaninemia due to defects in phenylalanine hydroxylase. It has recently been appreciated, however, that other biochemical defects can cause hyperphenylalaninemia (Eisensmith and Woo, 1992). As illustrated in this case report, these patients are important to identify because they have an atypical clinical course and do not respond to dietary therapy. Two types of defects in the metabolism of biopterin have been shown to be the cause of PKU in patients with normal amounts of phenylalanine hydroxylase activity. These patients have either a defect in biopterin biosynthesis or a problem in maintaining biopterin in its active, reduced form because of a deficiency of dihydropteridine reductase (Kaufman et al., 1975). All patients with hyperphenylalaninemia need to be screened for these disorders of biopterin metabolism by a screening test, such as the *Crithidia* test for biopterin. This test, like the Guthrie test, is a bioassay, and it depends on the growth of the protozoan *Crithidia luciliae*, whose growth depends upon biopterin in the patient's plasma specimen. Patients with defects in biopterin biosynthesis will have decreased levels of biopterin. In contrast, patients with dihydropteridine deficiency usually have elevated levels of biopterin, particularly the oxidized form (qBH_2). Another feature that distinguishes these two types of PKU is the response to biopterin loading; when patients with some defect in the pathway of biopterin biosynthesis are administered biopterin orally, their plasma phenylalanine levels markedly decrease and remain low. In contrast, patients with dihydropteridine reductase deficiency manifest only a minor and transitory decrease in their plasma phenylalanine concentration because they are unable to maintain biopterin in the active, reduced state; thus, any exogenously administered reduced biopterin (BH_4) can only act stochiometrically in lowering the plasma phenylalanine level.

Ultimately, to determine the precise biochemical defect in hyperphenylalaninemia, assays for enzymes known to be defective in phenylalanine catabolism must be performed. One problem with this approach, however, is that, unlike the other enzymes in the phenylalanine catabolic pathway, phenylalanine hydroxylase is expressed only in the liver, which renders the assay of this enzyme difficult, particularly in newborns. In such cases, a liver biopsy must be done and precludes intrauterine testing for PKU from cell cultures from amniotic fluid or chorionic villus cells. Because of this limitation, DNA-based testing is used to diagnose PKU (Woo et al., 1983; Wood et al., 1993). Unfortunately, the large size of the phenylalanine hydroxylase gene (approximately 90 kilobases) and the large number of mutations that have been described (>60) make direct DNA sequence analysis and other sequence-dependent approaches (e.g., allele-specific oligonucleotides) difficult to

perform. Currently, *in utero* restriction fragment length polymorphism (RFLP) analysis for predicting the chances of developing PKU, once a proband has been identified, is the only DNA type testing that is routinely performed.

MOLECULAR PERSPECTIVES

Because phenylalanine is an essential amino acid, and therefore is not endogenously produced, the only net source of phenylalanine is the diet (Fig. 28-1). Phenylalanine can also be released from protein breakdown, but it is also quickly reutilized for protein synthesis and does not cause a net change in total body phenylalanine. An acute change in protein turnover can transiently change the plasma phenylalanine concentration. The level of plasma phenylalanine is therefore largely dependent on the balance between the uptake of dietary phenylalanine and the rate of catabolism of phenylalanine. In PKU, the major route of catabolism begins with the conversion of phenylalanine to tyrosine (Scriver et al., 1989). This reaction is catalyzed normally by phenylalanine hydroxylase. In PKU, phenylalanine hydroxylase is defective (Fig. 28-1). Because of the decreased rate of phenylalanine catabolism in PKU, the level of plasma phenylalanine increases until the alternative pathway of catabolism is used. The alternative pathway normally does not significantly contribute to the catabolism of phenylalanine because the enzymes in this pathway have a much higher Michaelis constant (K_m) for phenylalanine than does phenylalanine hydroxylase.

The alternative pathway for the catabolism of phenylalanine is shown in Figure 28-2. All modifications of phenylalanine by this pathway occur only on the alanine side chain of the phenylalanine molecule. First is a transamination reaction that converts phe-

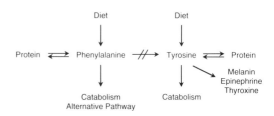

Figure 28-1. Metabolic pathways of phenylalanine and tyrosine metabolism.

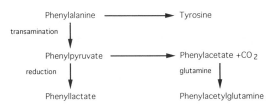

Figure 28-2. Alternative pathway for phenylalanine catabolism.

nylalanine to phenylpyruvate. Unlike the normal route of phenylalanine catabolism, the alternative pathway does not lead to complete breakdown and oxidation of phenylalanine. Instead, water-soluble compounds such as phenylpyruvate and phenylacetate accumulate and are excreted in the urine. The presence of phenylpyruvate in the urine can be detected by a simple, but nonspecific, ferric chloride test. The accumulation of phenylacetate is responsible for the musty odor that frequently occurs in PKU patients.

The first and the rate-limiting step in the normal pathway of phenylalanine catabolism is catalyzed by phenylalanine hydroxylase, which is a mixed-function oxygenase (Fig. 28-3). Mixed-function oxygenases split molecular oxygen and incorporate one of the oxygen atoms into the substrate while the other oxygen atom is reduced to water. To drive the reaction, reducing equivalents must be present as a source of energy. In the case of phenylalanine hydroxylase, phenylalanine serves as the substrate, and it is hydroxylated on the para position of the aromatic ring. The source of reducing equivalents in this

reaction is BH_4. Once BH_4 is oxidized, the resulting qBH_2 is converted back to BH_4 by dihydropteridine reductase and NADH. Both classic PKU and benign hyperphenylalaninemia are due to defects in phenylalanine hydroxylase. The difference between the two disorders lies in the relative amount of residual enzyme activity. In classic PKU, there is typically less than 2% residual phenylalanine hydroxylase activity. In benign hyperphenylalaninemia, the mutations in the phenylalanine hydroxylase protein do not cause as severe an effect on enzyme function. These patients typically have 10 to 25% residual activity, which is apparently enough to maintain the plasma phenylalanine level below its pathologic threshold.

The biosynthesis of biopterin occurs in three steps (Fig. 28-4). It begins with the conversion of guanosine triphosphate to dihydroneopterin by GTP-cyclohydrolase. The next step is catalyzed by pyruvoyltetrahydrobiopterin synthase and is the rate-limiting step. Two different enzymes that differ in their tissue distribution complete the biosynthesis of BH_4. Although defects in any of the four enzymes in the pathway could theoretically result in PKU, only defects in GTP-cyclohydrolase and pyruvoyltetrahydrobiopterin synthase have been described. In addition to BH_4, neopterin, a structurally related compound, can also be produced by a variation of this pathway. Neopterin has no known function, but it is specifically produced by activated T-cells and is used as a marker of immune activation.

An interesting feature of biopterin-defective PKU is that dietary treatment (e.g., phenylalanine-restricted diet) is ineffective in preventing neurologic disease.

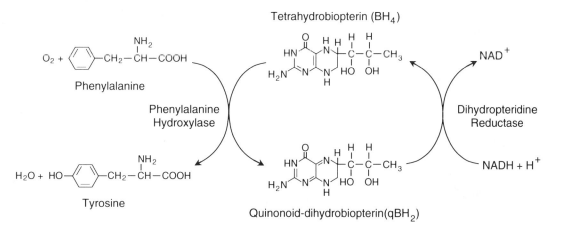

Figure 28-3. The conversion of phenylalanine to tyrosine by phenylalanine hydroxylase.

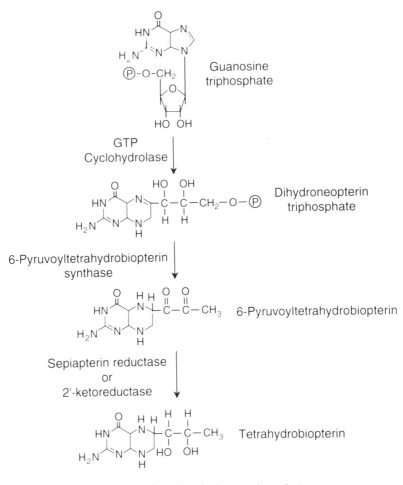

Figure 28-4. Pathway for biopterin biosynthesis.

Besides phenylalanine hydroxylase, several other mixed-function oxygenases, namely, tyrosine hydroxylase and tryptophan hydroxylase, use biopterin as a cofactor. All three enzymes are homologous and probably arose by gene duplication. Patients with defects in biopterin metabolism, therefore, have defects in not only phenylalanine hydroxylase activity but also in tyrosine and tryptophan hydroxylase activities. Tyrosine hydroxylase and tryptophan hydroxylase are important in the biosynthesis of several neurotransmitters, namely, dopamine, norepinephrine, epinephrine, and serotonin (Fig. 28-5). Abnormalities in the level of these neurotransmitters are probably responsible for the neurologic symptoms that are refractory to treatment by a low phenylalanine diet. These neurotransmitters are short-lived, and their production is usually inferred from the urine level of their more stable breakdown products. As in this case, homovanillic acid and vanillylmandelic acid are used to monitor dopamine and norepinephrine production, and 5-hydroxyindoleacetic acid is used to monitor serotonin production (Fig. 28-5).

An unresolved biochemical issue is identifying the mechanism for the neurologic abnormalities in classic PKU. Three main hypotheses have been proposed. One states that because tyrosine is only produced via hydroxylation of phenylalanine by phenylalanine hydroxylase, a deficiency of tyrosine is responsible for the neurologic abnormalities. Tyrosine, however, can also be obtained from the diet, and dietary tyrosine is usually sufficient to maintain plasma levels in the normal range. A related hypoth-

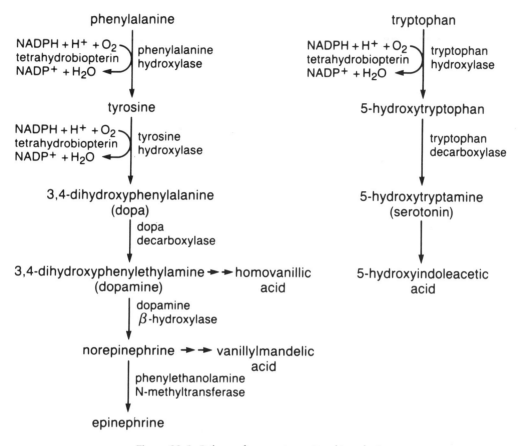

Figure 28-5. Pathways for neurotransmitter biosynthesis.

esis is that although extracellular levels of tyrosine may be normal, intracellular levels of tyrosine may be decreased. Phenylalanine competes with tyrosine and tryptophan for cellular uptake in the brain by the large, neutral amino acid uptake system. Because both tyrosine and tryptophan are important in neurotransmitter biosynthesis, the decreased intracellular levels of these amino acids may account for the neurologic symptoms. It has also been proposed that phenylalanine or an abnormal phenylalanine metabolite from the alternative pathway of catabolism is directly responsible for the symptoms. Numerous enzymatic reactions and cellular processes have been shown to be affected *in vitro* by elevated levels of phenylalanine and phenylalanine metabolites, but the *in vivo* relevance of these studies to the pathogenesis of PKU is unclear. In support of this model, the hypopigmentation one sees in PKU patients may occur by the inhibition of tyrosinase, an enzyme

involved in converting tyrosine to melanin, by the increased phenylalanine level or abnormal phenylalanine metabolites in PKU patients.

THERAPY

One reason why PKU was the first disease that was routinely screened for in newborns was that an effective therapy was available. It is one of the few genetic disorders that can be adequately treated by a modification of the diet (Clark, 1992). Because phenylalanine is an essential amino acid, the only source of phenylalanine is the diet. Unlike substances that are both present in the diet and endogenously produced (e.g., cholesterol), the level of plasma phenylalanine can be readily controlled by decreasing dietary phenylalanine. Phenylalanine, however, is relatively ubiquitous in our diet, and a significant modification in the diet must be made to reduce markedly the level of phenylalanine. In the PKU diet, about 70 to 90% of protein from natural sources is substituted with artificial protein that is low in phenylalanine. Because the diet is given to newborns and infants, the reduction in phenylalanine must be balanced with the need for phenylalanine for normal growth.

Originally, a low phenylalanine diet was used for children with PKU until they reached the age of 6 years, when brain development is mostly complete. If children are placed immediately on a low phenylalanine diet soon after birth, they appear to develop normally and can achieve a normal IQ. Because of the difficulty in complying with the diet, which is not very palatable, and concerns about a low growth rate, the diet was usually discontinued when children reached school age. It was recently observed, however, that some patients experience a deterioration of neurologic function once the diet is discontinued. Currently, there is no recommendation with regard to when, if ever, to discontinue the low phenylalanine diet in PKU patients (Potocnik and Widhalm, 1994).

Another factor favoring the prolonged use of dietary therapy is the recently described phenomena of maternal PKU (Koch et al., 1993). After the first female patients were successfully treated for PKU and had discontinued their diet, it was observed many years later that their children were born with a PKU-like disorder. These children suffered from the moment of birth mental retardation, microcephaly, and congenital heart malformations, and, *in utero,* intrauterine growth delay. These children were later shown not to have defects in phenylalanine catabolism but instead were suffering the consequences of *in utero* exposure to high levels of phenylalanine from the mother. If mothers with PKU are treated with a low phenylalanine diet throughout the pregnancy and, preferably, before conception, they can have normal children.

Unlike in classic PKU, dietary therapy alone is not sufficient for treating patients with defects in biopterin metabolism. The low phenylalanine diet does not correct the abnormalities in neurotransmitter biosynthesis. Neither does administration of BH_4 correct the neurologic abnormalities because BH_4 does not cross the blood–brain barrier. Instead, these patients are treated with L-dopa and 5-hydroxytryptophan, which cross the blood–brain barrier and are precursors to dopamine, epinephrine, and serotonin (Fig. 28-5). In addition, these patients, like those with Parkinson disease, are also given carbidopa, a dopamine carboxylase inhibitor that prevents the side effects arising from the conversion of L-dopa to dopamine in non-central nervous system tissues. Because patients with dihydropteridine reductase deficiency have been reported to be deficient in folate, they are also given folate supplements. It has been proposed that dihydropteridine reductase may play an auxiliary role in the metabolism of folate, a conjugated pterin that is structurally related to biopterin.

QUESTIONS

1. Using Michaelis-Menten kinetics, explain why the alternative pathway for phenylalanine catabolism is not used significantly under normal conditions.
2. Using the concepts of pathologic thresholds of biochemical metabolites and steady-state kinetics, explain why PKU is an autosomal recessive disease.
3. Explain why administration of BH_4 will lower plasma phenylalanine levels in patients with defects in biopterin synthesis but not significantly in patients with dihydropteridine deficiency.
4. Explain why defects in tyrosine metabolism can also lead to increased plasma phenylalanine levels.
5. Approximately one third of all mutations in the phenylalanine hydroxylase gene occur in exon 7. Discuss the possible reasons for the clustering of mutations in certain regions of genes.
6. Explain why the symptoms of PKU do not develop until several months after birth, whereas in the case of maternal PKU, infants are born with the manifestations of PKU.
7. Obligate heterozygotes of cross-reactive material-positive (CRM+) defects of phenylalanine hydroxylase frequently have significantly less than the expected 50% of residual activity. Given that phenylalanine hydroxylase is a multimeric enzyme, propose a mechanism for this unexpected gene-dosage effect.
8. Discuss possible alternatives to dietary therapy for treating PKU patients.

REFERENCES

Clark BJ: After a positive Guthrie-what next? Dietary management for the child with phenylketonuria. *Eur J Clin Nutr* **46:**S33–S39, 1992.

Eisensmith RC, Woo SL: Molecular basis of phenylketonuria and related hyperphenylalaninemias: mutations and polymorphisms in the human phenylalanine hydroxylase gene. *Hum Mutat* **1:**13–23, 1992.

Kaufman S, Holtzman NA, Milstien S, et al.: Phenylketonuria due to a deficiency of dihydropteridine reductase. *N Engl J Med* **293:**785–790, 1975.

Koch R, Levy HL, Matalon R, Rouse B, et al.: The North American collaborative study of maternal phenylketonuria. *Am J Dis Child* **147:**1224–1230, 1993.

O'Flynn ME: Newborn screening for phenylketonuria: Thirty years of progress. *Curr Prob Pediatr* **22:**159–165, 1992.

Potocnik U, Widhalm K: Long-term follow-up of children with classical phenylketonuria after diet discontinuation: a review. *J Am Coll Nutr* **13:**232–236, 1994.

Scriver CR, Kaufman S, Woo SLC: The hyperphenylalaninemias, *in* Scriver CR, Beaudet AL, Sly WS, Valle D: (eds): *The Metabolic Basis of Inherited Diseases.* New York, McGraw-Hill, 1989, pp. 495–546.

Woo SLC, Lidsky AS, Guttler F, et al.: Cloned human phenylalanine hydroxylase gene allows prenatal diagnosis and carrier detection of classical phenylketonuria. *Nature* **306:**151–155, 1983.

Wood N, Tyfield L, Bidwell J: Rapid classification of phenylketonuria genotypes by analysis of heteroduplexes generated by PCR-amplifiable synthetic DNA. *Hum Mutat* **2:**131–137, 1993.

PART IV

Steroids

29

Cushing's Syndrome

B. SYLVIA VELA

CASE REPORT

C.G., a 61-year-old man, has complained of weakness and generalized malaise for the last 4 to 5 months. Several months ago, he initiated a walking program and has lost 12 lbs. Despite the exercise, the weakness has progressed. Although the patient was pleased with his weight loss, he noticed that his face was becoming round and his cheeks fuller (Fig. 29-1A). On the other hand, the patient's arthritis had improved remarkably over the same period.

Past medical history is significant for a history of prostate cancer diagnosed 7 months before evaluation for which the patient had been treated with an *orchiectomy* (excision of the testicles) and a history of depression for which he had been treated with various antidepressants for the last one year. The patient is a nonsmoker and a social drinker. Currently, he was taking flutamide, an androgen antagonist for treatment of his prostate cancer.

On physical examination, his blood pressure was elevated at 193/105 mm Hg (normal <140/90), and his pulse was 80 beats per minute (normal 60–100). In general, he was *plethoric* (ruddy complexion) with a round, full face and central obesity. A dorsocervical fat pad was noticeable on his upper back as well as mild supraclavicular fullness (Fig. 29-1B). His lungs were clear and his cardiac examination unremarkable. The abdominal exam was made difficult by his obesity; however, the liver was palpably enlarged. Extremities had marked doughy pitting pedal edema or swelling. The skin was noticeably thin, and multiple *ecchymoses* (bruises)

were seen on the upper extremities. No hyperpigmentation or violaceous *striae* (stretch marks) was found. He had profound proximal muscle weakness with great difficulty getting out of a chair or climbing stairs.

Laboratory evaluation revealed a hemoglobin of 12 g/dL (normal, 14–18 g/dL), hematocrit of 36% (normal, 42–52%), white blood cell (WBC) count of 7,000/mm^3 (normal, 4,800–10,800/mm^3) with a prominent left shift or increased number of immature cells (88% neutrophils), and *lymphocytopenia*, or decreased numbers of lymphocytes (8% lymphocytes). Sodium was 131 mmol/L (normal, 135–148 mmol/L), potassium was decreased at 2.9 mmol/L (normal, 3.5–4.9 mmol/L), bicarbonate was elevated at 39 mmol/L (normal, 21–28 mmol/L), and glucose was 530 mg/dL (29.5 mmol/L) (normal, 3.9–6.1 mmol/L). Liver function tests were normal with the exception of a markedly elevated lactate dehydrogenase (LDH) of 4722 U/mL (normal, 213–618 U/ml). The electrocardiogram showed diffuse nonspecific changes. Chest roentgenogram revealed a thoracic vertebral crush fracture (Fig. 29-2). Lung fields were clear. A diagnosis of Cushing's syndrome or hypercortisolemia was suspected.

To document hypercortisolemia, a 1-mg overnight dexamethasone suppression test was performed and revealed an 8:00 AM cortisol >50 μg/dL (>1379 nmol/L) with normal being <5 μg/dL (138 nmol/L). To confirm the hypercortisolemia, a 24-hour urine free cortisol was collected and was markedly elevated at 12,200 μg with normal being <50 μg (33,500 nmol/day with normal <138 nmol/day).

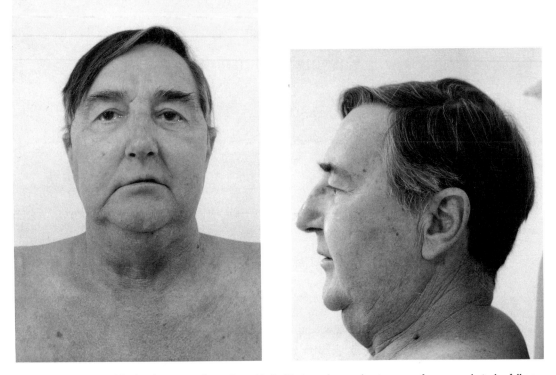

Figure 29-1. Abnormal fat distribution in index patient with Cushing's syndrome, showing moon face, supraclavicular fullness, and dorsocervical buffalo hump.

To determine the cause of the hypercortisolemia, a high-dose 8-mg overnight dexamethasone test revealed a baseline serum cortisol of 119 μg/dL (3282 nmol/L) and a post-dexamethasone cortisol of 170 μg/dL (4700 nmol/L). Plasma adrenocorticotropic hormone (ACTH) levels were elevated at 370 pg/mL with normal <50 pg/mL (18 pmol/L; normal, <2.4 pmol/L), confirming an ACTH-dependent process. Furthermore, the ACTH level was not suppressed with high-dose dexamethasone. These findings were considered most compatible with the ectopic ACTH syndrome. *Ectopic* refers to an aberrant or nonpituitary source of ACTH.

Computed tomography (CT) of the chest and abdomen revealed multiple hepatic masses and periaortic lymph nodes consistent with metastatic disease (Fig. 29-3). Also noted was bilateral adrenal hyperplasia, an expected consequence of excessive ACTH stimulation of the adrenal glands. Bone scan revealed multiple bony metastases in the ribs and spine (Fig. 29-4). To determine the tumor type, a CT-guided liver biopsy was performed and was compatible with metastatic small cell carcinoma of the lung.

During the patient's hospital stay, his mental status deteriorated significantly. He vacillated between periods of paranoia, confusion, mania, and psychosis. His hypertension and edema were treated and improved with spironolactone, an aldosterone antagonist. He was given supplements of potassium chloride, and his potassium level normalized; however, his metabolic alkalosis persisted. His blood glucose concentration was controlled by insulin administration. The patient was given ketoconazole, an inhibitor of cytochrome P450 enzymes involved in steroidogenesis, with marked improvement in his hypertension, hyperglycemia, and mental status. Repeat 24-hour urine free cortisol was 60 μg/24 h (166 nmol/daily), reflecting a marked reduction in his endogenous cortisol production. The patient's hypokalemia and alkalosis normalized, and his insulin and antihypertensive drugs were discontinued. His weakness was subjectively and objectively improved. He was given replacement doses of predni-

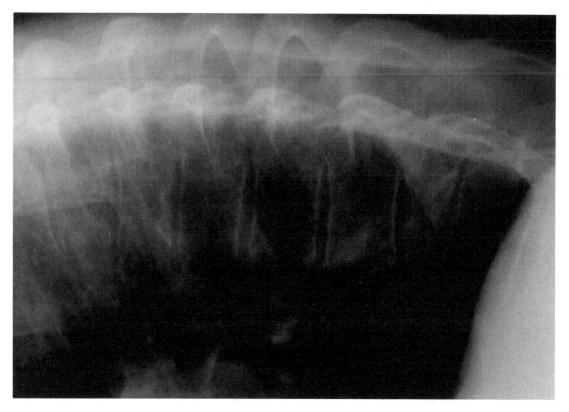

Figure 29-2. Lateral thoracic radiograph of subject with Cushing's syndrome demonstrating diffuse osteopenia of the axial spine with a wedge-shaped crush fracture of T-10 shown second from the bottom.

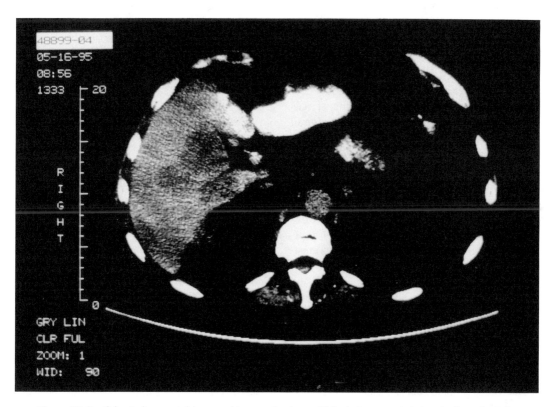

Figure 29-3. Abdominal computed tomographic scan showing multiple dark metastatic lesions in the patient's liver.

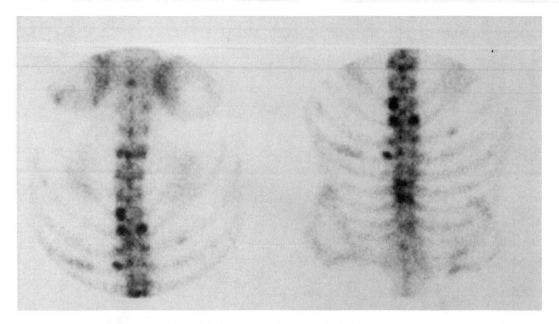

Figure 29-4. Technetium pyrophosphate-labeled bone scan showing multiple hot spots in the axial skeleton and rib cage consistent with metastatic disease to the bone.

sone (7.5 mg/day) and discharged from the hospital to the care of his family.

DIAGNOSIS

Definitions

Cushing's *syndrome* refers to a constellation of signs and symptoms associated with the chronic state of glucocorticoid excess in the circulation, without regard to etiology. Cushing's *disease* refers to glucocorticoid excess from overproduction of ACTH from the pituitary gland. Most commonly, this overproduction results from an ACTH-producing pituitary tumor. All patients with Cushing's disease have Cushing's syndrome, but the reverse is not always true, as many causes of cortisol excess are ACTH independent.

Clinical Features of Cushing's Syndrome

The clinical manifestations of Cushing's syndrome have not changed since they were first described by Harvey Cushing in 1932 (Fig. 29-5) (Cushing, 1932). Weight gain is the most common manifestation and initial symptom in most patients. It is classi-

cally described as "central obesity," referring to the fact that the face, neck, trunk, and abdomen are primarily affected, sparing the arms and legs. Generalized obesity may also be seen, however, especially in children. Weight loss, as seen in the present patient, is usually a harbinger of malignancy, either adrenal carcinoma or malignancy causing ectopic production of ACTH.

Several features of the fat distribution in Cushing's syndrome help distinguish it from simple obesity. Accumulation of fat in the face results in the classic "moon facies," which is usually plethoric because of thinning of the epidermis. Fat accumulation also occurs in the supraclavicular region, causing "supraclavicular fat pads," as well as in the posterior neck, known as the "buffalo hump" (Figs. 29-1A and B).

Skin changes include easy bruising, with a thinned, transparent appearance, and violaceous striae, usually over the abdomen, breasts, axilla, thighs, and buttocks resulting from thinning of the epidermis and the underlying connective tissue. Hyperpigmentation can be seen in patients with ACTH-dependent Cushing's syndrome, in which ACTH is overproduced either by the pituitary or from ectopic production from a malignancy, and binds to the melanocyte receptors in the skin. Acne and *hirsu-*

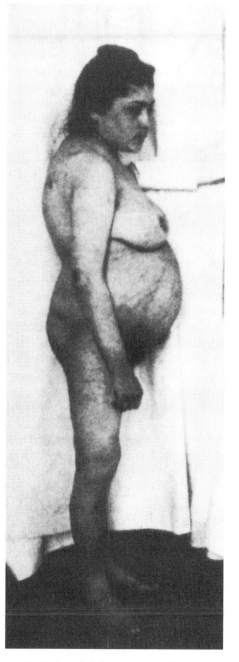

Figure 29-5. One of the patients originally described by Cushing in 1932. Note the central obesity, thinned extremities, abdominal striae, and moon face.

tism (excessive body/facial hair) can occur as a result of excess adrenal androgen production; however, severe hirsutism and virilization are strongly suggestive of an adrenal carcinoma.

Reproductive dysfunction is common due to excess androgens in females, causing amenorrhea and infertility. Excess cortisol in males causes suppression of gonadotropins, which leads to decreased *libido* (sex drive) and secondary or hypothalamo-pituitary *hypogonadism* (underproduction of gonadotropins and testosterone). Psychological disturbances range from mania, anxiety, depression, and loss of memory, to psychosis, paranoia, and suicide attempts. Proximal muscle weakness and osteoporosis occur commonly because of the effects of glucocorticoids on muscle and bone. Hypertension and atherosclerosis are present in 75 to 85% of patients and contribute to the excess morbidity and mortality seen in Cushing's syndrome. Diabetes or, more frequently, glucose intolerance is also commonly seen.

Differential Diagnosis

Iatrogenic Cushing's syndrome (a condition induced by the treatment itself) due to the administration of steroids to patients with inflammatory diseases is by far the most common type of Cushing's syndrome seen in medical practice. Noniatrogenic Cushing's syndrome is classified as either ACTH dependent or ACTH independent.

The ACTH-dependent types include Cushing's disease (ACTH overproduction from the pituitary gland) and ectopic ACTH syndrome, seen with certain types of malignancy that synthesize and secrete ACTH into the circulation. Most of these malignancies are derived from neuroendocrine cells histologically, such as medullary thyroid carcinoma, small cell carcinoma, carcinoids, pancreatic islet cell tumors, pheochromocytomas, and paragangliomas. In rare cases, these malignancies can secrete corticotropin-releasing hormone (CRH), which stimulates the pituitary to produce ACTH. In these disorders, the hypersecretion of ACTH causes bilateral adrenocortical hyperplasia with increased secretion of cortisol, androgens, and deoxycorticosterone, the precursor to cortisol.

In ACTH-independent Cushing's syndrome, adrenal neoplasms autonomously produce excess cortisol. The excess cortisol negatively feeds back to the pituitary and hypothalamus and suppresses further CRH and ACTH release. Hence, ACTH levels are usually low in ACTH-independent Cushing's syndrome and are critical in the diagnostic workup of all patients suspected of having Cushing's syndrome.

Cushing's disease is the most common cause of Cushing's syndrome, accounting for about 68% of all cases (Orth, 1995). ACTH-independent neoplasms, either adrenal carcinoma or adenoma, account for 15 to 20% of cases, and ectopic ACTH/CRH syndromes another 15%. Rare causes of Cushing's syndrome include micronodular hyperplasia, a genetic condition characterized by pigmented microscopic bilateral adrenocortical nodules, and macronodular hyperplasia, a condition thought to involve evolution from a pituitary-dependent disease to an adrenal-dependent process. Adrenal nodular hyperplasia accounts for 1% of cases.

Certain features often suggest a specific etiology. For example, women aged 20 to 40 years typically have Cushing's disease with all of the classic clinical manifestations of excess glucocorticoid as well as mild hirsutism. These features are generally slowly progressive. In Cushing's disease, the serum potassium level is usually normal, and peripheral edema is uncommon. Men aged 50 to 70 years predominate in the ectopic ACTH syndrome and frequently do not have classic manifestations of excess glucocorticoid. Instead, hypokalemia, peripheral edema, metabolic alkalosis, weakness, hyperpigmentation, hypertension and glucose intolerance are the most prominent manifestations, caused by equally elevated levels of glucocorticoid and mineralocorticoid. An elderly man with Cushing's syndrome should be considered to have ectopic ACTH syndrome until proved otherwise. The clinical picture in patients with adrenal adenomas is usually that of classic Cushing's syndrome with excessive glucocorticoid and gradual onset, whereas patients with adrenal carcinomas have glucocorticoid, mineralocorticoid, and androgen excess with a rapid onset.

A number of patients with alcoholism and depression can appear clinically to manifest signs and symptoms of hypercortisolemia, the so-called *pseudo-Cushing's syndrome*. These patients have elevated basal plasma levels of cortisol and both increased production rate and excretion of cortisol, such that they appear biochemically similar to patients with Cushing's disease. Alcoholism should therefore be considered in all patients suspected of hypercortisolemia. If a history of active excessive drinking is established, the workup for Cushing's syndrome should be postponed until the patient abstains.

Patients with depression, unlike patients with Cushing's disease, will usually suppress with low-dose dexamethasone testing or have normal urinary-free cortisol and can usually be distinguished on this basis; however, depression may also be a symptom of Cushing's syndrome, as in our index case. Other tests that may be useful in separating pseudo-Cushing's from true Cushing's are CRH and dexamethasone stimulation testing in sequence, naloxone testing, insulin-induced hypoglycemia, and cortisol circadian patterns (see below).

MOLECULAR PERSPECTIVES

The adrenal glands are small, approximately 5 g in weight, and are located above the kidneys on each side of the vertebral column. The cortex makes up most of the gland and consists of three histological zones: the zona glomerulosa, the zona fasciculata, and zona reticularis. The adrenal cortex produces three main steroid hormones: (1) mineralocorticoids, principally aldosterone, from the zona glomerulosa; (2) glucocorticoids, cortisol, and corticosterone, from the zona fasciculata and reticularis; and (3) adrenal androgens, dihydroepiandrosterone (DHEA), its sulfated form, and androstenedione from the zona reticularis. The adrenal medulla, a derivative of the sympathetic nervous system, produces the catecholamines epinephrine and norepinephrine.

Glucocorticoids

Glucocorticoids are 21-carbon-atom structures with a double bond at C-4 and hydroxyl groups at C-11 and C-21 (Fig. 29-6). Glucocorticoids, as their name implies, play a major role in glucose production and metabolism. They increase hepatic glycogen production and gluconeogenesis, and decrease glucose uptake and utilization in the periphery. In hypercortisolemia, the result can be hyperglycemia and frank diabetes, as seen in the patient presented or, more commonly, *glucose intolerance* (mildly elevated fasting glucose concentrations). Conversely, in adrenal insufficiency, hepatic glycogenolysis and glucose production are decreased, and sensitivity to insulin increases, resulting in hypoglycemia.

The effects of glucocorticoid on fat metabolism are demonstrated by the excess fat deposition (supraclavicular fat pads, moon face, buffalo hump) seen in patient's with Cushing's syndrome. Glucocorticoids increase lipolysis and the level of plasma free fatty acids. Augmentation of hepatic conversion of free fatty acids to ketones can lead to a mild *ketosis* (enhanced production of ketone bodies). There is also an increase in hepatic lipoproteins, for example, very low density lipoprotein (VLDL), low density lipoprotein (LDL) and high-density lipoprotein (HDL), with subsequent hyperlipidemia leading to accelerated atherosclerosis.

The glucocorticoids also effect protein, RNA, and DNA synthesis. In general, synthesis of RNA is stimulated in the liver and inhibited in the skin, adipose, muscle, bone, and lymphoid tissues. Protein breakdown in the skin and connective tissues leads to the violaceous striae, easy bruising, and thinned skin. In muscle, protein breakdown results in muscle wasting, most notably in the proximal muscle groups. In the patient presented herein, the proximal myopathy was exhibited in his inability to climb stairs or get up from a chair. His overall malaise is likely a consequence of his myopathy as well. Overall, the protein and muscle breakdown results in net nitrogen loss. Protein and collagen breakdown in bone can cause osteopenia and may result in fractures of the ribs or vertebral bodies, as seen in our index case. Glucocorticoid-induced osteoporosis is the most aggressive form of osteoporosis seen. In addition, glucocorticoids impair intestinal absorption of calcium and hypercalciuria, leading to negative calcium balance and secondary hyperparathyroidism, which exacerbates the bone loss.

The effects of glucocorticoids on the bone marrow include granulocytosis as well as a decrease in the number of lymphocytes, monocytes, eosinophils, and platelets. These effects are due to a redistribution of cells moving out of the circulation at an accelerated rate and into other compartments, such as bone marrow, spleen, and lymph nodes; this process is referred to as *demargination*. The mechanism for the thrombocytopenia is unclear.

Glucocorticoids are used pharmacologically to suppress inflammation and immune responses in inflammatory diseases. It is of interest that our patient's inflammatory arthritis improved over the course of his disease, undoubtedly due to his excessive hypercortisolemia. In Cushing's syndrome, however, these suppressive actions can be deleterious in that they can lead to immunosuppression and susceptibility to infection. The anti-inflammatory actions of glucocorticoids occur because of the inhibition of vasoactive agents and chemotactic factors, such as prostaglandins, kinins, and histamines, impairment of leukocyte migration to the site of infection, and impaired function of immunocompetent B and T cells.

Glucocorticoids affect the cardiovascular system, blood pressure, water excretion, and electrolyte balance, both through direct glucocorticoid actions and through mineralocorticoid-like actions, by binding to the mineralocorticoid receptor. Their important role in maintaining blood pressure is demonstrated by the fact that hypotension in patients who are adrenally insufficient cannot be reversed by fluids, sodium administration alone, or even by mineralocorticoids and is reversed only by the administration of glucocorticoid. Conversely in Cushing's syndrome, hypertension is common and not necessarily accompanied by edema, alkalosis, and hypokalemia as seen in mineralocorticoid excess. The mechanisms of these vascular effects are complex and involve direct action on vasculature smooth-muscle and endothelial cells, effects on the renin-angiotensin system, inhibition of vasodilators, and increases in the glomerular filtration rate and cardiac output.

Mineralocorticoids

Aldosterone, the predominant mineralocorticoid, contains an aldehyde at position 18 that is in equilibrium with the 11-hydroxyl function, forming a more stable, cyclic 11,18-hemiacetyl (Fig. 29-6). The mineralocorticoids, aldosterone and deoxycorticosterone, bind to the mineralocorticoid receptor and subsequently cause sodium reabsorption and potassium and hydrogen ion excretion in the collecting tubules of the kidney. In mineralocorticoid excess states, there are retention of sodium, resulting in hypertension; secretion of potassium, causing hypokalemia; and secretion of hydrogen ion, causing metabolic alkalosis as in our index case. Glucocorticoids can also bind mineralocorticoid receptors, although at a lower affinity. In states of excess glucocorticoid, however, such as in Cushing's syndrome, cortisol may occupy the mineralocorticoid receptor to a large extent and exert the same mineralocorticoid effects.

In the circulation, the affinity of the steroid for the receptor is the major immediate determinant of steroid activity, with the rate of clearance determining

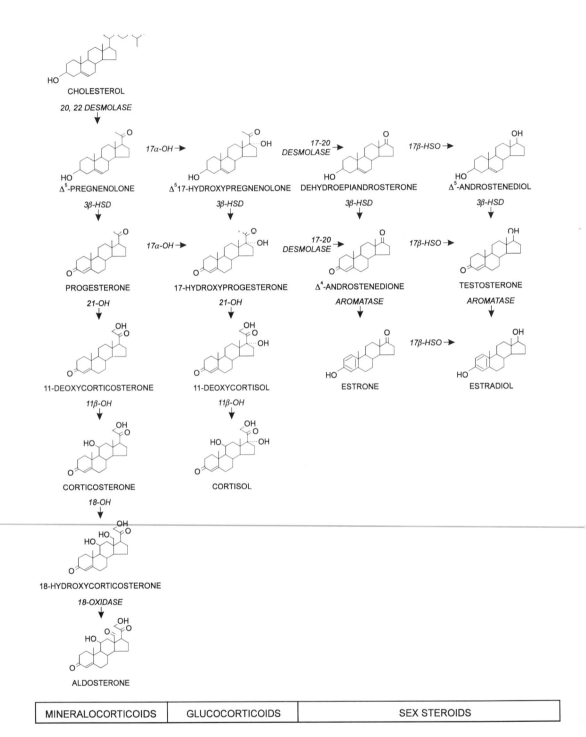

Figure 29-6. Steroid biosynthetic pathways.

the duration of the effect. Features associated with higher affinity include a reduced 4,5 or 1,2 double bond; a C-17 side chain; hydroxyl groups at positions 11, 17, and 21; C-3 and C-20 keto groups; and the presence of certain 16- and 17-substitutions.

Mineralocorticoids act by increasing the number of sodium channels in renal cells, increasing the renal $NADH/NAD^+$ ratio and the activities of mitochondrial enzymes involved in adenosine triphosphate generation, which may drive the sodium pump to stimulate sodium transport. Unfortunately, much less is known regarding the mechanisms of potassium and hydrogen ion secretion. Stimulation of potassium loss depends largely on sodium intake and sufficient delivery of sodium to the distal tubules. This in turn causes passive diffusion of potassium ion into the tubule from which it is excreted. Mineralocorticoids also affect sodium retention and potassium excretion in the gastrointestinal tract. Thus, patients with excess mineralocorticoid lose potassium in the stool.

Adrenal Androgens

The adrenal C-19 androgens, androstenedione, DHEA, and DHEA-sulfate, play a marginal role in sex steroid action in men; however, in women overproduction of these androgens can lead to hirsutism and virilization. After menopause, when the ovaries fail, the adrenal is the major site of adrenal androgen production. The adrenal C-19 androgens can be converted to C-18 estrogens in the periphery through the actions of the enzyme aromatase (Fig. 29-6).

Steroid Hormone Formation

All steroid hormones are derived from cholesterol. Most of the body's cholesterol if synthesized in the liver and carried to the steroid-producing cells in the form of LDL. The rate-limiting step of cholesterol synthesis is the cleavage of the side chain of cholesterol to yield pregnenolone by the cytochrome P-450_{scc} enzyme, one of the slowest enzymes known. Pregnenolone and all of its naturally occurring products contain 21 carbon atoms and hence are referred to as *C-21 steroids*. Once pregnenolone is produced, it may be converted to 17-hydroxypregnenolone or to progesterone by 3β-hydroxysteroid dehydrogenase (Fig. 29-6). Both

pregnenolone and progesterone can undergo 17α hydroxylation which, after scission of the C-17,20 carbon-carbon bond, yields DHEA and androstenedione. As the P450c17 enzyme has both 17α-hydroxylase activity and C-17,20 lyase activity, it is a key branch point in steroid hormone synthesis, determining whether pregnenolone is metabolized to mineralocorticoids, glucocorticoids, or sex steroids (Fig. 29-6).

Steroid Hormone Classification

The steroid hormones are classified on the basis of the receptors to which they bind. There are five major classes of steroid hormones: glucocorticoid, mineralocorticoid, estrogens, androgens, and vitamin D. Although vitamin D is not strictly a steroid, its receptor is considered a steroid receptor. In most cases, a single steroid mediates the action of a given class of receptors; but some receptors, such as the mineralocorticoid and androgen receptors, may bind several steroids with different affinities. After the steroid diffuses across the cell membrane, it associates with heat-shock proteins, forming a large complex. Binding of the complex to the receptor protein disassociates the heat-shock proteins, resulting in a steroid-dependent conformational change in the receptor, which then permits binding of the receptor to genomic DNA. This enabling of the receptor to bind DNA is known as *transformation* or *activation*. Binding of the receptor protein to the specific DNA sequence, known as the *hormone response element* (HRE), results in initiation of transcription, leading to biological effects.

Regulation of Steroid Hormone Synthesis

The primary regulation of the steroid hormones is through the hypothalamic-pituitary-adrenal axis. Corticotropin-releasing hormone is synthesized in the hypothalamus and is the primary and most potent physiologic regulator of ACTH release. It is a 41-amino acid peptide released by the paraventricular nucleus in the hypothalamus in response to stimuli such as stress. After release, CRH travels in the portal circulation to the anterior pituitary, where it results in the synthesis of ACTH. Other regulators of ACTH include arginine, vasopressin, and other hypothalamic agents.

ACTH is made in the anterior pituitary after cleavage from a precursor known as proopiomelanocortin (POMC), a large 241-amino acid peptide that can be processed post-translationally into ACTH, β-endorphin, β-lipoprotein, and other active peptides. In adrenocortical cells, ACTH increases the transcription of the genes for cytochromes $P450_{scc}$, $P450_{17\alpha}$, $P450_{21}$, and $P450_{11\beta}$, thereby stimulating the synthesis and release of cortisol and mineralocorticoids. Cortisol release occurs rapidly (within 2–3 minutes) and inhibits the biosynthesis and secretion of CRH and ACTH through negative feedback to the pituitary and hypothalamus. Coordinated effects of tropic hormones such as ACTH and growth factors result in hypersecretion and hypertrophy of the steroid-producing cells in the adrenal gland. With continued stimulation, ACTH receptors down-regulate and growth factors predominate, thereby inducing not only hypertrophy, but cell division as well. Consequently, adrenal hyperplasia develops and can be detected on CT scanning.

Protein Binding of Steroids

In the circulation, steroid hormones are either free or bound by glycoproteins made in the liver. Only free hormone is available for entering target cells, binding to receptors, and inducing a biological response. Bound steroids serve as a reservoir of hormone, which can be made available through dissociation. Cortisol-binding globulin binds cortisol and progesterone, whereas sex hormone-binding globulin binds testosterone and estradiol. The small fraction of free steroid hormone is in a constant equilibrium with the protein-bound fraction.

Structures of Steroid Hormone Receptors

Overall, the steroid hormone receptors have three domains. The amino-terminal domain is referred to as the *transactivation domain*. This region is heavily phosphorylated and enhances transcription. The middle portion contains the DNA binding domain, and the carboxy-terminal contains the hormone-binding domain.

Steroids bind reversibly and with high affinity to their receptors within minutes. Whereas the dissociation of the steroid with the receptor also occurs within minutes, the half-life of the mRNAs and pro-

teins produced are significantly longer, resulting in biological effects that may persist long after the signalling has been terminated. Some receptors bind more than one steroid. For example, the mineralocorticoid receptor has high affinities for both mineralocorticoid and glucocorticoid. Therefore, glucocorticoid excess can cause mineralocorticoid hypertension.

BASIS AND PRINCIPLES OF LABORATORY TESTS

Normally, cortisol is secreted in a circadian fashion, with levels highest in the morning, reflecting the response to high morning ACTH levels. Cushing's syndrome is characterized by loss of the normal circadian pattern of ACTH and cortisol secretion, impaired negative feedback of glucocorticoid secretion, and decreased response to hypoglycemia. Tests for the diagnosis of Cushing's syndrome include those for screening, confirmation of hypercortisolemia, and determination of the etiology of the hypercortisolemia (Fig. 29-7). Finally, imaging and functional studies are required to locate the source of hypercortisolism.

Screening Tests for Hypercortisolemia

The initial step in diagnosis is documentation of hypercortisolemia. The 1-mg overnight dexamethasone suppression test is popular for its simplicity and the fact that it can easily be done in an outpatient setting. One milligram of dexamethasone is given orally at 11:00 PM, followed by a serum cortisol determination at 8:00 AM the next morning. Normal persons suppress cortisol to a level below 5 μg/dL (138 nmol/L) in response to a 1 mg of dexamethasone. This suppression occurs because the exogenous glucocorticoid negatively feeds back to the hypothalamic-pituitary unit, thereby decreasing the synthesis of CRH, ACTH and cortisol (Fig. 29-8). Because the cortisol assay measures endogenous cortisol only (and not dexamethasone), cortisol levels are appropriately suppressed. The sensitivity of this test is 95%, but the specificity is poor, especially in obese, alcoholic, depressed, or acutely ill patients who may have "pseudo-Cushing's" syndrome. In addition, patients with high estrogen states will have increased cortisol-binding globulin (CBG) and therefore a falsely elevated cortisol level. Patients on

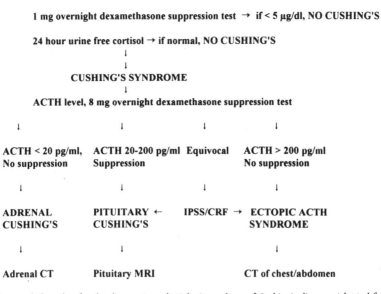

1 mg overnight dexamethasone suppression test → if < 5 μg/dl, NO CUSHING'S

24 hour urine free cortisol → if normal, NO CUSHING'S
↓
↓
CUSHING'S SYNDROME
↓
ACTH level, 8 mg overnight dexamethasone suppression test

↓   ↓   ↓   ↓

ACTH < 20 pg/ml, No suppression	**ACTH 20-200 pg/ml Suppression**	**Equivocal**	**ACTH > 200 pg/ml No suppression**
↓	↓	↓	↓
ADRENAL CUSHING'S	**PITUITARY ← CUSHING'S**	**IPSS/CRF →**	**ECTOPIC ACTH SYNDROME**
↓	↓		↓
Adrenal CT	**Pituitary MRI**		**CT of chest/abdomen**

Figure 29-7. Proposed algorithm for the diagnostic and etiologic work-up of Cushing's disease. *Adapted from* Kaye and Crapo, 1990.

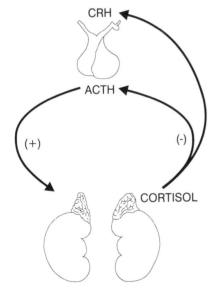

Figure 29-8. Hypothalamic-pituitary-adrenal axis. Corticotropin releasing hormone (CRH) is produced in the hypothalamus, travels down the pituitary stalk, and stimulates synthesis and release of adrenocorticotropic hormone (ACTH) from the pituitary gland. ACTH stimulates the formation of cortisol from the adrenal cortex, which in turn suppresses further release of ACTH and CRH in a classic "negative feedback loop" system.

dilantin (an anticonvulsant) or rifampin (a tuberculous drug) will metabolize dexamethasone rapidly and may exhibit a falsely normal test. For these reasons, a 24-hour collection of urine free-cortisol is preferred. The vast majority of patients with spontaneous Cushing's syndrome will have an elevated 24-hour urine free-cortisol level (see the following section).

Confirming Hypercortisolemia

Two tests are available to confirm spontaneous hypercortisolemia: 24-hour urine free-cortisol and the low-dose dexamethasone suppression test. A 24-hour urine collection for free cortisol is the simplest to obtain and is also the most reliable, practical index of cortisol secretion. Because ACTH and cortisol have a diurnal rhythm, the 24-hour collection allows integration of plasma free-cortisol concentrations. The mean rate of cortisol secretion in normal adults is 9.9 ± 2.7 mg per 24 hours (27 ± 7.5 μmol/24 h). Of this, approximately 10 to 40 μg (33–110 nmol) is excreted in the urine as free cortisol.

The classic confirmatory test for hypercortisolemia is the 2-day low-dose dexamethasone suppression test. This test involves the administration of 0.5 mg of dexamethasone every 6 hours orally for two consecutive days. Urinary free-cortisol or 17-hydroxy-corticosteroid (a cortisol metabolite) is collected at baseline and on day 2. A urinary free cortisol concentration >10 μg (28 μmol) per 24 hours or urinary 17-hydroxycorticosteroid value above 2.5 mg (6.9 μmol) per 24 hours confirms hypercortisolemia. Measuring dexamethasone at the conclusion of the test may be helpful in clarifying confusing results if noncompliance or the effects of drugs on dexamethasone metabolism are suspected as confounders.

Other tests to identify patients with pseudo-Cushing's syndrome due to depression include: (1) preservation of the evening nadir of cortisol; (2) CRH and low-dose dexamethasone stimulation testing in sequence; (3) naloxone stimulation; and (4) insulin-induced hypoglycemia (Orth, 1995). Depressed patients have a preserved evening nadir of cortisol, unlike true Cushing's patients, who do not. Consequently, a midnight plasma cortisol level >7.5 μg/dl (207 nmol/L) indicates the presence of Cushing's syndrome. A second, recently described test involves the administration of low-dose dexamethasone followed by CRH, the theory being that patients with Cushing's disease will respond to CRH with increased ACTH secretion, and patients with depression will suppress ACTH release with dexamethasone. Therefore, patients with depression will have low plasma cortisol levels, and patients with Cushing's syndrome will have higher cortisol levels. The naloxone test is based on the theory that depression is a state of stress in which CRH is increased, causing increased ACTH secretion and therefore increased cortisol production. Naloxone, an opioid antagonist, further stimulates CRH release in patients with depression but not in patients with Cushing's disease, who have suppressed CRH levels from glucocorticoid negative feedback. Finally, insulin-induced hypoglycemia can be used to distinguish depression from Cushing's disease. In depression, the hypercortisolism is usually mild, unlike Cushing's disease, and can be overcome by the stimulatory effect of hypoglycemia (a physiologic stress) on CRH secretion.

Determining the Etiology of the Hypercortisolism

Once hypercortisolemia has been confirmed, a search for etiology must be pursued. The two most useful tests to determine the cause of the Cushing's syndrome are the determination of the plasma ACTH level and the high-dose dexamethasone suppression test. The principle behind the high-dose dexamethasone suppression test is that, despite the fact that all patients with Cushing's syndrome have disordered regulation of the hypothalamopituitary-adrenal axis, pituitary tumors still retain some suppressibility in response to high doses of dexamethasone, whereas adrenal neoplasms and malignancies producing ectopic ACTH do not. Therefore, the high-dose dexamethasone suppression test is most commonly used to distinguish these conditions.

Several protocols for high-dose dexamethasone testing exist. The standard Grant Liddle protocol involves the administration of 2 mg of dexamethasone orally every 6 hours for two consecutive days, with measurement of 24-hour urine for the steroid metabolite 17-hydroxycorticosteroids or urine free-cortisol (Flack et al., 1992). A fall in 17-hydroxycorticosteroid excretion of more than 64%, or in urine free-cortisol of more than 90%, approaches 100% diagnostic specificity for pituitary Cushing's. A simpler approach is the 8 mg overnight dexamethasone suppression test in which a baseline cortisol level is obtained at 8:00 AM, 8 mg of dexamethasone is given at 11:00 PM, followed by another cortisol determination the following morning at 8:00 AM. Suppression >50% indicates a pituitary source of ACTH (Kaye and Crapo, 1990). Caution must be used in interpreting high-dose dexamethasone tests, however, because of incomplete sensitivity and specificity. Benign ectopic tumors (e.g., bronchial carcinoids) are notorious for suppressing in response to high-dose dexamethasone, unlike other tumors that are the cause of ectopic ACTH syndrome.

Analysis of plasma ACTH levels is also used to determine the source of Cushing's syndrome. If the plasma ACTH level is suppressed to below 20 pg/mL (0.95 pmol/L), the patient has ACTH-independent Cushing's syndrome, and an adrenal neoplasm should be sought with thin-cut CT or magnetic resonance imaging (MRI) of the adrenal glands. Adrenal carcinomas are more likely to be larger (>3 cm) and usually secrete adrenal androgens such as DHEA-S. If the plasma ACTH level is normal to moderately elevated (20–200 pg/mL or 0.95–9.5 pmol/L), Cushing's disease is likely and a dynamic pituitary MRI with gadolinium contrast should be obtained. If the plasma ACTH concentration is markedly elevated (>200 pg/mL or >9.5 pmol/L), ectopic ACTH syndrome is likely and a search for a malignancy should begin with a CT scan of the chest and abdomen if the malignancy is not already apparent.

Bilateral inferior petrosal sinus sampling (IPSS) with CRH simulation is proving to be an exceedingly reliable test for distinguishing pituitary from ectopic ACTH production (Oldfield et al., 1991; Findling et al., 1991). In many cases, this distinction is difficult because ACTH levels may overlap in the two conditions and because a pituitary microadenoma or ectopic tumor may both be occult. In this test, catheters are placed in the inferior petrosal sinuses, which drain the pituitary, thereby enabling simultaneous sampling of ACTH levels. Because each side of the pituitary gland drains into the ipsilateral petrosal sinus, venous samples must be obtained from both petrosal sinuses. Petrosal and peripheral samples are obtained both before and after the intravenous administration of CRH (1 μg/kg). In patients with Cushing's disease, a 2:1 ratio or greater exists for the petrosal and peripheral ACTH levels. In contrast, where there is ectopic ACTH production, there is an attenuated or absent response to CRH and the ratio is 1:1. This technique can lateralize the pituitary tumor to one side of the gland or the other, which can be very helpful to the neurosurgeon.

Pitfalls of the technique include the fact that the test cannot distinguish patients with Cushing's disease from those with pseudo-Cushing's syndrome. In addition, adrenal neoplasms may have IPSS results that can be confused with Cushing's disease. It is therefore imperative that only patients with true Cushing's syndrome that is ACTH-dependent be studied for reliable results (Orth, 1991).

The IPSS technique should be performed by experienced interventional radiologists to avoid the significant morbidity involved with the procedure (thrombosis, infection, hemorrhage) and to approach the sensitivity and specificity of 100% reported by centers with the greatest experience. Given its expense ($2500–5000) and the fact that CRH is not currently available for clinical use in this country without an Investigational New Drug exemption, IPSS with CRH cannot be recommended as a routine test in all cases.

Imaging Procedures

Tumors causing Cushing's disease tend to be small microadenomas less than 6 mm in diameter. Therefore, CT scans are not very sensitive in detecting these tumors, and dynamic MRI scanning is the test of choice. With dynamic MRI scans, gadolinium is used to perfuse the pituitary, and scans are obtained at short intervals to detect filling defects in the gland. Gadolinium, a member of the lanthanide group, is used as a contrast agent in MRI scanning.

Thin-section CT scanning of the abdomen is necessary to detect adrenal tumors. Carcinomas tend to be larger than adenomas and metastases may be present. Currently, there is no advantage to MRI scanning for adrenal tumors. For the detection of malignancies causing ectopic ACTH syndrome, CT scanning of the chest and abdomen are often required if the tumor is not clinically obvious.

In cases of ectopic ACTH syndrome where the tumor is occult, an indium-111-labeled octreotide scan often yields informative results. Most neuroendocrine tumors that can cause the ectopic ACTH syndrome are somatostatin-receptor-positive and can therefore be imaged (and sometimes treated) with ocetreotide. Octreotide scans can detect up to 86% of carcinoid tumors, which is comparable to results obtained with CT and MRI scans.

THERAPY

Available therapy for Cushing's syndrome depends on the cause. Both surgical and medical techniques are currently available for treatment.

Pituitary Surgery

Transphenoidal hypophysectomy is the procedure of choice for patients with Cushing's disease. Most of these tumors are small microadenomas (<6 mm) that can be successfully removed without damage to the remaining normal pituitary tissue. If the tumor cannot be located at the time of surgery, a near-total hypophysectomy should be performed. Another option would be to perform a hemi-hypophysectomy dictated by the lateralization of ACTH during IPSS. Remission rates of 80 to 90% are not uncommon. In the few cases of Cushing's disease due to macroadenomas, remission rates are significantly lower. The biochemical criteria for a cure should be undetectable plasma cortisol and an ACTH level <5 pg/mL (<1.1 pmol/L).

Hypertension and hyperglycemia should be controlled preoperatively. Perioperatively, stress doses of steroids should be given to prevent the onset of secondary adrenal insufficiency. Replacement doses of hydrocortisone or prednisone is often required for several months after surgery until the hypothalamic-pituitary-adrenal axis has recovered.

Radiation Therapy

Radiation in doses of 4500 to 4000 cGy (centigray) can lead to improvement in hypercortisolemia and shrinkage of pituitary tumors in as many as 45% of adults; however, the response can be delayed by many months or years, and cure rates are not as high as in pituitary surgery. Consequently, radiation therapy should be regarded as second-line therapy, or therapy to be used in conjunction with pituitary surgery. Complications of radiation therapy include panhypopituitarism, brainstem necrosis, and optic nerve atrophy.

Adrenal Surgery

Bilateral adrenalectomy is required in micronodular or macronodular adrenal hyperplasia. Unilateral adrenalectomy can be performed for adrenal neoplasms. Patients with benign adrenal adenomas removed surgically usually have excellent results, with the manifestations of Cushing's syndrome resolving quickly. Glucocorticoid replacement must be given post-operatively because the normal adrenal gland will be suppressed by the prolonged autonomous production of cortisol and may require many months to recover.

Surgery for adrenal carcinomas is not as successful. Many patients will have metastatic disease to the liver or lungs at the time of presentation and thus not be surgically cured. Others will have high recurrence rates that are not amenable to chemotherapy, irradiation, or surgical cure.

Nelson's syndrome can occur after adrenalectomy for pituitary Cushing's disease. In this setting, aggressive pituitary tumor growth occurs after surgery, presumably because of the lack of negative feedback by cortisol that would normally serve to suppress ACTH. Excessive tumor growth and ACTH secretion cause hyperpigmentation, a feature of the syndrome. These tumors must be treated aggressively with both surgery and radiation therapy. Patients who have undergone bilateral adrenalectomy need close follow-up for tumor recurrence and visual field defects.

Medical Therapy

Medical therapy should be considered for the following reasons: (1) to correct the metabolic consequences of hypercortisolemia, such as hypokalemia or hyperglycemia; (2) to improve the psychiatric disturbances, myopathy, and tissue fragility; (3) to palliate noncurable disease; and (4) to achieve remission in patients in whom surgery is contraindicated or unlikely to be successful. Hypercortisolism can usually be controlled with adrenal enzyme inhibitors such as ketoconazole, metyrapone, aminoglutethamide, or mitotane either alone or in combination (Miller and Crapo, 1993).

The imidazole derivative ketoconazole inhibits a variety of cytochrome p450 enzymes and induces a clinical and biochemical remission in 80% of patients. *In vitro* it is also a glucocorticoid receptor antagonist. Dosages range from 200 to 400 mg (orally) three times a day. Side effects include hepatitis within 60 days of initiating treatment, gynecomastia (breast tissue enlargement), and nausea in 8 to 15% of cases.

The pyridine derivative metyrapone, an 11 β-hydroxylase inhibitor, is unavailable in this country at this time; however, historically it has been quite effective in reducing cortisol levels.

The glutarimide derivative *p*-aminoglutethamide inhibits several cytochrome p-450 enzymes: the side-chain cleavage complex, 21-hydroxylase, 17α-hydroxylase, 11β-hydroxylase, and other enzymes. Use of aminoglutethamide causes dose-dependent side effects, including sedation (30%), nausea or anorexia (12%), and transient rash (18%). The mechanism of action of mitotane, an adrenolytic agent, is unknown. In combination with irradiation therapy, remission rates as high as 73% can be achieved. Despite its effectiveness, such therapy is complicated by several major side effects in 45 to 70% of patients, such as gastrointestinal distress, impaired mentation, and dizziness.

Therapy with any of these drugs can be monitored by measuring urine free-cortisol or plasma cortisol levels. Remission of hypercortisolemia can be achieved in 80% of cases. Caution is necessary, however, because these drugs can rapidly lead to adrenal insufficiency. Patients will likely need replacement doses of prednisone or hydrocortisone.

Other experimental approaches have been tried. Octreotide or synthetic somatostatin, by preventing the release of ACTH, has been successfully used to control ectopic ACTH secretion in neuroendocrine tumors that are somatostatin receptor-positive and visualized with indium-111 labeled octreotide. Reductions of ACTH secretion by 25 to 100% have been demonstrated.

Therapy for the ectopic ACTH syndrome, as in our index case, is perhaps the most difficult because the patient usually has metastatic disease at presentation. Because of the often severe hypokalemia, potassium chloride replacement is necessary. The metabolic alkalosis, however, remains unresponsive to chloride. The hypertension and edema can be treated with the potassium-sparing mineralocorticoid antagonist spironolactone. Spironolactone, by blocking the mineralocorticoid receptor, prevents the mineralocorticoid effects of hypertension and hypokalemia. Hyperglycemia should be treated with insulin, and the hypercortisolemia should be treated with one of the medical agents described above (e.g., ketoconazole, octreotide). In some cases, adrenalectomy should be considered, especially in patients with indolent, nonresectable tumors, such as bronchial carcinoids. Patients with ectopic ACTH-producing tumors and adrenal carcinoma often die of their malignancy.

Untreated Cushing's syndrome leads to significant morbidity and mortality. Patients are susceptible to thromboembolism, infection, atherosclerosis, and suicide. In addition, the hypertension and diabetes lead to cardiovascular and cerebrovascular disease. Equally distressing consequences include osteoporosis and psychosis.

QUESTIONS

1. Describe the rationale behind the high-dose dexamethasone suppression test for determining the etiology of Cushing's syndrome.

2. Name two factors that determine the activity of a steroid hormone.
3. How can glucocorticoids exert mineralocorticoid effects in Cushing's syndrome?
4. Describe the effects of glucocorticoids on protein, carbohydrate, and fat metabolism.
5. Explain which steroids account for the major clinical features of Cushing's syndrome, and describe how they exert their effects.
6. Describe when inferior petrosal sinus sampling with CRH should be performed in the workup of Cushing's syndrome.
7. Describe how the drug ketoconazole is useful in the therapy of Cushing's disease.

REFERENCES

Cushing H: The basophil adenomas of the pituitary body and their clinical manifestations. *Bull Johns Hopkins Hosp* **50:**137, 1932.

Findling JW, Kehoe ME, Shaker JL, Raff H: Routine inferior petrosal sinus sampling in the differential diagnosis of adrenocorticotropin dependent Cushing's syndrome: early recognition of the occult ectopic ACTH syndrome. *J Clin Endocrinol Metab* **73:**408–413, 1991.

Flack MR, Oldfield EH, Cutler GB Jr, et al.: Urine free cortisol in the high-dose dexamethasone suppression test for the differential diagnosis of the Cushing syndrome. *Ann Intern Med* **116:**211–217, 1992.

Kaye TB, Crapo L: The Cushing syndrome: an update on diagnostic tests. *Ann Intern Med* **112:**434–444, 1990.

Miller JW, Crapo L: The medical treatment of Cushing's syndrome. *Endo Rev* **14:**443–458, 1993.

Oldfield EH, Doppman JL, Nieman LD, Chrousos GP, et al.: Petrosal sinus sampling with and without corticotropin releasing hormone for the differential diagnosis of Cushing's syndrome. *N Engl J Med* **325:**897–905, 1991.

Orth DN: Differential diagnosis of Cushing's syndrome. *N Engl J Med* **325:**957–959, 1991.

Orth DN: Medical progress: Cushing's syndrome. *N Engl J Med* **332:**791–803, 1995.

30

Rickets Caused by a Vitamin D Deficiency

RUSSELL W. CHESNEY AND SHERMINE DABBAGH

CASE REPORT

A 13-month-old black girl was admitted to the hospital for growth failure. She was born after a full-term pregnancy to a gravida 3 (third pregnancy), para 2 (two viable births) mother from Nigeria. The patient's birth weight was 3650 g, and she left the hospital at age 3 days without any detected medical problems. Her motor and psychosocial development appeared normal until age 9 months when her parents noticed that, unlike her two older siblings, she could not pull up to stand. At the same time, her weight gain appreciably declined, and her weight increased only from 5 kg (11 lb) to 7.5 kg (16.5 lb) over the next 6 months.

The parents gave no history of fevers, seizures, infection, diarrhea, vomiting, loose stools, or steatorrhea. The patient received no medications. A dietary history revealed that she was exclusively breast-fed and that she refused all table food. Her mother's diet consisted almost entirely of eggs, cornflakes, potatoes, macaroni, and crackers; she rarely ate meat and infrequently ate green vegetables. Also, she generally avoided dairy products because of a lactase deficiency in family members (see Chapter 14).

The patient was confined to home with her parents and siblings and rarely left the house. When she was taken outside, both she and her mother were heavily clad with garments that effectively blocked out the sun.

On physical examination her height was 67.5 cm (26.6 in) (<5th percentile for chronological age or the 50th percentile), typical of a child aged 7 months,

her weight was 7.52 kg (<5th percentile, 50th percentile, typical of a child aged 7 months), and head circumference was 46 cm (18.1 in) (95th percentile for age). She was a small-appearing black girl in no acute distress. Her heart, lungs, and abdominal examinations were normal. She had a box-shaped head with frontal and occipital bossing (*protuberance*). She had a *rachitic rosary* (beading of the ribs) and bilateral flaring of the lower portion of the rib cage (*Harrison's groove*). She also had sharp, angular bowing of the arms and legs with double *malleoli* (rounded bony prominence) of the wrists and ankles. In addition, she had a potbelly. She also demonstrated a positive *Chvostek's sign* (spasm caused by tapping over the facial nerve).

Her laboratory findings, summarized in Table 30-1, included hypocalcemia, hypophosphatemia, an elevated immunoreactive parathyroid hormone (PTH) value, and markedly increased serum alkaline phosphatase activity, all suggestive of stage III rickets. Marked signs of rickets were present in radiograms of the long bones (Fig. 30-1a) with diffuse demineralization, fraying, and cupping of the metaphyseal ends of the long bones. She also had a nondisplaced fracture of the midshaft of the left ulna. Her bone age was markedly diminished; she had only five secondary centers of ossification, consistent with 1 SD below the mean for a 1-month-old child and 3 SD below the mean for her age (13 months).

Further laboratory evidence of nutritional rickets came from the finding of excessive urinary phosphate excretion, reduced tubular reabsorption of phosphate, generalized aminoaciduria (excessive

Table 30-1. Laboratory Data of Index Patient

Parameters	Patient Pretherapy	Posttherapy[a] (4 mos)	Normals[b] (Range)
Serum Levels			
Creatinine (mg/dL)	0.1	0.3	0.1–0.4
BUN (mg/dL)	10	14	5–20
Sodium (mEq/L)	138	135	135–145
Potassium (mEq/L)	3.8	4.2	3.5–5.0
Chloride (mEq/L)	106	100	98–104
Bicarbonate (Mm/L)	19	26	24–26
Calcium (mg/dL)	8.3	10.1	9.2–10.2
Phosphate (mg/dL)	1.4	5.2	5.0–6.2
Magnesium (mg/dL)	1.5	1.8	1.8–22
Albumin (g/dL)	3.9	3.7	3.0–4.5
Alkaline phosphatase (IU/L)	4431	658	150–280
25-Hydroxyvitamin D (ng/mL)	3	28	15–60
1,25-Dihydroxyvitamin D (pg/mL)	112	225	70–120
24,25-Dihydroxyvitamin D (ng/mL)	None detected	1.8	0.7–2.8
Immunoreactive parathyroid hormone (μlEq/mL)	120	42	<40
Urine			
Creatinine clearance (ml/min/1.73 m²)	98	102	80–120
Urinary calcium excretion (mg/24 h)	0	32	10–35
Tubular reabsorption of phosphate (%)	75	92	<85%
Magnesium excretion (%)	0.5	4.2	3–5
Aminoaciduria	Generalized, diffuse	No abnormalities	No abnormalities

BUN, blood urea nitrogen.

[a] Treatment consisted of feeding calcium-containing foods and giving vitamin D_2 at 5000 IU daily for 90 days and at 400 IU daily for 30 days.

[b] Mean ± SD.

urinary amino acid excretion), and the absence of calcium in the urine. The potbelly described in the physical examination is typical of the myopathy experienced by patients with vitamin D deficiency.

The patient was initially treated with calcium-containing foods such as yogurt, cheese, and green leafy vegetables, and vitamin D 5000 international units (IU) daily for 3 months and then 400 daily. She quickly gained muscle strength and achieved new motor milestones. The radiological appearance of her long bones improved, and the bowing was corrected without any surgical intervention (Fig. 30-1b). The laboratory values 4 months after the initiation of vitamin D therapy are shown in Table 30-1. The patient is now clinically well and is taking 400 IU/day of vitamin D, as well as eating calcium-containing foods.

DIAGNOSIS

The clinical presentation and features of this child suggest the bone disorder known as *rickets*. The primary defect in rickets is impaired mineralization of the cartilaginous portion of bone and bending or bowing of bone under weight. This failure of the osteoid to mineralize is termed *osteomalacia*, and it indicates that the crystalline mineral phase of hydroxyapatite and octacalcium phosphate are not being deposited in the collagen-containing osteoid. Osteomalacia occurs if either calcium or phosphate is not present in the extracellular fluid of bone in sufficient amount to permit mineral deposition. Thus, rickets can arise from either calcium or phosphate deficiency.

In this child the clues to calcium-deficient rickets

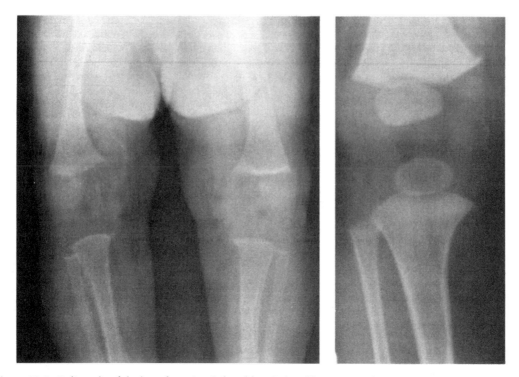

Figure 30-1. Radiographs of the legs of a patient before (a) and after (b) vitamin D_2 therapy, 5000 IU a day. In (a), note metaphyseal cupping and fraying, and a washed-out appearance to the bones. Moreover, the tibia on the right appears to be broken and bowed and there is considerable periosteal elevation with obvious unmineralized periosteum. In (b) the bone appears to be healing with rapid mineralization, and the metaphyses appear to be far more mineralized. In addition, there is evidence of mineralization of the epiphyses and of the periosteum. Thus, there is remarkable healing evident in (b) attributable to the therapy.

were the dietary history, the bone lesions associated with hypocalcemia, hypophosphatemia related to excessive urinary phosphate losses (Scriver, 1974), and an elevation of serum alkaline phosphatase activity. The radiological appearance of the long bones suggests sharp, angular bowing rather than the smooth bowing of primary hypophosphatemic rickets. In addition, this child has flaring at the ends of the ribs (the rachitic rosary) and an outward flaring at the lower end of the rib cage, termed *Harrison's groove*, as well as myopathy, aminoaciduria, and secondary hyperparathyroidism. All of these signs point to calciopenic rickets. Figure 30-2 shows a flow diagram indicating the diagnostic possibilities, and the differential diagnosis for this child is given in Table 30-2.

Several other features of this child's case establish a clear-cut diagnosis of nutritional rickets. First, the child developed bowing and myopathy at age 6 or 7 months, thereby excluding either the rickets of prematurity (which occurs at age 8–16 weeks) and

autosomal recessive vitamin D-dependency rickets, which usually occurs at age 2½ to 3 months. Second, the dietary history indicates that she has few dietary sources of calcium and vitamin D. Third, her exposure to sunshine is minuscule. Fourth, no history of malabsorption or hepatobiliary disease was evident. Finally, the parents reported no family history of rickets or other metabolic bone disease.

The laboratory studies indicate that this child has vitamin D deficiency (Chesney et al., 1981). Serum concentrations of vitamins D_2 and D_3, 25-$(OH)D_2$ and 25-$(OH)D_3$, and 24,25-$(OH)_2D$ are markedly reduced, and the concentration of 1,25-$(OH)_2D$ is in the "normal" range. The immunoreactive parathyroid hormone (iPTH) level in serum is elevated, as would be anticipated with hypocalcemia. The hypophosphatemia and elevated alkaline phosphatase values are other indicators of secondary hyperparathyroidism. A generalized tetany and aminoaciduria are evident along with the phosphaturia. Finally, the bone changes indicate that the concentration of

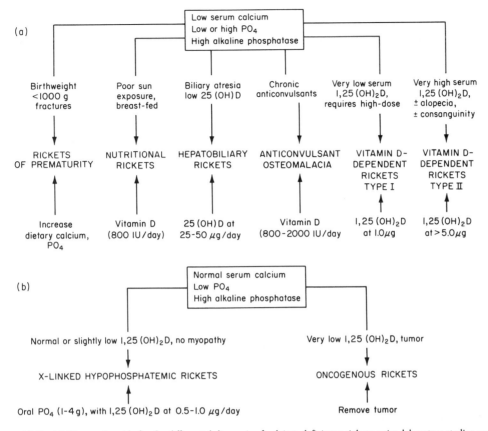

Figure 30-2. (a) Diagnostic guide for the differential diagnosis of calcium deficiency rickets, using laboratory studies as shown. The most prominent features of each of the calcium-deficient rachitic disorders are listed. (b) Major causes of phosphate deficiency rickets. Again, the most obvious and prominent features are indicated. Reproduced with permission from Chesney (1984).

ionized calcium in the extracellular fluid is reduced. Although the therapy in this case and for nutritional rickets in general will be discussed later, the finding that this patient responded to conventional vitamin D_2 at a relatively low daily dose indicates that she was not malabsorbing vitamin D, did not have a defect in the conversion of 25-(OH)D to 1,25-$(OH)_2D$, did not have a target organ resistance to the biological action of vitamin D, and did not have renal disease or pseudohypoparathyroidism. Finally, the laboratory changes after treatment indicate that a dose of 50,000 IU (125 μg) of vitamin D_2 caused an elevation in the concentration of circulating vitamins D_2 and D_3, 25-$(OH)D_2$ and D_3 and 24,25-$(OH)_2D$, and a remarkable increase in 1,25-$(OH)_2D$. Associated with these changes were increases in serum calcium and phosphate, a fall in alkaline phosphatase and iPTH, and reversal of aminoaciduria. The improvement in the radiological appearance of the bones demonstrates that bone is being remineralized and that a positive calcium (and phosphate) balance exists.

MOLECULAR PERSPECTIVES

The two principal minerals in the body are calcium and phosphorus, and their homeostases are maintained by integration affected by the vitamin D endocrine system (Chesney, 1984). Because 99% of whole-body calcium and 80 to 85% of phosphate are localized to bone, this organ system is both an important depot of these minerals and a reservoir for maintaining stable levels of these ions in the extracellular fluid. This function of bone explains why a

Table 30-2. Causes of Rickets Associated with Hypocalcemia Abnormalities of the Vitamin D System

Reduced intake

Reduced sunlight exposure

Reduced absorption—intestinal dysfunction

Hepatocellular disorders
  Impaired absorption of vitamin D
  Impaired synthesis of 25-hydroxyvitamin D [25-(OH)D]
  Impaired enterohepatic circulation

Enhanced metabolism of 25-(OH)D to inactive polar metabolites by phenobarbital, phenylhydantoins, ethanol (?), etc.

Reduced production of calcitriol [1,25-dihydroxyvitamin D (1,25-(OH)$_2$D)]:
  Renal insufficiency
  Autosomal-recessive vitamin D-dependency rickets

End-organ unresponsiveness to 1,25-(OH)$_2$D with rickets or vitamin D-dependency rickets, type II:
  With alopecia
  Rickets only

Appearance of rickets due to bone-responsive, renal nonresponsive pseudohypoparathyroidism

Rickets of prematurity:
  Maternal vitamin D deficiency
  Calcium deficiency   } due to limited intake
  Phosphate deficiency

---

deficiency of vitamin D, calcium, or phosphate will appear as a metabolic bone disease.

The main regulator of calcium and phosphate transport in the intestine and kidney is the vitamin D endocrine system (Deluca and Schnoes, 1984). This system begins with the photolysis of 7-dehydrocholesterol in the *stratum basalis* layer of the skin. UV radiation at 288 nm opens the B-ring of the steroid molecule to produce previtamin D$_3$, which then undergoes thermal conversion to vitamin D$_3$ (Fig. 30-3). Vitamin D$_3$ is transported in the blood to the liver by a specific molecular weight 52,000 vitamin D-binding protein (DBP). A hepatic cytochrome *P*-450 microsomal hydroxylase adds a hydroxyl group to C-25 of vitamin D, thereby generating 25-(OH)D.

This 25-(OH)D bound to DBP is the main circulating form of vitamin D at a normal concentration of 20–60 ng/mL. It is transported to the kidney, where a mitochondrial enzyme incorporates molecular oxygen at the 1α-position on the A-ring, yielding 1,25-(OH)$_2$D. Although the precise details of the regulation of 25-(OH)D 1 α-hydroxylase activity are not known, the circulating levels of 1,25-(OH)$_2$D appear to be increased by hypocalcemia, by an in-

crease in plasma iPTH, and by hypophosphatemia. In addition to its presence in the renal cortex, 1 α-hydroxylase is also found in the placenta of pregnant women and other mammalian species, which may account for the elevated serum 1,25-(OH)$_2$D values in pregnancy.

The renal cortex is also the main site of production of another vitamin D metabolite, 24,25-(OH)$_2$D. The enzyme that converts 25-(OH)$_2$D to 24,25-(OH)$_2$D is regulated reciprocally with the 1 α-hydroxylase such that 24,25-(OH)$_2$D is synthesized whenever the plasma concentrations of calcium and phosphate are normal, when plasma iPTH is normal, or when excessive amounts of vitamin D$_2$, D$_3$, or 25 (OH)$_2$D have been administered; 24,25 (OH)$_2$D circulates at 1 to 4 ng/mL, but serum levels are higher after high-dose vitamin D administration. Although both the intestine and bone produce this metabolite, the kidney is the main site of its synthesis. The biological function of this metabolite and its role in the vitamin D endocrine scheme are probably minimal; however, this metabolite disappears from the circulation under conditions of vitamin D deficiency when the activity of 25-(OH)D$_2$-24 hydroxylase falls to an immeasurable level. Because the serum values of 24,25-(OH)$_2$D are negligible in vitamin D deficiency, it has been suggested that this metabolite may be important in bone mineralization, but little evidence exists to support this contention. The vitamin D endocrine system regulates both calcium and phosphate economy, as indicated in Figure 30-4. A reduction in both total and ionized calcium results in increased PTH secretion, which in turn stimulates 1α-hydroxylase activity. 1,25-(OH)$_2$D combines with a specific receptor(s) in the intestine and stimulates the active transport of calcium from the lumen of the gut across the enterocyte into the bloodstream. It also augments intestinal phosphate absorption, This metabolite, which circulates at 20 to 60 pg/mL [~0.1% the level of 25-(OH)D], is the most biologically active form of vitamin D in terms of these intestinal functions. A role for 1,25(OH)$_2$D-dependent DNA-directed protein synthesis appears important, and clearly 1,25(OH)$_2$D directs the synthesis of an intestinal calcium-binding protein (CaBP); however, the gene product(s) of the 1,25-(OH)$_2$D-nuclear receptor complex are multiple and enhance intestinal calcium absorption.

In concert with PTH, 1,25-(OH)$_2$D promotes osteoclast-induced bone resorption with the release

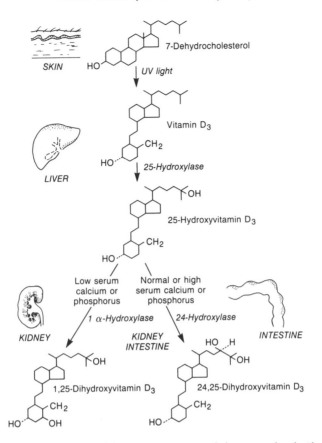

Figure 30-3. Factors regulating the production of the major vitamin D metabolites. Reproduced with permission from Chesney (1984).

of calcium into the extracellular fluid (DeLuca and Schnoes, 1984). The net result of 1,25-(OH)$_2$D action is to raise the calcium and phosphate concentrations in the blood, but the higher iPTH values result in renal proximal tubular events that promote phosphate excretion. Thus, on balance, serum calcium and phosphate levels normalize. PTH secretion and 1,25-(OH)$_2$D synthesis are then suppressed by the normal serum calcium concentration; thus, the synthesis of 1,25-(OH)$_2$D is feedback regulated. Because this metabolite is made at one site (the renal cortex) and acts on other organs (the intestine and bone) after transport via the bloodstream, 1,25-(OH)$_2$D should be considered a hormone rather than a vitamin. Wherever PTH secretion is reduced, as in hypoparathyroidism, or when its biological action is blocked, as in pseudohypoparathyroidism, plasma calcium will be low and plasma phosphate will be elevated. In addition, 1,25-(OH)$_2$D synthe-

sis will be reduced and the vitamin D endocrine system will not function.

The phosphate limb of the system (Fig. 30-4b) is stimulated by hypophosphatemia, which, *per se,* augments 1,25-(OH)$_2$D synthesis. Intestinal calcium and phosphate absorption are enhanced, raising the plasma levels of both. The kidney will excrete the excess calcium but will retain phosphate, because PTH levels are reduced. The higher serum phosphate concentration in turn suppresses 1,25-(OH)$_2$D synthesis. With a better understanding of both limbs of the vitamin D endocrine systems and its interplay involving bone and mineral metabolism, we can now appreciate why vitamin D deficiency has such profound effects on the skeleton. In the absence of sufficient 25-(OH)D, neither hypocalcemia nor hypophosphatemia will stimulate 1,25-(OH)$_2$D synthesis in sufficient quantities to promote intestinal mineral absorption.

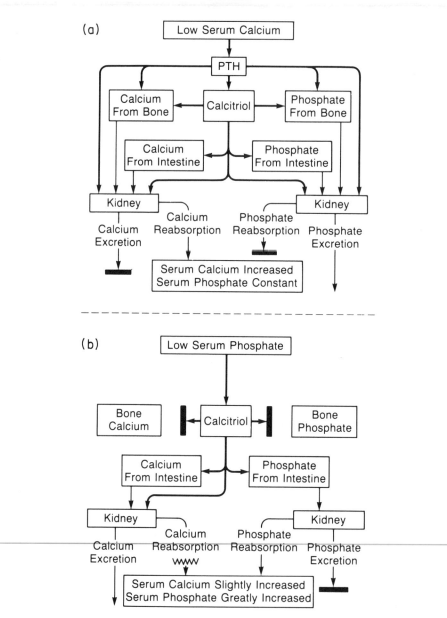

Figure 30-4. (a) The vitamin D endocrine system demonstrating the adaption to hypocalcemia. The term calcitriol is another chemical name for 1,25-$(OH)_2$D, and the arrows pointing to a given box indicate an increase in activity. For example, calcium from the intestine is increased because of the action of calcitriol. (b) The vitamin D endocrine system adaption to hypophosphatemia.

Rickets related to nutritional vitamin D deficiency is rare in North America because foodstuffs are supplemented with either vitamin D_2 (of plant origin) or vitamin D_3 (of mammalian origin). Each quart of milk or infant formula sold in the United States contains 400 IU (10 μg) of the prohormone. Thus, even in children living in the temperate zones of the United States, Canada, and Europe, where in winter sunlight exposure is limited, an adequate intake of vitamin D is assured. The ingested vitamin D is absorbed by the intestine in the same way as other fat-soluble vitamins, via the action of bile salt micelles that cross the intestinal wall and enter the portal circulation. Newly absorbed vitamin D then proceeds to the liver, where it is subjected to 25-hydroxylation.

Nutritional rickets due to vitamin D deficiency can occur when the dietary intake of the prohormone is low and there is a lack of exposure to sunshine (Bachrach et al., 1979). It is common in children whose parents' religious beliefs proscribe that they wear robes, which block virtually all exposure of the sun, or that they avoid all dairy products except human milk (Lubani et al., 1989). In Northern Europe and the British Isles, rickets is common among dark-skinned immigrants, particularly from India, Turkey, and the Middle East. This form of "Asiatic rickets" occurs because milk is not supplemented with vitamin D in Europe and because these latitudes receive less sunshine than the immigrant's native countries. At present, however, another reported cause of nutritional rickets is chronic use of anticonvulsants. Severely epileptic children are at great risk for developing vitamin D deficiency because they often stay indoors, do not ingest dairy products as a rule—and thus have a reduced intake of calcium, phosphate and vitamin D (as these are felt to lead to greater constipation)—and have accelerated hepatic inactivation of 25-(OH)D. The use of barbiturates and hydantoins stimulates the hepatic microsomal P450 system, causing 25-(OH)D to be rapidly metabolized to more polar, biologically inactive metabolites; the result is a lower serum 25-(OH)D concentration.

The pathophysiology of nutritional rickets begins with a reduction in total-body vitamin D stores: vitamins D_2 and D_3 in fat are depleted, 25-(OH)D_2 and D_3 levels fall, and 24,25(OH)$_2D_2$ and D_3 begin to disappear. As plasma calcium levels drop (stage 1), however, the parathyroid gland is stimulated to secrete PTH. The higher PTH level in turn stimulates: (1) increased excretion of phosphate in the urine with resultant hypophosphatemia; (2) more rapid bone turnover with excessive bone resorption and higher alkaline phosphatase activity; and (3) the synthesis of 1,25-(OH)$_2$D. In advanced rickets, the levels of 1,25-(OH)$_2$D are said to be "normal," but in reality they are low in view of the hypocalcemia, hypophosphatemia, and elevated iPTH values. Instead of the normal ratio of 25-(OH)D to 1,25-(OH)$_2$D of 1000:1, indicating stimulated synthesis of hormone, the ratios of PTH to 1,25-(OH)$_2$D, of calcium to 1,25-(OH)$_2$D, and of phosphate to 1,25-

(OH)$_2$D are all abnormal (Fig. 30-5), which further indicates that 1,25-(OH)$_2$D values are not normal but fail to be appropriately stimulated. Finally, as 25-(OH)D disappears from the blood, the levels of 1,25-(OH)$_2$D also begin to fall and vitamin D depletion is complete. This condition represents advanced rickets; the bone is so depleted of minerals that plasma calcium and phosphate concentrations are extremely low and no further mineral can be removed from bone.

After therapy with vitamin D_2 or D_3, the serum levels of 25(OH)D rise slowly into the normal range, the values of 24,25(OH)$_2$D appear after 7 to 10 days, and the 1,25-(OH)$_2$D concentration almost immediately rises to supranormal levels (>150 pg/mL). This rapid rise in 1,25-(OH)$_2$D probably reflects the availability of substrate for 1 α-hydroxylase as well as the high concentration of circulating iPTH. As shown in Figure 30-5, 1,25-(OH)$_2$D may remain elevated for several months.

The most remarkable changes in the patient treated with vitamin D are the improvement in myopathy and the loss of bone pain. Associated with this clinical improvement, over the next several weeks, serum calcium and phosphate concentrations normalize, reflecting improved intestinal absorption and positive mineral balance. The serum alkaline phosphatase value also begins to fall and the aminoaciduria disappears. The rachitic changes in bone films heal with calcification at the growth plate (*metaphyseal surface*) and disappearance of tra-

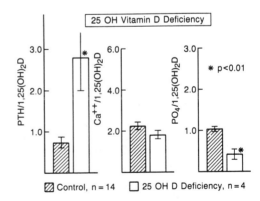

Figure 30-5. The ratio values of PTH to 1,25-(OH)$_2$D, total Ca^{2+} to 1,25-(OH)$_2$D, and PO$_4^{-2}$ to 1,25-(OH)$_2$D in four patients with nutritional rickets (empty bars). Controls, $n = 14$ (hatched bars). The patient ratio of PTH to 1,25-(OH)$_2$D is high, indicating poor production despite elevated iPTH values. Vertical bars, means $\pm$ SD. *$p<0.01$.

becular lesions (*endosteal surface*). By radiological examination, one can detect a transverse thin area of increased density, the so-called *growth arrest line,* indicating where the growth plate had been when vitamin D sufficiency was restored. Finally, over a period of months, the process of bone resorption and remodeling has caused much of the bowing to disappear. If the bowing is severe, an osteotomy may be needed to correct the irregular deformities.

If conventional therapeutic daily doses of vitamin D_2 or D_3, (2000–5000 IU) (50–125 μg), do not correct the biochemical or clinical features of vitamin D deficiency, it is likely that vitamin D is not being converted to $1,25(OH)_2D$ or that the $1,25$-$(OH)_2D$ is not influencing the target organs. The possibilities, shown in Table 30-2 and Figure 30-2, include vitamin D-dependency rickets, chronic renal insufficiency, and type I vitamin D dependency (Fraser et al., 1973). The activity of 1α-hydroxylase is reduced in vitamin D dependency and chronic renal insufficiency, in the latter case because of a reduction in renal mass; however, both disorders can be treated effectively with physiological doses of $1,25$-$(OH)_2D$ in the range of 0.5–1.0 μg/day. In type II vitamin D-dependency rickets, where there is a lack of receptors or receptor function is impaired, effective therapy requires extremely high doses (16–32 μg) of $1,25$-$(OH)_2D$.

Several features of vitamin D-deficiency rickets remain unexplained. The precise rose of vitamin D and its metabolites in the mineralization process within endochondral and chondrocytic bone is uncertain; we know only that the function of $1,25$-$(OH)_2D$ is to stimulate intestinal calcium and phosphate transport and to maintain levels of these minerals in the extracellular fluid at a concentration sufficient to permit mineralization. It seems that rickets and the other components of vitamin D deficiency appear when all the major circulating vitamin D metabolites are reduced, but the relative roles of each metabolite and their interplay are not understood. Finally, little is known about how much sun exposure is needed to prevent vitamin D deficiency in the child who is not receiving dairy products.

THERAPY

The therapeutic goals in the subject of the case report included the provision of adequate calcium

and phosphate intake and the use of a vitamin D preparation. The former can be achieved by urging the patient's parents to give the child commercially prepared milk or, if this is impossible due to allergy or religious beliefs, calcium supplements along with meat or other phosphate-containing foods. If the physician believes the case is one of nutritional rickets, vitamin D at 2000 to 5000 IU each day should be employed (Shah and Finberg, 1994). One can also administer 25-$(OH)D$ at 20–50 μg daily or even $1,25$-$(OH)_2D$ at 0.5 to 1.0 μg daily. In some patients, a large intramuscular dose of vitamin D, or so-called *stoss therapy* may be appropriate. Patients can be given up to 500,000 IU (12,500 μg). This therapy is indicated in patients in whom questions of compliance are raised. The patient should be evaluated at weekly intervals by observing the child's weight gain and muscle strength and by measuring serum calcium, phosphate, and alkaline phosphatase concentrations. One may also measure the concentration of vitamin D metabolites, as this will reveal if the child has autosomal-recessive vitamin D-dependency rickets (Fraser et al., 1973) or type II vitamin D-dependency rickets, which requires further therapy with either low-dose or high-dose $1,25$-$(OH)_2D$ or intravenous calcium.

The patient with nutritional rickets should be treated with high-dose vitamin D_2 and D_3 until the alkaline phosphatase value has returned to the normal range and the radiological appearance of the long bones shows signs of healing. At that point, the child can be maintained on a dose of 400 IU of vitamin D each day or, if anticonvulsants are also being given, 800–1,200 IU daily.

The patient described in the case report was treated with vitamin D_2 at 5000 IU (50 μg) per day along with increased calcium intake, which resulted in an increase in serum calcium and phosphate within 2 weeks. Within 10 weeks the alkaline phosphatase level had fallen to 400 IU/L, at which time the child's vitamin D dose was reduced to 400 IU daily. The prospect for a long-term cure of this disorder and its ultimate prognosis are excellent.

QUESTIONS

1. What is the mechanism of hypocalcemia in nutritional vitamin D deficiency?
2. A variety of factors can contribute to nutritional vitamin D-deficiency rickets, including a lack of sunshine expo-

sure, poor intake of calcium-containing foods and dairy products, wearing heavy clothes that block the sunshine, and the chronic use of anticonvulsants, particularly in institutionalized children. Defective 25-(OH)D, 1 α-hydroxylase activity has not been identified as a cause of nutritional rickets. Is the activity of this enzyme normal or reduced in nutritional rickets, and are there any disorders in which its enzyme activity is abnormal?

3. Each of the following factors may cause impaired conversion of 25-(OH)D to 1,25-(OH)$_2$D: (1) renal disease; (2) hypercalcemia; (3) an autosomal-recessive disorder consisting of reduced 1 α-hydroxylase activity in kidney cortex; and (4) hyperphosphatemia related to impaired renal function. What are some conditions that can stimulate 1 α-hydroxylase activity?

4. Rickets, hypocalcemia, and an elevated serum alkaline phosphatase activity are found in a child. Following therapy for 3 months with oral vitamin D$_2$ at 5000 IU (120 μg) daily, no clinical or biochemical improvement is noted. Of the following diagnostic possibilities, which is unlikely and why?
   (a) Chronic renal failure with a creatinine clearance of <10 mL/min/1.73m².
   (b) Nutritional vitamin D-deficiency rickets.
   (c) Primary hypophosphatemic rickets.
   (d) Autosomal-recessive vitamin D-dependency rickets.
   (e) Vitamin D-dependency rickets with alopecia and target organ resistance.

Acknowledgment: This work was supplied in part by NIH Grant DK 37223-08, Le Bonheur Chair of Pediatrics, the Center for Pediatrics Pharmacokinetics and Therapeutics, the Pediatric Pharmacology Research Unit, and the Crippled Children's Foundation Research Center.

REFERENCES

Bachrach S, Fisher J, Parks JS: An outbreak of vitamin D deficiency rickets in a susceptible population. *Pediatrics* **64**:871–877, 1979.

Chesney RW: Metabolic bone diseases. *Pediatr.* **5**:227–237, 1984.

Chesney RW, Zimmermann J, Hamstra A, et al.: Vitamin D metabolite concentrations in vitamin D deficiency. *Am J Dis Child.* **135**:1025–1028, 1981.

DeLuca HF, Schnoes HK: Vitamin D: Metabolism and mechanism of action. *Ann Rep Med Chem* **19**:179–190, 1984.

Fraser DS, Cooh SW, Kind HP, et al.: Pathogenesis of hereditary vitamin D-dependent rickets: An inborn error of vitamin D metabolism involving defective conversion of 25-hydroxyvitamin D to 1α, 25-dihydroxyvitamin D. *N Engl J Med* **289**:817–826, 1973.

Lubani MM, Al Shab TS, Al-Salch QA, et al.: Vitamin-D deficiency in Kuwait: The prevalence of a preventable disease. *Ann Trop Paediatr* **3**:134–139, 1989.

Scriver CR: Rickets and the pathogenesis of impaired tubular transport of phosphate and other solutes. *Am J Med* **57**:43–54, 1974.

Shah BR, Finberg L: Single-day therapy for nutritional vitamin D deficiency rickets: A preferred method. *J Pediatr* **125**:487–490, 1994.

Part V

Aspects of Infection
and Pharmacology

31

Management of Hypertension with Particular Attention to the Renin-Angiotensin System

YEHUDA TRAUB AND ALVIN P. SHAPIRO

CASE REPORTS

Case 1

A.B., a 31-year-old mother of two, had high blood pressure during the first trimester of her second pregnancy. Previously, she had been in good health, and except for her first pregnancy, she had never sought medical attention. Her family history was also negative except for her father having been hypertensive since the age of 55 years. The patient was given methyldopa (a centrally acting alpha-2 agonist) by the 22nd week of pregnancy, and her blood pressure (BP) was brought under reasonable control. At 39 weeks, she gave birth to a normal infant. Several months later, her BP again rose. The addition of hydrochlorothiazide (a diuretic) effectively lowered it to normal, but this was followed by *thrombocytopenia* (decreased number of blood platelets) on a routine blood count. At this stage, the patient's physician decided to submit her to extensive investigation, both because of her young age and the difficulties encountered in the first year of pharmacological management of her hypertension.

All medications were discontinued for 2 weeks, after which the patient was admitted to the hospital. Complete blood count, urinalysis, routine biochemical analyses, an electrocardiogram, and chest roentgenograms, were all within normal limits, as was a 24-hour urine collection for catecholamines. Because plasma renin activity (PRA) was almost twice the upper limit of normal, the patient underwent renal *arteriography* (roentgenographic visualization of an artery after injection of a radiopaque substance), which was normal, and blood sampling from both renal arteries and the inferior vena cava below the renal veins, for separate determinations of PRA. These studies did not exhibit any signs of lateralization; that is, PRA was equal in both renal veins and higher than in the inferior vena cava.

Based on the entire workup as well as on the patient's family history, it was believed that she had essential (primary) hypertension and that further attempts should be made to lower her BP by using drugs different from those used in the past. Because she had elevated PRA, captopril, an angiotensin-converting enzyme (ACE) inhibitor, 25 mg twice daily, was prescribed; within a week her BP fell from a previous average of 170/100 mm Hg to 130/85 mm Hg, and it remained at similar levels for the subsequent two years of follow-up without any subjective or laboratory adverse effects.

Case 2

D.M., a 68-year-old housewife, has been known to be hypertensive for more than 15 years. She had been treated with various drugs throughout the years, but her BP was never well controlled and she had claimed side effects from almost all the medications that had been prescribed, including diuretics, prazosin (an alpha-1-receptor blocking agent), clonidine, and methyldopa (central alpha-2 agonists). During the last 2 years, she received atenolol (a beta adrenergic blocking agent), but her BP remained elevated at around 180/105 mm Hg. She was then referred for further investigation and management.

A workup similar to that described in case 1 was undertaken after 2 weeks, during which time the patient had been kept free of antihypertensive medications. Urinalysis, blood count and blood chemistries, as well as a 24-hour urine collection for catecholamines, were within normal limits. The electrocardiogram showed signs of mild left ventricular hypertrophy, and this was confirmed by echocardiography. The chest roentgenogram showed borderline enlargement of the heart. Peripheral PRA was below the lower limit of normal, renal arteriography did not reveal any abnormalities, and renal vein PRA showed no signs of lateralization.

Accordingly, this patient was also labelled an essential hypertensive, and it was decided to treat her with some of the newer drugs. She was started on felodipine (a calcium channel blocker of the dihydropyridine class), 5 mg daily, and her BP dropped to 135/70 mm Hg after the first week of treatment.

However, after 1 month, the BP started to rise again, and by the end of the second month it leveled off at 165/100 mm Hg. Following another month of observation during which the blood pressure remained unchanged, the dosage of felodipine was increased to 10 mg daily, and within 3 days the BP dropped to 140/80 mm Hg. At the same time, however, bothersome ankle edema developed, and it was necessary to revert to the previous dose of felodipine, a step that was again followed by a significant rise in BP. At this point lisinopril (an ACE inhibitor), 10 mg daily, was added, and this combined therapy reduced the BP again to 130/70 mm Hg after 1 week. At the end of 6 months, the BP was still at about the same level, but by now the patient was complaining of a nagging dry cough, which was thought to be related to lisinopril. Several days after withdrawal of this drug, the cough subsided. Subsequently, an attempt to use another ACE inhibitor, enalapril, was soon followed by recurrence of the cough. Finally, atenolol, which had been well tolerated previously, was substituted for the ACE inhibitors, and over the past year the patient has been on this combined

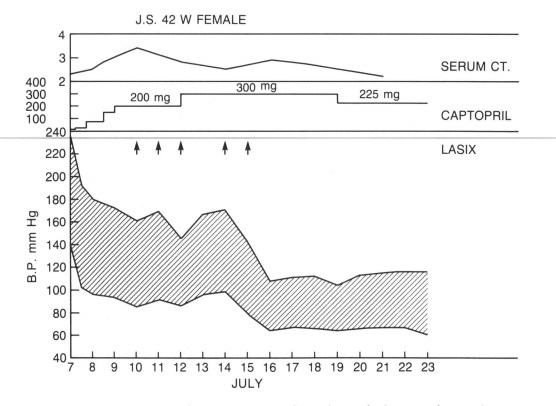

Figure 31-1. J.S.: patient with progressive systemic sclerosis. (See text for description of patient 3.)

(calcium and beta blockers) therapy with her BP remaining around 140/90 mm Hg.

Case 3 (Fig. 31-1)

J.S., a 42-year-old woman, has a 6-year history of scleroderma. She had done reasonably well, although she had experienced progressive skin involvement. While visiting in Pittsburgh to attend to the illness of a close relative, she developed severe headaches and blurring of vision and was admitted to the hospital; her blood pressure was 230/140 mm Hg. In addition, her fundi revealed edema of the optic discs with hemorrhages and exudates. She had no evidence of heart failure. Her serum creatinine concentration had been 1.0 mg/dL (normal, <1.4 mg/dL) with a normal blood pressure when seen by her own physician at home as recently as 1 month before admission to our hospital. On admission here, her creatinine concentration was 2.4 mg/dL and her PRA was 98.7 ng/mL/3 h (20 × ULN, upper limit of normal). She was immediately treated with captopril (an ACE inhibitor) and her blood pressure was quickly brought under control. Captopril, at a dosage of 100 mg three times a day, lowered blood pressure to levels of 110/70 mm Hg, and the headaches disappeared. The fundi showed gradual resolution of the hemorrhages and exudates and disappearance of her *papilledema* (swelling and protrusion of the blind spot of the eye caused by edema). The serum creatinine concentration continued to rise during the first few days of treatment, peaking at 3.3 mg/dL, but then it gradually declined such that after 3 weeks it was 2 mg/dL. She has maintained this improved condition with normal blood pressures on a reduced dose of captopril of 100 to 150 mg/day; at the same time, serum creatinine levels have fallen gradually to below 1.5 mg/dL. Apart from some slight taste disturbances, she has not experienced any problems with the captopril.

DIAGNOSIS

These case reports can provide a background for the discussion of *hypertension* (high BP), some of the mechanisms involved in its occurrence, as well as the general approach to workup and treatment of patients with this ailment. It is generally accepted that an adult person is hypertensive if BP is higher than 140/90 mm Hg on repeated measurements and on different occasions. Some 15 to 20% of the adult population in most countries are hypertensive by this definition. The first two case reports depict patients in whom extensive workup had been carried out, but no special cause of hypertension has been detected. This form is therefore called *essential* or *primary* hypertension, and it comprises more than 95% of all cases of hypertension.

Whereas both patients suffer from essential hypertension, they differ to some extent: The first woman is young, basically healthy, and has a high PRA, whereas the other is an elderly patient with a low PRA but some degree of end-organ involvement (a hypertrophied left ventricle of the heart). The BP of both patients responded favorably to ACE inhibitors; but the first patient received an ACE inhibitor alone, and her BP normalized throughout the entire 24 hours of the day, whereas the second patient received the ACE inhibitor in combination with another antihypertensive drug. Furthermore, the second patient developed a dry cough as an adverse effect of either of two different ACE inhibitors that she took.

Case 3 describes a patient with progressive systemic sclerosis (PSS) who was known to be normotensive and to have had normal renal function within a month of admission. She developed scleroderma renal crisis and malignant hypertension, a specific form of hypertensive disease related to marked activation of the renin-angiotensin system. Her BP rose and her renal function rapidly declined. Before an inhibitor of angiotensin II was available, patients with this sequence deteriorated and developed terminal renal failure despite reasonable control of BP with previously available drugs; they usually died of cardiac and cerebrovascular complications or required dialysis or even bilateral nephrectomy (performed after renal failure had ensued for "removal" of renin). This patient, however, had a dramatic improvement of her hypertension with the initiation of ACE inhibitor therapy, resulting in reversal of renal failure.

MOLECULAR PERSPECTIVES

Definition and Classification of Hypertension

Blood pressure, like many other quantitative characteristics, is a multifactorial trait that is determined by the interaction of multiple genetic and environmental factors (Kaplan, 1994). In essential hypertension, a variety of these factors play a role in raising the BP to levels we consider to be harmful. This is a disease of distorted homeostatic relationships among a number of mechanisms that ordinarily control BP within a relatively narrow range. It actually represents a discrepancy in the relationships between *blood flow* (cardiac output and fluid volume) and the caliber of the "space" (*vessels*) in which blood flow occurs (*peripheral resistance*). Each of these two components, blood flow and peripheral resistance, is influenced in turn by a finite number of mechanisms. Cardiac output is affected by stroke volume and heart rate and is under the control of the *inotropic* (influencing muscular contractility) and *chronotropic* (influencing heart rate) forces influencing the heart; vascular volume is a function of the intake of sodium and water, their output by the kidney, and their dispersion through the several compartments of fluid in the body. Peripheral resistance is a function of the intrinsic tone of arterial and arteriolar smooth muscle, the "set" of the autonomic nervous system, and the amount of local or circulating humoral vasopressor and vasodepressor materials (Fig. 31-2). Thus, the search for a single cause is inappropriate in this entity, which was realized many years ago by the "fathers" of modern research in hypertension, Sir George Pickering of England and Dr. Irvin Page of the United States.

A mechanism associating insulin resistance and hypertension was first proposed almost 30 years ago, but it was neglected until recently, when it was shown in epidemiologic studies that there is an impressive age-amplified overlap in diabetes, obesity, and hypertension and that patients with high BP are relatively hyperinsulinemic compared with persons with normal BP (Kaplan, 1989). Following this, there has been a surge of interest and research in the existence of such a relationship, which appears to be limited to patients with essential hypertension and does not involve patients with secondary forms of hypertension (see below). Although there is still no proof of a causal relationship, indirect evidence supports the hypothesis that insulin resistance and hyperinsulinemia may play a role in the causes of hypertension (Black, 1990). The mechanisms by which elevated plasma insulin concentration may be

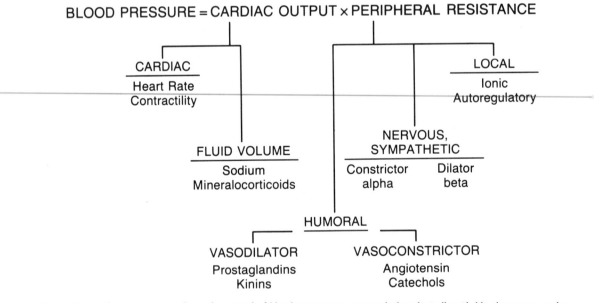

Figure 31-2. These sequences indicate the control of blood pressure as examined physiologically with blood pressure as the outcome of cardiac output times peripheral resistance. As discussed in the text, cardiac output is under the control of both direct cardiac factors as well as circulating volume; peripheral resistance is controlled by humoral, autonomic nervous system, and local factors. *From* Kaplan N: *Clinical Hypertension,* 3rd ed., Baltimore, Williams & Wilkins, 1982.

associated with increases in BP involve stimulation of catecholamine secretion, enhanced renal tubular reabsorption of sodium with a rise in fluid volume, increases in intracellular calcium, as well as the fact that insulin is a vascular growth factor. Insulin resistance is also linked with a number of other clinical and biochemical entities, such as non-insulin-dependent diabetes mellitus, *hypertriglyceridemia* (excess triglycerides in blood) and obesity, and the occurrence of several or all these entities in the same person is not uncommon. Recently, a number of investigators suggested that all these entities may represent various manifestations of a common disease or syndrome. Thus, Reaven coined the term *Syndrome X,* which includes insulin resistance, hyperinsulinemia, glucose intolerance, hyper-very low density lipoprotein (VLDL) triglyceridemia, decreased high-density lipoprotein (HDL) cholesterol concentration, and hypertension; Kaplan speaks of a "deadly quartet," including upper-body obesity, glucose intolerance, hypertriglyceridemia, and hypertension. It has even been proposed that a common "insulin resistance gene" may underlie this association. Nevertheless, this issue is far from settled, and more recent evidence suggests that significantly improving the insulin sensitivity of hypertensive persons does not lower their BP to any meaningful degree. Thus, decreased insulin sensitivity may be just epiphenomenon-associated but not etiologic. Other systemic humoral materials (e.g., atrial natriuretic peptide) as well as locally produced vascular substances (e.g., endothelin, nitric oxide) that act in either an *autocrine* (within the cell) or *paracrine* (cell to adjacent cell) manner have been described recently.

A probable basic mechanism is contained in the fact that a rise in intracellular calcium levels is the final step that brings about vascular smooth-muscle contraction. It has been hypothesized that in hypertensive persons a long-recognized increase in intracellular sodium concentrations may cause a permissive inhibition of the "sodium/calcium pump" in the cell membrane. In turn, the elevation of intracellular sodium concentration is presumably due to the inhibition of a sodium/potassium ATPase energy-dependent pump. The specific inhibitor of this pump is ouabain, a long known plant alkaloid, which turns out also to be a human steroid. Despite the enormous accumulation of knowledge regarding cardiac and vascular muscle contraction, however, the precise role and relative importance of the above-described mechanisms in essential hypertension have not yet been clearly elucidated.

Unlike essential hypertension, in a few patients a particular factor or mechanism is very specifically involved in the elevation of BP; the disease in these patients is labelled *secondary* hypertension (Table 31-1). In some such instances, removal of the specific cause of distortion of homeostasis (e.g., pheochromocytoma, primary aldosteronism, renal artery stenosis with renal ischemia) may lead to a "cure" of hypertension. Extensive investigation, such as was performed in the first two cases described above, is necessary either to confirm or to deny the presence of secondary hypertension, that is, a specific etiologic factor whose removal would normalize the BP. Such "curable" cases, however, represent fewer than 5% of the hypertensive population, and the clinical and financial burden of such extensive investigations for all hypertensives would be unjustified. Therefore, such workup is reserved for the relatively few patients in whom the medical history, physical examination, and a limited basic routine laboratory workup would indicate some suspicion for a special cause of their hypertension. It may also be worthwhile to perform such a workup in hypertensive patients who are very young or in those in whom reasonable control of BP cannot be achieved by pharmacological means.

The Renin-Angiotensin System in Hypertension

As outlined above and indicated in Figure 31-2, the mechanisms involved in regulating BP are numerous. Among them, the renin-angiotensin system (RAS) plays an important role and is a prominent example of the manner in which basic biochemical observations and research have contributed to clinical medicine and practice (Johnston, 1992). The activities of the RAS are mediated via the effector peptide angiotensin II (AII). *Angiotensinogen,* an alpha-globulin substrate synthesized primarily by the liver, is hydrolyzed by *renin,* a proteolytic enzyme released by the kidney, and transformed into a biologically inactive decapeptide, angiotensin I (AI). This, in turn, is converted by ACE into the physiologically active AII (Fig. 31-3).

Table 31-1. Major Secondary Hypertensions

Clinical Condition	Major Mechanism
Renal	
Renal parenchymal disease (RPD)	Volume and sodium
Glomerulonephritis	
Interstitial nephritis	
Polycystic kidney	
Diabetes mellitus	
Systemic lupus erythematous (SLE)	
Renal vascular	Humoral; renin-angiotensin
Renal artery stenosis (RAS)	
Scleroderma (PSS)	
Polyarteritis nodosa (PAN)	
Some cases of SLE	
Adrenal	
Primary aldosteronism	Volume (mineralcorticoids)
Pheochromocytoma	Sympathetic N.S. (catechols)
Cushing's syndrome	Volume and local peripheral resistance
Systolic hypertension	
Aortic atherosclerosis	Cardiac output
Hyperthyroidism	Cardiac output
Coarctation of aorta	Local peripheral resistance and humoral

N.S., nervous system.

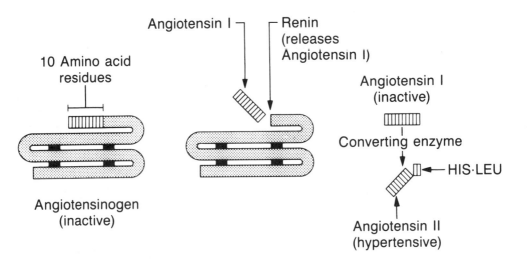

Schematic Representation of the Conversion of Angiotensinogen into Angiotensin II

Figure 31-3. Illustration of the sequences that follow after renin is released by the juxtaglomerular (JG) apparatus of the kidney and results in the elaboration of angiotensin II, which affects blood pressure through vasoconstriction and sodium retention through aldosterone release. Courtesy of Dr. Klaus Hofmann, University of Pittsburgh School of Medicine.

AII is a potent vasoconstrictor and the main promoter of the synthesis and secretion of aldosterone by the adrenal gland; in addition, AII enhances sympathetic nervous activity and is known also to induce hypertrophy of arterial smooth-muscle cells as well as cardiac hypertrophy, thereby further contributing to the complications of hypertension. Its role as a growth factor and a powerful stimulator of cellular hypertrophy is supported by the recent sequencing of the proto-oncogenes that respond to the AII signal and are responsible for new protein synthesis. In the kidney AII affects primarily the efferent glomerular arteriole, the constriction of which increases the intraglomerular pressure, which, in turn, may lead to increased filtration of fluid and certain substances, including protein. It has been postulated that increased glomerular filtration pressure may be a leading factor in the deterioration of renal function in diabetes, hypertension, and a variety of diseases of the kidney.

The vasoactive and other properties of AII are mediated by two subtypes of AII receptors: AT1 and AT2. These two subtypes can be recognized by selective antagonists; thus, the AT1 receptor, which seems to be responsible for almost all known actions of AII, is rendered inactive by dithiothreitol and can be selectively blocked by the recently developed oral nonpeptide drug used in clinical studies, losartan; the AT2 receptor, on the other hand, is insensitive to dithiotreitrol and to losartan, but it may be blocked by still investigational compounds. AT1 receptors in the cellular membrane exhibit an outward-pointing domain forming the binding site and a cytosolic domain connected through a GTP-binding protein (or G protein) to phospholipase C (PLC), the effector enzyme. Activation of this enzyme results in two end products, inositol-1,4,5-triphosphate and diacylglycerol, which represent the initial signals that lead to the release of calcium from the endoplasmic reticulum as well as to the entry of calcium through "receptor-dependent channels" from the extracellular space into the cytoplasm. The exact role of the AT2 receptors and the mechanism by which they may exert their effects have not yet been established, although they may be associated with modulation of renal function, vasopressin release, and prostaglandin synthesis.

ACE (or kininase II) is a large zinc-containing peptidase comprised of about 1300 amino acids.

ACE is relatively nonspecific and exerts its activities by cleaving two peptides from the carboxy-terminal of peptide substrates. Most notably, it converts the decapeptide AI into the octapeptide AII and, as kininase II in a rare example of "biochemical parsimony," it is a component of the kallikreinkinin system and catalyzes the breakdown of bradykinin (Fig. 31-4).

The release of renin from the kidney is regulated by a variety of factors, mainly in response to reduced renal blood blow, increased sodium load at the site of the distal tubule of the kidney, and sympathetic neural stimulation. Although measurements of PRA or of AII concentration may provide important information about certain types of hypertension, they probably do not define any specific type of essential hypertension. The concept of "high" or "low" renin hypertensive patients that has been expounded by some investigators and the argument that *renin profiling* (i.e., determination of whether the patient is a *high* or *low* renin type) should guide one's therapeutic approach has been confusing to clinicians. Note that case 1 (high renin) and case 2 (low renin) both responded to ACE, whereas case 3, a specific "very high" renin patient, responded most dramatically. Misconceptions stem from an oversimplification of the physiology of hypertensive disease and an attempt to place renin in a principal etiological role that may apply to PSS and renal artery stenosis is not in keeping with our present knowledge of essential hypertension. Renin's primary and phylogenetic role seems to be preservation of volume through the regulation of salt and water balance. It also has the role of producing arterial constriction and thus "decreasing the space" for a given volume to circulate. Although, as indicated above, the RAS can behave autonomously and produce a secondary type of hypertension (as in renal artery stenosis), the PRA level does not generally represent a "fingerprint" of a specific type of essential hypertension. Moreover, the level of PRA may vary with the severity of hypertension because of the secondary development of renal arterial disease, or it may be affected by various physiological stimuli or medications. Thus, in many patients, a high or low renin represents present physiological circumstances rather than any innate renin status. Furthermore, even the low renin patient can develop a renin response to marked sodium depletion, and even patients with primary

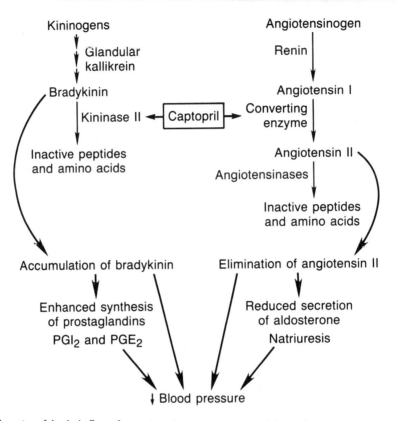

Figure 31-4. Illustration of the dual effects of an angiotensin-converting enzyme inhibitor, which prevents AI to AII conversion and also, as kininase II, prevents the breakdown of bradykinin, resulting in a two-fold effect on blood pressure control. *From* Kaplan N: *Clinical Hypertension,* 3rd ed., Baltimore, Williams & Wilkins, 1982.

aldosteronism can develop elevated PRA when given spironolactone.

To summarize, the following list includes factors that will affect renin secretion or activity one way or the other:

1. Sodium excess or depletion.
2. Posture (higher PRA with upright posture).
3. Sympathetic nervous system stimulation or inhibition.
4. Physical and emotional stress.
5. Age of the patient (higher in younger patients).
6. Diurnal variation (higher in the morning).
7. Renal injury (trauma or infarct).
8. Antihypertensive drugs (through effects on sodium or the sympathetic nervous system).
9. Arteriolar disease of the kidney (e.g., polyarteritis nodosa and progressive systemic sclerosis) (Traub et al., 1983).

Accordingly, whereas measurement of PRA need not be done routinely for "profiling" the patient, it can be of value in the following circumstances:

1. A high peripheral PRA may be suggestive of a renal artery stenosis if other reasons for elevation are absent; however, measurement of PRA in renal vein blood, to determine whether a difference in release from the two kidneys is present, is necessary to demonstrate significant unilateral renal ischemia (decreased arterial blood flow).
2. In the differential diagnosis of hypokalemia, a high PRA will generally rule out primary aldosteronism and suggest secondary aldosteronism (as in malignant hypertension) or the use of diuretics.
3. For the hypertension accompanying renal dis-

ease, differentiation can be made between hypertension due to retained sodium and volume in renal parenchymal disease, in which case PRA is low (*volume-dependent hypertension*), and that due to renal arteriolar disease, in which case PRA is high (*renin-dependent hypertension*).

Local Renin-Angiotensin Systems

The belief that the RAS is solely systemic and that AII acts only as a circulating hormone has been challenged by recent observations. There is rapidly accumulating evidence that most components of the RAS may be produced locally as well and that both the locally produced and the circulating components of the RAS may be physiologically active. Most compelling support for the existence of local tissue RASs comes from molecular biology studies in which the messenger RNA for components of the RAS has been demonstrated in a number of organs, such as the brain, kidney, heart, blood vessels, and other organs. AI may be produced intracellularly and then secreted and converted by circulating or locally produced ACE to AII at the level of the cell membrane. There is evidence of locally produced renin, angiotensinogen, ACE, AI, and AII in the brain, kidney, adrenal glands, endothelium, and smooth-muscle cells of blood vessels and in the heart. At each of these sites, the locally resulting effector substance (AII) may act in an autocrine or paracrine fashion. These autocrine and paracrine functions may be important cellular and tissue communication mechanisms that, among other things, govern vascular tone.

The finding that local production of the components of RAS can take place in the heart and the walls of small, medium, and large arteries is of particular relevance in the hemodynamics of hypertension. Thus, several potential physiologic and pathologic roles for the local vascular RAS have been proposed:

1. Regulation of regional vascular tone and blood flow.
2. Development of vascular hypertrophy.
3. Contribution to the vascular response to inflammation and injury.
4. Response to pharmacologic inhibitors of the RAS, even in the absence of enhanced systemic RAS activity (low PRA).

The possible cardiac manifestations of locally stimulated RAS may include:

1. Cardiac hypertrophy.
2. Potentiation of sympathetic nervous system activity with increased contractility, tachycardia, and a propensity toward arrhythmias.

Finally, it should be pointed out that fascinating discoveries have been made in recent years with regard to genetic aspects of the various components of the RAS. In most cases, however, no close relationship has been demonstrated between genotypic manifestations of RAS components and the occurrence of hypertension.

ANTIHYPERTENSIVE THERAPY

Brief Review of Classes of Agents

Effective antihypertensive drug therapy was introduced during the 1950s; subsequently, large-scale studies demonstrated that such treatment reduced the complications of essential hypertension, mainly stroke, cardiac and renal failure, and possibly coronary heart disease. Today a plethora of antihypertensive agents exists, and these can be divided into several major classes: thiazide diuretics, direct vasodilators; central alpha agonists; alpha-1 blockers; beta adrenergic blockers; calcium channel blockers; and inhibitors of the RAS. We are primarily interested in this article in the RAS inhibitors but will briefly review the other classes (Joint National Committee, 1993).

Thiazide diuretics (e.g., hydrochlorothiazide) and their congeners (e.g., chlorthalidone) have been used in the treatment of hypertension since the 1950s, and they are still among the most frequently prescribed drugs. They act by inhibiting sodium transport across the luminal membrane of the distal tubule in the kidney, whereby plasma and extracellular fluid volume are reduced and cardiac output falls. With chronic use, plasma volume tends to return toward normal, but at the same time arteriolar relaxation seems to ensue, peripheral resistance decreases and consequently the BP remains lowered. Treatment with diuretics may lead to a variety of adverse metabolic effects such as *hypokalemia* (a deficiency of K^+ in the blood), hyperglycemia, hyperlipidemia, and *hyperuricemia* (excess uric acid in the blood). Thrombocytopenia and pancreatitis are also rare but possible side effects. In addition, the reduction of plasma volume and BP is accompanied by powerful stimulation of the RAS.

Direct vasodilators (e.g., hydralazine and minoridil) act directly to relax the arteriolar smooth muscle, thereby decreasing peripheral resistance and BP; however, vasodilatation is almost immediately followed by an activation of compensatory mechanisms, mainly sodium retention by the kidneys and reflex stimulation of the sympathetic nervous system with increased cardiac output and renin secretion. These reflex mechanisms tend to offset the BP lowering effects unless they are counteracted by drugs with opposite effects (diuretics and beta blockers); thus, the direct vasodilators usually serve only as "third-step" agents.

Central alpha-2 agonists (e.g., methyldopa, clonidine, and others) act by decreasing sympathetic activity as reflected in the lower circulating levels of norepinephrine. Hemodynamically, they decrease BP by a modest diminution in both peripheral resistance and cardiac output. PRA is usually lowered, but this is not closely related to their antihypertensive effects. The administration of these agents is often followed by side effects related to the central nervous system, such as sleepiness, dry mouth, and impotence, as well as less frequently occurring "autoimmune" complications, such as methyldopa-induced drug fever, liver dysfunction, or hemolytic anemia.

Alpha-1-adrenergic receptor blockers (e.g., prazosin, doxazosin, terazosin) act as competitive antagonists of the postsynaptic receptors in blood vessels, thereby blocking their activation by circulating norepinephrine, an activation that would normally induce vasoconstriction. Consequently, both resistance vessels (*arterioles*) and capacitance vessels (*veins*) dilate, and peripheral resistance falls without major reflex changes in cardiac output. Moreover, these agents have been shown to have a favorable influence on blood lipids and insulin resistance; however, prazosin has a short half-life and frequent side effects (headache, drowsiness, fatigue and "first-dose" hypotensive syncope). Experience with the newer alpha-1 blockers is limited but suggestive of fewer side effects. These drugs also relieve urethral spasm and are useful in elderly male hypertensives with prostatic hypertrophy.

The competitive inhibition of beta-adrenergic activity by beta blockers (e.g., propranolol, atenolol, pindolol) produces numerous effects on functions that regulate the BP, including decreases in sympathetic nervous activity, cardiac output, renin release, and probably peripheral vascular resistance as well. Nevertheless, their exact mode of action still eludes us, despite their use since the early 1960s. The side effects of these drugs include asthmatic attacks in susceptible persons (by blockade of the bronchorelaxing effects of stimulated beta-2 receptors in the lungs) and cardiodepression, leading to fatigue and possible heart failure (by blockade of cardiac beta-1 receptors). The reduction in renin release is a result of blockade of beta-1 receptors in the kidney, thereby inhibiting the stimulatory effect of the sympathetic nervous system on renin production and release. Theoretically at least, the incidence of these side effects is influenced by whether the beta blocker is selective or nonselective (e.g., beta-1 alone or beta-1 and beta-2 blockade).

Calcium channel *antagonists* (blockers) have gained favor in the treatment of hypertension only in the last decade. They work by inhibiting the entry of calcium into cardiac and smooth-muscle cells through "channels" in the cell membrane. Because a rise in intracellular calcium is intimately involved in smooth-muscle contraction, these drugs act at the final, basic level to lower the BP. They may be subdivided into three major subgroups: verapamil, which affects primarily the cardiac muscle; diltiazem, which has a somewhat lesser effect on cardiac muscle, but also affects arteriolar smooth muscle; and the dihydropyridines (e.g., nifedipine, felodipine), which appear to have a greater effect on vascular smooth-muscle without significantly affecting the cardiac muscle. When given alone, any of these compounds will lower the BP of many hypertensive patients, the dihydropyridines being somewhat more effective than the others. Verapamil and diltiazem may have some cardiodepressive effects (bradycardia and diminished cardiac output), whereas the adverse effects of the dihydropyridines are related mainly to their vasodilating properties and thus comprise ankle edema, headache, facial flush, and other effects. None of these drugs has any major influence on the RAS.

The RAS offers at least four points at which therapeutic agents can be targeted (Fig. 31-5). Beta blockers, in addition to their effects on the central nervous system and the heart, reduce renin synthesis in the kidney and its release from it. Renin inhibitors

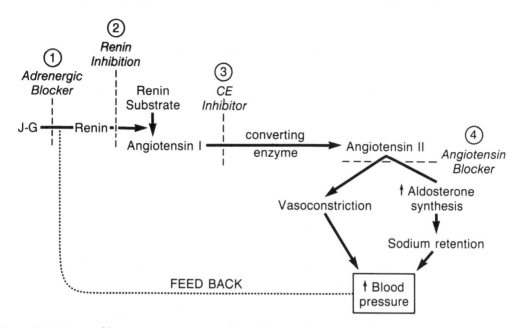

Figure 31-5. Diagram of the renin-angiotensin system indicating the points where renin production or the angiotensin II effect can be blocked: 1. prevention of release of renin by neuroblockade; 2. inhibition of renin action by immunological blockade; 3. inhibition of conversion of angiotensin I to angiotensin II; 4. blockade of the angiotensin II effect by competitive polypeptides. See text for further description. *From* Kaplan N: *Clinical Hypertension*, 3rd ed., Baltimore, Williams & Wilkins, 1982.

that impede the formation of AI are currently being developed. ACE inhibitors prevent the conversion of AI and thus the formation of the active peptide AII. Finally, the peptide (saralasin) and the recently developed nonpeptide (losartan) AII receptor (AT1) antagonists inhibit the action of AII by competing for its receptors on the target cell surface.

ACE Inhibitors

The history of ACE inhibitors is interesting, both in terms of their development and their use (Cushman and Ondetti, 1991). The first polypeptide ACE inhibitors were identified in the venom of the Brazilian viper, *Bothrops jararaca*. Teprotide, a nonapeptide, was developed for marketing. Teprotide, however, could be used only intravenously because it is rapidly degraded when given by oral route. The real breakthrough came with the development of captopril, the first oral ACE inhibitor. Captopril was synthesized two decades ago and first marketed in 1981 as the result of a rational drug program, specifically designed to produce an orally effective substrate that would bind ACE at the active site of the

enzyme (Fig. 31-6). Subsequently, more than two dozen orally active ACE inhibitors were developed (Materson and Preston, 1994). Of these, more than 10 have been marketed worldwide, seven in the United States. As shown in Table 31-2, captopril has a shorter half-life and duration of action, whereas all the newer ACE inhibitors can be given once daily. The route of elimination may also differ, most being excreted by the kidneys, some by the kidneys and liver, whereas spirapril, a newer ACE inhibitor, is eliminated only the hepatic route.

The history of the clinical use of ACE inhibitors is also noteworthy. When captopril was first marketed, the indications for its use, as approved by the Food

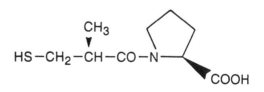

Figure 31-6. Structural formula of captopril, the prototype of an angiotensin converting enzyme inhibitor.

Table 31-2. Characteristics of Angiotensin-converting Enzyme Inhibitors

	Active Metabolite	Peak Effect (h)	Half-life (h)	Duration of Action (h)	Elimination
Captopril	−	1	1	8	Renal
Enalapril	+	4	5	24	Renal
Lisinopril	−	6	13	24	Renal
Benazepril	+	3	10	24	Renal/hepatic
Fosinopril	+	4	12	24	Renal/hepatic
Quinapril	+	2	3	24	Renal
Ramipril	+	5	12	24	Renal
Cilazapril	+	2	1.5	12	Renal
Trandolapril	+	6	3.5	24	Renal

h, hours.

and Drug Administration, included only severe hypertension resistant to multidrug therapy. In view of the drug's special design, it was administered primarily to hypertensives whose PRA was known to be enhanced, including patients with advanced renal disease, especially those with an autoimmune background (e.g., systemic lupus erythematosus, scleroderma, progressive systemic sclerosis, polyarteritis nodosa). These patients received large doses of captopril; a number of serious adverse effects, such as proteinuria and neutropenia, were probably results of these large doses. On the other hand, it was the experience in patients with scleroderma renal crisis (see below) that provided the first clue that ACE inhibition might have special implications for the preservation of renal function and structure. Only somewhat later did physicians begin to prescribe captopril in lower doses and, as its use increased, they began to appreciate its relative freedom from serious side effects. Finally, in 1985 the drug began to be used for all forms of hypertension, including mild and moderate hypertension. Accordingly, the major use of these agents today is in essential hypertensives; this group comprises the majority of all hypertensive patients.

Scleroderma renal crisis is a form of involvement of the kidneys in PSS, with malignant hypertension and marked activation of the RAS as its main features. Before the advent of ACE inhibitors, the outcome of this complication of PSS was lethal, whereas in the last decade most patients have survived with maintained renal function because of captopril and other drugs of this class. Today the principal use of ACE inhibitors is in essential hypertension, heart failure, left ventricular dysfunction in patients with isch-

emic heart disease, and diabetic nephropathy (especially when accompanied by proteinuria). Although the other drugs are equally important in the therapeutic armamentarium available to the hypertensive patient, the broad application of ACE inhibitors in cardiac medicine and the uniqueness of their biochemical development are deserving of their more comprehensive discussion.

The ACE inhibitors are a group of drugs that inhibit the conversion of AI to AII (Materson and Preston, 1994). They cause circulating levels of AII to diminish and PRA and angiotensin I levels to increase. Thus, to the extent that the maintenance of BP is dependent on the RAS, ACE inhibitors reduce BP by inhibiting several AII-dependent mechanisms, resulting in both a decrease in peripheral resistance by relaxation of the arterioles and a reduction in blood flow (volume and cardiac output) by suppression of aldosterone release from the adrenals. Because AII enhances sympathetic nervous activity, the reduction in BP by ACE inhibitors is not accompanied by reflex sympathetic stimulation. In addition, because AII is a potent growth factor, ACE inhibitors are the most effective antihypertensive agents in reversing cardiac hypertrophy and, possibly, arterial or arteriolar hypertrophy as well, even independent of BP reduction. Finally, ACE inhibition tends to lower glomerular filtration pressure in the kidney and thus delays the deterioration of renal function in diabetic kidney disease and perhaps in other diseases of the kidney as well. Furthermore, ACE inhibitors may increase insulin sensitivity, which may make them particularly attractive in view of the insulin resistance theory of essential hypertension.

The ACE inhibitors are more effective in patients

with enhanced PRA and elevated plasma AII concentrations than in those with low PRA and plasma AII; however, these agents can also lower BP in patients with low renin forms of hypertension (e.g., case 2). Because renin levels are often low in elderly hypertensive patients, initial skepticism about the antihypertensive efficacy of ACE inhibitors in this age group was reasonable. Experience has shown, however, that ACE inhibitors have effects that are similar to those of other antihypertensive agents on BP in the elderly. Such observations have led many to speculate that the activation of the kallikrein-kinin-prostaglandin system may be the explanation for this discrepancy between the BP effects of these drugs, their pharmacokinetic characteristics, and the levels of renin and other components of the RAS. A great deal of research, however, has not yielded data which support this mechanism with regard to the effect of ACE inhibitors on BP. The more recent discovery of the various tissue RASs provides an alternative concept that may better explain the above discrepancy, as ACE inhibitors may be working on an active tissue RAS, the existence of which has been demonstrated even in the absence of an active systemic RAS.

Common adverse effects of ACE inhibitors include hypotension, which may occur if a large first dose is administered to patients with enhanced PRA, such as in various edematous states or renal artery stenosis; rash, which may not be alleviated with a reduction in dose; and a dry, nocturnal, nagging cough, that usually appears several weeks after the initiation of treatment. Such a cough may occur with any of the ACE inhibitors in up to 10 to 20% of treated patients, and although its pathophysiologic mechanism is not well understood, it seems to be related to increased sensitivity of the cough centers or cough receptors in the midbrain or the tracheobronchial tree, respectively, due to enhancement of the bradykinin-prostaglandin system.

Angiotensin II Receptor Antagonists

The novel developments in the area of AII blockers deserve discussion in this chapter because they will probably assume increasing importance in the next decade. These agents prevent access of AII to its receptor, in contrast to ACE inhibitors, which prevent the formation of AII, the agonist (Kang et al., 1994).

Saralasin is an octapeptide similar in structure to the AII molecule, except that three amino acids have been substituted. This peptide has specific AII receptor (both AT1 and AT2) antagonistic activity. Although it had been available since the late 1960s, its usefulness has been limited by its short half-life, significant agonistic properties, and its lack of oral bioavailability. In recent years, a number of benzyl-substituted imidazoles were shown to have highly selective AII receptor blocking activities. Of these, losartan is the most potent orally active, specific, competitive nonpeptide AT1 receptor antagonist. Despite the as yet limited clinical experience with these agents and the fact that their relative efficacy versus ACE inhibitors remains unclear so far, they may offer an alternative for those patients who cannot tolerate ACE inhibitors because of their side effects (e.g., cough). Furthermore, AII receptor antagonists proved to be valuable pharmacologic models for research in the study of AII receptors in particular, as well as for the possibility of developing orally active antagonists to the growing number of peptide receptors in general.

CONCLUDING REMARKS

The development of a series of oral, therapeutically active ACE inhibitors and AII receptor antagonists represents the culmination of a course that has been steadily pursued in hypertensive disease for 40 years. This process has required an understanding of the mechanisms of BP control, elucidating their pathological distortions, and then developing pharmacological tools based on precise biochemical manipulations that can correct the distorted mechanisms of BP regulation. This sequential approach to a disease process has been the aim of research in cardiovascular disease in general and in hypertension in particular, and the introduction of ACE inhibitors and AII receptor antagonists represents significant advance toward the achievement of this goal.

QUESTIONS

1. Describe the steps in the production of angiotensin II, including the sites of synthesis of the enzymes and substrates involved.
2. Describe four different methods of inhibiting the synthesis or release of renin or its activity. Have these methods proved clinically effective? Why?

3. What other effects do inhibitors of the angiotensin-converting enzyme display? Are these effects likely to be helpful in blood pressure reduction?
4. From a knowledge of the homeostatic mechanisms involved in blood pressure control, and the sites of possible abnormalities in hypertensive individuals, describe four potential mechanisms for treating hypertensive patients. Discuss the possible advantages and disadvantages of these potential treatments.

REFERENCES

Black HR: The coronary artery disease paradox: The role of hyperinsulinemia and insulin resistance and implications for therapy. *J Cardiovasc Pharmacol* **15**(Suppl 5):S26–S38, 1990.

Cushman DW, Ondetti MA: History of the design of captopril and related inhibitors of angiotensin converting enzyme. *Hypertension* **17**:589–592, 1991.

Johnston CI: Renin-angiotensin system. *J Hypertens* **10**(Suppl 7):13–26, 1992.

Joint National Committee on Detection, Evaluation, and Treatment of High Blood Pressure: The fifth report of the Joint National Committee of Detection, Evaluation and Treatment of High Blood Pressure (JNC V). *Arch Intern Med* **153**:154–183, 1993.

Kang PM, Landau AJ, Eberhardt RT, Frishman WH: Angiotensin II receptor antagonists: A new approach to blockade of the renin-angiotensin system. *Am Heart J* **127**:1388–1401, 1994.

Kaplan NM: The deadly quartet: Upper-body obesity, glucose intolerance, hypertriglyceridemia, and hypertension. *Arch Intern Med* **149**:1514–1520, 1989.

Kaplan NM: *Clinical Hypertension*, 6th ed. Baltimore, Williams & Wilkins, 1994.

Materson BJ, Preston RA: Angiotensin-converting enzyme inhibitors in hypertension: A dozen years of experience. *Arch Intern Med* **154**:513–523, 1994.

Traub YM, Shapiro AP, Rodnan GP, et al.: Hypertension and renal failure (scleroderma renal crisis) in progressive systemic sclerosis: Review of a 25-year experience in 68 cases. *Medicine* **62**:335–352, 1983.

32

Chronic Granulomatous Disease

ADRIAN J. THRASHER AND ANTHONY W. SEGAL

CASE REPORT

A 2-year-old Asian girl was admitted to hospital for the evaluation of epilepsy. She was born in the United Kingdom of parents native to India. Both parents and two older siblings were well and had no significant history of illness. Neonatal and childhood development were uncomplicated until cervical *lymphadenopathy* (enlargement of the lymph nodes) and mild hepatosplenomegaly were detected at a routine health checkup at the age of 8 months. Tuberculous disease was considered and excluded. During investigation, a cutaneous abscess developed at a site of venepuncture from which *Staphylococcus aureus* was isolated. Treatment with antistaphylococcal agents resulted in healing of the cutaneous abscess and gradual resolution of cervical lymphadenopathy.

The patient failed to attend for follow-up investigations but was readmitted at the age of 2 years following onset of focal seizures. On examination she was afebrile and alert. Mild hepatosplenomegaly was noted as before. Reflexes were brisk on the right side, but both plantar responses were downgoing. Routine blood tests revealed a mild neutrophilia and *hypergammaglobulinaemia* (excess gamma globulins in the blood). The blood film was *microcytic* (abnormally small red blood cells) and, although hemoglobin was normal, serum iron and iron-binding capacity were low. Erythrocyte sedimentation rate (ESR) was within normal limits. Chest roentgenogram was normal. One day after admission, the right pupil became unreactive, and the right plantar response became upgoing. Computer tomography

scanning revealed a 3-cm lesion with surrounding edema in the posterior frontal convexity of the left cerebral hemisphere which enhanced with contrast. She was referred to neurosurgery and underwent a left frontoparietal *craniotomy* (surgical opening of the skull) and excision of the mass. At operation a firm mass was found in the frontoparietal convexity that leaked *caseous* (necrotic) material and was easily dissected from the brain to leave a smooth surface. Microscopically, there were numerous irregularly shaped *granulomata* (nodules of inflamed tissue) up to 30 mm in size lying within densely fibrous tissue that was infiltrated with plasma cells, some lymphocytes, and sparse calcific concretions. Most granulomata consisted of a palisade of epitheliod histiocytes mingled with some macrophages and multinucleated giant cells arranged around a core consisting predominantly of polymorphs and macrophages. Acutely branching septate hyphae typical of *Aspergillus* species were found in both the granulomata and in loose necrotic slough. There was no evidence of mycobacterial infection. The patient was administered amphotericin and made an uncomplicated recovery. Routine immunological investigations were normal; however, a nitroblue tetrazolium (NBT) slide test for neutrophil NADPH-oxidase activity was 100% negative. Maternal neutrophils were tested in a similar way and found to be normal. A provisional diagnosis of autosomal recessive chronic granulomatous disease (CGD) was made. Further investigation of NADPH-oxidase function confirmed the diagnosis and identified a deficiency of the cytosolic component p47^{phox}. She was continued on prophylactic co-trimoxazole and itroconazole, and one year after surgery was alive and well.

DIAGNOSIS

Any patient who has suffered from recurrent episodes of infection, infection at atypical sites, or infection by unusual organisms should be investigated for defects of host defense. A careful history, family history, and clinical examination may suggest a specific diagnosis and are important for focussing further investigation. Because neutrophil function defects are uncommon causes of increased susceptibility to infection, it is first necessary to exclude other more common conditions that involve deficiencies of complement, humoral, and cell-mediated mechanisms. Initial screening tests should include a full blood count, differential white cell count, immunoglobulin levels with subsets, complement levels, and skin testing with purified protein derivative and *Candida*. In persons deemed to be at risk, HIV infection should be excluded. Specific analysis of T-cell number, distribution, and function may also be indicated, particularly if the patient is *anergic* (inability to react to injected antigen). Morphologic evaluation of the leukocytes may also be useful. More specialized tests of white cell function can be performed if this initial evaluation fails to identify the cause, the nature of which will be guided by the clinical picture.

Chronic granulomatous disease is a heterogeneous group of disorders characterized biochemically by disordered function of a unique enzyme system present in phagocytic cells, the NADPH-oxidase (Segal, 1993). Clinically, CGD is characterized by recurrent bacterial and fungal infections that are relatively resistant to treatment by conventional means. In common with patients who are *neutropenic* (decrease in neutrophils), patients with qualitative disorders of neutrophil function are particularly susceptible to infection at tissue sites exposed to the environment that are easily colonized by microorganisms, such as skin, mucous membranes, and lungs. Dissemination and establishment of deep-seated infection are also frequently seen, however. The clinical response to infection is often delayed, and although fever, leukocytosis, elevated ESR, and appropriate inflammatory responses eventually appear, the infective disease process may be considerably advanced by this time. Lymphadenopathy occurs in more than 80% of patients and is the presenting feature in more than 40%. Similarly, hepatosplenomegaly is found in more than 60% of cases at some time during the course of the disease. One of the hallmarks of the clinical disease is that patients have particularly impaired microbicidal activity against *Staphylococcus aureus,* enteric Gram-negative rods, and *Aspergillus* species. The ability of a phagocyte to ingest and kill microorganisms, in particular *S. aureus* and *Candida,* forms the basis of an assay for phagocytosis and killing and is abnormal in CGD. The standard method for assessing activity of the phagocyte NADPH-oxidase system is the NBT slide test, in which the water-soluble yellow dye NBT is reduced to insoluble blue-staining formazan when the cell is stimulated. A negative test is indicative of CGD and can be followed up by quantitation of NADPH-oxidase activity and analysis of individual components of the system.

MOLECULAR PERSPECTIVES

Discovery of the NADPH-oxidase

A clinical syndrome characterized by recurrent life-threatening sepsis, hypergammaglobulinemia, and widespread chronic granulomatous infiltration was first recognized in the pediatric literature in the late 1950s. The pathological mechanisms responsible for this condition later became evident when it was demonstrated that neutrophils collected from a male patient were unable to kill *S. aureus in vitro* and that there was a primary abnormality of neutrophil function. At the same time, it was shown that neutrophils from patients with this familial granulomatosis, now called *chronic granulomatous disease* (CGD), failed to exhibit a characteristic increase of oxidative metabolism during phagocytosis called the *respiratory burst*. This phenomenon was initially attributed to increased production of energy during phagocytosis, and although known as "the extra respiration of phagocytosis," it was later shown to be resistant to conventional inhibitors of mitochondrial respiration. It was also shown that the necessary energy for phagocytosis and cytoplasmic degranulation was provided predominantly by the glycolytic pathway. The function of the respiratory burst remained obscure until it became apparent that the ability of phagocytic cells to kill certain bacteria *in vitro* was markedly diminished under anaerobic conditions and that cells obtained from patients with CGD, which were unable to mount this metabolic response, exhibited the same microbicidal deficiency in the presence of oxygen. Together, these observations indicated a crucial function for this system for host defense, although the mechanisms by which the respiratory burst mediate microbial killing remain the subject of some debate (Klebanoff, 1988).

The identity of the substrate for the reaction was the subject of considerable speculation, but the sharp increase in oxidation of glucose via the hexose monophosphate shunt (the purpose of which is to maintain cellular NADPH levels and the activity of which is controlled by the rate of oxidation of NADPH) coincident with neutrophil activation strongly suggested that NADPH was the most likely candidate molecule. In support of this, patients with severe glucose 6-phosphate dehydrogenase (G6PD) deficiency, in whom cellular replenishment of NADPH is diminished, show markedly diminished consumption of oxygen in response to stimulation. The enzyme complex responsible for the respiratory burst therefore became known as the NADPH-oxidase (Segal and Abo, 1993).

The Molecular Basis of the NADPH-oxidase

The molecular basis of the NADPH-oxidase was first uncovered in 1978, when the terminal electron transporting component, a membrane-bound flavocytochrome b_{558}, was purified from human neutrophils and shown to be missing in some patients with CGD. It later became clear, however, that additional cytosolic factors were necessary for activation. The *cell-free* system is an *in vitro* assay for NADPH-oxidase activity induced in broken cell preparations, and it has provided an important tool for the elucidation of many aspects of oxidase biology. When the substrate NADPH is added to broken preparations of resting cells, no activity is detectable; however, if the cells are activated before being disrupted, oxidase activity can be detected in the homogenate. A number of groups subsequently found that they could induce activity in a homogenate from inactive cells by the addition of amphiphiles, such as arachidonic acid or sodium dodecyl sulphate. Somewhat surprisingly, the particulate fraction of the homogenate, which was thought to be enriched for an exclusively membrane-bound NADPH-oxidase, could not be activated unless the soluble fraction consisting predominantly of cytosol was also present. Some patients with CGD have subsequently been shown to have normal levels of functional flavocytochrome b_{558} but deficiencies of this cytosolic activity, indicating the absence of proximal activating components.

Component Molecules and Function of the NADPH-oxidase

The NADPH-oxidase is most abundant in phagocytic cells, namely, neutrophils, eosinophils, and cells of the monocyte/macrophage lineage. It is now known to consist of a membrane-bound flavocytochrome b_{558} of two subunits, p22*phox* (the smaller α-subunit), and gp91*phox* (the larger β-subunit), although the stoichiometry of these is not clearly established (the suffix *phox* represents *ph*agocyte *ox*idase). In addition, three cytosolic factors are necessary for initiation of electron transport and translocation to the membrane on activation of the cell, namely p47*phox*, p67*phox*, and p21rac, a small GTP-binding protein (Fig. 32-1). In a cell-free system, NADPH-oxidase activity is reconstituted solely using these five recombinant proteins together with substrate and necessary defined cofactors. An additional component p40*phox* has been identified that is not essential for activation *in vitro,* but it seems to associate with p67*phox* and may therefore be important for stability or for directing the cellular localization of this molecule.

In resting neutrophils, the plasma membrane is devoid of flavocytochrome, which resides almost exclusively in specialized light-density intracellular vesicles and within the membranes of specific granules. When the cell is activated, the plasma membrane invaginates to form a phagocytic vacuole with which vesicles containing flavocytochrome b_{558} fuse. The cytosolic components form an activation complex that translocates to the membrane to associate with and induce electron transport through the flavocytochrome b_{558}. Binding sites for the substrates NADPH and FAD, which transfer electrons from NADPH to the heme, were recently identified on the flavocytochrome itself, indicating that flavocytochrome b_{558} constitutes the complete electron transporting system (Fig. 32-2).

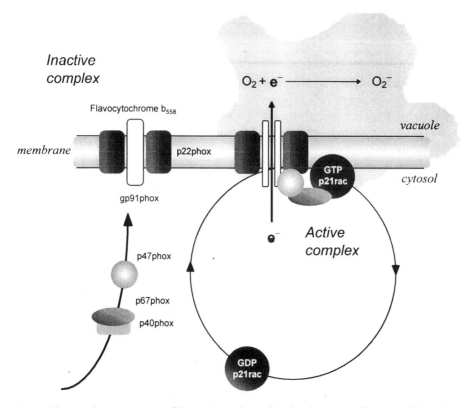

Figure 32-1. Schematic showing activation of the NADPH-oxidase. When the phagocytic cell is activated, the plasma membrane invaginates to form a phagocytic vacuole, and intracellular vesicles containing the flavocytochrome fuse with the plasma membrane, which in the resting state is relatively devoid of this complex. Induction of electron transport depends on translocation of the cytosolic components, p47*phox*, p67*phox*, p40*phox* and p21*rac* and interaction with the membrane-bound flavocytochrome. The phosphorylation status of the guanine nucleotide bound to p21*rac* may be essential for induction and termination of activation.

Products of Electron Transport and Antimicrobicidal Activity

Within the phagocytic vacuole of the neutrophil, as a result of electron transport through the membrane, one molecule of oxygen is reduced to a single molecule of superoxide anion (Klebanoff, 1988). Potentially deleterious cytosolic acidification is prevented by the simultaneous activation of a homeostatic hydrogen ion extrusion mechanism, including a unique hydrogen ion conductance, which seems to be dependent on normal assembly of oxidase components. Interaction between two molecules of superoxide in a dismutation reaction results in the formation of oxygen (O_2) and peroxide O_2^-. Spontaneous dismutation in the absence of superoxide dismutase (SOD) occurs optimally at pH 4.8 but is rapid at physiological pH and is followed by protona-

tion of peroxide to form hydrogen peroxide (H_2O_2). Although both H_2O_2 and O_2^- are produced in large amounts by stimulated phagocytes, and their concentrations reach the millimolar range in the phagocytic vacuole, the ability of these molecules to react directly with biological materials is probably limited. The generation of other more reactive oxygen-free radicals *in vivo*, such as the hydroxyl radical (HO·) or singlet oxygen ($^1O_2$), and more recently of radicals derived from nitric oxide, remains speculative. In particular, these processes are dependent on the presence of free metals such as copper and iron, which may themselves be sequestered by granule proteins such as lactoferrin and therefore be unavailable for reaction.

Myeloperoxidase, present in abundance in the primary granules of neutrophils and responsible for the yellow-green color of pus, is capable of using

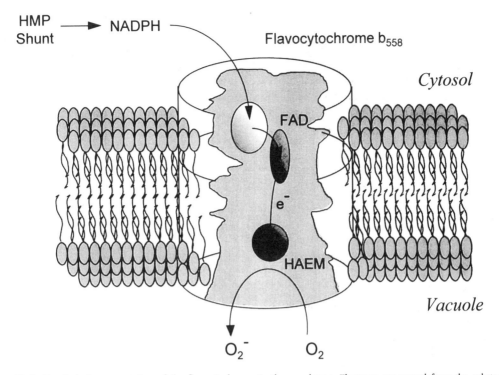

Figure 32-2. Topological representation of the flavocytochrome in the membrane. Electrons are passed from the substrate NADPH to FAD, both of which are bound to the β-subunit of the cytochrome itself, and finally to the terminal acceptor haem, the precise location of which in relation to either subunit is unknown. The midpoint potential for this molecule is the lowest recorded for any mammalian cytochrome b, and is low enough to induce direct reduction of oxygen to superoxide.

H_2O_2 as a substrate to catalyze the oxidation of halide ions to hypohalous acids. In the neutrophil, hypochlorous acid is the predominant reaction product, and it may interact with nitrogen-containing compounds to form reactive and potentially microbicidal chloramine species. The halogenation reaction is not necessarily the major or natural function of myeloperoxidase, which may be more important as a scavenging molecule. Myeloperoxidase deficiency occurs with a prevalence of 1 in 2000 in the population, yet only six patients with serious infections have been reported in the literature; four of these patients had disseminated or visceral candidiasis, and three of the four had concomitant diabetes mellitus. Furthermore, chicken neutrophils lack this enzyme. Myeloperoxidase has also been shown to reconstitute microbicidal activity of *cytoplasts* (neutrophils from which the granules and nuclei are removed, but are able to mount a respiratory burst) when introduced into the phagocytic vacuole.

The NADPH-oxidase may primarily influence microbial killing by other mechanisms. An important consequence of failure of the NADPH-oxidase is an unusually rapid and extensive fall in pH within the phagocytic vacuole (Segal et al., 1981). In a normal phagocytic vacuole, activation of electron transport and generation of H_2O_2 result in a dramatic consumption of protons and a rise in pH to 7.8 to 8.0 before this slowly falls back to neutral levels. This finding is important because many of the proteolytic enzymes released into the vacuole are maintained in the granules at a pH of about 5.0 but have a neutral pH optimum. Under normal circumstances, their release into the vacuole would coincide with an abrupt elevation in pH and killing and digestion of the microbe. In CGD or anaerobic cells, this initial alkalinization does not occur, and the excessively acidic environment leads to inefficient enzymatic killing of microbes and retention of undigested cellular debris. Because of its role in killing and digestion, it is interesting to speculate that the NADPH-oxidase is in some way involved in the processing of antigen, although direct evidence for this is lacking. Phagocytosis of bacteria without a mechanism for entry into the cytosol results in presentation of bacterial antigens by class I major histocompatibilty (MHC) molecules. This process is resistant to classic inhibitors of the class I processing pathway and suggests a novel pathway for the processing of exogenous phagocytic antigens, which could be partially dependent on NADPH-oxidase activity.

Molecular Pathology

The genes encoding both subunits of the flavocytochrome b_{558} and four cytosolic factors, p40$phox$, p47$phox$, p67$phox$, and p21rac, have been cloned, and molecular lesions resulting in CGD identified in all but p21rac and p40$phox$. The genetic loci for the first four components have been mapped to specific chromosomal locations. Large studies from the United States and Europe have identified the distribution of genetic lesions in CGD patients (Table 32-1) (Casimir et al., 1992).

Overall, about two thirds of patients have an X-linked defect of the β-subunit of the flavocytochrome b_{558}. The remaining patients have autosomal disease, with those exhibiting a deficiency of p47$phox$ being the most prevalent. Defects in the small α-subunit of the flavocytochrome b_{558}, and in p67$phox$ make up the remaining cases.

Flavocytochrome b_{558}-negative CGD

Expression of either component of the flavocytochrome b_{558} alone has not been reported, indicating that a mutual interaction is necessary for stability. Therefore, failure to express either subunit results in an absence of the entire heterodimer. gp91$phox$ is expressed almost exclusively in terminally differentiating myelomonocytic cells and was the first human gene to be cloned based on knowledge of its chromosomal location. Molecular lesions at the corresponding genetic locus on the X chromosome, CYBB, account for most cases of CGD. The mutations are particularly heterogeneous and are unique to individual families in more than 90% of the described cases. The most frequent encountered lesions are: missense mutations resulting in nonconservative amino acid substitutions; deletions in genomic DNA, which may be restricted to the gene locus or involve larger regions of the X chromosome; and mutations resulting in RNA splicing defects. Premature stop codons as a result of nucleotide insertions or missense mutations invariably lead to undetectable levels of flavocytochrome b_{558}. Some mutations in so-called *variant patients,* allow expression of protein but are functionally disruptive. Recently, two mutations in the gene promoter were shown to be associated with a variant form of CGD in which levels of immunoreactive protein and NADPH-oxidase activity are decreased.

The gene structure, chromosomal location, and identity of mutations in flavocytochrome b_{558}-negative autosomal recessive CGD were first described in 1990. Unlike other components of the NADPH-oxidase, the transcript for p22$phox$ is found ubiquitously; however, protein expression is restricted to cells in which gp91$phox$ is also expressed.

Table 32-1. Gene Structure and Distribution of CGD Patients

Component	gp91$phox$	p22$phox$	p47$phox$	p67$phox$
Genetic locus	CYBB	CYBA	NCF-1	NCF-2
Chromosomal location	Xp21.1	16q24	7q11.23	1q25
Gene/mRNA size (kb)	30/4.7	8.5/0.8	17–18/1.4	37/2.4
Exon number	13	6	9	16
Results of European CGD study of 56 families	X-linked inheritance X91 CGD[a]	Autosomal recessive A22 CGD[a]	Autosomal recessive A47 CGD[a]	Autosomal recessive A67 CGD[a]
No. of affected families and incidence (%)	X91⁰ 35 (63) X91⁻ 2 (4)	A22⁰ 3 (5)	A47⁰ 13 (23)	A22⁰ 3 (5)

CGD, chronic granulomatous disease.

[a]Accepted classification of CGD in which A or X denotes the inheritance pattern. This is followed by the molecular weight of the affected component in kD. The superscript refers to the level of detectable immunoreactive protein: (0) indicates no protein, (−) indicates diminished protein, and (+) indicates normal levels of defective protein.

Molecular lesions are again heterogeneous and have included both homozygous and missense compound heterozygous mutations, DNA deletions, and one homozygous donor splice site mutation.

Flavocytochrome b_{558}-positive CGD

The second most common cause of CGD is A47° CGD. The p47^{phox} gene is expressed exclusively in terminally differentiating myelomonocytic cells and, to a lesser extent, in some subgroups of lymphoid cells. In contrast to X91 CGD, a single lesion in the p47^{phox} gene accounts for more than 90% of mutant alleles. A GT dinucleotide deletion at a GTGT repeat at the boundary between the first intron and second exon results in a chain terminator at amino acid residue 51. The gene structure for p67^{phox} has also been described, but little is known about mutations arising in A67 CGD.

Functional Diagnosis of CGD

The diagnosis of CGD is confirmed by the demonstration of absent or markedly deficient respiratory burst activity in phagocytic cells. Other aspects of phagocyte function, including chemotaxis, adhesion, phagocytosis, and degranulation, are normal. The simplest and most widely available screening test for CGD is the NBT microscope slide test. This qualitative test assesses the ability of an activated cell to produce superoxide, the primary product of the NADPH-oxidase, by reduction of the yellow water-soluble NBT dye, to insoluble blue formazan, which precipitates on the activated cell. This test has the advantage of being able to detect the carrier state in female relatives of patients with X-linked CGD, in which cases there is a mixed population of NBT-positive and NBT-negative cells. Occasionally, preferential inactivation of the abnormal X-chromosome in carrier females results in an apparently normal NBT test, whereas preferential inactivation of the normal chromosome may result in a CGD phenotype. Carriers of autosomal types of CGD show little aberration of oxidase function, although reduced production of superoxide by neutrophils obtained from carriers of A47° and A67° CGD has been described. Variant CGD patients, so-called because of their ability to produce small amounts of superoxide (sometimes up to 30% of normal), and patients with severe glucose 6-phosphate dehydrogenase deficiency (in which cellular replenishment of NADPH is deficient) may produce a negative NBT test.

Quantitation of the respiratory burst is important to confirm the diagnosis in the case of an abnormal screening test or in cases where diagnosis is in doubt. This can be done either by direct measurement of oxygen consumption with an oxygen electrode or by measuring the products of electron transport. The most widely used measure of superoxide production is the superoxide dismutase (SOD)-inhibitable reduction of ferricytochrome c. Chemiluminescent assays, such as SOD-inhibitable reduction of lucigenin or catalyzed peroxidation of luminol, are less quantitative but are nonetheless more specific indicators of NADPH-oxidase activity and are much more sensitive. Activation *in vitro* is commonly produced by soluble stimuli, such as phorbol myristate acetate (PMA) and formyl-methionyl-leucyl-phenylalanine (fMLP), or particulate stimuli, such as opsonized bacteria or zymosan.

Prenatal diagnosis can be made by evaluation of neutrophil function in fetal blood samples obtained at 14 to 16 weeks' gestation. Increasingly, genetic analysis of fetal tissue obtained from chorionic villous sampling or cultured amniotic fibroblasts will replace functional assay on cord blood for families at high risk and obviates the need for second-trimester termination. This strategy is dependent on the identification of specific family-based mutations or on informative polymorphisms. As an alternative to genetic analysis, it may be possible to detect the presence of individual NADPH-oxidase components in chorion-derived macrophages with specific antibody.

Molecular Diagnosis of CGD

Immunoblotting for individual components of the NADPH-oxidase identifies the defective protein in most cases; however, molecular lesions in either component of flavocytochrome b_{558} usually result in an absence of the entire heterodimer. Although the site of mutation may be inferred from inheritance, it remains difficult to distinguish between males who may have acquired a new mutation of CYBB from the maternal germline and those with autosomal recessive deficiency of p22^{phox}. Identification of the defective component may also be difficult in rare individuals who express relatively normal levels of protein that is functionally deficient. In these cases, complementation studies in a cell-free system using recombinant protein or in whole cells by monocyte fusion or gene transfer may be helpful.

The Pattern of Clinical Disease

Between 1 in 500,000 and 1 in 1,000,000 persons are estimated to be affected by CGD, although it is probably underdiagnosed because of a general lack of awareness of the condition and also because some persons exhibit a mild clinical phenotype. Clinically, it is characterized by recurrent bacterial and fungal infections that are relatively resistant to treatment by conventional means. Most patients are now diagnosed before their second birthday, although some remain undiagnosed until later in childhood or even adult life. Phenotypic heterogeneity among patients with CGD is understandable in light of the diverse molecular pathology, but even those with identical genetic defects may exhibit quite different clinical patterns. The eldest recorded patient with CGD presented with his first serious infection at the age of 69 years. In contrast, a grandson died at the age of 5 years from *Pseudomonas cepacia* pneumonia. An often-stated dogma is that patients with X-linked CGD manifest the most severe clinical phenotype, and although this is probably true, it should not obscure the fact that some patients with autosomal inheritance patterns can be equally severely affected. Interestingly and somewhat surprisingly, *variant* patients, so-called because they retain partial activity of the NADPH-oxidase, may present with manifestations of classical disease no different from those with undetectable activity.

Infections usually predominate at epithelial surfaces in direct contact with the environment, in particular the skin, mucous membranes, lung, and gut. This is reflected in the most common presenting features: *lymphadenitis* (inflammation of lymph nodes), cutaneous infection and dermatitis, pulmonary infection, persistent fever, and diarrhea. Deepseated infections, such as *osteomyelitis* (infectious inflammatory disease of bone), visceral abscess formation, particularly in the liver, and septicemia are frequently encountered, and failure to thrive is a common response to chronic infection in childhood. Pulmonary infection with *Aspergillus* is not uncommon, is particularly difficult to eradicate, and is associated with a high mortality rate despite appropriate treatment. Gastrointestinal manifestations are

varied and often result in misdiagnosis and implementation of inappropriate treatment. These include diarrhea, often as a result of *Salmonella* infection, recurrent perianal abscess formation, and extensive *granulomatous enteritis* (inflammation of the intestines) which may be clinically and radiologically indistinguishable from Crohn's disease and may likewise be complicated by lumenal obstruction. Obstructive lesions are not restricted to the lower gut and have been associated with narrowing of the esophagus, gastric antrum, and ureteric orifices as a result of granulomatous cystitis. Hepatomegaly, splenomegaly, and dermatitis are other manifestations of the characteristic granulomatous reaction.

Pathological Features of Disease

The microbial organisms responsible for most infections are characteristic of this disorder; *S. aureus* and enteric Gram-negative rods such as *Salmonella*, *Klebsiella*, *Aerobacter*, *Serratia*, and *Pseudomonas* account for most bacterial pathogens, and *Aspergillus* species are the most commonly implicated fungi. Although numerous other pathogens have been described in association with CGD, the most striking feature of the common pathogens is that they produce a natural scavenging enzyme, catalase, which neutralizes H_2O_2. Catalase-negative organisms, such as *Streptococci*, do not appear to present particular problems. The most commonly cited explanation for this observation is that small amounts of H_2O_2 are generated by the microorganisms themselves within the phagocytic vacuole, which may be sufficient to activate some cellular microbicidal activity in the absence of a functional NADPH-oxidase but is effectively neutralized by catalase. Frequently, the pathogenic organism is not identified, and treatment remains empirical.

The characteristic histopathology is widespread granulomatous infiltration of tissues, probably as a result of inefficient cellular attempts to eliminate infectious agents and digest unwanted cellular debris. The granulomata are composed of numerous giant cells and lipid-laden histiocytes. The high levels of cytokines produced by and which maintain this inflammatory response contribute to the marked *cachexia* (physical wasting and malnutrition) seen in some patients and may be amenable to therapeutic manipulation. Patients are frequently anemic, usually as a consequence of chronic disease, but sometimes as a result of malabsorption syndromes, for example, of vitamin B_{12}, secondary to enteric disease. They are characteristically hypergammaglobulinemic, with a raised erythrocyte sedimentation rate even when apparently uninfected, and develop a leukocytosis during septic episodes.

Prognosis

Published retrospective studies suggest a survival rate at 10 years of 50 to 70%, although from the age of 20 years onward, survival is maintained at about 50%. The introduction of prophylactic therapy in the past few years, together with the availability of more powerful broad-spectrum antibiotics, has undoubtedly resulted in a greatly improved outlook and a reduction in associated morbidity and mortality.

TREATMENT

General Measures

The most important principles of treatment in this primary immunodeficiency syndrome are those of prevention and aggressive treatment of infection (Finn et al., 1990; Fischer et al., 1993). Patients with CGD are not overtly susceptible to viral infection, and routine childhood immunization against mumps, rubella, and measles is not contraindicated. Similarly, immunization with toxoids or capsular polysaccharide (as in Hib vaccines) can be given routinely. Vaccines against bacteria in which the immunogen is live, albeit attenuated (e.g., BCG and the recently available oral typhoid vaccine) should be avoided, however, except under exceptional circumstances. Skin wounds should be treated with topical antiseptic agents, and close attention be paid to dental hygiene, and to protection in particular of mucosal surfaces. Exposure to fungal spores in decaying plant material and wood chippings should be avoided. Nutrition should be adequately maintained and supplemented, if necessary, particularly in the presence of a malabsorption syndrome. If oral intake remains inadequate, consideration may be given to enteral or even parenteral feeding. Anemia of chronic disease responds well to subcutaneous erythropoietin in the presence of an adequate supply of hematinics and is associated with an improved sense of well-being, although it is not clear whether this influences the course of the

disease. Unfortunately, some patients with X-linked CGD have the rare Kell blood phenotype Mcleod, which should be determined before blood transfusion is contemplated.

Prophylactic Treatment

Although no prospective controlled trial has taken place, retrospective analyses of patient records from both the United States and Europe have shown that prophylactic antibiotics are effective in prolonging the period between major infections. In one study from the National Institutes of Health, prophylactic administration of trimethoprim-sulphamethoxazole to a group of 36 patients resulted in a decrease of nonfungal infection from 7.1 to 2.4 per 100 patient-months in patients with autosomal CGD and from 15.8 to 6.9 infections per 100 patient months in patients with X-linked inheritance. There is as yet no evidence that the frequency of fungal infection, in particular by *Aspergillus,* is reduced by prophylactic administration of antifungal agents, although itraconazole has shown promise in retrospective studies of neutropenic patients and is currently undergoing evaluation in CGD. Other antibiotics have not been formally evaluated.

Interferon-γ (IFN-γ) is an immunomodulatory cytokine secreted predominantly by TH (T-helper) cells following antigen-specific activation. It enhances MHC class II expression on antigen-presenting cells and contributes to late differentiation of B cells. It also acts as a potent macrophage-activating factor and synergizes with tumor necrosis factor (TNF) to enhance the susceptibility of target cells to T-cytotoxic (TC) and natural killer (NK) cells. On the basis of *in vitro* studies in which interferon (IFN-γ) resulted in partial restoration of NADPH-oxidase activity in neutrophils and monocytes from selected patients with X-linked CGD, four patients were treated with two consecutive subcutaneous injections of IFN-γ. Superoxide production increased in all four patients, peaking after 1 to 2 weeks in monocytes, and 2 to 3 weeks in granulocytes. This peak correlated with enhanced microbicidal activity 2 weeks after treatment and a modest increase in the levels of immunoreactive cytochrome b. The delayed peak of superoxide production after two consecutive doses of IFN-γ, however, is not consistent with the circulating half-life of neutrophils, which is measured in hours, and it has therefore been suggested that IFN-γ acts on progenitor cells rather than their differentiated progeny. These studies on selected patients with X-linked CGD, together with *in vitro* evidence for increased microbicidal activity of IFN-γ treated cells in the absence of enhanced respiratory burst activity, prompted a Phase III multicenter clinical trial. In this double-blind, placebo-controlled study, 128 patients with CGD were randomized to receive placebo or IFN-γ at a dosage of 50 g per m² administered subcutaneously three times per week. The primary endpoint was time before serious infection requiring hospitalization and treatment with parenteral antibiotics. The trial was prematurely terminated after 9 months, at which point IFN-γ-treated patients had experienced a 67% reduction in the relative risk of serious infection compared with the placebo group and had spent two thirds less time in the hospital. Children aged less than 10 years benefitted most from treatment, which was generally well tolerated; however, the frequency of infection in patients from some European centers receiving antibiotic prophylaxis alone was less than in the IFN-γ-treated trial group as a whole. Furthermore, IFN-γ did not reduce the rate of serious infections in the European patients who participated in the trial. Although the number of participating European patients does not permit statistical evaluation of this observation, the explanation for this difference is not clear, but it seems unlikely to arise from differences in patient groups.

In contrast to earlier studies, participants in the multicenter study and other groups have not demonstrated restoration of neutrophil NADPH-oxidase activity or increased expression of individual oxidase components. The mechanism of action of IFN-γ in most patients with CGD is therefore speculative, but it almost certainly reflects an influence on aspects of immunity divorced from the NADPH-oxidase. Nonetheless, IFN-γ appears to represent a useful therapeutic tool in CGD and perhaps should be administered prophylactically to identified patients at high risk of infection. The value of IFN-γ, when used to augment conventional treatment during septic episodes, is unknown, although there have been numerous anecdotal reports.

Some groups have investigated the ability of other cytokines to modulate the respiratory burst in cells derived from CGD patients, including one that reported enhanced superoxide production by CGD monocytes cultured in the presence of IFN-γ, TNF, IL-3, and IL-1. Recombinant GM-CSF was tested in a variant CGD patient with a hepatic abscess; despite a profound increase in the number of circulating leukocytes, there was no detectable improvement in oxidase function or clinical condition during the period of administration of the cytokine. Recombinant G-CSF has been used sporadically in septic CGD patients, but it is impossible to identify any potential benefit over conventional treatments.

Treatment of Active Infection

Conventional treatment of intervening sepsis in CGD focuses on aggressive antimicrobial chemotherapy initially directed at characteristic pathogens. In many cases, the pathogen is not isolated and treatment remains empirical. Modern drugs such as ceftazidime and ciprofloxacin, both of which have antipseudomonal activity, in combination with teicoplanin, which has broad-spectrum activity against Gram-positive organisms, have proved useful in resistant cases, particularly in the absence of an identified pathogen. Intravenous amphoteracin remains the mainstay of treatment for *Aspergillus* infection, although itraconazole, which is only available as an oral preparation, may be more effective and better tolerated. Corticosteroids carry an additional risk of immunosuppression but may be useful in situations where an intense granulomatous reaction has resulted in stricture formation and lumenal obstruction. Florid dermatitis may also respond to topical steroids but must be used in combination with appropriate antibiotics and topical antifungal agents. Neutrophils obtained from leukophoresed donors may be used as an adjunct to therapy, and can be given intravenously or even directly applied to the site of infection. Transfused neutrophils have been demonstrated in bronchoalveolar lavage fluids for up to 24 hours, and transfused monocytes may persist for longer periods. Pretreatment of donors with rhG-cerebrospinal fluid (CSF) can be used to increase the yield; however, difficulty with the purification and storage of adequate numbers of cells, potential transmission of viruses, and the possibility of graft-versus-host disease and the formation of allotypic antibodies all limit the use of transfused allogeneic neutrophils to cases resistant to conventional treatment.

Curative Therapy

As a primary immunodeficiency disorder, CGD is amenable to cure by haematopoietic stem cell transplantation. Allogeneic bone marrow transplantation (BMT), however, has been successful in only a small number of patients, and the risks associated with this procedure outweigh potential benefits in most cases. Morbidity and mortality relate to the high degree of immunosuppression required to achieve engraftment and to prevent graft-versus-host disease.

An alternative strategy to allogeneic BMT is somatic gene therapy. This therapy has the advantage of using autologous cells, which have been genetically manipulated, to repopulate the hematopoietic system. At the present time, hematopoietic gene transfer requires bone marrow to be harvested from the patient and manipulated *ex vivo* before reimplantation. In the future, it may be possible to deliver the genetic material *in vivo*. The need for cytoreductive conditioning before transplantation depends on the efficiency of gene transfer into multipotent hematopoietic stem cells but will clearly present increased risk to patients who are inherently immunosuppressed. On the basis of several *in vitro* studies, a Phase I clinical trial was recently initiated for the treatment of p47*phox*-deficient CGD by retrovirus-mediated gene transfer. The efficiency of gene transfer and the gene expression required to produce clinical benefit are currently unknown.

QUESTIONS

1. What are the clinical characteristics of CGD?
2. What are the biochemical characteristics of CGD?
3. Why may patients with severe G6PD-deficiency present with a similar immunodeficiency?
4. Why are CGD patients susceptible to infection by a relatively restricted range of microorganisms?
5. How does the NADPH-oxidase reduce oxygen in the phagocytic vacuole?
6. What are the potential mechanisms for NADPH-oxidase microbicidal activity?
7. What are the treatment options for CGD?

REFERENCES

Casimir CM, Chetty M, Bohler M, et al.: Identification of the defective NADPH-oxidase component in chronic granulomatous disease: a study of 57 European families. *Eur J Clin Invest* **22**:403–406, 1992.

Finn A, Hadzic N, Morgan G, Strobel S, Levinsky RJ: Prognosis of chronic granulomatous disease. *Arch Dis Child* **65**:942–945, 1990.

Fischer A, Segal AW, Seger R, Weening RS: The management of chronic granulomatous disease. *Eur J Pediatr* **152**:896–899, 1993.

Klebanoff SJ: Phagocytic cells: Products of oxygen metabolism, *in* Gallin JI, Goldstein IM, Snyderman R (eds): *Inflammation: Basic Principles and Clinical Correlates.* New York, Raven Press, 1988, p. 391.

Segal AW, Abo A: The biochemical basis of the NADPH oxidase of phagocytes. *TIBS* **18**:43–47, 1993.

Segal AW, Geisow M, Garcia R, Harper A, Miller R: The respiratory burst of phagocytic cells is associated with a rise in vacuolar pH. *Nature* **290**:406–409, 1981.

Thrasher AJ, Keep N, Wientjes F, Segal AW: Chronic granulomatous disease. *Biochim Biophys Acta* 1994; 1227:1–24.

Volkman DJ, Volpp BD, Nauseef WM, Clark RA: Two cytosolic neutrophil oxidase components absent in autosomal chronic granulomatous disease. *Science* **242**:1295–1297, 1988.

Index

Page numbers followed by *f* indicate figures.
Page numbers followed by *t* indicate tables.